# The Development of Sex Differences and Similarities in Behavior

# NATO ASI Series

## Advanced Science Institutes Series

*A Series presenting the results of activities sponsored by the NATO Science Committee, which aims at the dissemination of advanced scientific and technological knowledge, with a view to strengthening links between scientific communities.*

The Series is published by an international board of publishers in conjunction with the NATO Scientific Affairs Division

| | |
|---|---|
| **A Life Sciences**<br>**B Physics** | Plenum Publishing Corporation<br>London and New York |
| **C Mathematical**<br>   **and Physical Sciences**<br>**D Behavioural and Social Sciences**<br>**E Applied Sciences** | Kluwer Academic Publishers<br>Dordrecht, Boston and London |
| **F Computer and Systems Sciences**<br>**G Ecological Sciences**<br>**H Cell Biology**<br>**I  Global Environmental Change** | Springer-Verlag<br>Berlin, Heidelberg, New York, London,<br>Paris and Tokyo |

## NATO-PCO-DATA BASE

The electronic index to the NATO ASI Series provides full bibliographical references (with keywords and/or abstracts) to more than 30000 contributions from international scientists published in all sections of the NATO ASI Series.
Access to the NATO-PCO-DATA BASE is possible in two ways:

– via online FILE 128 (NATO-PCO-DATA BASE) hosted by ESRIN,
Via Galileo Galilei, I-00044 Frascati, Italy.

– via CD-ROM "NATO-PCO-DATA BASE" with user-friendly retrieval software in English, French and German (© WTV GmbH and DATAWARE Technologies Inc. 1989).

The CD-ROM can be ordered through any member of the Board of Publishers or through NATO-PCO, Overijse, Belgium.

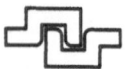

# The Development
# of Sex Differences
# and Similarities in Behavior

edited by

## Marc Haug
University Louis Pasteur,
Laboratory of Psychophysiology,
URA-CNRS 1295, Strasbourg, France

## Richard E. Whalen
Department of Psychology,
University of California,
Riverside, California, U.S.A.

## Claude Aron
University Louis Pasteur,
Institute of Histology,
Faculty of Medicine, Strasbourg, France

and

## Kathie L. Olsen
Neuroendocrinology Program,
National Science Foundation,
Washington, D.C., U.S.A.

Springer Science+Business Media, B.V.

Proceedings of the NATO Advanced Research Workshop on
The Development of Sex Differences and Similarities in Behavior
Château de Bonas, Gers, France
July 14-18, 1992

**Library of Congress Cataloging-in-Publication Data**


A C.I.P. Catalogue record for this book is available from the Library of Congress.




ISBN 978-94-010-4749-4        ISBN 978-94-011-1709-8 (eBook)
DOI 10.1007/978-94-011-1709-8

---

*Printed on acid-free paper*

---

# Contents

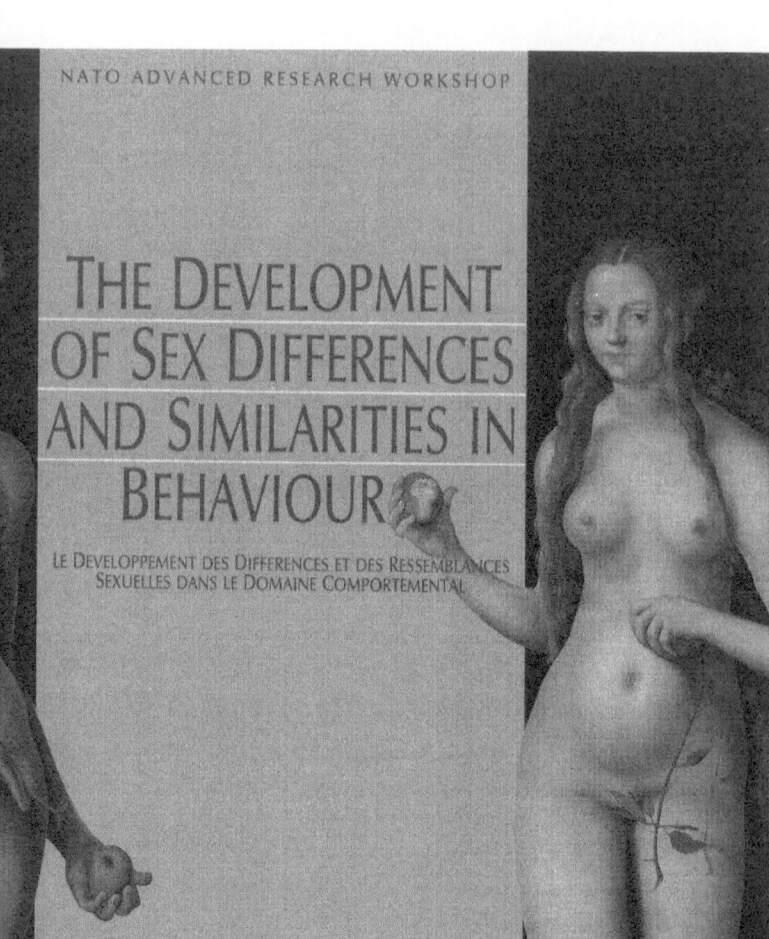

NATO ADVANCED RESEARCH WORKSHOP

# The Development of Sex Differences and Similarities in Behaviour

### Le Developpement des Differences et des Ressemblances Sexuelles dans le Domaine Comportemental

Château de Bonas, Gers, France
July 14-18, 1992

Directors:
Dr. M. Haug, Prof. R. Whalen, Prof. Cl. Aron, Dr. K. L. Olsen

# Preface

M. HAUG

*Université Louis Pasteur, Laboratoire de Psychophysiologie, URA 1295, 7, rue de l'Université, 67000 Strasbourg, France*

This varied and impressive volume is a record of the major presentations at the NATO sponsored Advanced Research Workshop on *The Development of Sex Differences and Similarities in Behaviour* held at the Chateau de Bonas, Gers, France July 14-18, 1992. It is fitting that a meeting evaluating masculine and feminine 'characteristics' was located in the Gascony region immortalised in Alexandre Dumas epic, macho tale of The Three Musketeers. It is even more satisfying that Marc HAUG the French Director (a D' Artagnan equivalent) was ably assisted by a US/French Consortium of three co-Directors (Drs. Richard E. WHALEN, Claude ARON and Kathie L. OLSEN).

The ARW also provided opportunities to explore the region around the Chateau, to appreciate the complex history of the area and to sample armagnac and other local gastronomic creations. A lively and varied cultural programme (classics to jazz) was also provided to maintain the interests and enthusiasms of the participants.

Although aspects of sex differences in human and animal behaviour have been recently extensively explored both academically (e.g. Haug et al., 1991a ; 1991b ; Bjorkquist and Niemela, 1992; Brain and Haug, 1992) and in popularised accounts (e.g. Diamond, 1992), it was felt that bringing scientists of diverse scholarly backgrounds together to explore questions of sex or gender differences in behavior was a most timely activity. The complex interplay between the various biological (e.g. genes, neural circuits, neurotransmitters, and hormones), political, psychological and sociological factors that account for *sex differences* has always been, and will continue to be, a source of infinite fascination and confusion to humans from all levels of education and training and in all parts of the globe.

The organizers brought together a powerful mixture of eminent scientists from most of the pertinent biological and social science areas. There was also an excellent mix of nationalities which led to some tempering of ethocentric tendencies. The intention (ably achieved) was to generate a creative interfacing between very different ways of looking at the genesis of sex differences in behavior in humans and other animals. It was also hoped that the various disciplines would gain new insights and increase their appreciation of their 'opponents' concerns and fears. This is especially necessary when journalistic imperatives create highly simplified (and often misleading) accounts of the neural origins of homosexuality, the generation of behavioral differences in male and female children and the origins of the differing relative mathematical skills of boys and girls. Immediacy and journalistic impact is a real problem when discussing complex phenomena which often require decades of detailed, wide-ranging and painstaking research.

The ARW explored many of the issues surrounding gender differences in behavior. For example, the biologically-orientated scientists re-evaluated the concepts concerning how hormones act during development to change the vectors (neural and somatic) of male and female "typical behavior". This was balanced by social scientists revealing current ideas on how societal factors exert influences on human behavior. A comparable discussion was largely led by the social scientists on the factors influencing human sexual identity. In this case, there was relevant input from the biologists.

What was exciting was that the foci changed during the Conference. For example, participants learned that aggression rather than being a "male-typical" behavior, is very situation-specific. Both biological and social scientists contributed to this changed viewpoint. Issues such as the recent Le Vay finding that the third interstitial nucleus of the hypothalamus is smaller (and more "female-like") in male homosexuals than in heterosexual males were raised. The status of such reports and its relevance to gender differences in behavior *in general* were explored at lenght. Certainly, an encouragingly different view of sexually "dimorphic" behaviors seems to be emerging with more emphasis on the flexibility of systems and less support being provided for simple deterministic viewpoints (this applied just as much to biologists as the social scientists). Further progress in understanding such phenomena clearly depends on enlightened and innovative cross-disciplinary approaches.

The organization and running of this outstandingly successful workshop were greatly facilitated by Cedric and Danielle Haug, Michèle Mauriac, Bernadette Malichat and Antoine Depaulis. The organizers also received valued financial support for the ARW from :-

The NATO Scientific Affairs Division
The National Science Foundation
L'Institut National de la Santé et de la Recherche Médicale (INSERM)
Kabi Pharmacia
Symbiose
University of California, Riverside
L'Université Louis Pasteur de Strasbourg
Le Conseil Régional Alsace

The book itself also benefited from Dr. P. F. Brain competent assistance with book editing, Marie Claire Hantch's excellent secretarial help, and Fabrice Perché painstaking help in making the chapters into a uniform format.

# References

BJorkqvist, K. and Niemela, P. (1992). *Of Mice and Women : Aspects of Female Aggression*, Academic Press, San Diego.
Brain, P. F. and Haug, M. (1992). Hormonal and neurochemical correlates of various forms of animal aggression. *Psychoneuroendocrinology*, **17** : 1-16.

Diamond, M. (1992). *Sex Watching : Looking Into the World of Sexual Behaviour*, Prion, London.

Haug, M., Brain, P. F. and Aron, C. (1991a). *Heterotypical Behaviour in Man and Animals*, Chapman and Hall, London.

Haug, M., Benton, D., Brain, P. F., Olivier, B. and Mos, J. (1991b). *The Aggressive Female*, CIP-Gegevens Koninklijke Bibliotheek, Den Haag.

# Contributors

**A. E. Ackerman** Department of Zoology and Neuroscience Program, Michigan State University, Natural Science Building, East Lansing, MI 48824, USA

**Y. Arai** Department of Anatomy, Juntendo University School of Medicine, Hongo, Tokyo 113, JAPAN

**C. Aron** Institut d'Histologie, 4, rue Kirschleger, 67085 Strasbourg, FRANCE

**J. Balthazart** Université de Liège, Laboratoire de Biochimie Générale et Comparée, 17, Place Delcour (bât. L1), B-4020 Liège, BELGIQUE

**M. J. Baum** Department of Biology, Boston University, 2, Cummington Street, Boston, MA 02215, USA

**C. P. Benbow** Department of Psychology, Iowa State University, Ames, IA 50011-3180, USA

**P. F. Brain** School of Biological Sciences, University College of Swansea, Swansea, SA2 8PP, Wales, UK

**T. Brand** Department of Endocrinology and Reproduction, Faculty of Medicine and health Sciences, Erasmus University, P.O. Box 1738, 3000 DR Rotterdam, THE NETHERLANDS

**L. G. Clemens** Department of Zoology and Neuroscience Program, Michigan State University, Natural Science Building, East Lansing, MI 48824, USA

**A. Chabli** Institut d'Histologie, 4, rue Kirschleger, 67085 Strasbourg, FRANCE

**D. Chateau** Institut d'Histologie, 4, rue Kirschleger, 67085 Strasbourg, FRANCE

**X. Chen** Center for Molecular Bioscience and Biotechnology, Mountaintop Campus 111, Lehigh University, Bethlehem, PA 18015, USA

**A. C. Clifford** Center for Molecular Bioscience and Biotechnology, Mountaintop Campus 111, Lehigh University, Bethlehem, PA 18015, USA

**M. Diamond** Department of Anatomy, University of Hawaii, School of Medicine, 1960 East-West Road, Honolulu, HI 96822, USA

**K. D. Döhler** Pharma Bissendorf Peptide GmbH, Karl-Wiechert Allee 3, 3000 Hannover 61, GERMANY

**A. H. Eagly** Department of Psychological Sciences, Purdue University, West Lafayette, IN 47907, USA

**A. Foidart** Université de Liège, Laboratoire de Biochimie Générale et Comparée, 17, Place Delcour (bât. L1), B-4020 Liège, BELGIQUE

**C. Ganzemüller** Department of Clinical Endocrinology, University School of Medicine, 3000 Hannover 61, GERMANY

**S. J. C. Gaulin** Department of Anthropology, University of Pittsburgh, Pittsburgh, PA 15260, USA

**B. A. Gladue** Department of Psychology, North Dakota State University, Fargo, ND 58105, USA

**R. Green** Department of Psychiatry and Biobehavioral Sciences, UCLA School of Medicine, 760 Westwood Plaza, Los Angeles, CA 90024-1759, USA

**A. Guillamon** Universidad Nacional de Education a Distancia, Departamento de Psicobiologia, P.O. Box, Apartado n° 50.487, Madrid, SPAIN

**M. Haug** Université Louis Pasteur, Laboratoire de Psychophysiologie, URA 1295, 7, rue de l'Université, 67000 Strasbourg, FRANCE

**M. Hines** Department of Psychiatry and Biobehavioral Sciences, UCLA School of Medicine, 760 Westwood Plaza, Los Angeles, CA 90024-1759, USA

**E. J. Houtsmuller** Department of Endocrinology and Reproduction, Faculty of Medicine and health Sciences, Erasmus University, P.O. Box 1738, 3000 DR Rotterdam, THE NETHERLANDS

**J. Juraska** Department of Psychology, University of Illinois, 603 E.Daniel Street, Champaign, IL 61820, USA

**M. Kail** Université René Descartes (Paris V), Laboratoire de Psychologie Expérimentale, URA 316, 23, rue Serpente, 75006 Paris, FRANCE

**E. B. Keverne**  University of Cambridge, Sub-Department of Animal Behaviour, Madingley, Cambridge CB3 8AA, UK

**S. F. Lu**  Center for Molecular Bioscience and Biotechnology, Mountaintop Campus 111, Lehigh University, Bethlehem, PA 18015, USA

**D. Lubinski**  Department of Psychology, Iowa State University, Ames, IA 50011-3180, USA

**M. Machida**  Department of Obstetrics and Gynecology, Juntendo University School of Medicine, Hongo, Tokyo 113, JAPAN

**S. E. McKenna**  Center for Molecular Bioscience and Biotechnology, Mountaintop Campus 111, Lehigh University, Bethlehem, PA 18015, USA

**W. H. Meck**  Department of Psychology, Columbia University, New York, NY 10027, USA

**M. Miyakawa**  Department of Anatomy, Juntendo University School of Medicine, Hongo, Tokyo 113, JAPAN

**J. Mos**  Duphar B.V., Department of Pharmacology, P.O. Box 900, 1380 DA Weesp, THE NETHERLANDS

**S. Murakami**  Department of Anatomy, Juntendo University School of Medicine, Hongo, Tokyo 113, JAPAN

**M. Nishizuka**  Department of Anatomy, Juntendo University School of Medicine, Hongo, Tokyo 113, JAPAN

**B. Olivier**  Department of Psycho-Pharmacology, Faculty of Pharmacy, State University of Utrecht, THE NETHERLANDS

**K. L. Olsen**  Neuroendocrinology Program, National Science Foundation, Rm 321, 1800 G. Street, Washington, DC 20550, USA

**P. Palanza**  Università Degli Studi di Parma, Dipartimento di Biologia e Fisiologia Generali, Sezione Zoologia, Viale delle Scienze, 43100 Parma, ITALY

**S. Parmigiani**  Università Degli Studi di Parma, Dipartimento di Biologia e Fisiologia Generali, Sezione Zoologia, Viale delle Scienze, 43100 Parma, ITALY

**L. F. Petrinovich**  Department of Psychology, University of California, Riverside, CA 92521, USA

**C. Schaeffer**   Institut d'Histologie, 4, rue Kirschleger, 67085 Strasbourg, FRANCE

**S. Segovia**  Universidad Nacional de Education a Distancia, Departamento de Psicobiologia, P.O. Box, Apartado n° 50.487, Madrid, SPAIN

**J. P. Signoret**  INRA, Station de Physiologie de la Reproduction, URA 1291, Centre de Recherches de Tours, 3738O Nouzilly, FRANCE

**N. G. Simon**   Center for Molecular Bioscience and Biotechnology, Mountaintop Campus 111, Lehigh University, Bethlehem, PA 18015, USA

**A. K. Slob**  Department of Endocrinology and Reproduction, Faculty of Medicine and  health Sciences, Erasmus University, P.O. Box 1738, 3000 DR Rotterdam, THE NETHERLANDS

**H. Sumida**  Research Laboratories, Nippon Kayaku Co. Ltd, Takasaki-City, Gumma 270-12, JAPAN

**H. Takeuchi**  Department of Obstetrics and Gynecology, Juntendo University School of Medicine, Hongo, Tokyo 113, JAPAN

**R. Unger**  Department of Psychology, Montclair State University, 124 Russ Hall, Upper Montclair, NJ 07043, USA

**C. Veit**  Department of Clinical Endocrinology, University School of Medicine, 3000 Hannover 61, GERMANY

**C. Wagner**  Institute of Animal Behavior, Rutgers University, 101 Warren Street, Newark, NJ 07102, USA

**R. E. Whalen**  Department of Psychology, University of California, Riverside, CA 92521, USA

**C. L. Williams** Department of Psychology, Barnard College of Columbia University, 3009 Broadway, New York, NY 10027, USA

**P. Yahr**  Department of Psychobiology, University of California, Irvine, CA 92717, USA

# Inherited and Environmental Determinants of Bisexuality in the Male Rat

C. ARON, D. CHATEAU, A. CHABLI and C. SCHAEFFER

*Institute of Histology, Faculty of Medecine, Louis Pasteur University, 67000 Strasbourg, France*

## Defining bisexual behavior

At the end of the last century Krafft-Ebing (1886) coined the term of bisexuality to characterize the gender of individuals adopting bisexual behavior and speculated the existence of a male/female brain within the brain of male and female individuals. Surprisingly bisexuality has long been a misunderstood phenomenon which was erroneously equated to homosexuality by researchers. Recent statistical data (Zinik, 1985) provide evidence that there is a significantly higher percentage of people who display bisexual behavior than exclusively homosexual behavior. The term of bisexuality must thus be used to designate human subjects who have sexual interactions with both males and females.

Sexual contacts between individuals of the same sex have been commonly observed in male and female mammals, but it is essential to define this kind of behavior in non-human species because we know nothing of the sexual motivation of either partner of an "homosexual" pair of animals.

However, we have known for some decades that female rats spontaneously mount other females with pelvic thrustings which characterize the copulatory pattern of a male which mounts a female. For their part, the males of certain strains of rats are capable, in the absence of any hormone treatment, of responding to male's mounts by the lordotic posture which represents the typical copulatory pattern of a female which is mounted by a male. The term "heterotypical" sexual behavior has been used to designate a kind of behavior, in both females and males, that is in disaccord with the genetic sex. In contrast homotypical sexual behavior will refer to the typical copulatory pattern of each sex.

We believe that female and male rats which display heterotypical behavior, i.e. the copulatory pattern of the opposite sex, may be said bisexual because most of the males which show lordosis in response to male mounts are also sexually vigourous copulators (Van de Poll and Van Dis, 1977; Schaeffer et al., 1990a; Chabli et al., 1991). Similarly the display of mounting  behavior by

1

*M. Haug et al. (eds.), The Development of Sex Differences and Similarities in Behavior, 1–18.*
© *1993 Kluwer Academic Publishers.*

female rats is often related to the state of estrous receptivity (see for review : Beach, 1968; Goy and Roy, 1991). Thus both males and females of some mammalian species possess a nervous and muscular organization compatible with the display of bisexual behavior.

It should, however, be recognized that spontaneous lordosis behavior represents a rather infrequent form of sexuality in non-hormonally treated male rats (Schaeffer et al., 1990a,b). On the contrary, the induction of lordosis behavior by either estrogen (Davidson, 1969; Aren-Engelbrektsson et al., 1970; Van De Poll and Van Dis, 1977; Chabli, et al., 1985) or estrogen associated with progesterone (Södersten, 1976 ; Van De Poll and Van Dis, op cit.; Chabli et al., op cit.; Södersten et al., 1983; Olster and Blaustein, 1988) has been clearly established in male rats castrated as adults and also in intact male rats (Van de Poll and Van Dis, 1977; Chabli et al., 1989; Schaeffer et al., 1990a, b).

Castrated males primed with ovarian hormones thus may be considered as an useful tool to determine whether 1. the olfactory system which fundamentally influences homotypical sexual interactions in the rat is also implicated in the control of heterotypical sexual interactions and 2. the activational mechanisms which are known to govern lordosis behavior in the female are also involved in the control of this behavior in the male.

This chapter is an overview of the most significant results obtained in our laboratory during the last past years. It has three objectives. The first objective is to study the involvement of olfactory cues and of the olfactory system on its own, in the regulation of lordosis behavior in the male rat. The second is to analyse the neuroendocrine mechanisms involved in the display of this behavior in the male. The third objective is to examine at the hypothalamic level the biochemical mechanisms of interaction between the hormonal and olfactory signals which control lordosis behavior in the male.

# Assessment of lordosis behavior in the male

## Animals

In all the experiments which will be reported below we used Wistar male rats from two strains (WI and WII) bred in our colony. They were castrated at 3-to-4 months after birth and given different subcutaneous doses of estradiol benzoate (EB) or EB associated with progesterone (P). The animals were kept until 1987 under a natural rhythm of natural lighting and later under controlled conditions of lighting (lights on 02.00-16.00 hr). Room temperature was maintained at 22°-24°C. The animals had free access to a commercial laboratory food and to tap water except for a group of them which was placed on a 23hr food deprivation cycle as to conduct more easily tests for anosmia.

## Sexual behavioral testing

Lordosis behavior of castrated male rats was tested for 10 min at the beginning of the dark period of either natural or the controlled lighting cycle by presenting them in a mating arena to two adult stimulus male rats selected from animals mounting vigourously highly receptive estrous females as male congeners. A 5 min period of adaptation of the stimulus males in the arena was allowed prior to the introduction of the castrated rats. Two paradigms were used for the evaluation of lordosis behavior in the castrated animals.

We determined the willingness of the males to display lordosis behavior as assessed by the proportion of animals in a given group that displayed at least one lordosis in response to male mounts. As in females, lordosis consisted of arching the back, extending the neck and deviating the tail to one side thus exposing the genital region. We also computed a lordosis quotient (LQ) in each castrated male rat by dividing the number of lordosis responses by the number of mounts and multiplying by 100. The mean LQ was calculated for each group of animals and served as a measurement of the sexual performance.

# Olfactory control of lordosis behavior in the male rat

## Influence of olfactory cues on lordosis behavior in the male rat

In rodents, olfactory cues play a major role when females are attractive to males or attracted by them. This led us some years ago (Schaeffer and Aron, 1981; Schaeffer et al., 1982) to speculate that olfactory cues provided by males would influence the display of lordosis behavior in castrated male congeners primed with ovarian hormones. Urine from adult intact male rats was selected as a source of pheromones.

Castrated WI male rats primed with 75 µg EB and 1 mg P at an interval of 39-40hr were placed on a grid 10 cm above the floor of their cages to prevent any licking of bedding. Lordosis testing was performed within 8-9hr after P injection. The animals were assigned to four experimental groups. The first group was exposed to bedding soiled by 5 ml urine at the time of P injection. Two other groups were submitted to either complete or anterior olfactory bulb removal 8 days prior to behavioral testing to study the influence of the olfactory system on it's own on lordosis. The last group comprised of animals which were neither operated nor exposed to urine and served as controls. We observed that the proportion of animals displaying lordosis was higher in rats exposed to the odor of male urine (19/30) than in the controls (22/60) ($P < 0.02$). Complete olfactory bulb removal mimicked the effects of olfactory cues (36/58). In contrast anterior olfactory bulb removal did not cause any changes in the proportion of rats showing lordosis as compared to the controls (18/75) ($P > 0.05$). No difference in LQ values was noted between the rats exposed to male urine odor and the controls ($47 \pm 6$ and $48 \pm 6$, respectively). Neither did LQ values differ in complete and anterior olfactory bulbectomized animals ($65 \pm 5$ and $58 \pm 7$, respectively). In combination these two last groups displayed high LQ values compared with animals exposed to male urine and controls ($P < 0.01$).

These results led to make a clear distinction between the two paradigms used for the evaluation of lordosis behavior in the male rats. They showed that the olfactory bulbs on their own inhibited the occurrence of lordosis in the male and that olfactory cues from the male released this inhibition. They also suggested that the accessory olfactory bulbs (AOB) which are located in the caudal part of the olfactory bulbs were involved in these inhibiting mechanisms. Finally the data allow the assumption that the main olfactory system controlled the sexual performance since both complete and anterior olfactory bulb removal increased LQ values. Further experiments were then conducted to verify these hypotheses.

## Accessory olfactory bulb lesions and lordosis behavior in the male

The castrated WI male rats used in this experiment (Schaeffer et al., 1986a) were assigned to three groups: 35 controls ; 53 rats in which AOB removal was attempted ; 27 sham-operated animals. The operated animals were allowed a postoperative period of 8-10 days. All the animals were given 75 µg EB s.c. and 1 mg P s.c. at an interval of 39hr and lordosis behavior was tested by 08.30 to 10.30hr after P injection. Because of high variations in size and shape of the AOB (Rehmer et al., 1970), preliminary studies were necessary to determine the most accurate coordinates for the placement of AOB lesions in WI rats. All the same, only 17 of the 53 operated animals exhibited AOB removal with no damage of the main olfactory bulb (Figure 1).

The proportion of animals which displayed lordosis behavior did not differ in controls (19/35) and sham operated (16/27) animals ($X^2 = 0.14$ ; $P > 0.7$). After AOB removal a significant rise in the number of animals showing lordosis behavior (15/17) was observed as compared to the two other groups taken as a whole ($X^2 = 4.79$ ; $P < 0.05$). LQ values did not differ in the three groups of animals (49 ; 58 ; 66 ; respectively) ($F_{(2,47)} = 1.67$, NS).

This study shows that AOB removal mimicked the effects of complete olfactory bulb removal by increasing the number of EB + P treated rats which displayed lordosis behavior as compared to control animals. This allows the assumption that the expression of lordosis behavior in the male is repressed by the action of the accessory olfactory system. Now the AOB may also be reasonably considered as the target for the olfactory cues from the male which have been shown, as mentioned above, to facilitate the occurrence of lordosis behavior. In that respect it is worthnoting that olfactory cues appeared to be efficient under distance exposure to male urine. Therefore the most plausible hypothesis is that airborne particles may reach the vomeronasal epithelium. Electrophysiological studies indicating that the vomeronasal organ may respond to some volatile compounds (Tucker, 1971; Muller, 1971; Meredith and O'Connell, 1979) provide support for this hypothesis. It is important to note that neither olfactory stimuli nor AOB removal affected LQ values. This provide support to the foregoing hypothesis that the main olfactory system conveyed olfactory cues which modulate the sexual performance. The experiments reported below were performed to investigate this problem.

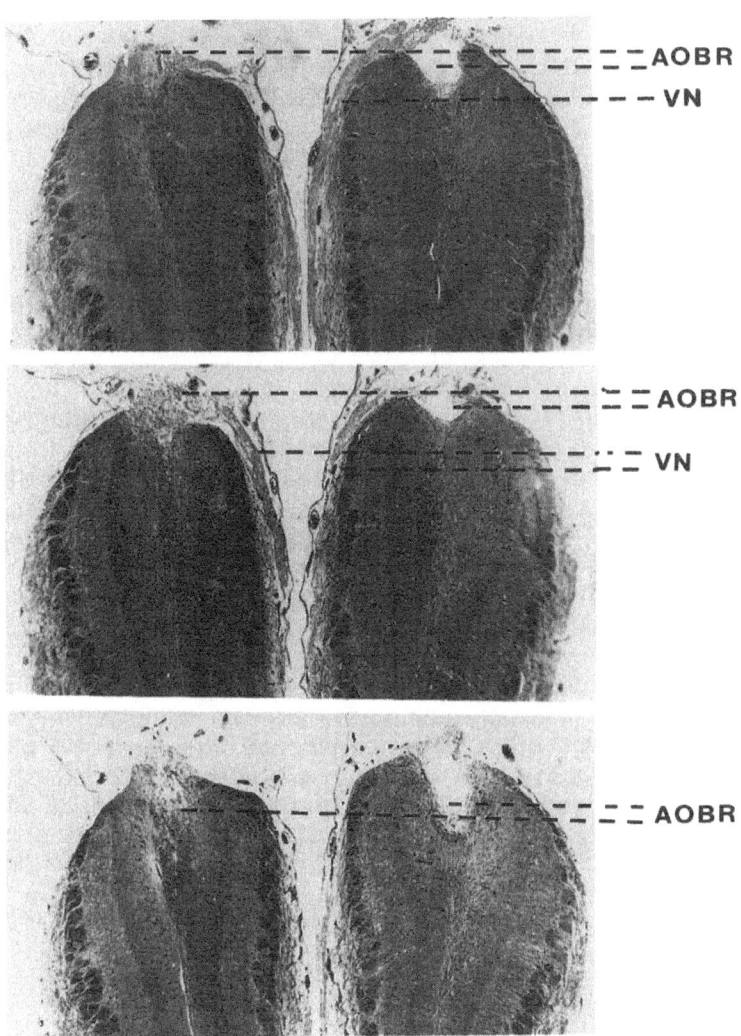

**Figure 1**  Representative horizontal sections of olfactory bulbs showing complete accessory olfactory bulb removal (AOBR) at three different levels. VN : Vomeronasal Nerve.(From Schaeffer et al., 1986a)

## Peripheral anosmia and display of lordosis behavior in the male

The aim of this experiment (Chateau and Aron, 1990) was to study the effects of peripheral anosmia caused by intranasal application of Zinc Sulfate (ZnSO4) on the display of lordosis behavior in W II castrated male rats given 25 μg EB at 10.00hr and 150 μg P 40hr later. All the animals had been placed on a 23hr food deprivation cycle and trained to locate a food pellet buried under fresh shavings once each day for 8 days. At the end of this training period they were assigned to four treatment conditions. A first and a second group were intranasally administered with either ZnSO4 or saline on the morning following EB injection. The day later they were tested for anosmia and 9 ± 1hr after P injection for lordosis behavior. After sexual behavior testing the ZnSO4 treated animals were tested for ability to locate buried food pellet once each day until the recovery of the sense of smell. Since pilot experiments showed that food deprivation might impair lordosis behavior in male rats a third group received intranasal ZnSO4 applications and a fourth group was given saline at the end of the training period and free access to food was then allowed for a week. At the end of this feeding period the animals were given ovarian hormones, ZnSO4 or saline and tested for lordosis as those of the first and second groups. Recovery of the sense of smell was tested as above.

The results shown in Table I indicate that ZnSO4 treatment significantly increased LQ values in both underfed and fed animals as compared to saline treated animals ($F_{(1,35)} = 41.29$ ; $P < 0.001$) but did not cause any changes in the number of fed animals showing lordosis behavior. They also show that irrespective of ZnSO4 treatment the number of animals displaying lordosis behavior was significantly reduced following food deprivation as compared to fed animals ($\varepsilon = 2.44$; $P < 0.02$).

Peripheral anosmia thus appeared to enhance the sexual performance as expressed by lordosis scores in castrated male rats feminized by ovarian hormones. Therefore it is reasonable to suppose that the main olfactory pathway conveys the olfactory cues which modulate sexual performance.

However peripheral anosmia did not affect the occurrence of lordosis behavior as compared with the controls. Regarding both the effects of AOB lesions and of anterior olfactory bulb removal it is likely that the main olfactory system regulates the sexual performance while the accessory olfactory system controls the willingness of the male to display lordosis behavior.

# Neuroendocrine mechanisms of lordosis behavior in the male rat

## The ventromedial nucleus is a primary center for the activation of lordosis behavior by ovarian hormones in the male

**Table I** Display of lordosis in castrated male rats primed with estradiol benzoate (EB) and progesterone (P) at an interval of 40hr. Effects of peripheral anosmia (ZnSO4) and/or food deprivation.

| Treatment | | Proportion of rats displaying lordosis behavior | Mean lordosis quotient ± S.E. in rats displaying lordosis |
|---|---|---|---|
| Food deprivation | Zn SO4 | 7/22† ≠(32 %) | 77.7 ± 5.1* |
| | Saline | 2/16† (12 %) | 49.0 ± 1.6 |
| Free access to food | Zn SO4 | 16/33 (48 %) | 85.2 ± 2.8 * |
| | Saline | 14/30 (47 %) | 47.5 ± 5.1 |

† Food deprivation vs Free access to food, $P < 0.02$; * Zn SO4 vs saline, $P < 0.001$; ≠ Zn SO4 vs saline, NS.

The hypothalamic ventromedial nucleus (VMN) is known to constitute a primary center for the activation of lordosis by ovarian hormones in the female rat (Carrer and al., 1973; Kennedy and Mitra, 1963; Pfaff and Sakuma, 1979). However the existence has been postulated (Okada and al., 1980; Yamanouchi and Arai, 1983) of a dual system facilitating female lordosis behavior, involving both the VMN and the pontine periventricular gray. It was therefore important to determine whether, in the male, the VMN also plays a key role in the display of lordosis behavior. This was suggested by experiments (Davis and Barfield, 1979) showing activation of lordosis behavior by implants of EB in the VMN of castrated male rats primed with estrogen. Yet the possibility that lordosis behavior might be displayed in the absence of the VMN remained to be explored. The following experiments (Chateau and Aron, 1987) were then carried out using WII castrated male rats which received 25 µg EB and 150 µg P, at an interval of 40hr, and were tested for lordosis behavior by 9 ± 1hr after P injection.

A week after castration was performed bilateral stereotaxic lesions were placed into the VMN, in a first group of animals, into the hypothalamic dorsomedial nucleus (DMN), in a second group, and sham operated animals served as non lesioned controls. Only the animals showing bilateral lesions of either the VMN or the DMN were taken into consideration. None of the VMN lesioned animals (0/16) displayed lordosis behavior as compared to the DMN lesioned and sham operated animals which showed lordosis responses in 50 % of the cases (8/16 and 8/16 respectively, $P < 0.01$). No differences in LQ values were noted in these last two groups of animals (36.9 ± 3.1 and 45.8 ±

11.9, respectively). The VMN may thus be considered as a target for ovarian hormones in the activation of lordosis behavior in the male rat as is the case in the female rat.

## Involvement of the amygdala in the control of lordosis behavior

The preceding results showing the role played by the olfactory system and the hypothalamic ventromedial nucleus in the control of lordosis behavior in the male led us to speculate that the amygdala also influences this kind of behavior. We have two good reasons to make this hypothesis. It is well known (Winans and Scalia, 1970; Scalia and Winans, 1975) that the corticomedial nucleus of the amygdala (CMN) receives afferent fibers from both the AOB and the main olfactory bulb, the former projecting fibers to the posteromedial region of the CMN and the latter to the anterolateral region. For its part the VMN receives projections via the stria terminalis from different amygdaloid nuclei (Winans and Scalia, 1970; Mac Lean, 1985). On the other hand, the interesting study by Masco and Carrer (1980) conclusively demonstrated that lesions placed in the corticomedial amygdaloid nucleus made female rats less receptive while lesions in the lateral amygdaloid nucleus had an opposite effect.

This encouraged us to examine the effects of lesions in different amygdaloid nuclei on lordosis behavior in male rats castrated as adults and primed with ovarian hormones.

### Effects of corticomedial nucleus lesions

The first experiment (Chateau and Aron, 1988) was designed to examine the effects of extended stereotaxic lesions of the CMN. One to two weeks after lesioning W II castrated male rats were given 25 µg EB and 150 µg P 40hr apart and tested for lordosis behavior $9 \pm 1$ hr after P injection. None of the lesioned animals (0/16) displayed lordosis in response to male mounts as compared to sham operated (8/16) and unoperated controls (8/16) (P < 0.01). Further experiments (Chateau and Aron, 1989) were performed to investigate the effects of lesions placed in different regions of the CMN. Stereotaxic lesions were placed into either the posterior part or the anterior part of the CMN. The schedule of hormone treatment and behavioral testing was the same as in the preceding group. Table II summarizes the results.

Posterior CMN lesions severely impaired the occurrence of lordosis with respect to sham operated and intact control animals ($X^2 = 10.3$ ; P < 0.01). LQ values did not differ in the three groups of animals. For their part, anterior CMN lesions did not induce any changes in the number of animals showing lordosis behavior as compared to sham operated animals but higher LQ values were observed in responding lesioned animals than in their sham operated counterparts ($F_{(1.30)} = 13.41$ ; P < 0.001).

**Table II** Effects of lesions of the anterior and posterior regions of the corticomedial amygdaloid nucleus (CMN) on lordosis behavior in castrated male rats primed with estradiol benzoate (EB) and progesterone (P).

| Treatment | Proportion of rats displaying lordosis | | Mean LQ in rats displaying lordosis ± SEM |
|---|---|---|---|
| **Experiment 1** | | | |
| Posterior CMN lesions | 3/32[†] | (9,3 %) | 31.0 ± 10.5 |
| Sham lesions | 10/24 | (41,7 %) | 48.8 ± 5.4 |
| Intact controls | 12/28 | (42,8 %) | 40.1 ± 4.0 |
| **Experiment 2** | | | |
| Anterior CMN lesions | 15/34 | (44,1 %) | 77.5 ± 2.6 [*] |
| Sham lesions | 17/42 | (40,5 %) | 48.0 ± 5.7 |

[†]P < 0.01 vs sham and controls ; [*] P < 0.001 vs sham.

## Effects of laterobasal nucleus lesions

We first examine the effects of extended lesions of the laterobasal nucleus of the amygdala (LN) on the display of lordosis behavior in W II castrated male rats given 25 μg EB and 100 μg P 40hr apart and tested for lordosis by 9 ± 1hr after P injection. A first behavioral testing was performed by 1 week after lesioning. Since pilot experiments suggested that extended lesions of the LN did not affect lordosis behavior at that time, a second test for lordosis was conducted by 4 weeks after lesioning under the same schedule of hormonal treatment as in the preceding test. In view of the observations of Masco and Carrer (1980) showing that posterior LN lesions specifically facilitated lordosis behavior in the female, lesions were placed into the posterior part and the anterior part of the LN respectively while sham-lesioned and unoperated animals served as controls. Concerning behavioral sessions, the same timing schedule as in the preceding experiments was used but the animals submitted to posterior LN lesions received 25 μg EB and 100 μg P and those lesioned in the anterior part of the LN 25 μg EB and 150 μg P before behavioral testing.

The results (Chateau and Aron, 1989) presented in Table III show that extended lesions of the LN neither affected the proportion of animals displaying lordosis behavior, nor caused any significant changes in LQ values by 1 and 4 weeks after surgery.

They also indicate that posterior LN lesions did not affect the display of lordosis behavior by 1 week after surgery. By contrast, the number of animals showing lordosis 4 weeks after surgery was significantly higher in lesioned animals than in their sham lesioned or unoperated counterparts ($X^2 = 16.4$ ; P < 0.001). As to LQ, the mean LQ values appeared higher in lesioned animals than in the two other groups in both the first and the second testing but the difference only appeared statistically significant in the second testing (F (1,27) = 8.21 ; P < 0.001).

Following lesioning in the anterior part of the LN, the number of animals showing lordosis behavior in both the first and the second testing was less in lesioned animals than in sham lesioned and unoperated animals but the difference only was significant in the first testing ($X^2$ = 6.82 ; P < 0.01).

## A tentative interpretation of the neuroendocrine mechanisms of lordosis behavior in the male rat

The present results show that an olfacto-amygdaloid pathway is involved in the display of bisexual behavior in the male rat. They support the view that the facilitatory control exerted by the VMN on the occurrence of lordosis is dependent on the caudal part of the CMN which itself is normally repressed by the action of the AOB; in addition, the data indicate that the rostral part of the CMN constitutes the target for the main olfactory system which modulates the sexual performance of the males displaying lordosis behavior. The CMN may then be considered as an heterogenous nervous structure exerting a dual control on the display of lordosis behavior in the male rat with a rostral region subserving inhibitory mechanisms probably related to satiety and caudal region regulating the willingness of males to display lordosis in response to mounts of male congeners.

As the VMN and the CMN, the LN represents a common neural substrate for the modulation of lordosis behavior in male and female rats. Our experiments in the male showed that lesions placed in the posterior part of the LN induced facilitation of the occurrence of lordosis and enhancement of the sexual performance. By contrast, lesions of the anterior part of the LN impaired the display of lordosis behavior. Since the anterior part of the LN projects fibers to the VMN (Kita and Oomura, 1982; Luiten et al., 1983), it constitutes a good candidate as a target for the inhibitory control exerted by the posterior part of the LN on lordosis behavior in the male. Alternatively the inhibitory effects may be mediated by the CMN which receives projections from the LN (Ottersen, 1982). Therefore extra-amygdaloid and intra-amygdaloid connections may explain the facilitation and inhibitory modulation of lordosis behavior in the male rat by a nervous structure which is not directly connected which the olfactory system.

# Mechanisms of interplay between the olfactory cues and the hormonal signals

Since the hypothalamic VMN constitutes in the male a target for the induction of lordosis by ovarian hormones, the question might be addressed whether the olfactory cues from the male interplay with the hormonal signals at the VMN level. This hypothesis had been suggested by our study (Chateau et al., 1987) showing that olfactory cues were inefficient in VMN lesioned W II male rats

**Table III** Effects of lesions of the laterobasal amygdaloid nucleus (LN) on lordosis behavior in castrated male rats primed with estradiol benzoate (EB) and progesterone (P).

| Treatment[a] | Proportion of rats displaying lordosis[b] | | Mean LQ ± SE in rats displaying lordosis | |
|---|---|---|---|---|
| | I | II | I | II |
| **Experiment 1** | | | | |
| Large LN lesions | 2/16 (12.5%) | 2/16 (12.5%) | 86.5 ± 3.5 | 76.5 ± 3.5 |
| Sham lesions | 6/24 (25.0%) | 7/24 (28.2%) | 51.8 ± 1.1 | 58.9 ± 5.0 |
| Intact controls | 6/24 (25.0%) | 8/24 (33.3%) | 49.0 ± 9.3 | 53.0 ± 7.5 |
| **Experiment 2** | | | | |
| LN posterior part lesions | 2/17[†] (11.8%) | 15/17* (88.2%) | 70.5 ± 15.5 | 70.0 ± 3.8** |
| Sham lesions | 5/24 (20.8%) | 7/24 (29.2%) | 35.6 ± 2.5 | 48.7 ± 6.8 |
| Intact controls | 6/24 (25.0%) | 8/24 (33.3%) | 49.0 ± 9.3 | 53.0 ± 5.7 |
| **Experiment 3** | | | | |
| LN anterior part lesions | 2/18** (11.1%) | 4.18 (22.2%) | 19.0 ± 0.9 | 28.2 ± 6.1 |
| Sham lesions | 11/24 (45.8%) | 11/24 (45.8%) | 37.4 ± 5.1 | 39.6 ± 4.8 |
| Intact controls | 11/24 (45.8%) | 12/24 (50.0%) | 30.0 ± 3.2 | 36.8 ± 3.7 |

[a] The animals received 25 µg EB (s.c.) at 16.00hr and either 100 µg P (s.c.) (experiment 1 and 2) or 150 µg P (s.c.) (experiment 3)
[b] Behavioral testing one week (I) and 4 weeks (II) after lesioning and 9 ± 1hr after P injection
[†] I vs II : P < 0.001. Lesions vs sham and controls * P < 0.01; ** P < 0.001

primed with EB and P. The hormone requirements for the facilitation of lordosis behavior by the olfactory cues in W II castrated animals had been previously clarified (Chabli et al., 1985). As shown in Table IV, the effects a dose of 25 µg, only capable *per se* of inducing lordosis behavior in a small number of animals, was not potentiated by exposure to the odor of male urine. It was also observed that P, in the absence of exposure to urine, was capable of enhancing the action of EB in a dose dependent manner.

A significant increase in the number of animals showing lordosis was noted in the males given 150 µg P compared to those given EB only or EB associated with 100 µg P. But the main fact which emerged from this study concerned the effects of a dose of 100 µg P which was uncapable as such to potentiate the effects of EB but became efficient under exposure to the odor of male urine. This led us to assume that an interaction between hormonal and sensory signals was involved in the facilitation of lordosis behavior in the male rat and to determine whether the facilitatory effects exerted by olfactory cues on lordosis behavior in the male rat were related to either changes in the amounts

**Table IV** Effects of exposure to the odor of urine collected from intact male rats on the display of feminine behavior in Wistar male rats (strain W II) castrated as adults and primed with estradiol benzoate (EB) (s.c.) combined or not with increasing doses of progesterone (P) (s.c.).

| Treatment | | Proportion of rats displaying lordosis responses [a] | | Mean LQ[b]± SE in rats displaying lordosis responses |
|---|---|---|---|---|
| 25 µg EB | No urine | 6/30 | (20.0%) | 52.2 ± 12.9 |
| | Urine | 5/30 | (16.7%) | 53.0 ± 13.7 |
| 25 µg EB | No urine | 4/28 | (14.3%) | 52.5 ± 3.8 |
| + 100 µg P[t] | Urine* | 20/30* | (66.7%) | 46.4 ± 6.0 |
| 25 µg EB | No urine | 12/29 | (41.3%) | 52.3 ± 8.3 |
| + 150 µg P[t] | Urine* | 13/16** | (82.2%) | 61.0 ± 8.0 |

[a] Testing with two vigorous males was performed by 48 ±1hr following EB injection.
[b] Lordosis quotient.
[t] By 39hr following EB injection and by 8hr before the behavioral session.
* Bedding soiled by 39hr after EB.
* P < 0.001 compared to no urine value ; ** P < 0.01 compared to no urine value.

of E2 and P receptors or in the binding capacity of estrogen to its receptors at the hypothalamic level.

Experiments were then conducted (Samama and Aron, 1989) in W II male rats which were castrated as adults and given either 25 µg EB alone or 25 µg EB + 100 µg P sequentially and exposed or not to the odor of male urine, as in Chabli's et al. (1985) experiments. Testing a first group of animals for lordosis behavior, 48hr after EB, confirmed previous results from Chabli et al. (1985). Exposure to the odor of male urine significantly increased the number of animals displaying lordosis only in those given EB + P (11/20 vs 2/20; P < 0.001). No difference appeared between the animals receiving EB only when exposed or not to the odor of urine (4/20 vs 1/20; P > 0.25). A second group was then killed 44hr after EB and used for E2 and P receptor assay in the mediobasal hypothalamus (MBH). Table V summarizes the results. Olfactory cues were shown to increase the number of E2 receptors in both the animals given EB or EB + P (P < 0.001) and P as such appeared to be capable of increasing the number (P < 0.001) and the rate of occupancy (P < 0.01) of E2 receptors.

A population of constitutive and estrogen inducible P receptors was detected in the MBH. Since only the animals given EB + P were shown to be sensitive to the facilitatory effects of male urine on lordosis behavior, it may be assumed that EB and P, on one hand, and olfactory cues on the other, exert cumulative effects at the level of the VMN and that both a high level and a high rate of occupancy of $E_2$ receptors are necessary for the olfactory cues to facilitate the display of lordosis behavior in the male rat.

**Table V** Estradiol ($E_2$) receptors in the mediobasal hypothalamus. Effects of exposure to the odor of male urine in castrated male rats given estradiol benzoate (EB) and progesterone (P) subsequently.

| Treatment [a] | Total nuclear and cytosolic $E_2$ receptors (fmol/mg DNA)[b] | Cytosolic $E_2$ receptors (fmol/mg DNA) | Nuclear $E_2$ receptors (fmol/mg DNA) | Percentage of nuclear $E_2$ receptors |
|---|---|---|---|---|
| Non injected controls | $184 \pm 3$ | $85 \pm 46$ | $99 \pm 48$ | $41 \pm 21$ |
| 25 µg EB   no urine | $186 \pm 18$ | $63 \pm 37$ | $123 \pm 38$ | $64 \pm 3$ |
|         urine[c] | $289 \pm 39$ | $140 \pm 84$ | $149 \pm 61$ | $63 \pm 4$ |
| 25 µg EB   no urine | $361 \pm 56$ | $136 \pm 69$ | $225 \pm 115$ | $93 \pm 4$ |
| + 100 µg P[d]  urine[c] | $829 \pm 30$ | $330 \pm 169$ | $499 \pm 172$ | $100 \pm 0$ |

[a] Removal of MBH, 44hr following EB
[b] The values represent the mean ($\pm$ SEM) of three experiments with duplicate determinations
[c] Bedding soiled by 10 ml urine 39hr following EB
[d] 39hr following EB

# Conclusions

Taken together the results presented here conclusively demonstrate that it is possible to induce lordosis behavior in Wistar male rats castrated as adults and given ovarian hormones. It is thus likely that the hypothalamic and limbic structures which underlie the display of lordosis in the male remain responsive to hormone treatment in adulthood despite the prenatal and neonatal effects of androgens secreted by the testes. However, it is important to note that strain differences in hormonal sensitivity exist in male rats. Overall, the males of the Wistar strain have been shown to be responsive to estrogens alone (Aren-Engelbrektsson et al., 1970; Van De Poll and Van Dis, 1977; Södersten et al., 1983; Chabli et al., 1985) or associated with P (Van De Poll and Van Dis, *op. cit.*;Chabli et al.,*op. cit.*; Schaeffer et al., 1986b). Long-Evans males appeared to be more responsive to hormone treatment in adulthood than Sprague-Dawley rats (Whalen et al., 1986) but progesterone failed to potentiate the effects of estrogen in Long-Evans (Davidson and Levine, 1969) and in Sprague-Dawley (Clemens and Gladue, 1978; Moreines et al., 1986) male rats by contrast with its facilitatory effects in the Wistar strain. The most plausible interpretation of these differences in lordosis potentials is that Wistar rats are less defeminized by their testes than those of the other strains and then more responsive to both estrogen and P.

A second point deserves attention. It concerns the neuroendocrine mechanisms governing sexual behavior in the male rat. The major finding of our studies is the demonstration, in both sexes, of a common neural substrate for the display of lordosis behavior. The fact that VMN lesions impaired the occurrence of lordosis in castrated male rats primed with EB + P clearly indicates that the VMN plays a key role in the control of bisexuality in the male rat. However this does not rule out at all the possibility that other nervous structures are also involved. According to Yamanouchi and Arai (1985) the pontine periventricular gray is implicated independently of the VMN in the activation of lordosis in the male as it does in the female rat (Yamanouchi and Arai, 1983).

It still remains to understand how the dimorphic structural organization of the nervous system in the male is compatible with the display of bisexuality. The vomeronasal organ (Segovia and Guillamon, 1982) and the AOB (Segovia et al., 1984; Roos et al., 1988, 1989) are sexually dimorphic structures controlled by the androgen present after birth. Androgens secreted by the testes shortly before birth may also affect in the male the organization of the preoptic area to promote the formation of the so-called sexual dimorphic nucleus (Gorsky et al., 1978). Both the preoptic area (see for review : Aron, 1984) and the AOB (Saito and Molz, 1986) are known to control the display of lordosis behavior in the male rat. By contrast preoptic lesions (Hennessey et al., 1986) and AOB lesions (Schaeffer et al., 1986) have been shown to facilitate the display of lordosis behavior in the male rat. It is then as though the nervous structures which facilitate masculine behavior in the male exert inhibitory effects on lordosis behavior. Similar mechanisms have been described (Kondo et al., 1990) showing in the male rat that the lateral septum potentiated the facilitatory effects of the medial preoptic area on mounting behavior but inhibited the dorsolateral preoptic area which facilitates the display of lordosis behavior.

The existence of repressive structures of bisexuality in the male rat probably accounts, in the absence of hormone treatment, for the very rare occurrence of lordosis, with the exception of a Danish strain of Wistar rats (Södersten et al., 1974), in the males of other strains. This means that both an appropriate hormone treatment and olfactory environment (Chabli et al., 1985; Schaeffer et al., 1986; Chabli et al., 1989) are necessary to counterbalance the influence of these inhibitory mechanisms thus allowing the activation of the nervous structures involved in the facilitation of lordosis behavior.

Taking the rat as an experimental model we are then led to assume that both inherited and environmental determinants are involved in the expression of bisexuality. Obviously we must keep in mind that the present knowledge in that field is based on the use of an artificial model. This raises the question of the ecological and physiological significance of the results. In that respect it is frustrating to realize that we only have a clear understanding of the mechanisms of bisexuality in manipulated male rats. We completely ignore those mechanisms which govern bisexuality in non-hormonally intact animals. The most convincing evidence is that blood estradiol and testosterone concentration did not differ in the males which spontaneously display lordosis behavior and those which do not (Södersten et al., 1974; Schaeffer et al., 1990a).

Notwithstanding, the males of the W I strain in which very few sexually inexperienced animals are capable of displaying spontaneous lordosis behavior may acquire this behavior (Chabli et al., 1991) following repeated sexual contacts with highly receptive females. Any interpretation of this phenomenon would be speculative at the present time. However these results suggest that the intact male rat possesses a nervous organization capable of mediating lordosis. Further experiments are then required to determine whether the occurrence of spontaneous lordosis by male rats is dependent either on neural sensitivity to the hormones present or on the capacity of the brain to aromatize androgens. This could be a stimulating approach for the study of bisexuality in the future.

# Acknowledgments

The authors thank Mr. Dujol for making the figure and Mrs. Matern and Machart for typing the manuscript.

# References

Aren-Engelbrektsson, B., Larsson, K., Södersten, P. and Wilhelmsson, M. (1970). The female lordosis pattern induced in male rats by estrogen. *Horm. Behav.*, **1** : 181-188.

Aron, C. (1984). La Neurobiologie du Comportement Sexuel des Mammifères. In: Delacour, J. (Ed.), *Neurobiologie des Comportements,* Hermann, Paris, pp. 57-108.

Beach, F. A. (1968). Factors involved in the control of mounting behavior by female mammals. In: Diamond, M. (Ed.), *Perspectives in Reproduction and Sexual Behavior,* Indiana Univiversity Press, pp. 83-131.

Carrer, H. F., Asch, G. and Aron, C. (1973). New facts concerning the role played by the ventromedial nucleus in the control of estrous cycle duration and sexual receptivity in the rat. *Neuroendocrinology,* **13** : 129-139.

Chabli, A., Schaeffer, C. and Aron, C. (1989). Lordosis inhibiting effects of endogenous progesterone in the male rat primed with estrogen. *Physiol. Behav.,* **45** : 1007-1010.

Chabli, A., Schaeffer, C. and Aron, C. (1991). Bisexual behavior in the male rat : influence of masculine sexual activity on the display of lordosis behavior. *Horm. Behav.,* **25** : 560-571.

Chabli, A., Schaeffer, C., Samama, B. and Aron, C. (1985). Hormonal control of the perception of the olfactory signals which facilitate lordosis behavior in the male rat. *Physiol. Behav.,* **35** : 729-734.

Chateau, D. and Aron, C. (1988). Heterotypic sexual behavior in male rats after lesions in different amygdaloid nuclei. *Horm. Behav.,* **22** : 379-388.

Chateau, D. and Aron, C. (1989). Lordosis behavior in male rats after lesions in different regions of the corticomedial amygdaloid nucleus. *Horm. Behav.,* **23** : 448-455.

Chateau, D. and Aron, C. (1990). Peripheral anosmia and display of lordosis behavior in the male rat. *Behav. Proc.,* **22** : 33-40.

Chateau, D., Chabli, A. and Aron, C. (1987). Effects of ventromedial nucleus lesions on the display of lordosis behavior in the male rat. Interactions with facilitory effects of male urine. *Physiol. Behav.,* **39** : 341-345.

Clemens, L. G. and Gladue, B. A. (1978). Feminine sexual behavior in rats enhanced by prenatal inhibition of androgen aromatization. *Horm. Behav.,* **11** : 190-201.

Davidson, J. M. (1969). Effects of estrogen on the sexual behavior of the male rats. *Endocrinology,* **84** : 1365-1372.

Davidson, J. M. and Levine, S. (1969). Progesterone and heterotypic sexual behaviour in male rats. *J. Endocrinol.,* **44** : 129-130.

Davis, P. G. and Barfield, R. J. (1979). Activation of feminine behavior in castrated male rats by intrahypothalamic implants of estradiol benzoate. *Neuroendocrinology,* **28** : 228-233.

Gorski, R. A., Gordon, J. H., Shryne, J. E. and Southam, A. M. (1978). Evidence for a morphological sex difference within the medial preoptic area of the rat brain. *Brain Res.,* **148** : 343-346.

Goy, R. W. and Roy, M. (1991). Heterotypic sexual behaviour in female mammals. In: Haug, M., Brain, P. F. and Aron, C. (Eds.), *Heterotypical Behaviour in Man and Animals,* Chapman and Hall, London, pp. 71-97.

Hennessey, A. C., Wallen, K. and Edwards, D. A. (1986). Preoptic lesions increase the display of lordosis behavior by male rats. *Brain Res.,* **370** : 21-28.

Kennedy, C. C. and Mitra, J. (1963). Hypothalamic control of energy balance and the reproductive cycle in the rat. *J. Physiol.,* **166** : 395-407.

Kita, H. and Oomura, Y. (1982). An HRP study of the afferent connections to rat medial hypothalamic region. *Brain Res. Bull.,* **8** : 53-62

Kondo, Y. Shinoda, A., Yamanouchi, K. and Arai, Y. (1990). Role of septum and preoptic area in regulating masculine and feminine sexual behavior in male rats. *Horm. Behav.,* **24** : 421-434.

Krafft-Ebting, R. V. (1931). *Psychopathia Sexualis,* 16 th and 17th German ed. rewritten by Moll, A. (translation by Lolstein, R.), 906p. Payot, Paris.

Luiten, P. G. M., Ono, T., Nishimo, H. Y. and Fukuda, M. (1983). Differential input from the amygdaloid body to the ventromedial hypothalamic nucleus in the rat. *Neurosci. Lett.,* **35** : 253-258.

Mac Lean, P. D. (1985). Fiber systems of the forebrain. In: Paxinos, G. (Ed.), *The Rat Nervous System* **Vol. 1,** Academic Press, New York, pp. 417-440.

Masco, D. H. and Carrer, H. F. (1980). Sexual receptivity in female rats after lesion or stimulation in different amygdaloid nuclei. *Physiol. Behav.,* **24** : 1073-1080.

Meredith, M. and O'Connell, R. (1979). Efferent control of stimulus access to the hamster vomeronasal organ. *J. Physiol. (London),* **286** : 301-316.

Moreines, J., McEwen, B. and Pfaff, D. (1986). Sex differences in reponse to discrete estradiol injections. *Horm. Behav.,* **20** : 445-451.

Muller, N. (1971). Vergleichende elektrophysiologische untersuchungen an den sinnesepitheliendes jacobsonchen organs und der nase von amphibien (Rana), reptilien (Lacerta) und saügetieren (Mus). *Z. Vergl. Physiol.,* **72** : 370-385.

Okada, R., Yamanouchi, K. and Arai, Y. (1980). Recovery of sexual receptivity in female rats with lesions of the ventromedial hypothalamus. *Exp. Neurol.,* **68** : 595-600.

Olster, D. H. and Blaustein, J. D. (1988). Progesterone facilitation of lordosis in male and female Sprague-Dawley rats following priming with estradio' pulses. *Horm. Behav.,* **22** : 294-304.

Ottersen, O. P. (1982). Connections of the amygdala in the rat. IV. Corticoamygdaloid and intraamygdaloid connections as studied with axonal transport of horseradish peroxydase. *J. Comp. Neurol.,* **205** : 30-48.

Pfaff, D. K. and Sakuma, Y. (1979). Deficit in the lordosis reflex of female rats caused by lesions in the ventromedial nucleus of the hypothalamus. *J. Physiol. (London),* **228** : 203-210.

Rehmer, H., Schulz, E. and Schönheit, B. (1970). Variabilität der form und grösse des bulbus olfactorius der erwachsenen weissen laboratte. *J. Hirnforsch.,* **12** : 111-122.

Roos, J., Roos, M., Schaeffer, C. and Aron, C. (1988). Sexual differences in the development of accessory olfactory bulbs in the rat. *J. Comp. Neurol.,* **270** : 121-131.

Roos, J., Roos, M., Schaeffer, C. and Aron, C. (1989). Prepubescent hormonal control of the development of accessory olfactory bulbs in the male rat. *Develop. Brain Res.,* **47** : 309-312.

Saito, T. R. and Moltz, H. (1986). Copulatory behavior of sexually naive and sexually experienced male rats following removal of the vomeronasal organ. *Physiol. Behav.,* **37** : 507-510.

Samama, B. and Aron, C. (1989). Changes in estrogen receptors in the mediobasal hypothalamus mediate the facilitory effects exerted by the male's olfactory cues and progesterone on feminine behavior in the male rat. *J. Steroid Biochem.,* **32** : 525-529.

Scalia, F. and Winans, S. S. (1975). The differential projections of the olfactory bulb and accessory olfactory bulb in mammals. *J. Comp. Neurol.,* **161** : 31-56.

Schaeffer, C. and Aron, C. (1981). Studies on feminine sexual behavior in the male rat : influence of olfactory stimuli. *Horm. Behav.,* **15** : 377-385.

Schaeffer, C., Roos, J. and Aron, C. (1986a). Accessory olfactory bulb lesions and lordosis behavior in the male rat feminized with ovarian hormones. *Horm. Behav.,* **20** : 118-127.

Schaeffer, C., Chabli, A. and Aron, C. (1986b). Endogenous progesterone and lordosis behavior in male rats given estrogen alone. *J. Steroid Biochem.,* **25** : 99-102.

Schaeffer, C., Chabli, A. and Aron, C. (1990a). Lordosis behavior in gonadally intact male rats : correlation with blood progesterone concentration but not with blood testosterone and 17β-estradiol values. *Biol. Behav.,* **15** : 53-61.

Schaeffer, C., Roos, J. and Aron, C. (1990b). Lordosis behavior in intact male rats : effects of hormonal treatment and/or manipulation of the olfactory system. *Horm. Behav.,* **24** : 50-61.

Schaeffer, C., Al Satli, M., Kelche, C. and Aron, C. (1982). Olfactory environment and lordosis behavior in the female and male rat. In : Breipohl, W. (Ed.), *Olfaction and Endocrine Regulation,* IRL Press Limited, London, pp. 115-126.

Segovia, A. and Guillamon, S. (1982). Effects of sex steroids in the development of the vomeronasal organ in the rat. *Dev. Brain Res.,* 5 : 209-212.

Segovia, A., Orensanz, L. M., Valencia, A. and Guillamon, A. (1984). Effects of sex steroid on the development of the accessory olfactory bulb in the rat: a volumetric study. *Dev. Brain Res.,* **16** : 312-314.

Södersten, P. (1976). Lordosis behaviour in male, female and androgenized female rats. *J. Endocrinol.,* **70** : 409-420.

Södersten, P., Petterson, A. and Eneroth, P. (1983). Pulse administration of estradiol 17β cancels sex difference in behavior estrogen sensitivity. *Endocrinology,* **112** : 1883-1885.

Södersten, P., De Jong, F. H., Vreeburg, J. T. M. and Baum, M. J. (1974). Lordosis behavior in intact male rats : absence of correlation with mounting behavior or testicular secretion of estradiol 17β and testosterone. *Physiol. Behav.,* **13** : 803-808.

Tucker, D. (1971). Non olfactory responses from the nasal cavity : Jacobson organ and the trigeminal system. In: Beidler, L. M. (Ed.), *Handbook of Sensory Physiology : Chemical Senses,* **Vol.1**, Springer Verlag, New York, pp. 151-181.

Van De Poll, N. E. and Vand Dis, H. (1977). Hormone induced lordosis and its relation to masculine sexual activity in male rats. *Horm. Behav.,* **8** : 1-7.

Whalen, R. E., Gladue, B. A. and Olsen, K. L. (1986). Lordotic behavior in male rats : genetic and hormonal regulation of sexual differentiation. *Horm. Behav.,* **20** : 73-82.

Winans, S. S. and Scalia, F. (1970). Amygdaloid nucleus new afferent input from the vomeronasal organ. *Science,* **170** : 330-332.

Yamanouchi, K. and Arai, Y. (1983). Forebrain and lower brainstem participation in facilitatory and inhibitory regulation of the display of lordosis in female rats. *Physiol. Behav.,* **30** : 155-159.

Yamanouchi, K. and Arai, Y. (1985). Presence of neural mechanisms for the expression of female sexual behaviors in the male rat brain. *Neuroendocrinology,* **40** : 393-397.

Zinik, G. (1985). Identity conflict or adaptative flexibility ? Bisexuality reconsidered. *J. Homosex.,* **1**: 7-19.

# A Sexually Dimorphic Motor Nucleus : Steroid Sensitive Afferents, Sex Differences and Hormonal Regulation

**L. G. CLEMENS, C. K. WAGNER[1] and A. E. ACKERMAN**

*Department of Zoology and Neuroscience Program, Michigan State University, East Lansing, Michigan, 48824 USA*

[1] *Present Address : Institute of Animal Behavior, Rutgers University, 101 Warren St., Newark, New Jersey, 07109 USA*

In the past two decades we have seen the development of numerous models for studying sexual differentiation of the nervous system. These include the sexually dimorphic area (SDA) of the hypothalamus in the rat (see Gorski, 1991 for review), ferret (Tobet et al., 1986) and gerbil (Commins and Yahr, 1984), the vocal control system in song birds (Notebohm and Arnold, 1976; see also Arnold, 1985 and Konishi, 1985 for reviews) and the sexually dimorphic motor nuclei of the lower lumbar cord (see Rand and Breedlove, 1988 for review). Each model offers specific advantages and each comes with its own limitations. We have chosen to focus on the sexually dimorphic motor nuclei of the lower lumbar cord, the spinal nucleus of the bulbocavernosus (SNB) and the dorsolateral nucleus (DLN). The SNB has served as an excellent model for the study of sexual differentiation in the central nervous system because the SNB is sexually dimorphic, motoneurons of the male SNB concentrate androgens, and the development of the SNB is dependent on the presence of gonadal steroids during perinatal life. In addition, the SNB contains a limited number of cells that can be easily identified, counted and labelled. In this regard, examining the supraspinal afferents to the SNB as a model for sexual dimorphism in the CNS is important to the understanding of neural circuits involving steroid sensitive neurons and how they may regulate sexually dimorphic behaviors.

The SNB is part of a neural circuit that has the potential to modulate penile responses through its innervation of the bulbocavernosus muscle (BC). Recent findings from our laboratory suggest that the androgen sensitive cells of the SNB are part of a larger steroid hormone-sensitive neural circuit in which both efferent target tissues as well as the afferent components of the circuit are sensitive to gonadal steroid hormones.

*M. Haug et al. (eds.), The Development of Sex Differences and Similarities in Behavior, 19–31.*
© 1993 *Kluwer Academic Publishers.*

# Sexual differentiation of the SNB

In the rat, the SNB is a sexually dimorphic motor nucleus located in the lower lumbar spinal cord (Breedlove and Arnold, 1980). Larger in the male than in the female, it provides somatic efferent innervation to the bulbocavernosus (BC) (bulbospongiosum) muscle. The SNB also innervates the levator ani and the external anal sphincter (Rand and Breedlove, 1988; McKenna and Nadelhaft, 1986). Studies of the SNB have shown that it develops under the influence of gonadal hormones during early development.

During perinatal development, the motoneurons of the SNB share a common population of cells with the DLN (Sengelaub and Arnold, 1986). Between embryonic day 22 and postnatal day 10, the cells of the SNB migrate medially toward the dorsomedial region of the ventral horn. The sex difference in the number of SNB motoneurons is not yet present during this cell migration. In both males and females, the number of motoneurons continues to increase until the day before birth, at which time the number of cells exceeds that of an adult male (Sengelaub and Arnold, 1986). A critical period of differential cell death occurs from the day before birth to postnatal day 10. It is during this time that sexual differentiation occurs in motoneuron number and in the masculinization of perineal musculature. In the absence of circulating androgens, females lose a greater number of motoneurons due to cell death, and their perineal musculature begins to atrophy as compared to males. However, cell loss is reduced in developing females treated with androgens and induced in males treated with the anti-androgen, flutamide (Sengelaub and Arnold, 1986; Nordeen et al., 1984; Breedlove and Arnold, 1983a; Breedlove and Arnold, 1983b). In adulthood, the SNB of males contains five times more motoneurons than females (Breedlove and Arnold, 1980; Arnold, 1984; Breedlove, 1984).

# Afferents to the SNB

While the projections of the motoneurons in the SNB have received considerable attention, less is known concerning the afferent input to this nucleus. Studies of afferent input can be used to test and expand hypotheses concerning the functional relation of the SNB to both behavior and other neural mechanisms. We were particularly interested in possible afferents from the hypothalamus to the SNB since many areas of the hypothalamus are steroid sensitive and play an important role in male copulatory behaviors. The paraventricular nucleus of the hypothalamus (PVN) became a good candidate for several reasons. It had been shown that the PVN is involved in the modulation of penile reflexes. Lesions of the PVN abolish penile reflexes that are induced by the central administration of oxytocin, or the dopamine agonist apomorphine (Argiolas et al., 1987). PVN projects to all levels of the spinal cord, including lumbar levels (Armstrong et al., 1980; Schwanzel-Fukuda et al., 1984). We tested the idea that the PVN was a possible afferent to the SNB by injecting the retrograde tracers wheatgerm agglutinin conjugated-horseradish peroxidase (WGA-HRP) or Fluorogold into the lower lumbar spinal cord. Following such injections labelled cells were found in the dorsal and lateral parvocellular (lp) subnuclei of the PVN (Wagner and Clemens, 1991). Labelled cells were also seen in the lateral hypothalamus and dorsal area of the hypothalamus, but no cells were labelled in the medial preoptic area. Since Fluorogold is not known to cross synapses, these findings suggested a direct projection from the PVN to the L5-L6 region of the spinal cord containing the sexually dimorphic motor nuclei.

While the functional significance of this projection requires further analysis, it is important to note that the PVN is the chief source of oxytocin in the CNS (Hawthorne et al., 1985; Lang et al., 1983). Since oxytocin also plays an important role in male sexual responses (Argiolas et al., 1987; Melis et al., 1986), it is likely that the projections of the PVN to the lower lumbar cord are involved with these oxytocin effects. If oxytocin from the PVN is involved with supraspinal modulation of the SNB, one would expect to find oxytocin and related peptides in the projections from PVN to the SNB. Our studies show that immunoreactivity for both oxytocin and its co-product, neurophysin, are present in fibers in the L5-L6 region of the cord. In males, many fibers, appearing to enter the ventral horn by running adjacent to the central canal, were found among the motoneuron cell bodies of the SNB (Figure 1). These fibers in the ventral horn were located only within the rostro-caudal extent of the SNB motor nucleus, suggesting that these fibers play a role specific to the functioning of this nucleus. Fibers were rarely found in the region of the DLN.

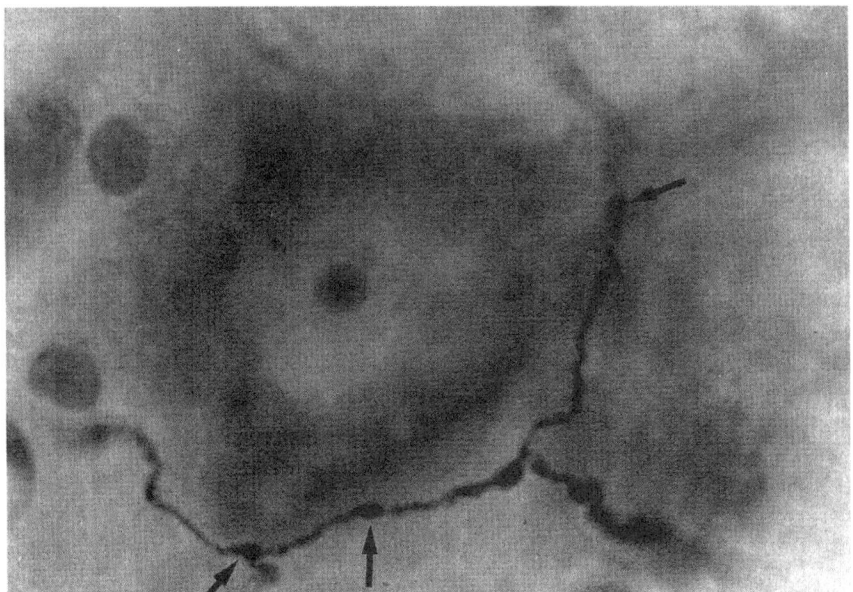

**Figure 1** Neurophysin containing fibers and putative terminals (arrows) that appear to contact the soma of and SNB motoneuron.

22

Two additional studies provide further support for the notion that fibers containing neurophysin and/or oxytocin originate in the PVN. First, lesions in the PVN abolished neurophysin immunoreactivity (ir) in the lower lumbar cord. Few if any neurophysin-ir fibers could be found in the region of the SNB subsequent to lesions that destroyed the lp subnucleus of PVN (Wagner and Clemens, unpublished). In a second study, a double labelling paradigm was used to show that some of the cells in the PVN that project to the SNB contain neurophysin-ir or oxytocin-ir. When PVN cells were retrogradely labelled with Fluorogold following injections into the lower lumbar spinal cord, then reacted with antisera for neurophysin, we found that more that approximately 20 % of the Fluorogold labelled cells in PVN contained neurophysin-ir (Wagner and Clemens, unpublished). Nearly 70 % of cells containing both Fluorogold and neurophysin-ir were located in the lp subnucleus of PVN. Within the lp, 30 % of the Fluorogold-labelled cells contained neurophysin-ir. Work in progress has also shown that some of the cells in PVN that project to lower lumbar spinal cord also contain oxytocin-ir (Ackerman and Clemens, 1992).

One characteristic of the neural substrates that mediate copulatory behavior is their responsiveness to gonadal hormones. This is evident in the SNB both during development and in the adult. During development gonadal steroids play a major role in the regulation of the dendritic arborization of SNB motoneurons (Goldstein et al., 1990). In the adult, castration reduces synaptic coverage of SNB motoneurons, an effect that is reversed by testosterone replacement (Leedy et al., 1987; Matsumoto et al., 1988). Taken together these findings support the idea that steroid hormones modulate the relation between SNB motoneurons and their afferent input. We next addressed the hypothesis that steroid sensitive neural circuits exist, in which neurons of all nuclei within a circuit contain steroid receptors. Because these circuits are the target of steroid hormone action, the activity of these pathways may play a key role in the display of sexually dimorphic behavior.

Specifically we wanted to know if PVN neurons that project to the region of the SNB contain nuclear steroid receptors. Previous literature had documented that there are relatively few androgen receptor-containing neurons in the PVN of male rats (Sar and Stumpf, 1975; Lisciotto and Morrell, personal communication). In the male, testosterone can be metabolized to estradiol by the P450 enzyme aromatase. We therefore examined the PVN for neurons containing receptors for estrogen. This was achieved using retrograde fluorescent tract tracing in conjunction with steroid hormone autoradiography (Wagner et al., unpublished).

While estradiol-concentrating cells were found throughout the PVN of the male, the majority were located in the anterior and lp subnuclei. The majority of double labelled cells, those containing Fluorogold and concentrating estradiol, was found in the lp subnucleus and very few in other subnuclei. Approximately 30 % of the neurons in the lp subnucleus that project to the lower lumbar cord concentrate estradiol. Nearly 50 % of the estrogen-concentrating cells in the lp subnucleus project to the lower lumbar spinal cord. This study, providing the first evidence that steroid hormone-sensitive hypothalamic neurons send axons to the spinal cord, strengthens the concept that the PVN and SNB are components of a larger steroid hormone-sensitive neural circuit mediating male reproductive behavior.

The finding that 30 % of the neurons in the lp subnucleus that project to the lumbar cord also concentrate estradiol suggests that some of these steroid hormone-concentrating cells may also contain oxytocin. In support of this hypothesis are results demonstrating that in the female rat some estrogen-sensitive PVN neurons are also neurophysin-producing cells (Rhodes et al., 1981).

The functional roles played by these populations of estrogen concentrating and oxytocin producing cells in PVN that project to lower lumbar spinal cord in the male is not clear. However, the function of the SNB/BC neuromuscular system (i.e. penile reflexes) is dependent upon gonadal steroid hormones (Hart, 1973; Rodgers and Alheid, 1972; Davidson et al., 1978; Bradshaw et al., 1981). Castration abolished penile reflexes which were restored by testosterone replacement (Gray et al., 1980). While administration of estrogen failed to facilitate penile response in the *ex copula* situation, estrogen did restore penile responses and copulatory behavior in castrated males during mating tests with females (Meisel et al., 1984; O'Hanlon et al., 1981). It is possible that the elicitation of penile reflexes *ex copula* involves only local lumbosacral spinal circuity, whereas the display of these reflexes in the context of copulation involves hypothalamic circuits as well. If so, the ability of estrogen to restore penile responses only during copulation may require supraspinal levels of neural function that are important in the display of male copulatory behavior. One mechanism by which estrogen may restore penile reflexes during copulation is by acting on the estrogen-sensitive pathway from the PVN to the region of the SNB.

# Male and female comparisons

Neurophysin-containing fibers have been found in several regions of the lower lumbar spinal cord in both male and female rats (Wagner and Clemens, unpublished). In both sexes, neurophysin-containing fibers were seen in the region dorsal to the central canal in laminas X and IV and in the intermediolateral cell column. In addition, fibers were also found in the apex of the dorsal horn in laminas II and III. Rarely were fibers found in the ventral horn, with the exception of the region of the male SNB.

In general, the distribution of neurophysin-containing fibers in the lower lumbar spinal cord of the female is similar to that seen in the male. However, there appeared to be some degree of sexual dimorphism. The density of fibers in the region dorsal to the central canal (lamina X) was greater in females compared to males. In contrast, there was a smaller number of fibers in the apex of the dorsal horn (laminas II and III) in the female compared to the male. The most dramatic sex difference in the distribution of neurophysin fibers was seen in the ventral horn. Whereas neurophysin fibers were found throughout the SNB of males, there was a virtual absence of fibers in the region of the SNB in females. The fibers in the ventral horn of females were generally located in the ventral funiculus and not in the gray matter and were found in fewer and more rostral sections in the female than in the male.

In addition to the PVN, the region of the SNB also receives input from a variety of other brain areas. Using retrograde tracers it has been shown that one of the heaviest sets of input come from the lateral vestibular nucleus, and the gigantocellular reticular nucleus (including the ventral and alpha divisions) (Shen et al., 1990). Cells were also found in the medullary raphe nuclei, the ventral medullary nucleus, and the spinal vestibular nucleus. In the pons, cells were found in the locus coeruleus, nucleus subcoeruleus, and the caudal pontine reticular nucleus.

Afferent input from the paragigantocellular reticular nucleus has been shown to mediate a tonic, inhibitory influence on spinal coital reflexes (Bors and Comarr, 1960; Hart, 1967; Hart, 1968; Hart and Kitchell, 1966; Higgins, 1979; Riddoch, 1917; Sachs and Garinello, 1980). In the male, these reflexes consist of penile erection, contraction of striated perineal muscles, and ejaculation. In the female, coital reflexes are characterized by contractions of striated perineal muscles and rhythmic contractions of the vagina and uterus. Both sets of reflexes are elicited by urethral stimulation following spinal transection, indicating a descending, inhibitory control (Chung, 1988).

Bilateral electrolytic and neurotoxic lesions in the region of the paragigantocellular reticular nucleus were effective in removing the inhibition (Marson and McKenna, 1990). Using retrograde and anterograde tracers, these investigators reported that projections from the paragigantocellular reticular formation surround motoneurons in the DLN, the SNB and lamina X in lower lumbar spinal cord. The lamina X in lower lumbar cord has been shown to integrate visceral and somatic information (Honda, 1985).

## Studies of the SNB in the house mouse

In order to expand the comparative base for this model we carried out several experiments using the house mouse. As in the rat, the SNB in the house mouse is sexually dimorphic, containing more cells in the male than in the female (Wee and Clemens, 1987).

The SNB can be characterized by the size of its motoneurons, the number of cells present in the nucleus and by the projections of these cells. Examination of the anatomical organization of the SNB neuromuscular system in the mouse revealed a specificity that differed somewhat from the rat. Using the retrograde tracer, cholera toxin-bound horseradish peroxidase, we found that motoneurons innervating the BC were located in the SNB, (Wagner and Clemens, 1989a) as well as in the ventral nucleus (V) and in the mid-region of the ventral horn (MVH). Following injections of retrograde tracers into the ischiocavernosus muscle (IC), labelled neurons were found in the DLN, as well as in V, DM and MVH. Cells innervating the external anal sphincter in both males and females were located in the SNB, as well as in the V and MVH. An elaborate network of dendrites extended between all labelled nuclei (Wagner and Clemens, 1989a).

Using quantification methods of Breedlove and Arnold (1980), we found that in the house mouse, the number of SNB motoneurons is influenced by genotype. Using sections stained with the Nissl stain thionin, the number and size of SNB motoneurons were determined in three inbred strains of mice C57B1/6J (C57), DBA/2J (DBA) and the B6D2F1 (F1) hybrid resulting from a cross between a C57 female and a DBA male. While no strain differences were seen in the size of SNB cells, DBA males had significantly fewer SNB motoneurons than either the C57 or F1 males (Wee and Clemens, 1987).

# Hormonal control of the mouse SNB in adulthood

The influence of gonadal hormones on cell size and the number of thionin stained cells in the SNB of the mouse varies with genotype. Castration of C57 adult males significantly reduced the number of thionin stained SNB motoneurons but did not alter soma area. In the DBA, castration reduced soma area, but did not affect neuronal number. In the F1, both neuronal number and soma area were reduced by castration (Wee and Clemens, 1987).

Further analysis of the steroid hormone effects on the SNB of the F1 mouse was undertaken. The decrease in the number of SNB cells in thionin stained tissue following castration in adulthood in F1 mice, was dramatically different from results obtained in studies using rats. SNB cell number is unaffected by castration in adulthood in rats (Breedlove and Arnold, 1981). There were at least two explanations for the decrease in cell number in mice. One possibility was that the decrease in cell number following castration reflected a loss of cells due to cell death resulting from the abence of androgens. Another possibility, was that castration altered the Nissl staining properties of some SNB cells.

To rule out the possibility that the decrease in SNB cell number after castration was due to neuronal degeneration, the retrograde tracer cholera toxin-bound horseradish peroxidase (CT-HRP) was injected into the BC muscle of castrate and intact male mice. In contrast to the thionin stained material, castration did not affect the number of CT-HRP labelled motoneurons in the region of the SNB (Wagner and Clemens, 1989b). Based upon these observations we suggest that castration of the adult mouse did not result in SNB cell loss, but instead castration altered the thionin staining properties of some SNB motoneurons.

Thionin, a Nissl stain, reacts with DNA in the nucleus and RNA in the cytoplasm. Therefore, Nissl stains can serve as a crude marker of protein synthetic activity in neurons. In the mouse, castration may result in a decrease in protein synthetic activity of some SNB motoneurons and thereby result in a decrease in the accumulation of thionin stain in the cytoplasm. This would result in a decrease in the number of neurons reaching the level of detectability. The decrease in cell size following castration in F1 mice is also consistent with the idea that cell activity is being altered in the absence of gonadal steroid hormones.

# Effects of steroid hormones during development in the mouse

The sex difference in the SNB of the mouse appears to result from differential exposure to gonadal steroids during early development (Wagner and Clemens, 1989b). Male mice castrated on the day of birth had significantly fewer SNB motoneurons than sham-castrated males when examined at 30 or 60 days of age. Soma area of SNB motoneurons was not different in castrates and non-castrates at 30 days of age, but was significantly larger in shams when examined in 60 day-old adults.

Thus while cell number was altered by testosterone during early neonatal life, soma area was influenced later, between 30 and 60 days of age. This later effect probably resulted from an increase in testosterone that occurs around the time of puberty.

The effect of testosterone on cell number was also seen following prenatal treatment of females. Testosterone propionate administered during early prenatal (days E11-14) or late prenatal (days E14-17) development significantly increased SNB cell number in adult females when compared to oil treated controls (Wagner and Clemens, 1989b). Testosterone treatment on postnatal days 1, 3 and 5 also increased SNB cell number whereas testosterone exposure on postnatal days 7, 9 and 11, did not increase cell number.

Sexual differentiation of the SNB in the mouse also differs from the rat. Whereas the gonadal steroid hormones had their effect on SNB cell number both prenatally and postnatally in the mouse, the effects in the rat were limited to prenatal exposure only. Further comparisons of characteristics of the sexually dimorphic neuromuscular system between the mouse and the rat are summarized in Table 1.

# Summary

The SNB can be seen as part of a polysynaptic, steroid hormone-sensitive neural circuit. We can sketch this circuit broadly as one in which androgen-sensitive SNB motoneurons innervate the BC muscle, which also contains androgen and estrogen receptors (Krieg et al., 1974; Dube et al., 1976; Dionne et al., 1979). Motoneurons of the SNB appear to be innervated by E-concentrating neurons of the PVN. The PVN, in turn, receives input from the medial preoptic area (Silverman et al., 1981) which is known to contain androgen and estrogen concentrating neurons important for male sexual behavior (Sar and Stumpf, 1975; Stumpf et al., 1975). As we look at this expanded circuit it appears as though neurons in different locations within the circuit may be sensitive to different hormones. Thus we have a model in which several different hormones are needed to fully activate the entire circuit. Such models bring us closer to the kinds of systems that accomodate the complexity

**Table I** Species differences in the sexually dimorphic neuromuscular system

|  | MOUSE | RAT |
|---|---|---|
| **INNERVATION :** |  |  |
| Bulbocavernosus Muscle | SNB, VN | SNB |
| Ischiocavernosus Muscle | DLN, SNB, MVH | DLN |
|  |  |  |
| **SEXUALLY DIMORPHIC ?** | Yes | Yes |
|  |  |  |
| **DEVELOPMENT :** |  |  |
| Day I Castration in male | ↓ Adult Cell # | No Effect |
| Prenatal TP to female | ↑ Adult Cell # | ↑ Adult Cell # |
| Postnatal T to female | ↑ Adult Cell # | No Effect |
|  |  |  |
| **CASTRATION IN ADULTHOOD :** |  |  |
| Cell Number (Nissl) | ↓ | No Effect |
| Cell Size | ↓ | ↓ |
| Cell Number (CT-HRP) | No Effect | ? |

of the effects that hormones have on behavior. Studies of the SNB in other species such as the house mouse provide important insights into the generality and genetic variability of this model.

# Acknowledgement

This work support by NSF Grant : BNS 9109292.

# References

Ackerman, A. and Clemens, L. G. (1992). Oxytocin projections from the paraventricular nucleus of the hypothalamus to lower lumbar spinal cord and the distribution of oxytocin fibers in the region of the spinal nucleus of the bulbocovernosus in male and female rats. *Neurosci. Abstr.,* **152** :14.

Argiolas, A., Melis, M. R., Mauri, A., and Gessa, G. L. (1987). Paraventricular nucleus lesion prevents yawning and penile erection induced by apomorphine and oxytocin but not by ACTH in rats. *Brain Res.,* **421** : 349-352.

Armstrong, W. E., Warach, S., Hatton, G. I. and McNeill, T. H. (1980). Subnuclei in the rat hypothalamic paraventricular nucleus : a cytoarchitectural, horseradish peroxidase and immunocytochemical analysis. *Neuroscience*, **5** : 1931-1958.

Arnold, A. P. (1984). Androgen regulation of motor neuron size and number. *Trends Neurosci.*, **7** : 239-242.

Arnold, A. P. (1985). Gonadal steroid-induced organization and reorganization of neural circuits involved in bird song. In: Cotman, C. W. (Ed.), *Synaptic Plasticity*, Guilford, New York, pp. 263-285.

Bradshaw, W. G., Baum, M. J. and Awh, C. C. (1981). Attenuation by a 5-alpha-reductase inhibitor of the activational effect of testosterone propionate on penile erections in castrated male rats. *Endocrinology*, **109** : 1047-1051.

Bors, E. and Comarr, A. E. (1960). Neurological disturbances of sexual function with special reference to 529 patients with spinal cord injury. *Urol. Surv.*, **10** : 191-222.

Breedlove, S. M. and Arnold, A. P. (1980). Hormone accumulation in a sexually dimorphic motor nucleus in the rat spinal cord. *Science*, **210** : 564-566.

Breedlove, S. M. and Arnold, A. P. (1981). Sexually dimorphic motor nucleus in the rat lumbar spinal cord : response to adult hormone manipulation, absence in androgen-insensitive rats. *Brain Res.*, **225** : 297-307.

Breedlove, S. M. and Arnold, A. P. (1983a). Hormonal control of a developing neuromuscular system. I. Complete demasculinization of the male rat spinal nucleus of the bulbocarvenosus using the antiandrogen flutamide. *J. Neurosci.*, **3** : 417-423.

Breedlove, S. M. and Arnold, A. P. (1983b). Hormonal control of the developing neuromuscular system. II. Sensitive periods for the androgen-induced masculinization of the rat spinal nucleus of the bulbocavernosus. *J. Neurosci.*, **3** : 424-432.

Breedlove, S. M. (1984). Androgen forms sexual dimorphic spinal nucleus by saving motorneurons from programmed death. *Soc. Neurosci. Abstr.*, **10** : 927.

Chung, S. K., McVary, K. T. and McKenna, K. E. (1988). Sexual reflexes in male and female rats. *Neurosci. Let.*, **91** : 343-348.

Commins, D. and Yahr, P. (1984). Adult testosterone levels influence the morphology of a sexually dimorphic area in the mongolian gerbil brain. *J. Comp. Neurol.*, **224** : 132-140.

Davidson, J. M., Stefanick, M. L., Sachs, D. and Smith, E. R. (1978). Role of androgen in sexual reflexes of the male rat. *Physiol. Behav.*, **21** : 141-146.

Dionne, F. T., Dube, J. Y., Lesage, R. and Tremblay, R. R. (1979). In vivo androgen binding in rat skeletal and perineal muscles. *Acta Endocrinol.*, **91** : 362-372.

Dube, J. Y., Lesage, R. and Tremblay, R. R. (1976). Androgen and estrogen binding in rat skeletal and perineal muscle. *Can. J. Biochem.*, **54** : 50-55.

Goldstein, L. A., Kurz, E. M. and Sengelaub, D. R. (1990). Androgen regulation of dendritic growth and retraction in the development of a sexually dimorphic spinal nucleus. *J. Neurosci.*, **10** : 935-946.

Gorski, R. A. (1991). Sexual differentiation of the endocrine brain and its control. In : Motta, M. (Ed.), *Brain Endocrinology*, Raven Press, New York.

Gray, G. D., Smith, E. R. and Davidson, J. M. (1980). Hormonal regulation of penile erection in castrate male rats. *Physiol. Behav.*, 24 : 463-468.

Hart, B. L. (1967). Sexual reflexes and mating behavior in the male dog. *J. Comp. Physiol. Psych.*, 64 : 388-399.

Hart, B. L. (1968). Sexual reflexes and mating behavior in the male rat. *J. Comp. Physiol. Psych.*, 65 : 453-460.

Hart, B. L. (1973). Effects of testosterone propionate and dihydrotestosterone on penile morphology and sexual reflexes of spinal male rats. *Horm. Behav.*, 4 : 239-246.

Hart, B. L. and Kitchell, R. L. (1966). Penile erection and contraction of penile muscles in the spinal and intact dog. *Am. J. Physiol.*, 210 : 257-262.

Hawthorne, J., Ang, V. T. Y. and Jenkins, J. S. (1985). Effects of lesion in the hypothalamic paraventricular, supraoptic and suprachiasmatic nuclei on vasopressin and oxytocin in rat brain and spinal cord. *Brain Res.*, 346 : 51-57.

Higgins, G. E. Jr. (1979). Sexual response in spinal cord injured adults : a review of the literature. *Arch. Sex. Behav.*, 8 : 173-196.

Honda, C. N. (1985). Visceral and somatic afferent convergence onto neurons near the central canal in the sacral spinal cord of the cat. *J. Neurophysiol.*, 54 : 1059-1078.

Konishi, M. (1985). Birdsong : from behavior to neuron. *Ann. Rev. Neurosci.*, 8 : 125-170.

Krieg, M., Szalay, R. and Voight, K. D. (1974). Binding and metabolism of testosterone and 5α-dihydrotestosterone in bulbocavernosus/levator ani (BCLA) of male rats : *in vivo* and *in vitro* studies. *J. Steroid Biochem.*, 5 : 453-459.

Lang, R. E., Heil, J., Ganten, D., Hermann, K., Rascher, W. and Unger, T. (1983). Effects of lesions in the paraventricular nucleus of the hypothalamus on vasopressin and oxytocin contents in brainstem and spinal cord of rat. *Brain Res.*, 260 : 326-329.

Leedy, M. G., Beattie, T. S. and Bresnahan, J. S. (1987). Testosterone-induced plasticity of synaptic inputs ot adult mammalian motoneurons. *Brain Res.*, 424 : 386-390.

Marson, L. and McKenna, K. E. (1990). The identification of a brainstem site controlling spinal sexual reflexes in male rats. *Brain Res.*, 515 : 303-308.

Matsumoto, A., Micevych, P. E. and Arnold, A. P. (1988). Androgen regulates synaptic input ot motoneurons of the adult rat spinal cord. *J. Neurosci.*, 8 : 4168-4176.

McKenna, K. E. and Nadelhaft, I. (1986). The organization of the pudendal nerve in the male and female rat. *J. Comp. Neurol.*, 248 : 532-549.

Meisel, R. L., O'Hanlon, J. K. and Sachs, B. D. (1984). Differential maintenance of penile responses and copulatory behavior by gonadal hormone in castrated male rats. *Horm. Behav.*, 18 : 56-64.

Melis, M. R., Argiolas, A. and Gessa, G. L. (1986). Oxytocin induced penile erection and yawning : site of action in the brain. *Brain Res.*, 398 : 259-265.

Nordeen, E. J., Nordeen, K. W., Sengelaub, D. R. and Arnold, A. P. (1984). Ontogeny of sexual dimorphism in a rat spinal nucleus. I. Hormonal control of neuron number. *Soc. Neurosci. Abstr.*, 10 : 453.

Notebohm, F. and Arnold, A. P. (1976). Sexual dimorphism in vocal control areas of the songbird brain. *Science*, **194** : 211-213.

O'Hanlon, J. K., Meisel, R. L. and Sachs, B. D. (1991). Estradiol maintains castrated male rats' sexual reflexes in copula, but not ex copula. *Behav. Neural Biol.*, **32** : 269-273.

Rand, M. N. and Breedlove, S. M. (1988). Progress report on a hormonally sensitive neuromuscular system. *Psychobiology*, **16** : 398-405.

Rhodes, C. H., Morrell, J. I. and Pfaff, D. W. (1981). Distribution of estrogen concentrating, neurophysin-containing magnocellular neurons in the rat hypothalamus as demonstrated by a technique combining steroid autoradiography and immunohistochemistry in the same tissue. *Neuroendocrinology*, **33** : 18-23.

Riddoch, G. (1917). The reflex functions of the completely divided spinal cord in man, compared with those associated with less severe lesions. *Brain*, **40** : 264-402.

Rodgers, C. H. and Alheid, G. (1872). Relationship of sexual behavior and castration to tumescence in the male rat. *Physiol. Behav.*, **9** : 581-584.

Sachs, B. D. and Garinello, L. D. (1980). Hypothetical spinal pacemaker regulating penile reflexes in rats : evidence from transection of spinal cord and dorsal penile nerves, *J. Comp. Physiol. Psychol.*, **94** : 530-535.

Sar, M. and Stumpf, W. E. (1975). Distribution of androgen concentrating neurons in rat brain. In: Stumpf, W E. and Grant, L. D. (Eds.), *Anatomical Neuroendocrinology*, S. Karger-Basal, Munchen, pp. 120-133.

Schwanzel-Fukuda, M., Morrell, J. I. and Pfaff, D. W. (1984). Localization of forebrain neurons which project directly to the medulla and spinal cord of the rat by retrograde tracing with wheat germ agglutinin. *J. Comp. Neurol.*, **226** : 1-20.

Sengelaub, D. R. and Arnold, A. P. (1986). Development and loss of early projections in a sexually dimorphic rat spinal nucleus. *J. Neurosci.*, **6** : 1613-1620.

Shen, P. Arnold, A. P. and Micevych, P. E. (1990). Supraspinal projections to the ventromedial lumbar spinal cord in adult male rats. *J. Comp. Neurol.*, **300** : 263-272.

Silverman, A. J., Hoffman, D. L. and Zimmerman, E. A. (1981). The descending afferent connections of the paraventricular nucleus of the hypothalamus (PVN). *Brain Res. Bull.*, **6** : 47-61.

Stumpf, W. E., Sar, M. and Keefer, D. A. (1975). Atlas of estrogen target cells in rat brain. In: Stumpf, W. E. and Grant, L. D. (Eds.), *Anatomical Neuroendocrinology*, S. Karger-Basal, Munchen, pp. 104-119.

Tobet, S. A., Zaniser, D. J. and Baum, M. J. (1986). Sexual dimorphism in the preoptic/anterior hypothalamic area of ferrets : effect of adult exposure to sex steroid. *Brain Res.*, **364** : 249-257.

Wagner, C. K. and Clemens, L. G. (1989a). Anatomical organization of the sexually dimorphic perineal neuromuscular system in the house mouse. *Brain Res.*, **499** : 93-100.

Wagner, C. K. and Clemens, L. G. (1989b). Perinatal modification of a sexually dimorphic motor nucleus in the spinal cord of the B6D2F1 house mouse. *Physiol. Behav.*, **45** : 831-835.

Wagner, C. K. and Clemens, L. G. (1991). Projections of the paraventricular nucleus of the hypothalamus to the sexually dimorphic lumbosacral region of the spinal cord. *Brain Res.*, **539** : 254-262.

Wee, B. E. F. and Clemens, L. G. (1987). Characteristics of the spinal nucleus of the bulbocavernosus are influenced by genotype in the house mouse. *Brain Res.*, **424** : 305-310.

# Neonatal Programming of Adult Partner Preference in Male Rats

## T. BRAND, E. J. HOUTSMULLER and A. K. SLOB

*Department of Endocrinology and Reproduction, Faculty of Medicine and Health Sciences, Erasmus University, P.O. Box 1738, 3000 DR Rotterdam, The Netherlands*

Estradiol, derived from aromatization fo testosterone (T), is essential during a critical period around the time of birth for masculinization and defeminization of adult sexual behavior in male rats (e.g. Baum, 1979). The role of estradiol in organizing adult sexual orientation, as indicated by partner preference behavior, has received relatively little attention (Adkins-Regan, 1988). Recently we have published that neonatal treatment with the aromatase inhibitor ATD (1,4,6-androstatriene-3,17-dione) significantly affected adult partner preference behavior of male rats (Brand et al., 1991). Compared to control males these ATD males showed a significantly lower preference for the estrous female partner. These findings prompted us to assume that T, through its metabolite estradiol, plays a role in the organization of adult partner preference in male rats.

The effects of neonatal Atamestan (1-methyl-1,4-androstadiene-3,17-dione, another aromatase inhibitor) on partner preference and sexual behavior in adult male rats was investigated in Experiment 1.

In Experiment 2, the ontogeny of partner preference behavior of males rats was investigated in neonatal ATD and cholesterol treated males before, during and after puberty.

It has been suggested that the volume of the sexual dimorphic nucleus of the preoptic area (SDN-POA) is organized by the estradiol metabolite of testosterone (Döhler, 1984). Perinatal treatment with ATD could therefore affect the SDN-POA volume in male rats. This was investigated in Experiment 3.

## General method

### Animals

Experimental animals were Wistar albino rats ; stimulus animals were F1 hybrids of two inbred Wistar strains (R x U). They were housed two to four to a cage with food and water available *ad lib* and kept in a 14hr light 10hr dark cycle (lights on : 5:30 PM to 7:30 AM). Temperature in the animal room ranged from 20 to 22°C.

*M. Haug et al. (eds.), The Development of Sex Differences and Similarities in Behavior, 33–49.*
© 1993 *Kluwer Academic Publishers.*

## Treatments

Three experiments are reported (see also Table I for a comprehensive overview of the various experimental designs).

**Table I** Overview of the various experimental designs to study of perinatal endocrine manipulations on sexual orientation of adult male rats.

| Number exept | Treatment | | Number of litters | Number of male young used | Number of adult behavioral tests (age at time of testing : weeks (w) or days (d)) | | | |
|---|---|---|---|---|---|---|---|---|
| | Prenatal injection | Neonatal Silastic implant | | | Partner preference tests (F vs M) ; with sexual interaction : | | Sexual pair tests vith : | |
| | | | | | prevented | allowed | estrous F | active M |
| 1* | - | empty | 5 | 12 | | | | |
| | - | ATD | 8 | 11 | 1(12 w) | 3(14,16,17 w) | 4(18,20,22,29w) | 1(19 w) |
| | - | Atamestan | 2 | 14 | | | | |
| 2* | - | cholesterol | 4 | 9 | 9(32-60 d) | 2(88,90 d) | - | - |
| | | | | 9 | 7(63-84 d) | 2(89,91 d) | - | - |
| | - | | 8 | 19 | 9(32-60 d) | 2(88,90 d) | - | - |
| | | ATD | | 20 | 7(63-84 d) | 2(89,91 d) | - | - |
| 3* | solvent | empty | 4 | 14(55)# | | | | |
| | ATD | empty | 4 | 12(5)# | 7 | 6 | 1 | 1 |
| | ATD | ATD | 6 | 18(5)# | (11-19 w) | (20-25 w) | (27 w) | (26 w) |

* all animals were left intact ; # 5 males out of each group were used for SDN-POA study ; Atamestan = 1-methyl-1,4-androstadiene-3,17-dione ; AZTD=1,4,6-androstatriene-3,17-dione ; M (male) ; F (female)

Female rats were timed mated (Day of mating = day 0 of pregnancy) and parturition occurred 22 days later.

Prenatal treatment (Experiment 3) consisted of daily injections to the mothers with ATD (1,4,6-androstatriene-3,17-dione ; 5 mg/day) or solvent (propylene glycol ; O.1 ml/day) from days 10-22 of pregnancy.

Neonatal treatment consisted of implantation (between 3 and 9 hours after birth s.c. in the back, under ice anaesthesia) of a Silastic capsule filled with ATD, Atamestan (1-methyl-1,4-androstadiene-3,17-dione), cholesterol or with nothing (Experiment 1-3). The implants were removed when the pups were 21 days of age. Pups were weaned at 21 days of age and housed two to four to a cage of same sex and treatment. The animals were left undisturbed until the onset of behavioral testing.

Stimulus animals were sexually active male and ovariectomized female rats. The latter were brought into estrus with 30 µg estradiol benzoate (EB) 24-48h prior to testing followed by 2.5 mg progesterone (P) 3-4h before testing.

# Behavioral testing

## Three-compartment partner preference test

A test box (Figure 1) made of gray perspex with a transparent front was used (Slob et al., 1987) which had three compartments (60 x 30 x 40 cm each) with a small opening (13 x 12 cm) in both partitions near the front window.

These openings could be closed by a sliding door. Stimulus animals could be put in the left and right compartments. The incentives, an estrous female and a sexually active male, wore either a leather harness which was attached with a stainless-steel string to the rear of the compartment or no harness when placed behind a wire mesh separation halfway down the lateral compartment. Tethered animals had a limited action radius. They were adapted to the tethering device during 1hr in the week before testing. When physical interaction was prevented by wire mesh, the experimental animal could only see, smell, and hear the incentives.

Behavioral tests lasted 15 minutes. Before testing all three animals (one experimental, two incentives) were put in the box, one in each compartment, with the sliding doors closed, for 15-20 min of adaptation. At the beginning of the test the sliding doors were removed and the experimental animal could freely move around and interact with the stimulus animals or sit before the wire mesh separation. Time spent in each compartment was recorded. To quantify partner preference, a preference score was calculated for each test by subtracting time spent in the compartment containing the sexually active male from time spent near the estrous female (the prevailing method in our laboratory, adopted from Edwards and Pfeifle, 1983). Thus, a positive score indicates preference for the estrous female ; a negative score indicates preference for the sexually active male. In the tests in which interaction was possible, the sexual behaviors with the incentives were also scored. Only ejaculation frequencies are presented.

## Pair test with estrous female

In these tests, lasting 15 minutes, semicircular cages measuring 62 x 40 x 36 cm were used. Before the test the experimental animal was put in the cage for a 5-minutes adaptation period. At the beginning of the test an estrous female was put in the cage. Various behaviors were scored. For this report the number of ejaculations were analysed.

## Pair test with sexually active male

For these tests, carried out also in semicircular cages, sexually active males were used. After a 5-minutes adaptation period of the stud males, the experimental males were put in the boxes. The lordosis responses of the experimental male to the mounting of the stud male were recorded. The test lasted until the experimental male had received 10 mounts or, at the longest, 10 minutes. Since many males were not very attractive and did not receive 10

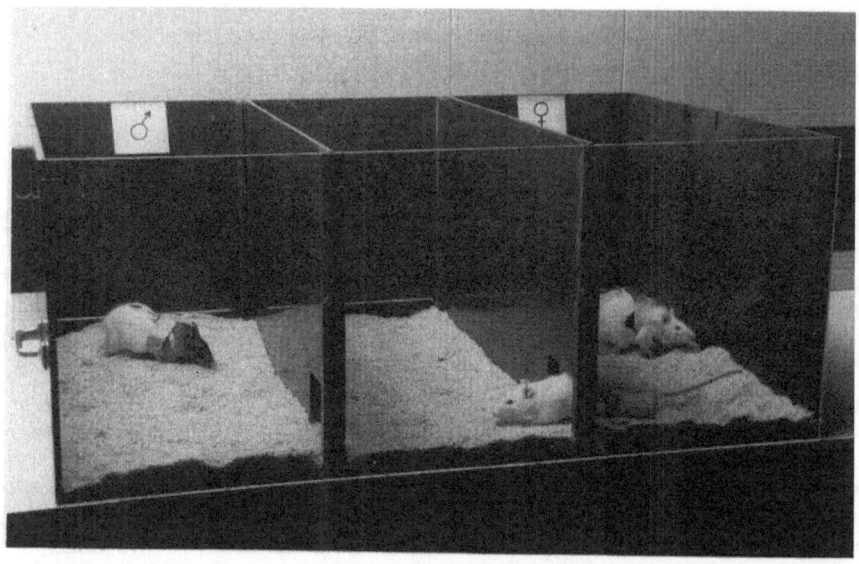

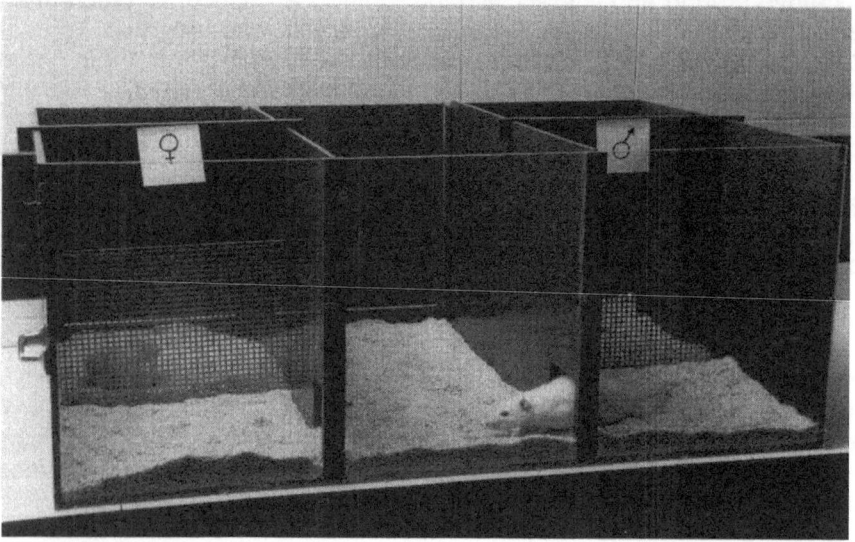

**Figure 1** Three-compartment-boxes. The lateral compartments contain the stimulus animals, an estrous female and a sexually active male. The incentives were tethered (top) or were placed behind wire mesh (bottom). The experimental male could freely move around. Sexual interaction with the incentives was possible (top) or prevented by wire mesh (bottom).

mounts, we have included in the analyses the lordosis quotients of those experimental males that received three or more mounts.

## Hormone assay

Blood was collected for testosterone assays in Experiments 1 and 2. Testosterone concentrations were estimated in serum by radioimmunoassay, without chromatography using the prevailing method in our laboratory (e.g. Baum et al., 1988). The interassay and intraassay coefficents of variation were 13.4 % and 5.6 %, respectively. In Experiment 2 also the estradiol concentrations were measured. Intra- and interassay coefficients of variation were less than 15 % and less than 19 % for the estradiol assay (e.g. Kwekkeboom et al., 1990).

## Statistics

Most data were analysed using One- or Two-way ANOVA (Perlman, 1986). For further analysis the least significant difference (LSD) procedure (Kirk, 1968) was used.
The numbers of animals displaying some type of behavior were analysed using Fisher exact two-tailed probability analysis or the Binomial test when appropriate. The data of Experiment 3 were analysed using Kruskall-Wallis or Mann-Whitney analysis.

# Experiment 1

## Test procedure

The males were subjected to four consecutive partner preference test (see Table I). In test 1, sexual interaction was prevented by wire mesh ; in tests 2-4 sexual interaction with the tethered stimulus animals was possible. The experimental males received a s. c. injection with progesterone (0.5 mg) which was given 4-7h prior to preference test 4. Also, four pair tests with an estrous female were carried out (S1-S4) ; tests S1 and S4 without any pretreatment, test S2 after 3 s. c. daily injections with 20 $\mu$g EB/day, test S3, 25-30 minutes after one i. p. injections with 2 mg/kg Yohimbine, an $\alpha^2$-adrenoreceptor blocker with sexual behavior stimulating properties (e.g. Clark et al., 1984). Lordosis behavior was studied in a pair test with a sexually active male (test L), without any treatment. Blood was collected from the orbital plexus under light ether anaesthesia following the last pair test (30 weeks of age).

## Partner preference behavior

Partner preference scores are depicted in Figure 2.

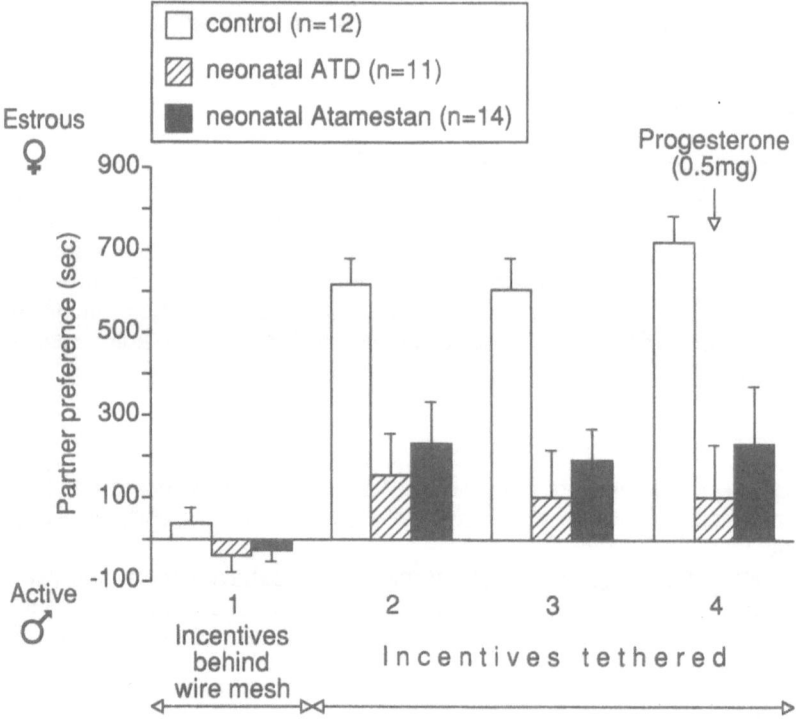

**Figure 2** Mean (± SEM) preference (seconds) for an estrous female over a sexually active male of intact adult male rats after neonatal ATD, Atamestan or control treatment. See also text and Table I for experimental details.

One-way ANOVA of test 1 did not show a significant group difference (F(2/34) = 1.44, n.s.). Two-way ANOVA of tests 2-4 revealed a significant group difference (F(2/34) = 11.32, P < 0.0005), no significant effect of tests (F(2/68) = 0.41, n.s.), and no significant groups x tests interaction (F(4/68) = 0.28, n.s.). Further analysis of the group difference (LSD(5 %) = 233.2 sec.) showed that control males had significantly higher preference scores for the estrous female than neo-ATD and neo-ATA males ; the latter two groups did not differ.

## Sexual behavior with estrous female

Ejaculation behavior during partner preference and pair testing is shown in Figure 3.

Fisher's two-tailed probability analysis, performed on the total number of males ejaculating at least once during partner preference tests 2, 3 and 4 (combined), showed that a lower number of neo-ATD and neo-ATA males ejaculated than controls (control vs neo-ATD : P < 0.001 ; control vs neo-ATA : p < 0.02). Neo-ATD and neo-ATA males did not differ.

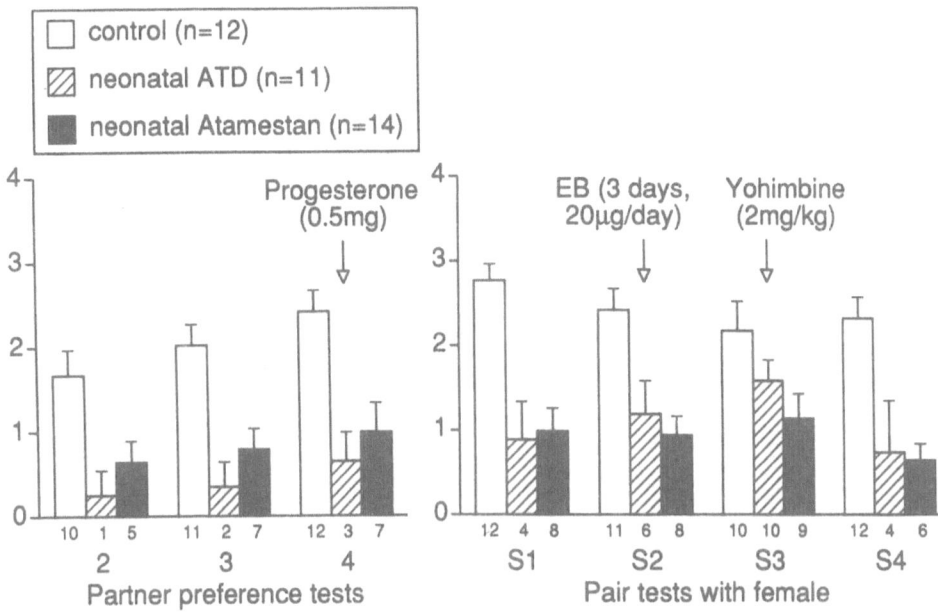

**Figure 3** Mean (± SEM) ejaculation frequency during partner preference tests (2-4) and pair tests with an estrous female (S1-S4) of intact adult male rats after neonatal ATD, Atamestan or control treatment. The digits below the bars indicate the number of males per group ejaculating during the test. For details see text and Table I.

Two-way ANOVA of the ejaculation frequencies displayed during pair testing, showed a significant group difference ($F_{(2/34)} = 17.66$, $P < 0.0005$), no significant effect of tests ($F_{(3/102)} = 1.70$, n.s.), and no significant interaction ($F_{(6/102)} = 1.27$, n.s.). Further analysis of this group difference (LSD(5 %) = 0.65 ejac.) showed that neo-ATD males and neo-ATA males had lower ejaculation frequencies than controls in all 4 pair tests.
Yohimbine only increased the number of neo-ATD males that ejaculated : after a single injection (test S3) almost all ATD-males ejaculated (10 of 11), whereas in tests before (S1) and after Yohimbine (S4) only 4 of 11 males ejaculated (10 of 11 vs 4 of 11, $p < 0.001$, binomial test). Such stimulatory effect of Yohimbine was not found in neo-ATA and control males. Adult treatment with EB had no effect in any group.

## Lordosis behavior with active male

Lordosis data are shown in Figure 4.
In this experiment many males were not very attractive, i.e. they were not readily mounted by the stimulus male.

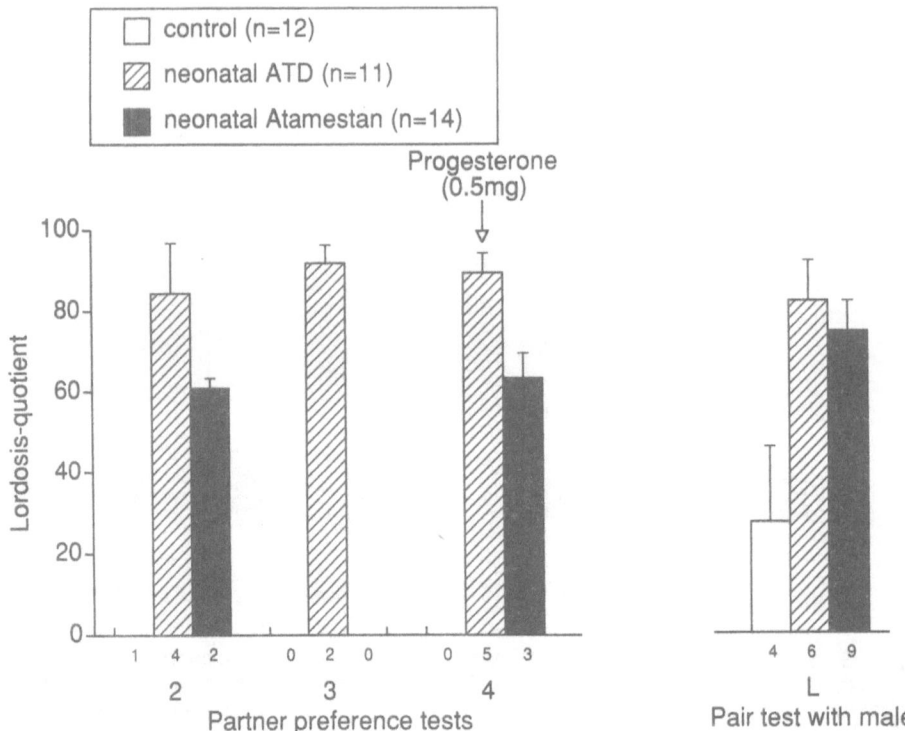

**Figure 4**  Mean (± SEM) lordosis quotients of intact male rats during partner preference tests 2-4 and pair test with a sexually active male (test L) after neonatal ATD, Atamestan or control treatment. The digits below the bars indicate the number of males per group that were mounted by the sexually active male and that contributed to the calculated lordosis quotients. Test 4 was carried out 4-7h after a s.c. injection with 0.5 mg progesterone.

The number of males that had received 3 or more mounts by the stimulus male in at least one of the partner preference tests 2-4 were : control : 1 of 12, ATD 6 of 11, and Atamestan : 3 of 14. Fisher's exact two-tailed probability analysis did not show differences between groups (control vs neo-ATD, P = 0.07 ; control vs neo-ATA, P = 1.00 ; neo-ATD vs neo-ATA, P = 0.11). It is remarkable that neo-ATD and neo-ATA males that were receptive, showed fairly high lordosis quotients ; the one control male allowing mounts from the stimulus male during partner preference testing did not show lordosis.

Fisher's exact two-tailed probability analysis of the number of males being mounted 3 times or more by the sexually active male (during test L) did not reveal statistically significant differences. One-way ANOVA of the lordosis quotients (of the responders) in test L showed a significant group difference ($F_{(2/16)}$ = 5.95, P < 0.02). Further analysis (LSD(5%) = 35.8) showed that controls had lower lordosis quotients than neo-ATD and neo-ATA males ; the latter two groups did not differ.

## Hormone data

Testosterone levels at 30 weeks of age can be seen in Table II.

One-way ANOVA of the serum T levels showed no significant group difference ($F(2/30 = 1.75$, n.s.). From these data it appears that neonatal ATD or Atamestan treatment had no effect on adult endogenous testosterone levels in these gonadally intact males.

**Table II** Blood serum levels (mean ± SEM) of testosterone and estradiol in male rats during 2 experiments.

| Number expt | Neonatal treatment (Silastic implant) | Age in weeks (w) or days (d) | Number of animal samples | T-levels (nmol/1) | $E_2$-levels (pmol/1) |
|---|---|---|---|---|---|
| 1* | empty | | 11 | 7.3 + 1.0 | - |
| | ATD | 30 w | 9 | 5.2 + 0,3 | - |
| | Atamestan | | 13 | 5.2 + 0.7 | - |
| 2* | cholesterol | 60 d | 6 | 19.6 + 3.2 | 58.3 + 4.3 |
| | ATD | 60 d | 13 | 18.4 + 2.6 | 56.4 + 5.5 |
| | cholesterol | 90 d | 17 | 14.4 + 1.5 | 58.2 + 5.3 |
| | ATD | 90 d | 36 | 26.1 + 2.7 | 54.1 + 1.3 |

* All animals were left intact ; Atamestan = 1-methyl-1-1,4-androstadienen-3,17-dione ; ATD = 1,4,6-androstatiene-3,17-dione

# Experiment 2

In Experiment 1, clear effects were found of neonatal treatment with aromatase inhibitors on adult 'sexual orientation' and sexual behavior. In Experiment 2, the ontogeny of these effects was investigated.

## Test procedure

Firstly, the animals were tested for partner preference behavior with sexual interaction prevented by wire mesh. Half of the males was tested 9 times between days 32-60 (group 1), the other half, 7 times between days 63-90 (group 2). Both groups then received two tests in which sexual interaction with the tethered stimulus animals was possible (see also Table I).

## Partner preference behavior

The preference data are shown in Figure 5.

Tests without sexual interaction were analysed separately from tests in which sexual interaction was possible. Tests 1-9 from group 1 were analysed

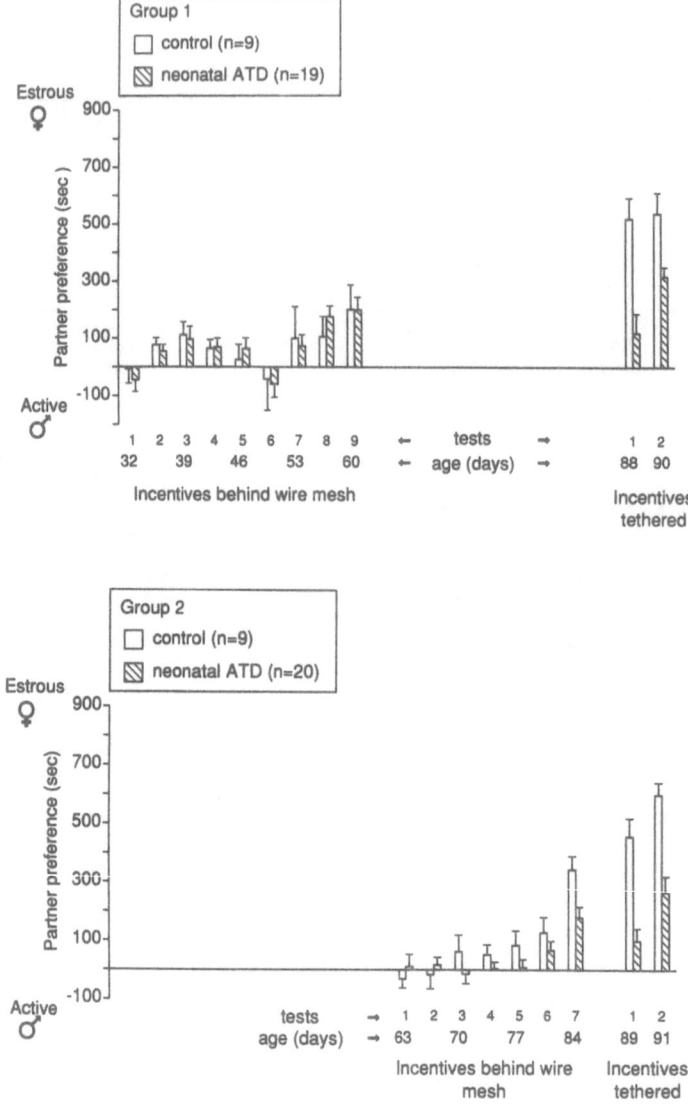

**Figure 5** Mean (± SEM) preference for an estrous female over a sexually active male of male rats neonatally treated with ATD or cholesterol. The animals were tested with incentives behind wire mesh or with tethered incentives with sexual interaction possible (see also Table I for details).

separately from tests 1-7 from group 2. Two-way ANOVA of tests 1-9 of group 1 revealed no statistically significant group difference (F(1/26) = 0.001, n.s.), a significant effect of tests (F(8/208) = 6.16, P < 0.0005), and no significant interaction (F(8/208) = 0.26, n.s.). Further analysis of the difference between tests (LSD(5 %) =89.6 sec.) showed a significant increase in preference for the estrous female between tests 1 and 2, as well as between tests 7 and 9. Between tests 2 and 7 the preference scores were similar. Surprisingly, however, the preference scores in test 6 were quite different from the other tests. In test 9 (60 days of age) neo-ATD and control males both showed a similar preference for the etrous female partner.

The preference scores of group 2 (test 1-7) are depicted in Figure 5 (bottom). Overall, there were gradually increasing preference scores for the estrous female. Two-way ANOVA showed no significant group difference (F(1/28) = 2.34, n.s.), a significant effect of tests (F(6/168) = 13.24, P < 0.0005) and a borderline significant interaction (F(6/168) = 2.08, P < 0.06). Further analysis of this interaction (LSD(5 %) = 96.05 sec.) indicated that only during test 7 (84 days of age) ATD males had significantly lower preference scores than controls.

The preference scores of groups 1 and 2 of the tests in which sexual interaction was possible are also shouwn in Figure 5 (right and side). Two-way ANOVA revealed a significant difference between groups (F(3/53) = 15.92, P < 0.0005), a significant effect of tests (F(1/53) = 16.72, P < 0.0005), and no significant interaction (F(3/53) = 0.90, n.s.). The preference scores of test 2 are significantly higher than those of test 1. Further analysis of the difference between groups (LSD (5 %) = 136.3 sec.) showed that both ATD-groups (not different from each other) had lower preference scores than both control groups. The control groups did not differ.

## Sexual behavior with estrous female

Sexual behavioral data during the two partner preference tests in which sexual interaction was possible are shown in Figure 6.

Since only a few ATD males ejaculated, the number of the males that ejaculated at least once during tests 1 and 2 (combined) was used. Fisher's exact two-tailed probability test showed that less ATD males ejaculated than controls in groups 1 and 2 (P < 0.002).

## Hormone levels

Mean testosterone and estradiol levels are shown in Table II. Samples of Experiment 1 and 2 were analysed separately in assays approximately 6 months apart.

One-way ANOVA of the T-levels at 90-91 days of age showed a significant group difference (F(1/51) = 8.11, P = 0.006), i.e. ATD males had higher T-levels than controls. Two-way ANOVA of the T-levels of those males that were bled both at 60 and 90-91 days of age revealed a significant group difference

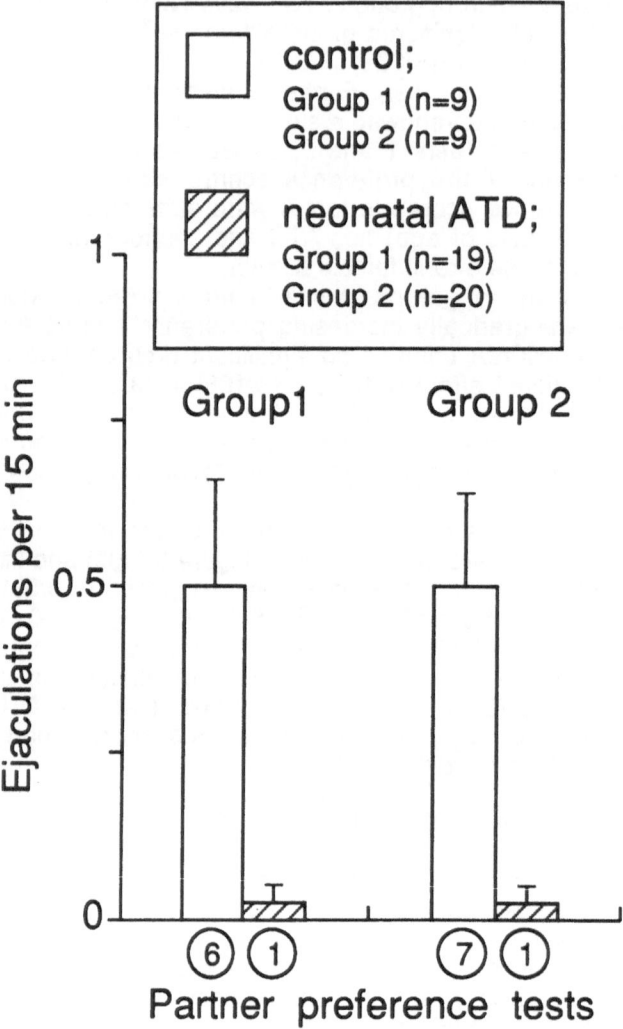

**Figure 6** Mean (± SEM) ejaculation frequencies during partner preference tests in which sexual interaction was possible of the same males as in Figure 5. The digits below the bars indicate the number of males that ejaculated at least once during one of those tests.

(F(1/17) = 7.00, P < 0.02), a significant effect of age (F(1/17) = 6.91, P < 0.02), and a significant interaction (F(1/17) = 8.95, P = 0.008). Further analysis of this interaction (LSD(5 %) = 13.79 nmol/1) showed that at 60 days of age the levels of T did not differ. At 90-91 days of age the T-level in the ATD males was significantly higher than the control males.

One-way ANOVA of the E2-levels at 90-91 days of age did reveal no difference (F(1/51) = 1.00, n.s.). Two-way ANOVA of the E2-levels of those males that were bled both at 60 and 90-91 days of age showed no significant difference between groups (F(1/17) = 0.20, n.s.) or age (F(1/17) = 0.29, n.s.) and no significant interaction (F(1/17) = 0.005, n.s.).

# Experiment 3

We published recently about the effects of perinatal endocrine manipulations, using ATD, on adult partner preference and sexual behavior in male rats (Brand et al., 1991). The SDN-POA of a representative sample of these animals was studied in Experiment 3 (Houtsmuller et al., 1992).

## Previous experimental procedure (Brand et al., 1991)

Three experimental groups were used : (1) control (n=14), (2) prenatal ATD (pre-ATD ; n=12), (3) pre- and neonatal ATD (preneo-ATD ; n=18).

From 11 weeks onward, the males were subjected to 13 weekly partner preference tests. In tests 1-7 sexual interaction was prevented. In tests 8-13 sexual interaction with the tethered incentives was possible. In tests 6, 10 and 12, 8-OH-DPAT (a serotonin agonist) was injected 30 minutes prior to testing. In tests 4, 5, 9, 11 and 13 saline (2 ml/kg) was injected 30 minutes before testing.

One and 2 weeks following the last partner preference test the males were pair tested with a sexually active male or with an estrous female.

## Present experimental procedure

Detailed data will be presented elsewhere (Houtsmuller et al.,1992). At 28 weeks of age, 5 males of each group were randomly chosen for histological examination of the SDN-POA. They were injected with pentobarbital (Nembutal, O.5 ml/rat i. p.). All males were then perfused intracardially with saline followed by 500 ml fixative (4 % paraformaldehyde, pH = 7.2). The brains were removed and stored in fixative at 4°C for one day. Subsequently the brain was dehydrated and embedded in paraffin. Serial 6 $\mu$m frontal sections were cut according to the coronal plane of the atlas of the rat brain by Paxinos and Watson (1986), mounted upon chrome-aluminium-coated slides and stained with thionin.

## Morphometry

Area measurements of the SDN were performed bilaterally by means of a Calcomp 2000 digitizer connected to a VAX 1/780 computer, using a Zeiss microscope with x10 and x40 (plan) objectives respectively, and x12.5 plan oculars. The volume of the SDN was determined by integrating area measurements from the first to the last cell-containing sections. These measurements were taken twice. The mean of these two volumes was calculated and used in the statistical analysis (Kruskall-Wallis and Mann-Whitney U).

## SDN-POA data

The SDN-data are shown in Figure 7.

## SDN volume

The three groups differed significantly (Kruskall-Wallis, $P = 0.007$). The SDN of the control group was significantly (Mann-Whitney) larger than the SDN of the pre-ATD ($P = 0.036$) or preneo-ATD males ($P = 0.009$). The SDN of pre-ATD males was larger than the SDN of the preneo-ATD males (M-W, $P = 0.047$).

## Summary of behavioral data

Detailed behavioral data of these animals will be presented elsewhere (Houtsmuller et al., 1992). In summary the results are as follows. Male rats perinatally treated with ATD had significantly lower preference scores for the estrous female than pre-ATD or control males. The latter 2 groups did not differ. In pair tests with an estrous female none of the 5 preneo-ATD males ejaculated, whereas 4 of 5 controls and pre-ATD males did. In a pair test with a sexually active male, all 5 preneo-ATD males were mounted (mean lordosis quotient 78 ± 9 %), whereas 2 of 5 pre-ATD and 0 of 5 control males were mounted.

# General discussion

In the first experiment, carried out in gonadally intact male rats, the effects of neonatal ATD treatment on adult partner preference found earlier (Brand et al., 1991) were replicated : neonatally ATD treated males had significantly lower preference scores for an estrous female than controls. Neonatal treatment with Atamestan had similar effects on adult partner preference behavior of male rats. Thus, the present study confirms the hypothesis from our laboratory (Brand et al., 1991; Brand and Slob, 1991) that estradiol derived from testosterone plays a significant role in programming adult male rat partner preference behavior.

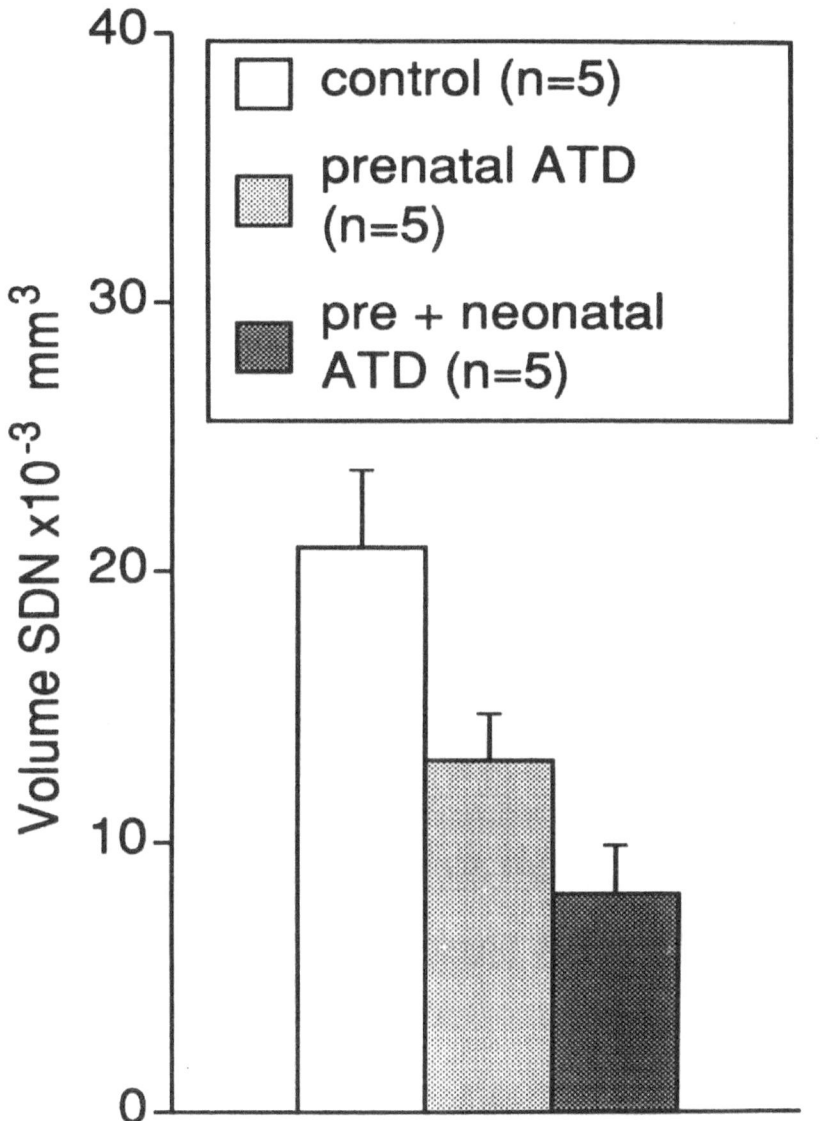

**Figure 7**   Mean (± SEM) volume of sexually dimorphic nucleus of the preoptic area (SDN-POA) of adult male rats after perinatal ATD or control treatment.

Similarly to the altered adult sexual partner preference, sexual behavior with an estrous female or with a sexually active male was affected by the neonatal ATD or Atamestan treatment. Neo-ATD and neo-ATA males displayed "bisexual" behavior, i.e. they responded complementary to the partner : displaying mounts and intromissions when paired with the estrous female and lordosis behavior when mounted by the stud male. Neo-ATD and neo-ATA males showed significantly lower ejaculation frequencies than controls, in partner preference tests and in pair tests. Thus, neo-ATD and neo-ATA males are less 'masculinized' and less 'defeminized' in adulthood.

In the second experiment the ontogeny of partner preference behavior was investigated. It appeared that the different partner preference behavior of neo-ATD males (a lower preference for the estrous female) first became apparent at the age of around 84 days, i.e. postpubertally. This suggests that testicular hormones play a significant role in the expression of this behavior. Future research into the effects of castration and subsequent subtitution with testicular hormones could support or reject this supposition.

In the third experiment it was found for the first time that the volume of the SDN-POA was larger in control males than in pre-ATD and preneo-ATD males. The SDN-POA volume of the pre-ATD males was also larger than the SDN-POA volume of preneo-ATD males. It thus seems that neonatal as well as prenatal E2 has a programming effect on the volume of the SDN-POA. Whether there is a causal relationship between the altered volume of the SDN and the altered partner preference and sexual behavior is not clear. However, the smaller volume of the SDN following perinatal ATD treatment is in line with the hypothesis that E2 programs the volume of this nucleus (Döhler et al., 1984).

In conclusion, neonatal estradiol programs adudlt partner preference and sexual behavior in male rats. The difference between ATD treated and control males becomes apparent after puberty (around 80 days of age) and is presumably dependent on the activating action of endogenous testicular hormones. The volume of the SDN-POA, a sex-dimorphic nucleus, is programmed by pre- as well as neonatal E2. Whether there is a causal relationship between the volume of this nucleus and partner preference and sexual behavior remains to be investigated.

# Acknowledgements

Thanks are due to J. van Ophemert, S. M. Haensel, M. Koolen and F. Jonker for support with animal testing and maintenance. Dr. F. H. de Jong is thanked for supervising the hormone assays and Professor J. J. van der Werff ten Bosch for reading and commenting on an earlier version of this manuscript. Mr. A. Houba, Schering Ned. Inc, is thanked for providing the aromatase inhibitor Atamestan.

# References

Adkins-Regan, E. (1988). Sex hormones and sexual orientation in animals. *Psychobiol.*, **16** : 335-347.

Baum, M. J. (1979). Differentiation of coital behavior in mammals : a comparative analysis. *Neurosci. Biobehav. Rev.,* **3** : 265-284.

Baum, M. J., Brand, T., Ooms, M., Vreeburg, J. T. M. and Slob, A. K. (1988). Immediate postnatal rise in whole body androgen content in male rats : correlation with increased testicular content and reduced body clearance of testosterone. *Biol. Reprod.,* **38** : 980-986.

Brand, T., Kroonen, J., Mos, J. and Slob, A. K. (1991). Adult partner preference and sexual behavior of male rats affected by perinatal endocrine manipulations. *Horm. Behav.,* **25** : 323-341.

Brand, T. and Slob, A. K. (1991). Neonatal organization of adult partner preference behavior in male rats. *Physiol. Behav.,* **49** : 107-111.

Clark, J. T., Smith, E. R. and Davidson, J. M. (1984). Enhancement of sexual motivation in male rats by yohimbine. *Science,* **225** : 847-849.

Döhler, K. D., Srivastava, S. S., Shryne, J. E., Jarzab, B., Sipos, A. and Gorski, R. A. (1984). Differentiation of the sexually dimorphic nucleus in the preoptic area of the rat brain is inhibited by postnatal treatment with an estrogen antagonist. *Neuroendocrinol.,* **38** : 297-301.

Edwards, D. A. and Pfeifle, J. K. (1983). Hormonal control of receptivity, proceptivity and sexual motivation. *Physiol. Behav.,* **30** : 437-443.

Houtsmuller, E. J., Brand, T., de Jonge, F. H., Joosten, R., van de Poll, N. E. and Slob, A. K. (1992). Effects of perinatal exposure to the aromatase inhibitor ATD on differentiation of the sexually dimorphic nucleus of the preoptic area (SDN-POA), sexual orientation and sexual behavior in male rats. Submitted for publication.

Kirk, R. E. (1968). Experimental Design : *Procedures for the Behavioral Sciences,* Brooks/Cole, Belmont, CA.

Kwekkeboom, D. J., de Jong, F. H., van Hemert, A. M., Vandenroucke, J. P., Valkenburg, H. A. and Lamberts, S. W. J. (1990). Serum gonadotropins and $\alpha$-subunit decline in aging normal postmenopausal women. *J. Clin. Endocrinol. Metab.,* **70** : 944-950.

Paxinos, G. and Watson, C. (1986). *The Rat Brain in Stereotaxic Coordinates,* Academic Press, Sydney.

Perlman, G. (1986). *The UNIX/STAT Handbook : Data Analysis Programs on Unix and MSDOS,* Wang Institute, Tyngsboro.

Slob, A. K., Deklerk, L. W. L. and Brand, T. (1987). Homosexual and heterosexual partner preference in ovariectomized female rats : Effects of testosterone, estradiol and mating experience. *Physiol. Behav.,* **41** : 571-576.

# Neural Bases of Behavioral Sex Differences in Quail

J. BALTHAZART and A. FOIDART

*Laboratory of General and Comparative Biochemistry, University of Liège, 17 Place Delcour, B-4020 Liège, Belgium*

Many behaviors of vertebrates are sexually differentiated. This dimorphism concerns in particular reproductive behaviors. The existence of such differences in behavior raises two major questions: 1. how do they develop during ontogeny? and 2. what are the central mechanisms underlying their expression in adults. At one time, it was thought that the type of hormone determined the kind of behavior observed in an animal and that the substrate the hormone acted on was irrelevant (Steinach, 1940). It is now well established that the condition of the substrate the hormone is acting on (i.e. the brain), which is determined by such factors as the animal's sex, age, experience, and condition of rearing, has profound effects on the type of behavior an animal will exhibit in response to steroid treatment (Beach, 1948; Feder, 1981; Leshner, 1978). Understanding the biochemical nature of the sex differences in this neural substrate is one of the major challenges facing behavioral endocrinology today.

For the past ten years, research in my laboratory has been largely devoted to these two broad questions. The Japanese quail has been used as a model in all these studies because its reproductive behavior is extremely differentiated. We have obtained in this period of time a detailed answer to the first of these questions: the sex difference in male reproductive behavior develops essentially under the influence of early steroids (in particular estradiol) and we have established the time-course of this process. The mechanism of sexual differentiation of male copulatory behavior is now well known in quail so that we can manipulate it *ad libitum* and produce genetic males that have a female behavioral phenotype but also genetic females with a male phenotype.

On the other hand, the search for the brain mechanisms underlying the sex differences in quail behavior has been more frustrating. Although copulatory behavior is extremely dimorphic in this species (complete qualitative difference; the behavior is always present in males and almost always absent in females irrespective of the adult hormonal milieu), the brain in the two sexes is extremely similar. A number of morphological or biochemical sex differences have been detected in the brain of adult males and females. However many of these disappeared when the endocrine condition was made similar in both sexes. In a few instances, some stable differences (still present when endocrine milieu is similar) have been observed. Even if they cannot, at the present time,

51

*M. Haug et al. (eds.), The Development of Sex Differences and Similarities in Behavior, 51–75.*
© 1993 *Kluwer Academic Publishers.*

be directly related to the sex difference in behavior, they are connected in an obvious way to the control of behavior. The second part of the present chapter is devoted to the review of these data.

## Testosterone and the sex dimorphism in quail reproductive behavior

In most vertebrate species, castration leads to complete elimination of male reproductive behaviors and associated morphological phenomena (Feder, 1984; Leshner, 1978) (see however Crews and Moore, 1986 for exceptions). This relationship is well illustrated by studies of sexual behavior in the Japanese quail. When presented to a female, male quail show a stereotyped behavioral sequence including neck-grab of the female (NG), mount attempts (MA), mount (M) and cloacal contact movement (CCM) which often results in a successful copulation. Males also show a pre- or post-copulatory display called strutting and have a specific call, the crow. These behaviors are androgen-dependent. They disappear completely after castration and are restored by testosterone (T) treatment (Beach and Inman, 1965; Sachs, 1969; Adkins and Adler, 1972; Balthazart et al., 1983; Schumacher and Balthazart, 1983).

These effects of T are sexually differentiated. The androgen-dependent behaviors are never seen in intact females and additionally, some of them (e.g. CCM) cannot be elicited in ovariectomized females even in the presence of pharmacological doses of T (Adkins, 1975; Schumacher and Balthazart, 1983; Balthazart et al., 1983). This sex difference in behavior is, therefore, not only a function of the different endocrine condition of intact males and females (i.e. ovaries not secreting enough T to activate the behavior). This dimorphism is a phenomenon of the central nervous system. Circulating levels of androgens are only slightly lower in female than in male quail (Doi et al., 1980; Balthazart et al., 1983; Balthazart et al., 1987). There is enough overlap between male and female values such that plasma T levels should be adequate in some females to activate male behavior. This would be the case, if these females were not showing a form of androgen-insensitivity. Secondly, treatment of ovariectomized females with doses of T ten times higher than those required to activate sexual behavior in males still does not induce male-type sexual behavior (Adkins and Adler, 1972; Adkins, 1979; Balthazart et al., 1983). It has also been demonstrated that silastic implants filled with T produce similar levels of T in gonadectomized males and females so that the differential response to the hormone treatment cannot be attributed to a different peripheral catabolism of the hormone (Schumacher and Balthazart, 1986; Balthazart et al., 1987). Taken together, these data indicate that the behavioral dimorphism in quail is not solely a consequence of the different circulating levels of T but rather depends on differential properties of the brain areas involved in the control of behavior. Our search for sex differences in the quail brain has therefore been focussed on those morphological or physiological differences that do not simply reflect the sexually dimorphic endocrine condition of the adult.

However, not all reproductive behaviors are so extremely differentiated. Females are not in all cases completely insensitive to androgen. After being treated with exogenous T, they will show struts and produce crows, although with frequencies lower than those observed in males. Sexual dimorphism in quail is thus quite specific: it is qualitative (yes/no) for the copulatory behavior and quantitative for other variables such as crow, strut, and aggressive behavior. As a consequence, one might expect specific correlates of this dimorphism to be reflected at the neural level. In that the dimorphic behaviors under study are all androgen-dependent a mechanism underlying this brain dimorphism probably consists of a differential responsiveness to the activating effects of T.

# The ontogeny of sex differences in behavior

In quail and in chicken, it is clearly established that the behavioral dimorphism is not only the direct consequence of genetic differences between the sexes but mainly results from the early exposure to a different hormonal milieu. Based on experiments carried out mostly in the laboratory of Dr. E. Adkins during the seventies, it has been largely admitted that the absence of male-type sexual behavior in adult females results from their early exposure to estrogens (Adkins, 1978; Adkins-Regan et al., 1982; Adkins-Regan, 1983). Females would be demasculinized by embryonic estrogens in galliforms. Our more recent assays of circulating concentrations of estradiol ($E_2$) during quail ontogeny are also consistent with this model (higher plasma levels of $E_2$ were found in females; Schumacher et al., 1988). It is important to notice, however, that this model of quail sexual differentiation is based only on indirect evidence. It has been shown very convincingly that injections of estrogens in male embryos demasculinize their copulatory behavior (Adkins, 1975; Adkins, 1979; Schumacher et al., 1989) but this effect might well be of a pharmacological nature. There is no or little direct proof that the same mechanism is responsible for the demasculinization of females under physiological conditions. One study only addressed this question. Adkins injected female embryos with an antiestrogen (CI-628) and showed that this treatment increased the proportion of adult females mounting a stimulus animal after treatment with T (Adkins, 1976). Presumably, the demasculinization of behavior by endogenous steroids had been blocked by the antiestrogen. However, these treated females were partly demasculinized since only 3 out of 9 experimental females showed the full copulatory sequence. In addition, the intensity of the behavior exhibited by these CI-628-treated females (frequency and latency to first behavior) was clearly different from that observed in normal males. Therefore, these data were in agreement with the notion that estrogens demasculinize female quail during ontogeny but could not be taken as conclusive evidence that this was the only process implicated in the sexual differentiation of reproductive behavior in quail.

These experiments also demonstrated that the demasculinization of male quail by exogenous estrogens was restricted to a critical period of the embryonic life. It was shown that EB injections into male embryos demasculinized copulatory behavior only if they were performed before the 12th day of incubation (Adkins, 1979; Adkins-Regan, 1983; Schumacher et al., 1989). Delayed injections were without effect. This suggested that in females, the behavioral demasculinization was also completed before incubation day 12 under the influence of endogenous, presumably ovarian, estrogens. Yet experiments in females suggested that their behavioral demasculinization was not completed even at hatching (day 17 of incubation). Neonatally ovariectomized females showed a weak masculine sexual behavior in response to T-treatment in adulthood (Hutchison, 1978; Schumacher and Balthazart, 1984a). This behavior was seen only in a fraction of the birds tested in optimal conditions but since it was completely absent in females ovariectomized later in life, this indicated that the demasculinization of females was in progress but not fully completed at the time of hatching. Ovarian estrogens were apparently able to complete the behavioral demasculinization of these females during the first 4 weeks post-hatch (Balthazart and Schumacher, 1984). There was therefore an apparent discrepancy between results showing that male quail were demasculinized by exogenous estrogens only if the treatment was applied before day 12 of incubation and results showing that the demasculinization of females was not completed at hatching. This suggested that the time course of the differentiation process in females could be different from the expectation based on the results of hormonal manipulations of males.

We recently reassessed the mechanisms underlying the sexual differentiation of behavior in quail with the help of a new very potent aromatase inhibitor (Wouters et al., 1989; De Coster et al., 1990) with great specificity. Aromatase inhibitors represent an alternative to antiestrogens for the physiological study of estrogen-dependent events: instead of blocking estrogens action at the receptor level, their synthesis is suppressed in the gonads and in other potential sources of steroid. The triazole derivative, R76713 (6-[(4-chlorophenyl)(1H-1,2,4-triazol-1-yl)methyl]-1-methyl-1H-benzotriazole) had previously been used to block the T-induced copulatory behavior and preoptic aromatase activity in castrated male quail (Balthazart et al., 1990a). The same compound was used here to suppress estrogen production in quail embryos and study the behavioral long-term effects of this treatment (Balthazart et al., 1992a).

In a series of 4 experiments, embryos were injected with 10 μg R76713 at various ages (days 6 [D6], 9 [D9], 12 [D12] or 15 [D15]) to prevent the production of endogenous estrogens. Controls were injected with the vehicle solution on day 6 All birds were then gonadectomized at the age of 3-4 weeks post-hatch. When adult, all subjects received subcutaneous silastic implants filled with T, a hormonal treatment sufficient to restore sexual behavior in castrated males and the effects of this steroid on male copulatory behavior were quantified during standard presentations to sexually mature females. Behavioral frequencies were analyzed by a two way ANOVA (age at injection and sex as factors) which revealed significant effects of the sex and of the interaction sex by age. The Fisher protected least significance test was used for additional comparisons of the groups two by two (see Figure 1; $^*P < 0.05$ compared to control birds of the same sex; $^\#P < 0.05$ compared to males submitted to the same treatment).

When injected before day 12 of incubation, R76713 completely blocked the behavioral demasculinization of females without affecting the behavior of the males. After the T treatment in adulthood, almost all R76713-treated females (26 out of 27) showed a masculine copulatory behavior that was undistinguishable from the behavior of intact males. By comparison none of the females (n = 15) that had received a control injection in egg showed cloacal contact movements.

Injections of R76713 during the early phases of incubation (day 6 or 9) blocked the female demasculinization to the same extent but the injections performed in the late phase of the incubation (day 12 or 15) only maintained a weak or no copulatory behavior in females. Males were unaffected by all treatments. This confirmed that the behavioral demasculinization in quail takes place mainly though not exclusively during the early stages of ontogeny.

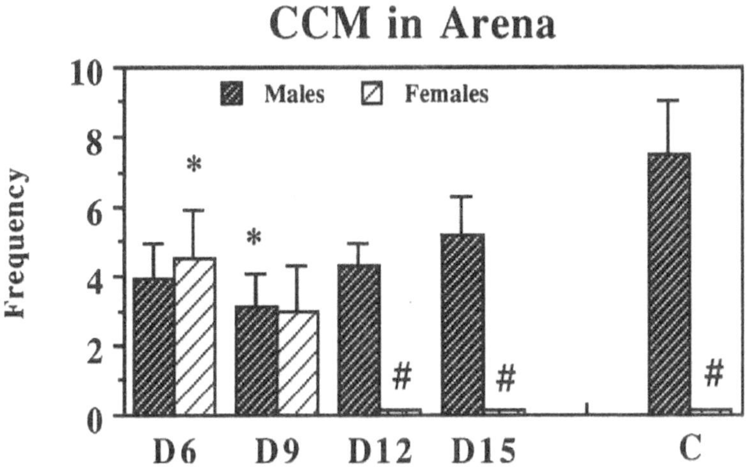

## CCM in Arena

**Figure 1** Effects embryonic treatment with the aromatase inhibitor, R76713 on the frequency of male copulatory behavior (cloacal contact movements; CCM) observed in adulthood after activation by exogenous testosterone. Redrawn from data in Balthazart et al. (1992a).

In a subsequent experiment, the R76713 injections in egg (10 µg on day 9) were combined in some birds with an injection of estradiol benzoate (EB; administered on day 9 also). The effects of the aromatase inhibitor were fully reversed by the injection of EB demonstrating that the effects of R76713 were specifically due to the suppression of endogenous estrogens. Once again, the aromatase inhibitor had no visible effect on the development of behavior in males but EB alone or in combination with R76713 completely blocked the development of the male copulatory behavior.

In a last experiment, we combined an early R76713 treatment (10 µg on day 9) with an injection of EB (25 µg) either on day 9 or on day 14 of incubation. Control birds were injected with the oil vehicle. Behavioral frequencies were analyzed by a three way ANOVA (age at injection of EB, EB versus oil and sex as factors) which revealed significant effects of the three main factors as well as significant interactions of EB with age and of EB with sex with age (secondary interaction). The Fisher protected least significance test was used for additional comparisons of the groups two by two (see Figure 2; *P < 0.05 compared to control birds of the same sex (R76/Oil); # P < 0.05 compared to males submitted to the same treatment; ΔP < 0.05 compared to birds of the same sex treated with EB on day 9).

This experiment showed that the sensitivity to differentiating effects of estrogens varies with age in a sexually differentiated manner. As shown previously, the EB injection on day 9 demasculinized both male and female embryos. If this injection was delayed until day 14, it was no longer effective in males but still caused a partial demasculinization of females).

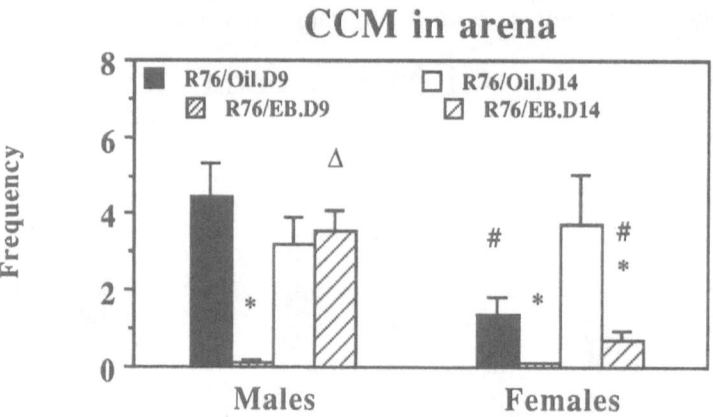

**Figure 2** Effects of embryonic treatment with the aromatase inhibitor, R76713 combined or not with estradiol benzoate (EB) on the frequency of male copulatory behavior (cloacal contact movements; CCM) observed in adulthood after activation by exogenous testosterone. Redrawn from data in Balthazart et al. (1992a).

Taken together, these studies demonstrate that masculine sexual behavior is lost in females during embryonic life under the influence of estrogens. This was suggested by the effect of exogenous estrogens in male embryos but this model receives here a direct confirmation since it is possible to maintain copulatory behavior in females by blocking estrogen synthesis during embryonic life with a potent aromatase inhibitor such as R76713. These experiments also show that estrogens are presumably the only hormonal stimulus that is responsible for the behavioral demasculinization of females since the blockade of their synthesis results in adult females which have a behavioral phenotype indistinguishable from that of normal males.

R76713 was also used as a tool to determine the time-course of the sensitive period for sexual differentiation in quail. The evolution in time of the female demasculinization was analyzed by injecting female embryos with the aromatase inhibitor on different days during incubation (Figure 1). It was shown that early treatments are the most effective. Day 12 appears to be a critical age in this respect: if the differentiation is interrupted at that age by injection of the aromatase inhibitor, females are only partly demasculinized. Some of them are active at low frequency while others are not. The weak activity is clearly enhanced when a more appropriate test situation (Schumacher and Balthazart, 1984a) such as the home cage is used (Balthazart et al., 1992a; data not shown here). A treatment with R76713 performed on day 15 is much less effective. Female demasculinization has progressed too far and/or the amount of estrogens that have been accumulated in the egg is already too high so that intense masculine behavior can no longer be elicited even if the synthesis of new estrogens is interrupted. However, some residual activity (mount attempts) is still present and will persist until the first few days after hatching. It will be revealed in optimal testing conditions. These data therefore show that the sexual differentiation of female behavior is a progressive phenomenon and that the most active phase for this process takes place between days 9 and 15 of incubation. This in fact corresponds well with the period during which plasma levels of estradiol are increased in female embryos (Schumacher et al., 1988). This phenomenon is driven by estrogens as revealed by the blockade following injection of an aromatase inhibitor and the restoration following the treatment with exogenous estrogens.

To obtain the sexual differentiation of behavioral or morphological characteristics, the appropriate hormonal stimulus (estrogen) must be present during the period when the embryo is sensitive to its action (critical period). The differentiation and its evolution in time as described by the injection of R76713 at different ages (figure 1) result from the summation of these two factors. Data presented in figure 2 reveal in addition that, in quail, the sensitivity to the differentiating action of estrogens is in itself a process that varies in time and that is sexually differentiated. In this experiment, the differentiation of females was blocked by an injection of R76713 on day 9 of incubation and the effect of exogenous estrogens was subsequently tested. This confirmed that male embryos are no longer sensitive to estradiol effects after day 12 of incubation. The injection of EB on day 9 completely suppressed copulatory behavior in males but had absolutely no effect on day 14. By contrast, in females, the sensitivity to estrogens was not lost so abruptly. A treatment with EB on day 14 still produced a partial but nevertheless significant demasculinization. The evolution in time of the sensitivity to estradiol is therefore sexually differentiated in quail embryos. Females retain a partial sensitivity longer than the males. This is in agreement with previous results from this laboratory that showed that a post hatching treatment with estradiol was able to complete the demasculinization of neonatally ovariectomized females but had no effect in neonatally castrated males (Balthazart and Schumacher, 1984).

It appears therefore that differentiation in quail takes place during two distinct stages: an early phase when the sensitivity to estrogens becomes differentiated and a latter phase during which the behavioral demasculinization is established by estrogens. The notion that hormones might act in a biphasic manner during ontogeny to first sensitize brain cells and subsequently differentiate them has been proposed more than 10 years ago (Weisz and Ward, 1980; Harlan et al., 1979). Circumstantial evidence suggests that this two-step model might be applicable to several experimental systems in both mammals and birds (Baum et al., 1990; Rhees, 1990; Schumacher and Balthazart, 1985; Balthazart and Schumacher, 1987). The present data provide strong experimental evidence showing that the sensitivity to differentiating effects of estrogens is sexually differentiated during the late phase of the incubation in quail. The hormonal bases of the sexual differentiation in estrogen sensitivity are unknown and should now be investigated. This could be done using the aromatase inhibitor, R76713 as an experimental tool. It should indeed be possible to inhibit estradiol production very early on in female embryos (before day 9) and then to test their sensitivity to estrogens. It is quite possible that if they are never exposed to estrogens, females embryos will then react like male embryos to experimental manipulations performed later in the embryonic or early post-hatching life.

# Central mechanism underlying the activation of copulatory behavior in adult quail

A major part of our recent research efforts has been devoted to the identification of sexual brain dimorphisms that could potentially explain the sex differences in quail behavior. As a prerequisite to these studies, it was however necessary to identify the neuroanatomical and neurochemical substrate underlying the activation of copulatory behavior in the male. We shall briefly review the results obtained in these studies before analyzing in more detail the sex differences observed in the quail brain.

## Testosterone metabolism, and sexual behavior in the Japanese quail

In the brain of Japanese quail, and in other avian species, T can be aromatized into estradiol ($E_2$) or estrone ($E_1$) (Callard et al., 1978; Callard, 1984; Steimer and Hutchison, 1980; Schumacher et al., 1984) and this process plays an important role in the activation of reproductive behavior. In male quail for example, T-induced copulation is blocked by the antiestrogens, CI-628 or tamoxifen (Adkins and Nock, 1976; Alexandre and Balthazart, 1986) and by the aromatase inhibitors, ATD or R76713 (Adkins et al., 1980; Balthazart et al., 1990a; Balthazart et al., 1990c). Thus $E_2$ derived from T aromatization is involved in the control of copulation. This behavior can, in fact, be activated by T as well as by $E_2$ (Adkins and Adler, 1972; Schumacher and Balthazart, 1983; Balthazart et al., 1985). In addition it should be pointed out that androgens *per se* can contribute to the activation of copulatory behavior in quail (Balthazart et al., 1985; Alexandre and Balthazart, 1986; Balthazart and Surlemont, 1990b) so that the hormonal determinants of this behavior include both androgen- and estrogen-sensitive mechanisms.

The aromatase activity (AA) in the quail preoptic area (POA) seems to be a limiting factor in the activation by T of male copulation. The induction of AA by T in the POA is dose- and time-dependent. The minimal dose of T (10 mm silastic implant) which reliably restores copulatory behavior approximately doubles the AA in the POA. A significant increase in AA is observed within 16 hours after the start of the treatment with T and the induction is maximal after 48 hours. Activation of copulatory behavior follows a similar time-course but occurs with a delay of 24-48 hours. In addition, if T-treated birds receive at the same time silastic implants filled with ATD, the activation of behavior is suppressed for at least one week. This behavioral inhibition is, as expected, accompanied and very probably caused by the inhibition of the aromatase activity in the preoptic area and anterior hypothalamus (Balthazart et al., 1990c).

## The sexually dimorphic nucleus of the quail POA

A second phase of this study consisted in the identification of the important brain site(s) for T action on behavior. Our research focussed on the POA because, previous studies carried out on birds and mammals had shown that this region was binding sex steroids (Morrell et al., 1975; Pfaff, 1976; Morell and Pfaff, 1978; Stumpf and Sar, 1978) and that T action in the POA was usually sufficient to activate sex behavior in castrated males (Kelley and Pfaff, 1978).

Morphometric studies of Nissl-stained sections in the POA of quail were undertaken in collaboration with Italian neuroanatomists of the University of Torino (Drs G.C. Panzica and C. Viglietti-Panzica). This led to the identification of a sexually dimorphic nucleus (SDN) in the POA. It was found that the medial preoptic nucleus (POM) of the quail is significantly larger in males than in females (Viglietti-Panzica et al., 1986; Adkins-Regan and Watson, 1990). This structure is also T-sensitive: its volume regresses after castration and increases following T treatment (Panzica et al., 1987; Panzica et al., 1991). POM volume therefore provides a morphological signature of T action in the POA.

These data indicated that POM might be implicated in the control of male copulatory behavior. Electrolytic lesions and stereotaxic implantation of steroids, aromatase inhibitors and steroid receptor antagonists were therefore undertaken to test the role of POM in the activation of male behavior. Previously published studies indicated that stereotaxic implants of T in the POA located in or near POM were able to activate sexual behavior in castrated male quail (Watson and Adkins-Regan, 1989a; Watson and Adkins-Regan, 1989b) but these did not permit a precise delineation of the active area since fairly large amounts of steroids had been implanted and they had possibly diffused over a wide area. Smaller amounts of hormone contained in 27 g needles were stereotaxically implanted in the POA of castrated male quail. This confirmed that T implants must be within the boundaries of the POM as defined in Nissl-stained material in order to activate behavior (Balthazart and Surlemont, 1990a; Balthazart et al., 1992d). In addition, electrolytic lesions aimed at the POA produced deficits in the T-induced copulatory behavior of castrated males that were proportional to the amount of the nucleus that had been destroyed (Balthazart and Surlemont, 1990a). These experiments therefore indicated that the SDN of the quail POA was a necessary and sufficient site for T action on behavior.

A series of studies in which synthetic androgens or estrogens, antiandrogens, antiestrogens and aromatase inhibitors were stereotaxically implanted in the POM of castrated male quail also demonstrated that T must be aromatized and the synthesized estrogens must interact locally in the nucleus with estrogen receptors in order to produce a significant behavioral activation (Balthazart and Surlemont, 1990b; Balthazart et al., 1990a). Implantation of aromatase inhibitors such as ATD or R76713 or of the antiestrogen tamoxifen into the POM inhibited the copulatory behavior activated in castrates by a systemic treatment with T. In addition, implants of the synthetic estrogen, diethylstilbestrol into the dimorphic nucleus were also able to activate male sexual behavior in castrates.

The quail POM therefore appears as a unique model structure for the study of the activation of masculine sexual behavior by steroids in that it is a T-sensitive sexually differentiated nucleus which is at the same time a sufficient site for the induction of behavior by T. It is also clear that the effects of T in this nucleus are mediated through local aromatization.

# Sex differences in the adult brain

## Catecholamines concentration, turnover and receptors

Since the POA/POM appears to be key site in the activation of male copulatory behavior, detailed biochemical and morphological studies of possible sex dimorphisms in this region have been carried out. These have concerned in part the concentration, turnover and receptors of the catecholamines, norepinephrine (NE) and dopamine (DA).

Sex differences in the baseline concentration and/or in the turnover of both NE and DA were originally identified in the POA of sexually mature quail (Ottinger and Balthazart, 1987; Ottinger et al., 1986). Subsequent studies in which NE and DA were assayed by HPLC and electrochemical detection in microsamples dissected by the Palkovits punch technique (Palkovits, 1973; Palkovits and Brownstein, 1983) confirmed that these sex dimorphisms were present within the POM (Balthazart et al., 1992b). These sex differences, however, usually disappeared in birds that were exposed to the same hormonal conditions (gonadectomized subjects treated or not with T) suggesting that they resulted only from a differential regulation by steroids in the adult. One noticeable exception to this rule concerned the DA turnover in POM that appeared to be lower in females than in males irrespective of the endocrine condition (Balthazart et al., 1992b). It is established that the dopaminergic system plays an important role in the control of copulatory behavior in mammals (Meyerson and Malmnas, 1978; Bitran and Hull, 1987; Crowley et al., 1989; Blackburn et al., 1992) but comparable data are still lacking in birds. Since DA appears to stimulate male sex behavior in mammals, it can be speculated that the lower DA turnover in female quail compared to males may be responsible for their lack of behavioral responsiveness to T treatment. This interesting possibility should be experimentally tested.

Noradrenergic ($\alpha_1$, $\alpha_2$, $\beta_1$, $\beta_2$ subtypes) and dopaminergic (D1 and D2 subtypes) receptors have also been studied in the quail POA by quantitative autoradiography in collaboration with Dr. G. F. Ball (The Johns Hopkins University, Department of Psychology). With one noticeable exception ($\alpha_2$ receptors), all these binding sites appear to be extremely rare in the POA (Ball et al., 1989; Balthazart et al., 1989; Casto et al., 1991; Ball and Balthazart, unpublished data) and it appears quite unlikely that sex differences in receptor densities could be observed in that region by quantitative autoradiography. By contrast, $\alpha_2$ adrenergic receptors are extremely abundant in the quail POA and they specifically outline the sexually dimorphic nucleus, POM (Ball et al., 1989; Balthazart and Ball, 1989). Although our first experiment (Ball et al., 1989) suggested that $\alpha_2$ adrenergic binding sites could be slightly more numerous in the female than in the male POM, no confirmation of this sex difference was obtained in a subsequent more detailed study (Balthazart et al., 1991b). No specific relationship can therefore be established between the distribution of catecholamine receptors in the quail POA and the sex difference in reproductive behavior. If catecholamines contribute to the explanation of the behavioral dimorphism, it is probably through their differential turnover rates rather than through a differentiated receptor system.

## The cytoarchitectonic organization of the POM

We had established that the POM volume was significantly larger in sexually mature male quail than in females (Viglietti-Panzica et al., 1986). It was found later that this gross dimorphism in volume resulted from a differential activation by T in adulthood. Gonadectomy significantly reduced POM volume in both males and females. After a treatment with a same dose of T, large preoptic medial nuclei similar to those of sexually mature males were observed in both sexes (Panzica et al., 1987; Panzica et al., 1991). Parallel changes in staining density were observed (Balthazart et al., 1991b). This suggested that organizational effects of hormones were probably playing little or no role in the control of the POM volume dimorphism. This conclusion was supported by experiments showing that embryonic treatment of male quail with estradiol benzoate (EB), at doses which completely suppress the capacity to exhibit male copulatory behavior (Adkins, 1979; Schumacher et al., 1989), did not affect the total volume of POM (Panzica et al., 1987).

A more interesting sex dimorphism was however detected during the analysis of the cytoarchitectonic organization of the nucleus. We found that neurons in the dorso-lateral part of the POM were consistently larger than the more medial ones. These dorso-lateral neurons increased in size following treatment with T of castrates (Panzica et al., 1991). This increased cell size was observed only in the lateral but not in the medial POM. Interestingly, it was present in castrated males but not in ovariectomized females treated with T. This suggests two important conclusions. First the increase in POM volume observed in both sexes after a same treatment with T may reflect cellular processes that are substantially different (e.g. change in neuronal size vs variation in cell spacing vs modification of the glial components) and this interesting possibility is currently studied by quantitative morphometry on semi-thin sections in the laboratory of Drs Panzica and Viglietti-Panzica. Second, since T action on the dorsolateral neurons is different in adult males and females, organizational effects of hormones may actually take place at this level, even if they are not reflected in measures of the overall POM volume.

Initial support to this hypothesis comes from a recent experiment in which the effects of an embryonic treatment with EB on the T-induced copulatory behavior and on the neuronal size in POM were studied (Aste et al., 1991). This study confirmed that when male embryos are treated with EB on day 9 of incubation, they are usually completely demasculinized (see above). In parallel, the size of the neurons in the dorsolateral part of the POM in these birds was significantly reduced. This effect was quite specific since it was not observed in the medial part of the POM nor in birds which had been treated with EB on day 14 of incubation, which is too late to affect behavior (Adkins, 1979; Schumacher et al., 1989). The correlation with behavior could also be strengthened by exploiting the natural variance present in the data. A few males treated with EB on day 9 had not been fully demasculinized and they showed a weak sexual behavior during the experimental tests. Interestingly, the neurons in the dorsolateral POM of these birds had not been affected by EB and were therefore significantly larger than in the demasculinized males. These correlative data therefore strongly support the notion that POM constitutes a part of the brain circuitry controlling male sex behavior. This is also suggested by experimental manipulations (electrolytic lesions and stereotaxic implantation of T) of this sexually dimorphic nucleus (Balthazart et al., 1992d) and by correlative studies relating the effects of T and its metabolites on the male sexual behavior on one hand and on the size of the dorso-lateral POM neurons on the other side (Aste et al., 1992).

## The preoptic aromatase activity

As discussed above, the behavioral responses to T are sexually differentiated in quail. Considering the important role played by T metabolism, it was hypothesized that the insensitivity to androgens observed in females could be related to a differential T metabolism in their brains. These could for example produce insufficient amounts of active metabolites such as E2. Aromatase activity was therefore assayed in discrete areas of male and female brains obtained by a free-hand microdissection or by the Palkovits punch technique (Palkovits, 1973; Palkovits and Brownstein, 1983). In several brain nuclei, a marked sexual dimorphism was revealed: aromatase was more active in males than females throughout the hypothalamus and especially in the preoptic area (POA) (Schumacher and Balthazart, 1984b; Schumacher and Balthazart, 1986). Male brains produced in larger quantities than female brains metabolites such as E2 that are involved in the activation of copulation. It is therefore possible that the insensitivity of females to T is causally related to a metabolic deactivation of the hormone.

However, these studies were all performed on intact birds so that the observed differences may have been induced by the different circulating gonadal hormones in males and females. This experiment was thus repeated in order to assess enzymatic differences not only in intact but also in gonadectomized males and females and in birds treated with T at doses which restore sexual behavior in males but not in females. The reactions to castration and T replacement were strikingly dissimilar for the different T-metabolizing enzyme ($5\alpha$- and $5\beta$-reductase, aromatase) and have been described in detail (Schumacher and Balthazart, 1986). The preoptic aromatase was the only enzyme to show sex differences that were resistant to gonadectomy and steroid treatment. This enzymatic activity was much higher in intact males than females. This sexual dimorphism disappeared in castrated birds. The enzymatic activity was then induced in both sexes by T but the extent of this induction was significantly different in the two sexes. In males, T treatment restored aromatase activity to its pre-castration level in all parts of the hypothalamus while the same treatment in females resulted in more limited induction of enzymatic levels, similar to those seen in intact females (Schumacher and Balthazart, 1986; Balthazart, 1989b; Balthazart et al., 1990c). This induction by T was sexually differentiated. This sex difference in enzymatic activity presumably contributes to the differential sensitivity of males and females to the activating effects of T on behavior. It cannot however be taken as the sole responsible of the behavioral dimorphism since treatment of females with large doses of estrogens (which should bypass the enzymatic limiting factor) still fails to activate a strong copulatory behavior (Schumacher and Balthazart, 1983).

## Aromatase-immunoreactive neurons in the POA

These studies strongly suggested that aromatase activity was sexually differentiated in the quail POA and that this dimorphism might be causally related to the sex differences in behavior. A number of questions concerning the anatomical organization of this neurochemical sex difference could however not be studied by the enzymatic assay of aromatase activity. Several mechanisms could for example be implicated in existence of a higher enzymatic activity in males: higher concentration of enzymes in a similar number of cells, presence of a larger number of aromatase-containing cells, differential distribution of the positive cells in the POA or even differential regulation of a same amount of enzyme. These possibilities are presented in a schematic mode in Figure 3. At the top, the situation in the POM (ovoid nucleus) of a male is shown: many cells contain many aromatase molecules. Aromatase activity can be lower in females with no associated change in concentration of the enzyme (regulation of the activity in the molecules that are already present; A) or because the aromatase concentration in each cell is lower (B) or because fewer cells contain the enzyme (C) or because the distribution of positive cells is different so that these are spread out in the preoptic area (D). These different mechanisms are in addition not exclusive.

The precise anatomical organization of the aromatase-containing system was also unknown and this prevented the study of the neural circuitry mediating T action on behavior. The recent development of an immunocytochemical procedure to visualize aromatase-containing cells in the quail brain (Balthazart et al., 1990b; Balthazart et al., 1990f) has allowed us to begin the study of these questions. The technique is based on a polyclonal antibody raised in rabbit against human placental aromatase (Harada, 1988). Biochemical, immunological and physiological criteria confirm that this antibody specifically recognizes the enzymatically active aromatase molecule in the quail brain (Balthazart et al., 1990b; Balthazart et al., 1990d).

Aromatase-immunoreactive (ARO-ir) cells were detected in all brain areas that had been shown previously by product-formation assays to contain AA, namely:

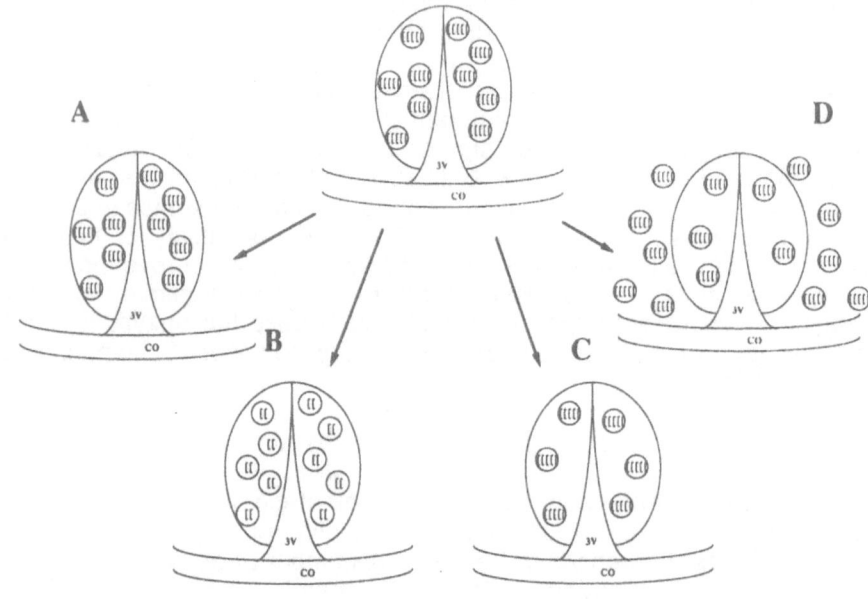

**Figure 3** Diagram illustrating the mechanisms that could potentially explain a sex difference in aromatase activity in the medial preoptic nucleus (POM).

the medial POA, the area under the lateral ventricles from the level of the nucleus accumbens to the level of the nucleus striae terminalis and the tuberal hypothalamus at the level of the nucleus infundibuli hypothalami (Balthazart et al., 1990b; Balthazart et al., 1990f). In the POA, the ARO-ir cells were a specific marker for the POM. These immunoreactive cells outlined the borders of the nucleus throughout its rostral to caudal extent (see Figure 4, top and middle panels). At the level of the anterior commissure (Figure 4, middle panel), another group of immunoreactive cells could also be observed dorsally under the lateral ventricles. At the caudal end of POM, the group of ARO-ir cells located dorsally under the lateral ventricles merged with the POM cell group to form a V-shaped arrangement of immunoreactive perikarya that corresponds to the full extent of the nucleus striae terminalis (Figure 4, bottom panel).

65

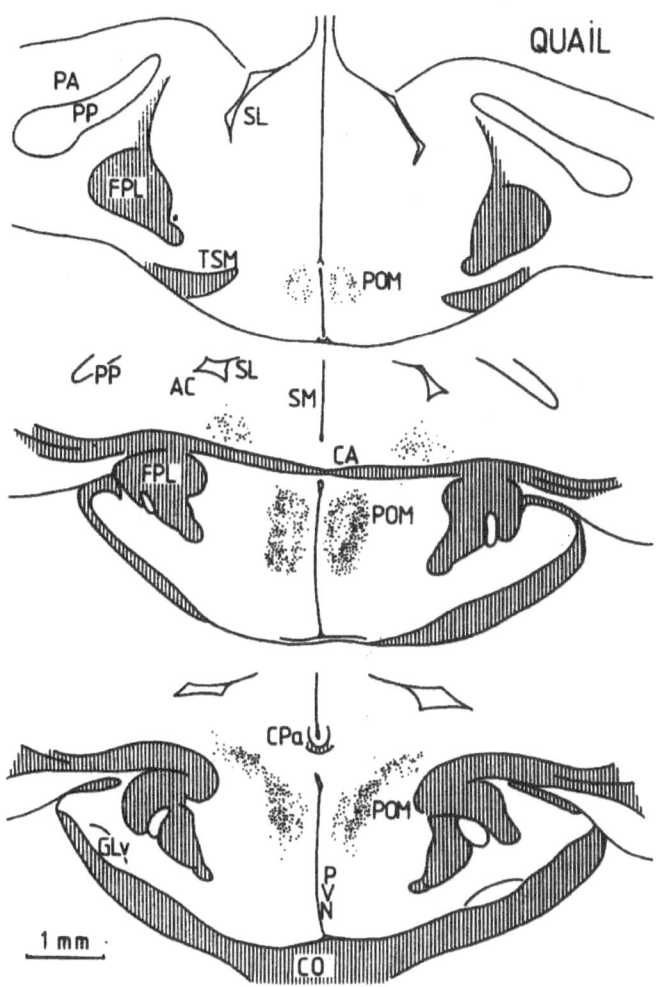

**Figure 4** Camera lucida drawing illustrating the distribution of ARO-ir cells in the preoptic area of the quail brain.
Three successive levels in the rostral to caudal order are shown from top to bottom. AC: nucleus accumbens, CA: commissura anterior, CO: chiasma opticum, CPa; commissura pallii, FPL: fasciculus prosencephali lateralis, GLv: nucleus geniculatus lateralis pars ventralis, PA: paleostriatum augmentatum, POM: nucleus preopticus medialis, PP: Paleostriatum primitivum, PVN: nucleus paraventricularis magnocellularis, SL: nucleus septalis lateralis, SM: nucleus septalis medialis, TSM: tractus septomesencephalicus. Magnification bar= 1 mm.

66

Immunocytochemistry was then used to study at a cellular level the sex difference of AA that had been previously identified in the POA. Serial sections were collected every 100 μm throughout the rostral to caudal extent of the POM and stained for aromatase. Immunoreactive cells were then counted in six pairs of sexually mature males and females compared in males and females by a t-test ([**]P < 0.01). The position of the sections in different birds was standardized by reference to the anterior commissure (see Figure 5, top panel).

The POM of males contained more ARO-ir perikarya than the POM of females. This difference was, however, restricted to a limited portion of the nucleus just under and before the anterior commissure (significant in levels labelled 6-7 in the figure). In the more rostral parts, females had actually more immunoreactive cells than males. Experimental data (electrolytic lesions and stereotaxic implantation of T; Balthazart et al., 1992d) suggest that the dimorphic region located just before the anterior commissure is specifically implicated in the control of male behavior.

These immunocytochemical studies clearly indicated that the overall distribution of ARO-ir cells was similar in males and females (they are in both sexes located within the boundaries of the POM) but that these cells were present in larger number in males suggesting therefore that the concentration of aromatase was higher in this sex. This sex difference in the number of ARO-ir cells and in the concentration of aromatase may be implicated in the causal network responsible for the behavioral sex dimorphism.

To further test this idea, the distribution of ARO-ir cells was investigated in the POA of male and female quail that had been gonadectomized and treated with T. These hormonal manipulations produce subjects that have in essence the same endocrine milieu (in particular plasma T levels are identical) (Schumacher and Balthazart, 1986; Balthazart et al., 1987) but strongly differ in their behavior (males show the copulatory sequence while the females do not; see above). The neurochemical dimorphism that had been observed in intact sexually mature birds was no longer found in males and females exposed to the same concentration of T (see Figure 5, lower panel). This somehow contradicts our earlier studies (Schumacher and Balthazart, 1986; Balthazart, 1989a) showing that aromatase activity is significantly higher in castrated T-treated males than in ovariectomized T-treated females. Several interpretations may be proposed to explain this discrepancy. Either aromatase concentration (and therefore number of ARO-ir cells) is similar in both sexes but the activity of the enzyme differs due to sex specific regulations or aromatase concentration is really higher in males than in females but this difference is too subtle to be detected by a simple count of immunoreactive cells. It is also possible that sex specific patterns in the distribution of ARO-ir cells are present but that these were obscured in the present analysis in which all immunoreactive cells located at a same rostro-caudal level have been pooled. In particular, a specific analysis of the ARO-ir cells located in the dorso-lateral part of POM (the region where cell size is affected by T in males but not in females) should now be carried out.

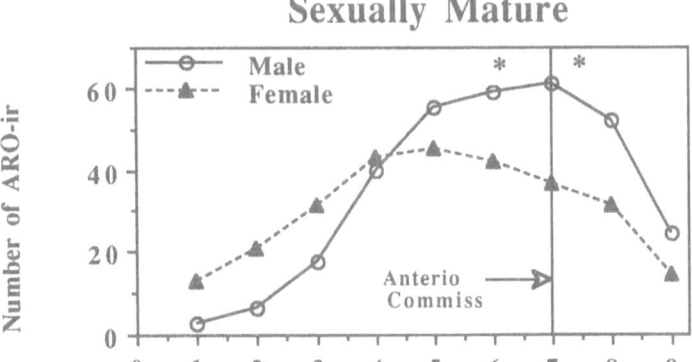

## Sexually Mature

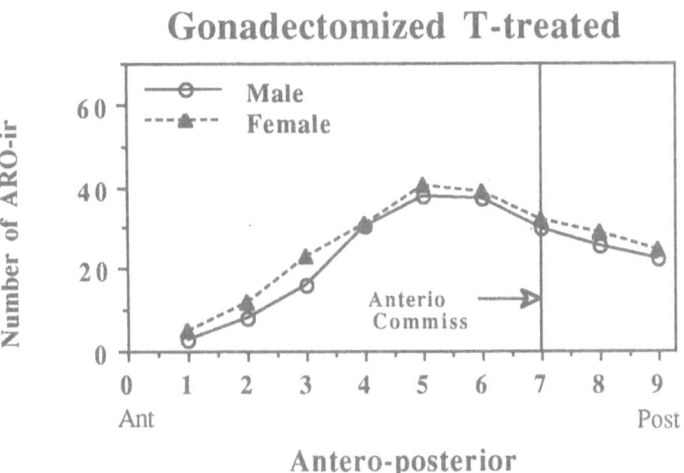

## Gonadectomized T-treated

**Figure 5** Sex difference in the distribution of ARO-ir cells in the POM of adult sexually mature quail (top panel) and in gonadectomized birds treated with exogenous testosterone (bottom panel).

# Conclusions

In the course of the last five years decisive progresses have been made in the understanding of the neuroendocrine mechanisms underlying male copulatory behavior and its sexual dimorphism. The quail has been a very useful animal model in this context. The hormonal mechanisms that are responsible for the development of behavioral sex differences have been identified and they can now be manipulated *ad libitum*. Critical progress has also been made in the understanding of the brain mechanisms controlling copulatory behavior in the adult bird. In particular, a sexually dimorphic nucleus has been identified in the quail POA and it represents a necessary and sufficient site of T action for the activation of male copulation. The role of T aromatization in this process has been well established and the dimorphic nucleus of the POA appears to be the location of the behaviorally relevant central aromatization of T. An immunocytochemical technique to visualize aromatase has also become available. It has been demonstrated that the dimorphic nucleus contains all preoptic ARO-ir cells and that their number varies as a function of the sex and hormonal condition of the birds.

A number of morphological or neurochemical sex dimorphisms have now been identified in the quail brain. However, many of them appear to be induced by the dimorphic endocrine milieu of adult males and females and they cannot therefore be invoked to explain the behavioral dimorphism that is observed when gonadectomized birds of both sexes are submitted to a same hormonal replacement therapy with T. In a more limited number of cases (dopamine turnover in POM, aromatase activity in the POA, neuronal size in the lateral POM), brain sex differences have been detected in gonadectomized T-treated birds. Their nature or anatomical localization suggest that they may be causally implicated in the control of the behavioral dimorphism. The magnitude of these brain dimorphisms is however always limited and it appears, at present, unlikely that one single of these differences in brain structure or functioning will be able to account for the qualitative sex dimorphism in copulatory behavior. Complex interactions will have to be invoked to reach this goal.

The quail now appears to be a very useful and promising model for the understanding of the web of causal interactions mediating the development and activation of reproductive behavior and its sexual differentiation. The availability of an immunocytochemical technique to visualize ARO-ir cells allows the study of this enzyme at a cellular level. Sex differences in the number of immunoreactive cells have already been observed in specific subregions of the sexually dimorphic nucleus. In addition, we are now able to study the anatomical relationships between aromatase-containing cells and estrogen (Balthazart et al., 1991a) or androgen, (Balthazart et al., 1992c) receptors. The subcellular distribution of the aromatase enzyme has been analyzed by electron microscopy and this has shown that the estrogen synthetase is found in the cell perikarya but also at the level of the presynaptic terminals (Naftolin et al., 1990; Balthazart et al., 1990e). The role played by estrogens produced in the vicinity of the synaptic membranes has now to be establish. ARO-ir cells are, in all probability, embedded in the circuitry controlling male copulatory behavior. By combining aromatase-immunocytochemistry with anterograde and retrograde tracing techniques, it will now become possible to map this neuronal network and analyse its sexually differentiated aspects both from an anatomical and neurochemical point of view. This should lead, in a near future, to a better understanding of the neural bases of the sexual dimorphism in quail behavior.

# Acknowledgments

The recent work described in this review was supported by grants from the Belgian FRFC (Nbr. 2.9003.91 and 9.4601.90) and the University of Liège (Fonds Spéciaux pour la Recherche). I thank the late Professor E. Schoffeniels for his continued interest and support of my research. I also would like to thank all my collaborators in Liège and in other laboratories who have been of an invaluable help in collecting the data presented here, namely C. Surlemont, M. Schumacher, A. De Clerck and L. Evrard (Laboratory of General and Comparative Biochemistry, University of Liège), F. Naftolin and C. Leranth (Department of Obstetrics and Gynecology, Yale University), G.C. Panzica, C. Viglietti-Panzica and N. Aste (Department of Human Anatomy and Physiology, University of Turin), N. Harada (Molecular Genetics, Fujita Health University, Toyoake) and G.F. Ball (Department of Psychology, Johns Hopkins University). Collaboration with G.F. Ball was supported by a NATO Collaborative Research Grant (CRG910526).

# References

Adkins, E. K. and Adler, N. T. (1972). Hormonal control of behavior in the Japanese quail. *J. Comp. Physiol. Psychol.*, **81** : 27-36.

Adkins, E. K. (1975). Hormonal basis of sexual differentiation in the Japanese quail. *J. Comp. Physiol. Psychol.*, **89** : 61-71.

Adkins, E. K. (1976). Embryonic exposure to an antiestrogen masculinizes behavior of female quail. *Physiol. Behav.*, **17** : 357-359.

Adkins, E. K. and Nock, B. L. (1976). The effects of the antiestrogen CI-628 on sexual behavior activated by androgen and estrogen in quail. *Horm. Behav.*, **7** : 417-429.

Adkins, E. K. (1978). Sex steroids and the differentiation of avian reproductive behavior. *Amer. Zool.*, **18** : 501-509.

Adkins, E. K. (1979). Effect of embryonic treatment with estradiol or testosterone on sexual differentiation of the quail brain. *Neuroendocrinol.*, **29** : 178-185.

Adkins, E. K., Boop, J. J., Koutnik, D. L., Morris, J. B. and Pniewski, E. E. (1980). Further evidence that androgen aromatization is essential for the activation of copulation in male quail. *Physiol. Behav.*, **24** : 441-446.

Adkins-Regan, E. (1983). Sex steroids and the differentiation and activation of avian reproductive behaviour. In: Balthazart, J. and Gilles, R. (Eds.), *Hormones and Behaviour in Higher Vertebrates*, Springer-Verlag, Berlin, pp. 219-228.

Adkins-Regan, E. and Watson, J. T. (1990). Sexual dimorphism in the avian brain is not limited to the song control system of birds: a morphometric analysis of the brain of the quail *(Coturnix japonica)*. *Brain Res.*, **514** : 320-326.

Adkins-Regan, E. K., Pickett, P. and Koutnik, D. (1982). Sexual differentiation in quail : conversion of androgen to estrogen mediates testosterone-induced demasculinization of copulation but not other male characteristics. *Horm. Behav.*, **16** : 259-278.

Alexandre, C. and Balthazart, J. (1986). Effects of metabolism inhibitors, antiestrogens and antiandrogens on the androgen and estrogen induced sexual behavior in Japanese quail. *Physiol. Behav.*, **38** : 581-591.

Aste, N., Panzica, G. C., Viglietti-Panzica, C. and Balthazart, J. (1991). Effects of in ovo estradiol benzoate treatments on sexual behavior and size of neurons in the sexually dimorphic medial preoptic nucleus of Japanese quail. *Brain Res. Bull.*, **27** : 713-720.

Aste, N., Panzica, G. C., Aimar, P., Viglietti-Panzica, C., Foidart, A. and Balthazart, J. (1992). Implication of testosterone metabolism in the control of the sexually dimorphic nucleus of the quail preoptic area. (submitted)

Ball, G. F., Nock, B., McEwen, B. S., and Balthazart, J. (1989). Distribution of $\alpha_2$-adrenergic receptors in the brain of the Japanese quail as determined by quantitative autoradiography: Implications for the control of sexually dimorphic reproductive processes. *Brain Res.*, **491** : 68-79.

Balthazart, J., Schumacher, M., and Ottinger, M. A. (1983). Sexual differences in the Japanese quail: behavior, morphology and intracellular metabolism of testosterone. *Gen. Comp. Endocrinol.*, **51** : 191-207.

Balthazart, J. and Schumacher, M. (1984). Estradiol contributes to the postnatal demasculinization of female Japanese quail (*Coturnix coturnix japonica*). *Horm. Behav.*, **18** : 287-297.

Balthazart, J., Schumacher, M., and Malacarne, G. (1985). Interaction of androgens and estrogens in the control of sexual behavior in male Japanese quail. *Physiol. Behav.*, **35** : 157-166.

Balthazart, J. and Schumacher, M. (1987). A two-step model for sexual differentiation. In: Komisaruk, B. R., Siegel, H. I., Cheng, M. F. and Feder, H. H. (Eds.), *Reproduction: a Behavioral and Neuroendocrine Perspective*, Annals of the New York Academy of Sciences, New York, pp. 308-324.

Balthazart, J., Delville, Y., Sulon, Y. and Hendrick, J. C. (1987). Plasma levels of luteinizing hormone and of five steroids in photostimulated, castrated and testosterone-treated male and female Japanese quail *(Coturnix coturnix japonica)*. *Gen. Endocrinol. Life Sci. Adv.*, **5** : 31-36.

Balthazart, J. (1989a). Correlation between the sexually dimorphic aromatase of the preoptic area and sexual behavior in quail: effects of neonatal manipulatons of the hormonal milieu. *Arch.I nt. Physiol. Bioch.*, **97** : 465-481.

Balthazart, J. (1989b). Steroid metabolism and the activation of social behavior. In: Balthazart, J. (Ed.) *Advances in Comparative and Environmental Physiology, vol 3*, Springer Verlag, Berlin, pp. 105-159.

Balthazart, J. and Ball, G. F. (1989). Effects of the noradrenergic neurotoxin DSP-4 on luteinizing hormone levels, catecholamine concentrations, $\alpha_1$-adrenergic receptor binding, and aromatase activity in the brain of the Japanese quail. *Brain Res.*, **492** : 163-175.

Balthazart, J., Ball, G. F. and McEwen, B. S. (1989). An autoradiographic study of $\alpha_1$-adrenergic receptors in the brain of the Japanese quail *(Coturnix coturnix japonica). Cell.Tissue Res.*, **258** : 563-568.

Balthazart, J., Evrard, L. and Surlemont, C. (1990a). Effects of the non-steroidal aromatase inhibitor, R76713 on testosterone-induced sexual behavior in the Japanese quail *(Coturnix coturnix japonica). Horm. Behav.* , **24** : 510-531.

Balthazart, J., Foidart, A. and Harada, N. (1990b). Immunocytochemical localization of aromatase in the brain. *Brain Res.*, **514** : 327-333.

Balthazart, J., Foidart, A. and Hendrick, J. C. (1990c). The induction by testosterone of aromatase activity in the preoptic area and activation of copulatory behavior. *Physiol. Behav.*, **47** : 83-94.

Balthazart, J., Foidart, A., Surlemont, C. and Harada, N. (1990d). Preoptic aromatase in quail: behavioral, biochemical and immunocytochemical studies. In: Balthazart, J. (Ed.), *Hormones, Brain and Behavior in Vertebrates. 2. Behavioral Activation in Males and Females - Social Interactions and Reproductive Physiology,* Comp. Physiol. Vol 9, Karger, Basel, pp. 45-62.

Balthazart, J., Foidart, A., Surlemont, C., Harada, N., Leranth, C. and Naftolin, F. (1990e). Immunocytochemical localization of aromatase and estrogen receptors in the brain. *Soc. Neurosci. Abstr.*,**16** : 1313.

Balthazart, J., Foidart, A., Surlemont, C., Vockel, A. and Harada, N. (1990f). Distribution of aromatase in the brain of the Japanese quail, ring dove, and zebra finch: an immunocytochemical study. *J. Comp. Neurol.*, **301** : 276-288.

Balthazart, J. and Surlemont, C. (1990a). Copulatory behavior is controlled by the sexually dimorphic nucleus of the quail POA. *Brain Res. Bull.*, **25** : 7-14.

Balthazart, J. and Surlemont, C. (1990b). Androgen and estrogen action in the preoptic area and activation of copulatory behavior in quail. *Physiol. Behav.*, **48** : 599-609.

Balthazart, J., Foidart, A., Surlemont, C. and Harada, N. (1991a). Neuroanatomical specificity in the co-localization of aromatase and estrogen receptors. *J. Neurobiol.*, **22** : 143-157.

Balthazart, J., Sante, Ph. and Ball, G. F. (1991b). Testosterone effects on the staining density and autoradiographic investigations of the $\alpha_2$-adrenergic receptor in the medial preoptic nucleus of the Japanese quail: relationship to the activation of reproductive behavior. *Arch. Int. Physiol. Bioch.*, **99** : 385-392.

Balthazart, J., De Clerck, A. and Foidart, A. (1992a). Behavioral demasculinization of female quail is induced by estrogens: studies with the new aromatase inhibitor, R76713. *Horm. Behav.*, **26** : 179-203.

Balthazart, J., Foidart, A., Sante, P. and Hendrick, J. C. (1992b). Effects of a-methyl-para-tyrosine on monoamine levels in the Japanese quail: sex differences and testosterone effects. *Brain Res. Bull.*, **28** : 275-288.

Balthazart, J., Foidart, A., Wilson, E. M. and Ball, G. F. (1992c). Immunocytochemical localization of androgen receptors in the male songbird and quail brain. *J. Comp. Neurol.*, **317** : 407-420.

Balthazart, J., Surlemont, C. and Harada, N. (1992d). Aromatase as a cellular marker of testosterone action in the preoptic area. *Physiol. Behav.*, **51** : 395-409.

Baum, M. J., Erskine, M. S., Kornberg, E. and Weaver, C. E. (1990). Prenatal and neonatal testosterone exposure interact to affect differentiation of sexual behavior and partner preference in female ferrets. *Behav. Neurosci.*, **104** : 183-198.

Beach, F. A. (1948). *Hormones and Behavior*, Paul B. Hoeber, Inc., New York.

Beach, F. A. and Inman, N. G. (1965). Effects of castration and androgen replacement on mating in Japanese quail. *Proc. Natl. Acad. Sci. USA*, **54** : 1426-1431.

Bitran, D. and Hull, E. M. (1987). Pharmacological analysis of male rat sexual behavior. *Neurosci. Biobehav. Rev.*, **11** : 365-389.

Blackburn, J. R., Pfaus, J. G. and Phillips, A. G. (1992). Dopamine functions in appetitive and defensive behaviours. *Prog. Neurobiol.*, **39** : 247-279.

Callard, G. V., Petro, Z. and Ryan, K. J. (1978). Conversion of androgen to estrogen and other steroids in the vertebrate brain. *Amer. Zool.*, **18** : 511-523.

Callard, G. V. (1984). Aromatization in brain and pituitary: an evolutionary perspective. In: Celotti, F., Naftolin, F. and Martini, L. (Eds.), *Metabolism of Hormonal Steroids in the Neuroendocrine Sructures*, Raven Press, New York, pp. 79-102.

Casto, J. M., Ball, G. F. and Balthazart, J. (1991). Dopamine receptors in the song control system: area X is defined by the D2 but not the D1 dopamine receptor subtype. *Soc. Neurosci. Abstr.*, **17** : 1053.

Crews, D. and Moore, M. C. (1986). Evolution of mechanisms controlling mating behavior. *Science*, **231** : 121-125.

Crowley, W. R., O'Connor, L. H. and Feder, H. H. (1989). Neurotransmitter systems and social behavior. In: Balthazart, J. (Ed.), *Molecular and Cellular Basis of Social Behavior in Vertebrates*, Springer Verlag, Berlin, pp. 162-208.

De Coster, R., Wouters, W., Bowden, C. R., Vanden Bossche, H., Bruynseels, J., Tuman, R. W., Van Ginckel, R., Snoeck, E., Van Peer, A. and Janssen, P. A. J. (1990). New non-steroidal aromatase inhibitors: focus on R76713. *J. Steroid Biochem.*, **37** : 335-341.

Doi, O., Takai, T., Nakamura, T. and Tanabe, Y. (1980). Changes in the pituitary and plasma LH, plasma and follicular progesterone, and estradiol, and plasma testosterone and estrone concentrations during the ovulatory cycle of the quail *(Coturnix coturnix japonica)*. *Gen. Comp. Endocrinol.*, **41** : 156-163.

Feder, H. H. (1981). Perinatal hormones and their role in the development of sexually dimorphic behaviors. In: Adler, N. (Ed.), *Neuroendocrinology of Reproduction*, Plenum Press, New York, pp. 127-158.

Feder, H. H. (1984). Hormones and sexual behavior. *Ann. Rev. Psychol.*, **35** : 165-200.

Harada, N. (1988). Novel properties of human placental aromatase as cytochrome P-450: purification and characterization of a unique form of aromatase. *J. Biochem.*, **103** : 106-113.

Harlan, R. E., Gordon, J. H. and Gorski, R. A. (1979). Sexual differentiation of the brain: implications for neuroscience. In: Schneider, D. M. (Ed.), *Review of Neuroscience, vol 4*, Raven Press, New York, pp. 31-71.

Hutchison, R. E. (1978). Hormonal differentiation of sexual behavior in Japanese quail. *Horm. Behav.*, **11** : 363-387.

Kelley, D. B. and Pfaff, D. W. (1978). Generalizations from comparative studies on neuroanatomical and endocrine mechanisms of sexual behaviour. In: Hutchison, J. B. (Ed.), *Biological Determinants of Sexual Behaviour*, John Wiley and Sons, Chichester, pp. 225-254.

Leshner, A. I. (1978). *An Introduction to Behavioral Endocrinology*, Oxford University Press, New York.

Meyerson, B. J. and Malmnas, C. O. (1978). Brain monoamines and sexual behaviour. In: Hutchison, J. B. (Ed.), *Biological Determinants of Sexual Behaviour*, John Wiley and Sons, Chichester, pp. 521-554.

Morell, J. I. and Pfaff, D. W. (1978). A neuroendocrine approach to brain function: localization of sex steroid concentrating cells in vertebrate brains. *Amer. Zool.*, **18** : 447-460.

Morrell, J. I., Kelley, D. B. and Pfaff, D. W. (1975). Sex steroid binding in the brain of vertebrates. In: Knigge, K. M., Scott, D. E., Kobayashi, H., Miura, S. and Ishii, S. (Eds.), *Brain-Endocrine Interactions II*, Karger, Basel, pp. 230-256.

Naftolin, F., Leranth, C. and Balthazart, J. (1990). Ultrastructural localization of aromatase immunoreactivity in hypothalamic neurons. *The Endocr. Soc. Abstr.*, 669 : 192.

Ottinger, M. A., Schumacher, M., Clarke, R. N., Duchala, C. S. and Balthazart, J. (1986). Comparison of monoamine concentrations in the brains of adult male and female Japansese quail. *Poultry Sci.*, **65** : 1413-1420.

Ottinger, M. A. and Balthazart, J. (1987). Brain monoamines in Japanese quail: effects of castration and steroid replacement therapy. *Behav. Proc.*, **14** : 197-216.

Palkovits, M. (1973). Isolated removal of hypothalamic or other brain nuclei of the rat. *Brain Res.*, **59** : 449-450.

Palkovits, M. and Brownstein, M. J. (1983). Microdissection of brain areas by the punch technique. In: Cuello, A. C. (Ed.), *Brain Microdissection Techniques*, Wiley, New York, pp. 1-36.

Panzica, G. C., Viglietti-Panzica, C., Calcagni, M., Anselmetti, G. C., Schumacher, M. and Balthazart, J. (1987). Sexual differentiation and hormonal control of the sexually dimorphic preoptic median nucleus in quail. *Brain Res.*, **416** : 59-68.

Panzica, G. C, Viglietti-Panzica, C., Sanchez, F., Sante, P. and Balthazart, J. (1991). Effects of testosterone on a selected neuronal population within the preoptic sexually dimorphic nucleus of the Japanese quail. *J. Comp. Neurol.*, **303** : 443-456.

Pfaff, D. W. (1976). The neuroanatomy of sex hormone receptors in the vertebrate brain. In: Anand Kumar, T. C. (Ed.), *Neuroendocrine Regulation of Fertility*, Karger, Basel, pp. 30-45.

Rhees, R. W., Shryne, J. E. and Gorski, R. A. (1990). Termination of the hormone-sensitive period for differentiation of the sexually dimorphic nucleus of the preoptic area in male and female rats. *Dev. Brain Res.*, **52** : 17-23.

Sachs, B. D. (1969). Photoperiodic control of reproductive behavior and physiology of the male Japanese quail *(Coturnix coturnix japonica)*. *Horm. Behav.*, **1** : 7-24.

Schumacher, M. and Balthazart, J. (1983). The effects of testosterone and its metabolites on sexual behavior and morphology in male and female Japanese quail. *Physiol. Behav.*, **30** : 335-339.

Schumacher, M. and Balthazart, J. (1984a). The postnatal demasculinization of sexual behavior in the Japanese quail. *Horm. Behav.*, **18** : 298-312.

Schumacher, M. and Balthazart, J. (1984b). Sexual dimorphism of the hypothalamic metabolism of testosterone in the Japanese quail *(Coturnix coturnix japonica)*. *Prog. Brain Res.*, **61**: 53-61.

Schumacher, M., Contenti, E. and Balthazart, J. (1984). Partial characterization of testosterone-metabolizing enzymes in the quail brain. *Brain Res.*, **305** : 51-59.

Schumacher, M. and Balthazart, J. (1985). Sexual differentiation is a biphasic process in mammals and birds. In: Gilles, R. and Balthazart, J. (Eds.), *Neurobiology: Current Comparative Approaches*, Springer-Verlag, Berlin, pp. 203-219.

Schumacher, M. and Balthazart, J. (1986). Testosterone-induced brain aromatase is sexually dimorphic. *Brain Res.*, **370** : 285-293.

Schumacher, M., Sulon, J. and Balthazart, J. (1988). Changes in serum concentrations of steroids during embryonic and post-hatching development of male and female Japanese quail *(Coturnix coturnix japonica)*. *J. Endocrinol.*, **118** : 127-134.

Schumacher, M., Hendrick, J. C. and Balthazart, J. (1989). Sexual differentiation in quail: critical period and hormonal specificity. *Horm. Behav.*, **23** : 130-149.

Steimer, Th. and Hutchison, J. B. (1980). Aromatization of testosterone within a discrete hypothalamic area associated with the behavioral action of androgen in the male dove. *Brain Res.*, **192** : 586-591.

Steinach, E. (1940). *Sex and Life,* Viking Press, New York.

Stumpf, W. E. and Sar, M. (1978). Anatomical distribution of estrogen, androgen, progestin, corticoid and thyroid hormone target sites in the brain of mammals: phylogeny and ontogeny. *Amer. Zool.*, **18** : 435-445.

Viglietti-Panzica, C., Panzica, G. C., Fiori, M. G., Calcagni, M., Anselmetti, G. C. and Balthazart, J. (1986). A sexually dimorphic nucleus in the quail preoptic area. *Neurosci. Lett.*, **64** : 129-134.

Watson, J. T. and Adkins-Regan, E. (1989a). Activation of sexual behavior by implantation of testosterone propionate and estradiol benzoate into the preoptic area of the male Japanese quail *(Coturnix japonica)*. *Horm. Behav.*, **23** : 251-268.

Watson, J. T. and Adkins-Regan, E. (1989b). Testosterone implanted in the preoptic area of male Japanese quail must be aromatized to activate copulation. *Horm. Behav.*, **23** : 432-447.

Weisz, J. and Ward, I. L. (1980). Plasma testosterone and progesterone titers of pregnant rats, their male and female fetuses, and neonatal offspring. *Endocrinology*, **106** : 306-316.

Wouters, W., De Coster, R., Krekels, M., Van Dun, J., Beerens, D., Haelterman, C., Raeymaekers, A., Freyne, E., Van Gelder, J., Venet, M. and Janssen, P. A. J. (1989). R 76713, a new specific non-steroidal aromatase inhibitor. *J. Steroid Biochem.*, **32** : 781-788.

# Animal Sexual Differentiation The Early Days and Current Questions

R. E. WHALEN

*Department of Psychology, University of California Riverside, CA 92521, USA*

In 1959, Phoenix and colleagues published a trailblazing paper entitled *"Organizing action of prenatally administered testosterone propionate on the tissues mediating mating behavior in the female guinea pig"*. In that study they gave testosterone to pregnant guinea pigs and later examined the mating patterns of their offspring. The male offspring were mostly unaffected. The female offspring were substantially inhibited in the display of lordosis, a concave arching of the back that characterizes sexual receptivity in many animals. This was true even when the females were ovariectomized and treated with estrogen and progesterone in doses that induce receptivity in normal females.

When Phoenix et al. treated their "androgenized" females with testosterone in adulthood they showed substantially more male-typical mounting responses than control females.

These findings led to what I have termed the Linear Model of Sexual Differentiation - the presence of testosterone during development makes the organism more male-like and less female-like. We will return to this concept.

In 1962 Harris and Levine published an abstract showing similar effects when female rats were treated with testosterone shortly after birth. Their full report appeared in 1965 (Harris and Levine, 1965).

As an aside I should note that it is now well established that these treatment effects are time-limited. They can be produced at specific developmental periods, usually called "sensitive periods".

In the two decades following the original report there was a great deal of controversy about the nature of the differentiation process because different investigators studied different species each of which has its own sensitive period or periods. These sensitive periods are not either prenatal or postnatal - they may be both - and the effects of treatments and their timing depend upon the output behavior being studied.

Since I was studying rats at the time, I was particularly fascinated by the Harris and Levine report. A graduate student working with me, Ronald Nadler, and I

77

*M. Haug et al. (eds.), The Development of Sex Differences and Similarities in Behavior, 77–86.*
© 1993 *Kluwer Academic Publishers.*

decided to add another component to the picture drawn by Harris and Levine. We treated newborn female rats with the ovarian hormone estradiol. Much to our surprise, this treatment yielded female rats that would not mate spontaneously nor when given estradiol and progesterone (Whalen and Nadler, 1963). We had no idea why this should be so.

Later work by others and in my laboratory (e.g. Whalen and Luttge, 1971) led to the "aromatization hypothesis" of differentiation. In several tissues, including the brain, testosterone, secretred by the testes, is metabolically converted to estradiol by aromatizing enzymes. Thus, today, it is thought that sexual differentiation is brought about by estradiol as a metabolic product of testosterone. But, I must emphasize that while this may be true for the differentiation of sexual behavior in rats, it may not be true for the differentiation of other sex-specific behaviors or for the differentiation of sexual behavior in other species. Evolution seems to work to achieve certain functional goals, such as the ability and desire to reproduce, but does not utilize the same pathway in every genome.

In the early 1960's it seemed to me that if the treatment of newborn female rats with testosterone prevented the display of lordosis in adulthood, it may be possible to "preserve" the potential for lordotic behavior in male rats by removing their testosterone at birth. I started castrating newborn male rats. It worked. But I was not alone in this line of thinking. Harvey Feder, who was a postodoctoral researcher in William Young's laboratory, had the same idea. I told Young about my findings and he told me about Harvey's. Young recommended that we publish together. We did (Feder and Whalen, 1965) and the resulting paper was more powerful than if we had each pubished alone. In subsequent research in my laboratory I found that in our hands male rats must be castrated with 96 hours of birth to retain the potential to respond to estradiol and progesterone in adulthood with the display of lordosis.

Note that Aron (this volume) reports the display of lordosis in "normal" male rats. I have never seen this and believe that the difference represents yet another example of a genetic difference, here within a single species. Many want to deny this, yet it is quite the case. When I was a graduate student, I had the opportunity to study the sexual behavior of the so-called "maze-bright" and "maze-dull" rats that Tryon had developed at the University of California, Berkeley in his studies of the inheritance of learning ability (Whalen, 1961). I found significant quantitative differences in the mating patterns of these two strains, even though they had not be selectively bred on the basis of their mating behavior. Simon (this volume) also reports on significant differences in the attack behavior of three strains of mice that we studied (Simon and Whalen, 1986) and on their differential responsiveness to hormones. We must be circumspect in our generalizations from research on a particular group of organisms given the vast genetic diversity that surrounds us.

I have given you a few caveats about our ability to find "truth". But let us return to the data.

My second graduate student, David Edwards, and I, in the mid-1960's decided that we needed more information in order to be able to generate some concepts on the sexual differentiation of rats. We initiated a large study

(Whalen and Edwards, 1967) in which we reared normal male rats were castrated in adulthood (our control group). Other males and females were gonadectomized at birth ; some were treated simultaneously with either testosterone or estradiol and some were untreated.

When these animals were adult, we treated them with testosterone and tested them for the display of male-typical mounting behavior and then they were treated with estradiol and progesterone and their propensity to display lordosis was studied.

The treatments had little effect on the display of male-typical mounting behavior. When given testosterone, the females mounted less frequently than did the males, but their behavior was independent of neonatal treatment. Neonatal castration of males did not reduce their mounting behavior.

What was striking were the effects of our treatments on the ability of our animals to respond to ovarian hormones with the display of lordosis. Simply put, the presence of endogenous hormones or the presence of exogenous hormones at birth suppressed the potential to display lordosis. Males castrated in adulthood or castrated and hormone treated at birth did not display lordosis. Females given either testosterone or estradiol at birth did not display lordosis. Males castrated at birth, normal females and females ovariectomized at birth did show equivalent levels of lordosis when given estradiol and progesterone.

# A new model

The guinea pig studies suggested the Linear Model - more male, less female. Our study sugested that "maleness" and "femaleness" are quite independent. Edwards and I hypothesized that sexual differentiation *in the rat* is characterized by an inhibition of the potential to show female-typical behavior and not by an enhancement of male-typical behavior.

We introduced the term "defeminization". We suggested that early hormonal stimulation in the rat makes the animals less female rather than more male. Of course, we were only partially correct.

Joseph DeBold, one of my graduate students, and I decided to study hamsters because others had shown that female hamsters (unlike female rats) rarely show male-typical mounting responses, even when given large doses of testosterone in adulthood. Male hamsters (unlike male rats) do show some lordotic responses when given estrogen and progesterone. These species differences are a product of a differential timing of the sensitive periods in these species and upon the developmental state of each at the time of birth. The guinea pig is a long gestation species (69 days) and newborn guinea pigs can to some extent fend for themselves. The rat is a relatively short gestation species (21 days) and they require their dam's attention. Hamsters are a very short gestation species and are much less developed at birth than are rats.

DeBold and I (DeBold and Whalen, 1975) reported that testosterone given 24 hours after birth caused a dose-dependent (1 μg-250 μg) reduction in lordosis potential in our female hamsters. However, a very small dose of testosterone (1 μg) maximized their adult potential to show male-typical mounting behavior.This was another dissociation between the hormonal regulation of the enhancement of male-typical and the inhibition of female-typical sexual behavior.

In 1974, I proposed an alternative to the model which I called the "Orthogonal" model. In this model "male-typical" and "female-typical" are orthogonal or independent dimensions of sexuality. The dimensions proposed were "male-non-male" and "female-non-female". What I wrote was:

*"The orthogonal model states that masculinity and femininity are not unitary processes, but reflect many behavioral dimensions that can be independent. The model further states that during development hormones can defeminize without masculinizing and masculinize without defeminizing and that hormones can defeminize one behavioral system (e.g., mating) while masculinizing another system".* (Whalen, 1974, p. 469).

# Another behavior

Early in my career, without conscious thought of the future, I decided to study another sexually differentiated system, aggression. Following the research of the French scientist Karli, I introduced mice into the home cage of male rats. That study (unpublished) terminated when one morning I opened the rat's cage to find the mouse happily asleep on the rat's head. Nonetheless, my interest in aggression remained.

David Edwards was ready to begin his doctoral dissertation research. We discussed possibilities and he suggested studies of the sexual differentiation of aggression in mice. I was excited by that idea.

Beeman, in 1947, showed that if you put a group of male mice together they fight until a stable social order is established. When she castrated males she found that such aggression was reduced. Grouped female mice did not fight. A dynamic sex difference.

So Edwards (1968) gave testosterone to newborn female mice. They became much more male-like in their attack behavior. He later showed that male mice, castrated at birth, were less likely to show attack behavior.

About this time, industry developed radioactively labeled steroids. Reproductive biologists were showing that tritium labeled estradiol was selectively accumulated by the uterus, an estrogen sensitive tissue, and that the prostate selectively accumulated androgen.

At that time I had in my laboratory a graduate student, William Luttge, who had training in biochemistry. He, Richard Green and I decided to study the accumulation of 3H-testosterone in the brain of rats. It was hilarious. We had to learn how to prepare the tissues (in those days one had to digest them in an ugly solvent) and we had to learn how to use the scintillation counter. Basically, you place your digested tissue into a vial with a fluid which contains a fluorescent material. When tritium is released from the tissue it contacts the fluorescent material which then emits a photon. The machine counts photons.

What we did was to take our samples to the machine and very carefully shake them to ensure a good mixing. When we returned to look at the tape output from the counter we found these wonderful numbers - millions of counts per sample. The joke was on us. We should have kept the samples undisturbed in the dark. We did not know of the phenomenon of chemoluminescence. Shaking the samples in the light caused an enormous release of photons unrelated to the selective accumulation of the androgen.

Later, my students and I (Whalen et al., 1973) published a report comparing methods and proposing one method that maximizes the reliability of measuring the selective accumulation of radioactive gonadal hormones in the brain. We did learn our lesson.

Since our behavioral data had suggested that the difference between male and female rats was that the presence of hormone during the sensitive period makes the rat insensitive to estrogen, I turned my attention to the estrogen response system in the brain.

My first thought was that the male brain, unlike the female brain, would respond like a non-target tissue for estradiol, that is, that it would not accumulate 3H-estradiol. We did the study, but found no differences between the sexes (Green et al., 1969).

Luttge and I thought that there might be sex specific hormone metabolism. We gave tritium labelled estradiol and chromatographically separated the metabolites. Males and females generated the same amount of estrone and estriol (Luttge and Whalen, 1970).

At that time, biochemical and autoradiographic data were showing that when estradiol enters a cell in a target tissue it becomes attached to a protein, called a receptor and that the receptor translocates the hormone into the cell nucleus where the hormone-receptor complex interacts with the DNA to generate the production of regulatory proteins. (Note : This view has been modified over the years, but it was the hypothesis current in the 1970's. For a current view, see Lauber and Pfaff, 1990).

Clearly, the total hypothalamic accumulation of estradiol did not distinguish between the sexes. I thought that we might possibly see differences at the intracellular level. Working with a superb technician, Jose Massicci, we examined the accumulation of estradiol by hypothalamic cell nuclei. We found that in males nuclear estradiol levels rose for two hours and then declined. In females the levels continued to increase over a four hour period. Overall, nuclear accumulation of estradiol was greater in females than males (Whalen and Massicci, 1975).

We had our first clue that the sex difference in estrogen action was in the cell nucleus.

Later, working with my graduate student, Kathie Olsen, we went to the nuclear chromatin level. This involves stripping off some of the proteins that protect the DNA. We found substantially greater binding of 3H-estradiol to hypothalamic chromatin from female than from male rats. We also found a male-female difference in the kinetics of binding -male chromatin lost estradiol more rapidly than female chromatin (Whalen and Olsen, 1978), which could account for estradiol's relative ineffectiveness in male brains.

Olsen and I also examined the hypothalamic chromatin binding of estradiol in male and female rats hormonally manipulated at birth. As I noted earlier, males castrated at birth do show lordotic behavior in adulthood when given estradiol and progesterone ; females given hormone at birth do not. The results were as we hoped. Males castrated at birth showed a greater chromatin binding of estradiol than did males castrated after the sensitive period. Females androgenized at birth showed reduced binding (Olsen and Whalen, 1980).

My last attack on the biochemistry of sex differences in male and female rat brains came with my research with my graduate student Andrea Lauber. Evidence had been accumulating that sex differences existed in neurotransmitter function. Moreover, studies were beginning to appear that showed that pharmacological manipulation of neurotransmitter function could alter estradiol binding in the brain.

We chose to study the cholinergic system not because we believed that the cholinergic system was the only neurotransmitter system that controlled lordosis, but because it is a system that is easily manipulated pharmacologically. Indeed, it has become clear that even a relatively simple sexually differentiated reflex like lordosis is under multiple neurotransmitter control.

Lauber examined the effect of cholinergic agonists and antagonists on he abundance of hypothalamic estrogen receptors. She administered the agonist bethanechol to female rats and found that it increased hypothalamic estradiol binding sites in a dose-dependent fashion. Moreover, when she gave the cholinergic antagonist, atropine, before the bethanechol, the effect was eliminated.

Lauber also found that bethanechol treatment does not increase the level of estradiol binding in the brain of male rats (Lauber and Whalen, 1988).

An interesting feature of her research is that she utilized an early finding by Barraclough and Gorski (1962) that a high dose of testosterone given neonatally would cause both an inhibition of ovulation (anovulatory sterility) and an inhibition of the potential to show lordosis ; a low dose of testosterone given neonatally would inhibit ovulation, but not lordosis. This is yet another demonstration that components of reproductive function are differentially susceptible to the actions of hormones during sensitive periods of development.

Lauber found that female rats treated with a high dose of testosterone neonatally responded to the cholinergic agonist like males, that is, with no increase in estradiol binding. Females treated with a low dose of testosterone neonatally, that is females which were anovulatory, but still capable of showing lordosis responded like females - bethanechol caused an increase in estrogen receptor density in the hypothalamus (Lauber, 1988).

These data indicate that neuronal activity in the cholinergic system can modulate estradiol binding in females, but not in males. It is possible that changes in cholinergic neuronal activity enhance estradiol binding in females thereby facilitating the induction of lordosis by estradiol. But, as I have noted, the data do not show that the cholinergic system is the only neurotransmitter system involved in the control of lordosis. We have much to learn.

Not only do we have much to learn about how gonadal hormones interact with neurotransmitter systems, we are in desperate need of an integrating hypothesis.

While Lauber was pursuing her doctoral research on hormone-neurotransmitter systems, Frank Johnson joined my laboratory as a graduate student.

I had recently read Marc Haug's studies. In 1972 Haug reported that when three female mice are housed together they would attack a lactating female which was introduced into their territory, but they would attack a non-lactating intruder much less. When Haug painted ovariectomized females with urine from lactating females, these females were attacked. Again, I was excited. Female mice attack. This was not as Beeman had described in 1947.

We all knew that postpartum females would attack intruders, but it was widely believed that virgins would not.

Haug and Brain (1979) demonstrated that attack behavior does not even require gonadal hormones. They showed that gonadectomized male and female mice would attack lactating female mice. This is a very interesting finding.

Frank Johnson and I replicated the Haug and Brain findings using a different procedure. Male mice were housed singly to establish their territory and then were given, on alternate tests either another male whose olfactory bulbs had been removed (such males elicit attack, but they do not fight back) or a lactating female. The resident males attacked the intruder males, but not the lactating females. When the resident males were castrated most showed a clear reduction in their attack of intruder males. However, our resident, now castrated males, began to attack the lactating female intruders. We found no overall change in the frequency of attack, but we did find a major change in who our residents attacked.

As formerly demonstrated by Haug and Brain (1979), treatment of the castrates with testosterone led to an inhibition of attack against the lactating females (Whalen and Johnson, 1987).

These findings indicate that gonadal hormones do not merely regulate "motivation" or the need or desire to attack, the hormones regulate the selective response to potential attack stimuli.

## Sex differences in aggression

In 1974 Svare and colleagues demonstrated that female mice will attack male intruders if they are given testosterone chronically. Johnson and I (Whalen and Johnson, 1988) found that chronic testosterone treatment did not make the females male-like ; females so treated began to attack both male and lactating female stimuli. In males, testosterone inhibits the attack of lactating females.

For his doctoral dissertation Johnson returned to the sexual differentiation model. He treated female mice with testosterone prenatally, postnatally or both pre-and postnatally. When they were aduldt they were housed singly and were presented with a male or lactating female intruder on alternate tests.

He found that for postnatally treated females there was a dose dependent increase in attack behavior. However, these mice attacked both male and female intruders. They were not made male-like.

Prenatally treated females did not show an increase in attack behavior against males. However, their attack of lactating females was increased. Pre-and posnatally treated females showed moderate levels of attack, but did not discriminate.

Females treated with testosterone both pre- and postnatally and given testosterone in adulthood were the only animals in which testosterone treatment in adulthood caused both an increase in attack against males and a decrease in attack against lactating females. Thus, prenatal plus postnatal treatment with testosterone made these females more male-like. (see Whalen and Johnson, 1990 for a summary of these findings).

We see in these studies that gonadal hormones can have powerful effects both during periods of differentiation and in adulthood on the perceptual mechanisms that regulate behavior.

This was my final venture into research on the sexual differentiation of animal behavior.

The Phoenix et al. paper fired the imagination of a generation of investigators. Even now, 23 years later, we have barely tilled the soil. I expect that this garden will grow for many years into the future.

# References

Barraclough, C. A. and Gorski, R. A. (1962). Studies on mating behavior in the androgen-sterilized female rat in relation to the hypothalamic regulation of sexual behavior. *J. Endocr.*, **25** : 175-182.

Beeman, E. A. (1947). The effect of male hormone on aggressive behavior in mice. *Physiol. Zool.*, **20** : 373-405.

DeBold, J. F. and Whalen, R. E. (1975). Differential sensitivity of mounting and lordosis control systems to early androgen treatment in male and female hamsters. *Horm. Behav.*, **6** : 197-209.

Edwards, D. A. (1968). Mice : fighting by neonatally androgenized females. *Science*, **161** : 1027-1028.

Feder, H. H. and Whalen, R. E. 1965). Feminine behavior in neonatally castrated and estrogen-treated male rats. *Science*, **147** : 306-307.

Green, R., Luttge, W. G. and Whalen, R. E. (1969). Uptake and retention of tritiated estradiol in brain and peripheral tissues of male, female and neonatally androgenized female rats. *Endocrinology*, **85** : 373-378.

Harris, G. and Levine, S. (1865). Sexual differentiation of the brain and its experimental control. *J. Physiol.*, **181** : 379-400.

Haug, M. (1972). Phenomènes d'agression liés a l'introduction d'une femelle étrangère vierge ou allaitante au sein d'un groupe de souris femelles. *C.R. Acad. Sci. (D) (Paris)*, **275** : 2729-2732.

Haug, M. and Brain, P. F. (1979). Effects of treatments with testosterone and oestradiol on the attack directed by groups of gonadectomized male and female mice towards lactating intruders. *Physiol. Behav.*, **23** : 397-400.

Lauber, A. H. (1988). Behanechol-induced increase in hypothalamic estrogen receptor binding in female rats is related to capacity for estrogen-dependent reproductive behavior. *Brain Res.*, **456** : 177-182.

Lauber, A. H. and Whalen, R. E. (1988). Muscarinic cholinergic modulation of hypothalamic estrogen binding sites. *Brain Res.*, **443** : 21-26.

Lauber, A. H. and Pfaff, D. (1990). Estrogen regulation of mRNAs in the brain and relationship to lordosis behavior. *Cur. Top. Neuroendocrinol.*, **10** : 115-147.

Luttge, W. G. and Whalen, R.E. (1970). Regional localization of estrogenic metabolites in the brain of male and female rats. *Steroids*, **15** : 605-612.

Olsen, K. L. and Whalen, R. E. (1980). Sexual differentiation of the brain : effects on mating behavior and (3H)-estradiol binding by hypothalamic chromatin in rats. *Biol. Reprod.*, **22** : 1068-1072.

Phoenix, C. H., Goy, R. W., Gerall, A. A. and Young, W. C. (1959). Organizing action of prenatally administered testosterone propionate on the tissues mediating mating behavior in the female guinea pig. *Endocrinology*, **65** : 369-382.

Simon, N. G. and Whalen, R. E. (1986). Hormonal regulation of aggression : evidence for a relationship among genotype, receptor binding and behavioral sensitivity to androgen and estrogen. *Aggres. Behav.*, **12** : 225-266.

Svare, B., Davis, P. G. and Gandelman, R. (1974). Fighting behavior in female mice following chronic androgen treatment during adulthood. *Physiol. Behav.*, **12** : 399-403.

Whalen, R. E. (1961). Strain differences in sexual behavior of the male rat. *Behaviour*, **18** : 199-204.

Whalen, R. E. (1974). Sexual differentiation : models, methods and mechanisms. In: Friedman, R. C., Richart, R. M. and Van de Wiele, R. L. (Eds.), *Sex Differences in Behavior*, John Wiley and Sons, pp. 467-481.

Whalen, R. E. and Nadler, R. D. (1963). Suppression of the development of female mating behavior by estrogen administered in infancy. *Science*, **141** : 273-274.

Whalen, R. E. and Edwards, D. A. (1967). Hormonal determinants of the development of masculine and feminine behavior in male and female rats. *Anat. Rec.*, **157** : 173-180.

Whalen, R. E. and Luttge, W. G. (1971). Perinatal administration of dihydrotestosterone to female rats and the development of reproductive function. *Endocrinology*, **89** : 1320-1322.

Whalen, R. E., Gorzalka, B. B. and Luttge, W. G. (1973). Steroid extraction and tissue digestion in the assay of radioactivity in rat brain following tritiated estradiol-17β. *Steroids*, **21** : 219-232.

Whalen, R. E. and Massicci, J. (1975). Subcellular analysis of the accumulation of estrogen by the brain of male and female rats. *Brain Res.*, **89** : 255-264.

Whalen, R. E. and Olsen, K. L. (1978). Chromatin binding of estradiol in the hypothalamus and cortex of male and female rats. *Brain Res.*, **152** : 121-131.

Whalen, R. E. and Johnson, F. (1987). Individual differences in the attack behavior of male mice : a function of attack stimulus and hormonal state. *Horm. Behav.*, **21** : 223-233.

Whalen, R. E. and Johnson, F. (1988). Aggression in adult female mice: : chronic testosterone treatment induces attack against olfactory bulbectomized male and lactating female mice. *Physiol. Behav.*, **43** : 17-20.
Whalen, R. E. and Johnson, F. (1990). To fight or not to fight : the question is 'whom' ? In: Balthazart, J. (Ed.),*Hormones Brain and Behaviour in Vertebrates* **2**. *Behavioural Activation in Males and Females - Social Interaction and Reproductive Endocrinology* , Basel, Karger, pp.201-212.

# Consequences of Gender Differences in Mathematical Reasoning Ability and Some Biological Linkages

## C. P. BENBOW and D. LUBINSKI

*Iowa State University, Department of Psychology, W112 Lagomarcino Hall, Ames, IA 50011-3180, USA*

Gender differences in cognitive abilities and achievement are not new. They have been reported for several decades. Yet what is new is that recent reports seem to indicate that these differences are steadily diminishing in normative samples. That is, males and females apparently are converging toward a common mean on a variety of abilities, including mathematics (Feingold, 1988; Hyde et al., 1990; Rosenthal and Rubin, 1982). Hyde et al. (1990), for example, in their meta-analytic review of 100 studies, reported that the average effect size for the gender difference in mathematics was only .14 for studies published in 1974 or later compared to .31 for studies published earlier. Feingold (1988) studied scores on two test batteries over a 30-year period and also concluded that females have been catching up with males. Such findings have led several individuals to conclude that research on gender differences is better referred to as research on sex similarities (Connell, 1987; Riger, 1992). Some investigators have been more flippant, asserting that gender differences in cognitive functioning are decreasing "faster than the gene can travel".

Although such conclusions are encouraging and consonant with the current *Zeitgeist* (Halpern, 1992), they are perhaps misleading. Stanley et al. (1992) have noted that, for at least the past 20 years, some test publishers have attempted to minimize what some would call "gender bias" by discarding, from one revision to the next, items that show the greatest gender disparities. So meta-analytic reviews in this area are difficult to interpret ; and further, not all studies have documented a decline in gender differences (Benbow, 1988; Lubinski and Benbow, 1992). Firm conclusions are still unavailable. What we do know, however, is that gender differences vary as a function of a variety of variables, including age, ability-level of sample surveyed, ethnicity, and the ability itself. For example, Hyde et al. (1990) revealed that girls showed a slight

*M. Haug et al. (eds.), The Development of Sex Differences and Similarities in Behavior, 87–109.*
© 1993 *Kluwer Academic Publishers.*

superiority in computation in elementary and middle school with no gender differences in problem-solving at those stages. Differences favoring males emerged in high school and in college but only on tests measuring problem-solving or mathematical reasoning ability. Similarly, Aiden (1986,1987) concluded that the largest gender disparities occur for mathematical reasoning ability, and favor males ; Marshall and Smith (1987) have substantiated these claims in a study of third-graders. Third-grade girls surpass boys in computation, while third-grade boys show superiority in solving word problems and on geometry and measurement problems.

Obtaining picture of the magnitude and nature of the many ability parameters on which the genders may differ is complex ; but more definitive conclusions are desperately needed. This need arises from the stubborn and pronounced gender differences in mathematical reasoning ability, plus other key nonverbal abilities such as spatial and mechanical reasoning abilities, which are consistently observed among the most intellectually able students. These are the abilities most critical for educational and career excellence in math/science domains. Further, mathematical reasoning ability is correlated with a number of important personal preferences relevant to making and maintaining a commitment to physical science disciplines. Among the most intellectually able women, there is a tendency for interests in aesthetic and social areas to compete with interests in the physical sciences, while this phenomenon does not appear to operate much in gifted males. Thus, gender differences in personal preferences important for the expression of intellectual talent in nontechnical aesthetic and social domains appear to compound gender differences in mathematical reasoning to exacerbate gender disparities in math/science achievement across a number of disciplines. Although many observers find gender differences in math/science achievement among the gifted perplexing, now that so many educational barriers have been removed for women, our examination of a number of key ability *and* nonability attributes reveals that these disparities are quite understandable.

In this chapter, we will discuss those gender differences in cognitive abilities and preferences that have special significance as determinants of disparate male/female proportions all along the math/science pipeline. We will then frame our review in the context of a theory of vocational adjustment to better understand their psychological implications more fully. Some biological correlates of these gender differences also will be reviewed. Following this, suggestions for future research aimed at underlying biological mechanisms possibly responsible for generating these phenotypic differences at the behavioral level will be offered. But first, because most of our review draws on the research conducted by the Study of Mathematically Precocious Youth (SMPY), it will be useful to describe in some detail this planned 50-year longitudinal study, its goals, and the sample of individuals being tracked over the course of their entire lives.

# Study of mathematically precocious youth

SMPY was founded by Julian C. Stanley at Johns Hopkins University in 1971 and predicated on the philosophy of conducting research through service to intellectually talented students. SMPY was interested in first identifying adolescents who possess exceptional intellectual abilites and, then, uncovering the factors that contribute to their optimal educational and vocational development. Special attention has alsways been devoted to math/science disciplines. One intervention, implemented from the start, was to provide these students with better opportunities to develop their already exceptional quantitative skills. Studying at the college level was one form of acceleration offered to these students, which, from the beginning, generated remarkable success (cf. Stanley, 1977; Stanley and Benbow, 1986). To facilitate the uncovering of other beneficial interventions and to answer basic research questions about intellectual giftedness more generally, SMPY established, at Iowa State University in 1986, a 50-year longitudinal study. Through this study, which currently includes about 5,000 talented individuals identified over a 20-year period, SMPY is beginning to bring into focus the factors that contribute to gifted student' educational, intellectual, personal, and vocational development.

Participants in SMPY were identified through a talent search, a concept developed by Stanley (cf. Cohn, 1991; Keating and Stanley, 1972; Stanley et al., 1974). The concept of a talent search has been refined over the last 20 years, but the basic premise remains the same : students in 7th or 8th grade (12 to 13 year-olds), who are already known to have scored in the top 3 % (on national norms) on standardized achievement tests (e.g., the Iowa Test of Basic Skills) administered routinely by american schools, are invited to take the College Board Scholastic Aptitude Test (SAT) at a regular administration[1].The SAT measures mathematical reasoning (SAT-M) and verbal reasoning (SAT-V) ability and is designed for 11th and 12th graders who are planning to attend college. (This form of assessment is known as above-level-testing, inasmuch as the SAT was designed for subjects 4 to 5 years older than SMPY participants, see Stanley, 1990). Nonetheless, the score distributions manifested by these gifted 7th or 8th graders are similar to those observed in random samples of high school students (Benbow, 1988; Keating and Stanley, 1972). It is through this mechanism that the SMPY subject pool for the longitudinal study was formed ; all 5000 subjects, except one group, are drawn from the talent search on the basis of high SAT scores that place them in at least the top 1 % in intellectual ability. (For more detailed reading on this exceptional sample, including case histories of their many remarkable achievements, see Note 1 in Lubinski and Benbow, 1992).

# Gender differences in cognitive abilities

In the process of identifying the first group of students to be included in SMPY, the gender difference in mathematical reasoning ability was discovered unexpectedly. It was then reaffirmed in every annual talent search conducted since 1972. To date, annual talent searches organized by Duke, Iowa State, Johns Hopkins, Northwestern, and University of Denver have tested well over 1 million gifted students (approximately equal numbers of males and females) across the United States. Among these students, there are no gender differences in SAT-V scores. The males, however, score almost one-half standard deviation higher than the females on SAT-M and display greater

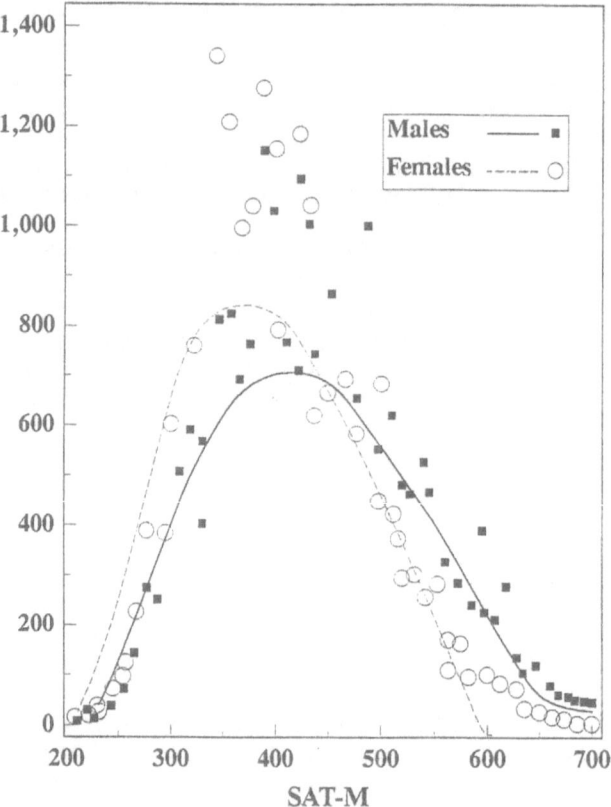

**Figure 1** Distribution of SAT-Math scores for participants in the 1980-1982 CTY talent searches by sex (males = 19,833 ; females = 19,937) ; adapted from Benbow (1988).

dispersion of SAT-M scores; a typical score distribution is illustrated in Figure 1

(Benbow, 1988). The resulting proportion of males and females at various cutting scores on the SAT-M is approximately as follows : SAT-M > 500 (average score of college-bound 12th-grade male), 2:1 ; SAT-M > 600, 4:1 ; and SAT-M > 700 (top 1 in 10,000 for 7th-graders), 13:1 (Benbow and Stanley, 1983). These disparate ratios have remained relatively stable over the past 20 years, have now been observed among gifted students in third grade, cross-culturally (but are smaller in Asian populations, see Benbow, 1988), and have profound implications for the math/science pipeline (Benbow, 1992). That is, there are far fewer females than males who qualify for advanced training in disciplines that place a premium on mathematical reasoning (e.g., engineering and the physical sciences).

The picture intensifies when other cognitive abilities are examined, which are salient covariates of SAT-M and contribute to achieving advanced educational credentials in the physical sciences. Mathematically talented students, whether male or female, tend to have highly developed spatial and mechanical reasoning abilities. There are, however, substantial gender differences in those abilities (e.g., Benbow et al., 1983; Benbow and Minor, 1990; Humphreys et al., in press; Lubinski and Benbow, 1992; Lubinski and Humphreys, 1990a). Table I, which is taken from Lubinski and Benbow (1992), exemplifies these differences.

It contains data on abilities (and values) on students tested through SMPY at Iowa State University from 1988-1991. Gender differences in mathematical reasoning ability are consistently observed, paralleling findings described above for the entire nation. Although there are non meaningful differences in SAT-V or Advanced Raven Progressive Matrices scores, there are substantial gender differences in spatial and mechanical reasoning abilities, not unlike those observed 20 years by SMPY. (In 1992 mechanical reasoning was again assessed by SMPY and a gender difference in standard score units of .77 was revealed). These data have further implications for the math/science pipeline because highly developed mechanical and spatial abilities are among the most distinguishing psychological features of physical scientists (Humphreys et al., in press).

Moreover, in select samples as well as in the SMPY sample, gender differences favoring males also are observed on achievement tests in physics, chemistry, computer science, european history and mathematics taken at the end of high school or when in college, and these differences have been stable from at least 1982 to 1991 (Benbow and Minor, 1986; Benbow and Stanley, 1982; Stanley et al., 1992; Stanley, personal communication, 1992). The magnitude of these differences for the select samples studied by Stanley et al. (1992) are illustrated in Figures 2, 3, and 4. It should be noted that the pattern of differences was consistent across many kinds of tests and grade levels and large enough to have a profound effect on admission to (as well as keeping up with the curriculum in) selective universities in the United States.

In sum, gender differences in mathematical reasoning ability among the gifted are accompanied by gender differences in spatial and mechanical reasoning abilities, as well as in subsequent math/science achievement test scores.

92

| YEAR | GENDER | | AGE-ADJUSTED | | | | | ADVANCED RAVEN'S | | | MENTAL ROTATION TEST | | | BENNETT MECHANICAL REASONING | | | STUDY OF VALUES | | | | | | | | | | | | | | | | | |
|---|---|---|---|---|---|---|---|---|---|---|---|---|---|---|---|---|---|---|---|---|---|---|---|---|---|---|---|---|---|---|---|---|---|---|---|
| | | | SAT-M | | | SAT-V | | | | | | | | | | | THEORETIC | | | SOCIAL | | ECONOMIC | | AESTHETIC | | POLITICAL | | RELIGIOUS | |
| | | | N | X̄ | SD | X̄ | SD | N | X̄ | SD | N | X̄ | SD | N | X̄ | SD | N | X̄ | SD | X̄ | SD | X̄ | SD | X̄ | SD | X̄ | SD | X̄ | SD |
| 1991 | M | ● | 68 | 532 | 101 | 426 | 78 | 68 | 25.1 | 3.9 | 68 | 29.9 | 8.1 | | | | 68 | 47.7 | 7.0 | 37.1 | 7.3 | 41.6 | 7.2 | 36.4 | 8.2 | 42.9 | 6.6 | 34.2 | 10.4 |
| | F | ● | 51 | 480 | 87 | 418 | 87 | 51 | 25.8 | 4.3 | 51 | 25.1 | 10.2 | | | | 51 | 42.0 | 6.8 | 43.2 | 8.1 | 37.8 | 6.9 | 42.6 | 7.1 | 39.0 | 7.2 | 35.4 | 10.2 |
| | M | ■ | 107 | 579 | 101 | 413 | 81 | 92 | 25.2 | 4.2 | 95 | 30.0 | 8.1 | | | | 77 | 47.6 | 6.9 | 37.1 | 7.0 | 41.8 | 6.9 | 36.5 | 8.3 | 43.1 | 6.8 | 33.8 | 10.1 |
| | F | ■ | 67 | 472 | 85 | 418 | 80 | 58 | 25.9 | 4.2 | 63 | 24.1 | 10.0 | | | | 57 | 41.7 | 7.0 | 43.8 | 8.3 | 37.5 | 7.0 | 42.8 | 7.5 | 38.7 | 7.0 | 35.6 | 10.3 |
| 1990 | M | ● | 69 | 537 | 100 | 415 | 79 | 69 | 24.5 | 6.5 | 69 | 29.2 | 9.1 | | | | 69 | 46.6 | 8.8 | 38.4 | 7.8 | 40.4 | 8.2 | 38.4 | 8.4 | 42.5 | 6.9 | 33.4 | 11.4 |
| | F | ● | 48 | 487 | 74 | 422 | 76 | 48 | 25.3 | 4.4 | 48 | 22.5 | 9.7 | | | | 48 | 40.3 | 8.0 | 44.0 | 8.0 | 35.8 | 7.1 | 42.1 | 6.4 | 40.1 | 6.7 | 37.5 | 8.1 |
| | M | ■ | 87 | 545 | 96 | 415 | 79 | 82 | 24.6 | 6.8 | 80 | 29.8 | 8.8 | | | | 73 | 46.6 | 8.7 | 38.3 | 7.6 | 40.4 | 8.1 | 37.8 | 8.7 | 42.7 | 6.8 | 33.9 | 11.3 |
| | F | ■ | 61 | 487 | 71 | 419 | 80 | 57 | 25.1 | 4.1 | 56 | 21.6 | 9.4 | | | | 51 | 40.7 | 8.0 | 43.6 | 8.1 | 35.3 | 7.2 | 42.8 | 7.1 | 40.1 | 6.6 | 37.1 | 8.4 |
| 1989 | M | ● | 20 | 585 | 86 | 441 | 98 | 20 | 27.3 | 4.4 | 20 | 24.9 | 9.9 | 20 | 40.2 | 9.4 | 20 | 49.3 | 7.4 | 35.4 | 5.9 | 40.3 | 9.4 | 37.3 | 8.0 | 45.0 | 7.8 | 30.8 | 11.1 |
| | F | ● | 11 | 505 | 80 | 449 | 96 | 11 | 24.7 | 5.1 | 11 | 17.8 | 4.1 | 11 | 35.6 | 8.0 | 11 | 39.0 | 9.1 | 42.3 | 9.1 | 41.1 | 9.6 | 40.6 | 5.2 | 40.4 | 9.3 | 36.6 | 12.5 |
| | M | ■ | 43 | 593 | 95 | 446 | 78 | 21 | 27.0 | 4.4 | 40 | 23.8 | 9.7 | 42 | 42.2 | 10.0 | 43 | 50.0 | 6.8 | 34.8 | 7.5 | 42.2 | 8.2 | 37.0 | 7.7 | 44.1 | 8.2 | 30.9 | 10.7 |
| | F | ■ | 34 | 514 | 82 | 455 | 79 | 11 | 24.7 | 5.1 | 34 | 21.8 | 7.9 | 32 | 35.2 | 9.4 | 34 | 41.8 | 7.4 | 41.2 | 8.3 | 39.6 | 7.7 | 43.9 | 8.2 | 39.2 | 7.2 | 34.3 | 10.9 |
| 1988 | M | ● | 57 | 562 | 81 | 435 | 59 | 57 | 26.6 | 3.8 | | | | | | | 57 | 48.0 | 8.5 | 34.4 | 7.8 | 44.9 | 7.6 | 35.3 | 8.1 | 45.2 | 8.2 | 32.4 | 12.8 |
| | F | ● | 32 | 491 | 65 | 424 | 80 | 32 | 25.1 | 5.3 | | | | | | | 32 | 42.3 | 7.5 | 40.7 | 8.0 | 38.2 | 7.5 | 43.6 | 8.4 | 40.1 | 6.2 | 34.9 | 10.3 |
| | M | ■ | 72 | 571 | 85 | 440 | 62 | 66 | 26.8 | 3.7 | | | | 8 | 39.3 | 6.5 | 61 | 48.3 | 8.5 | 34.5 | 7.6 | 44.7 | 7.4 | 35.0 | 8.0 | 44.9 | 8.3 | 32.9 | 12.7 |
| | F | ■ | 39 | 500 | 64 | 425 | 76 | 36 | 25.3 | 5.3 | | | | 9 | 29.0 | 7.2 | 33 | 42.5 | 7.4 | 40.9 | 8.0 | 38.0 | 7.5 | 43.4 | 8.4 | 40.0 | 6.2 | 35.2 | 10.2 |

● Students who took all of the tests

■ All students who took any one test

**Table I** Ability/preference profiles of intellectually gifted students (top 5%) attending a summer academic program across four separate years by gender.[1]

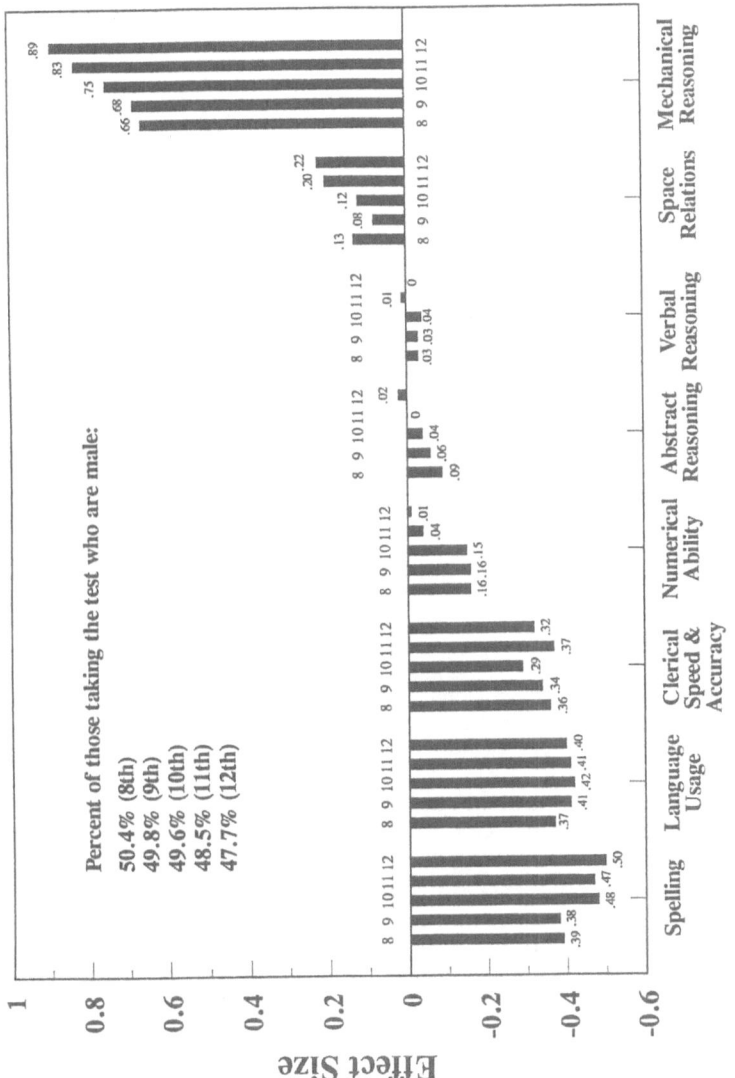

**Figure 2** Effect sizes for differential aptitude tests (DAT). Effect sizes represent the standard deviation difference between the genders in the ability in question (it is computed by subtracting the female mean from the male mean and dividing by the pooled standard deviation). (Adapted from Stanley et al., 1992).

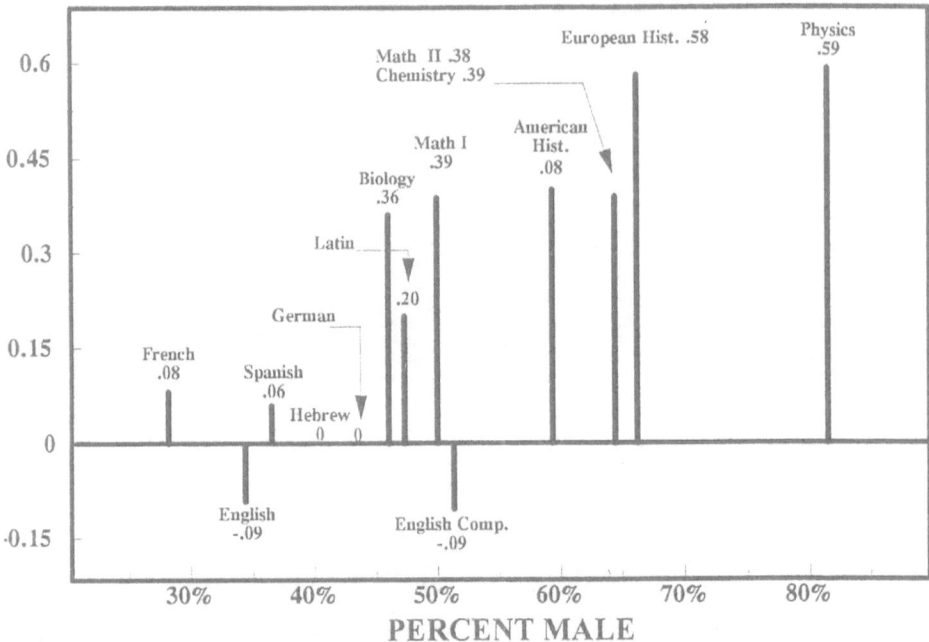

**Figure 3** Average standardized gender differences on each of the 14 college board achievement tests for the years 1982-85, plotted against the medial percent of those taking the test who were male (r = 78). (Adapted from Stanley et al., 1992).

Contrary to the claims made in recent reports, there is no evidence that these differences are diminishing among the gifted. Rather, they have remained rather stable over the past 20 years. An often overlooked explanation for these findings, even if contemporary meta-analytic reviews are accurate about the genders converging toward a common mean on most abilities, is the following. Males tend to be more variable on measures of cognitive functioning, even on tests for which females have *higher* means (Feingold, 1992; Lubinki and Dawis, 1992; Stanley et al., 1992). As a result, males are more frequently found at the extremes, both in the retarded and talented tails of ability distributions (Lubinski and Benbow, 1992; Lubinski and Dawis, 1992). Consumers of meta-analytic reviews *must* keep in mind that overall effect sizes assess only gender differences in group means. If there are also gender differences in dispersion (or variability), male/female proportions at high levels of an attribute can, and often do, differ markedly. This, we believe, is one of the most under-appreciated points in the assessment of gender differences in human abilities.

# Preferences : values and interests

Abilities are only one important class of variables that affect educational and career decisions. Preferences for certain environments and occupational reinforcers are another. In this section, we illustrate how gender differences in mathematical reasoning are accompanied by gender differences in values and interests. Two of the more useful schemes for analyzing interests and values are Holland's (1985) hexagon (consisting of investigative, artistic, social,

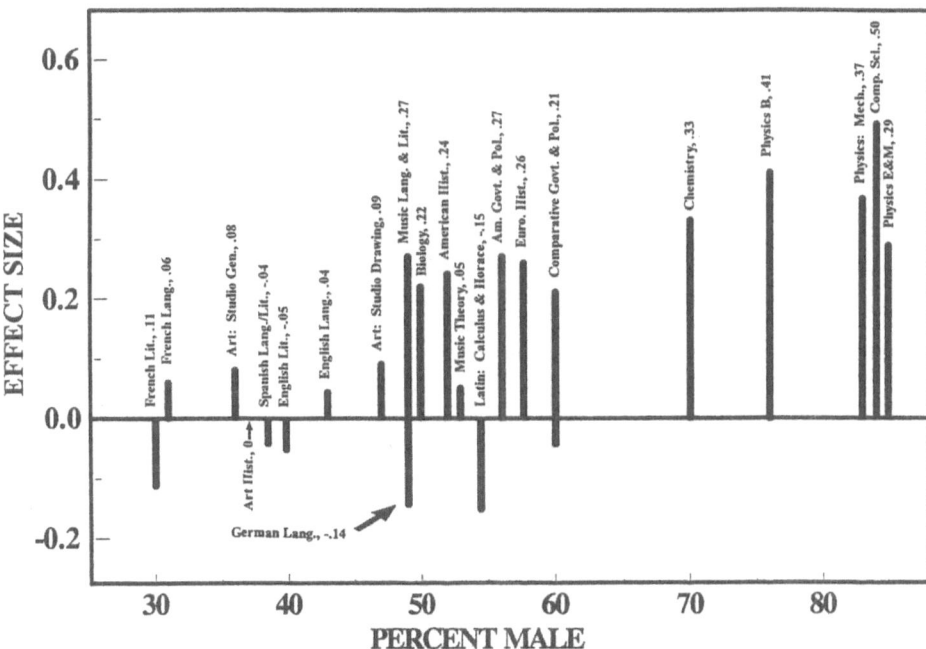

**Figure 4** Average standardized gender differences on each of the 26 college board advanced placement program examinations for the years 1984-86 (1987 for american government and politics, and comparative government and politics), plotted against the median percent of those taking the examination who were male (r = .75). (Adapted from Stanley et al. 1992).

enterprising, conventional and realistic vocational interest themes) and the Allport et al. (1970) Study of Values (SOV), six value dimensions based on Spranger's (1928) *Types of Men* and sharing appreciable overlap with Holland's model. The SOV "evaluative attitudes" are theoretical, aesthetic, social, economic, religious, and political. (Readers interested in more detailed discussions of these critical preferences for structuring contrasting educational choices and career paths are referred to Lubinski et al., in press).

Vocational interests and personal value orientation function to determine the focal content domain of one's academic area of concentration. Investigative interests and theoretical values are among the most salient personal preferences of physical scientists. Moreover, a high theoretical complemented by a high aesthetic orientation is correlated with scientific creativity (MacKinnon, 1962; Southern and Plant, 1968). Table I reveals how theoretical values, which are characteristic of physical scientists, are much more characteristic of gifted males than females. Social values, which are negatively correlated with interests in physical science, are more characteristic of gifted females than males. Benbow and Lubinski (1992) presented similar data on Holland's vocational interest themes. They found for mathematically talented students (top .5 %) that there were no gender dfferences in investigative interests. Nonetheless, an interesting pattern of gender differences emerged : males' interests were primarily focused around investigative careers (i.e., preference for academic pursuits involving math and science) and secondarily in realistic areas (a strong preference for working with things or gadgets). The interest pattern of gifted females', in contrast, was more evenly distributed across investigative, artistic (writing and artistic forms of self- expression), and social areas (considerable people contact or social service). These findings seem to reflect gender differences on one of the most celebrated dimensions of individual differences, "people versus things" (Thorndike, 1911). Mathematically talented females tend to gravitate toward the former, while mathematically talented males gravitate toward the latter (cf. Lubinski and Humphreys, 1990b). Might it be more precise to say that gender differences in vocational preferences are structured around organic versus inorganic content domains ? Regardless, this dimension of individual differences has predictive utility for familiar educational and occupational categories.

Although students are not formally selected for advanced training based on their theoretical values, their investigative interests, or their spatial and mechanical reasoning abilities (but they are on mathematical reasoning ability), students appear to self-select areas of concentration based on all of these attributes, whether they are explicitly aware of their abilities and preferences or not. Gender differences in mathematical reasoning are, therefore, compounded by gender differences in spatial visualization and mechanical reasoning, and disparate male/female proportions in math/science achievement created by these abilities are intensified by gender differences in values and interests critical for forming a commitment to these disciplines. In addition, at least one other factor exacerbates these disparities ; for intellectually gifted subjects, there are huge gender differences in commitment to full-time work : 95 % of the males versus 55 % of the females say they plan to work full-time until retirement (Benbow and Lubinski, 1992). This finding must be taken into account when addressing all forms of gender differences in achievement and career advancement ; as long as the genders differ so markedly in their commitment to full-time work, marked differences in achievement and promotion are sure to remain, even among males and females whose relevant ability/preference profiles are equivalent.

# Gender differences in math/sciences career choices

The data in Table II show the current gender discrepancy in math and science educational credentials for a sample of SMPY participants in the top 1 % of mathematical ability. More males than females are entering math/science career tracks, especially the ("inorganic") nonbiological/behavioral sciences ones, and they hold higher educational aspirations. Yet perhaps the most startling finding in Table II is that less than 1 % of females in the top 1 % of mathematical ability are pursuing doctorates in mathematics, engineering, or physical science. Approximately 8 % of such males are doing so. Similar discrepancies were reported by Benbow and Lubinski (1992) for two other cohorts of mathematically talented students surveyed in the 1980's/1990's. Among students with mathematical abilities in at least the top .5 %, Benbow and Lubinski reported that 12 % of females compared to 27 % of males were pursuing doctorates in mathematics, engineering, and physical science. Even among 18 year-old students in the top 1 in 10,000 in mathematical ability (SAT-M > 700 before age 13), we find 77 % of these males but only 47 % of the females pursuing bachelor degrees in mathematics, physical science, and engineering. As the following theoretical discussion will reveal, as long as gender differences in critical ability/preference profiles remain stable, as they have over at least the past 20 years for the gifted, corresponding disparities along the math/science pipeline are predicted to continue. Moreover, given the nature of the gender differences (larger means and standard deviations for males in relevant abilities, plus larger mean differences favoring males on relevant interests and values), gender differences in achievement should be expected to become more pronounced at higher educational levels.

# Educational and vocational decision making and adjustment

It is helpful to organize the above findings around a well-known model of vocational adjustment. This model is useful for several reasons. One especially attractive feature is that it is readily extended to critical antecedents of vocational adjustment, such as choosing a college major. According to the Theory of Work Adjustment (TWA), one's psychological adjustment to any given educational or career track is a joint function of two broad dimensions of correspondence, *satisfaction* and *satisfactoriness* (Dawis and Lofquist, 1984; Lofquist and Dawis, 1991). The latter is defined by the extent to which abilities correspond to the ability requirements of a given occupation, and the former is defined by correspondence between one's personal preferences (interests, needs, values) and the rewards offered by the discipline or occupation.

| Highest Degree / Major | Bachelor | | Advanced Less than Doctorate | | Doctorate | | Total Across Degrees | |
|---|---|---|---|---|---|---|---|---|
| | Males | Females | Males | Females | Males | Females | Males | Females |
| **Math and Science** — Mathematics | 3.4 | 3.5 | 0.3 | 0.7 | 0.5 | 0.0 | 4.2 | 4.2 |
| Engineering | 16.2 | 7.6 | 7.9 | 3.0 | 3.4 | 0.7 | 27.5 | 11.3 |
| Physical Science | 2.2 | 1.5 | 0.5 | 0.4 | 3.7 | 0.2 | 6.4 | 2.1 |
| Biology | 2.2 | 5.4 | 0.3 | 0.4 | 1.1 | 1.5 | 3.6 | 7.3 |
| Medicine | | | | | 8.7 | 5.9 | 8.7 | 5.9 |
| Social Science | 4.8 | 6.1 | 0.4 | 2.0 | 1.9 | 0.9 | 7.1 | 9.0 |
| Humanities | 2.5 | 5.0 | 0.1 | 2.4 | 0.8 | 1.7 | 3.4 | 9.1 |
| Law | | | | | 6.4 | 4.1 | 6.4 | 4.1 |
| Business | 7.1 | 11.1 | 4.5 | 5.0 | 0.8 | 0.7 | 12.4 | 16.8 |
| **Total** — All Majors | 42 | 52 | 15 | 17 | 28 | 17 | 85 | 86 |
| Math/Science Majors | 24 | 18 | 9 | 5 | 18 | 9 | 51 | 32 |

**Table II** Longitudinal data for mathematically talented students (top 1%), identified by a SMPY talent search at age 13. Percentages reflect students' current level of educational attainment or pursuit (at age 23) by gender.[2]

Correspondence between both of these dimensions is critical for an individual to be adjusted to a particular educational or work environment (see Figure 5).

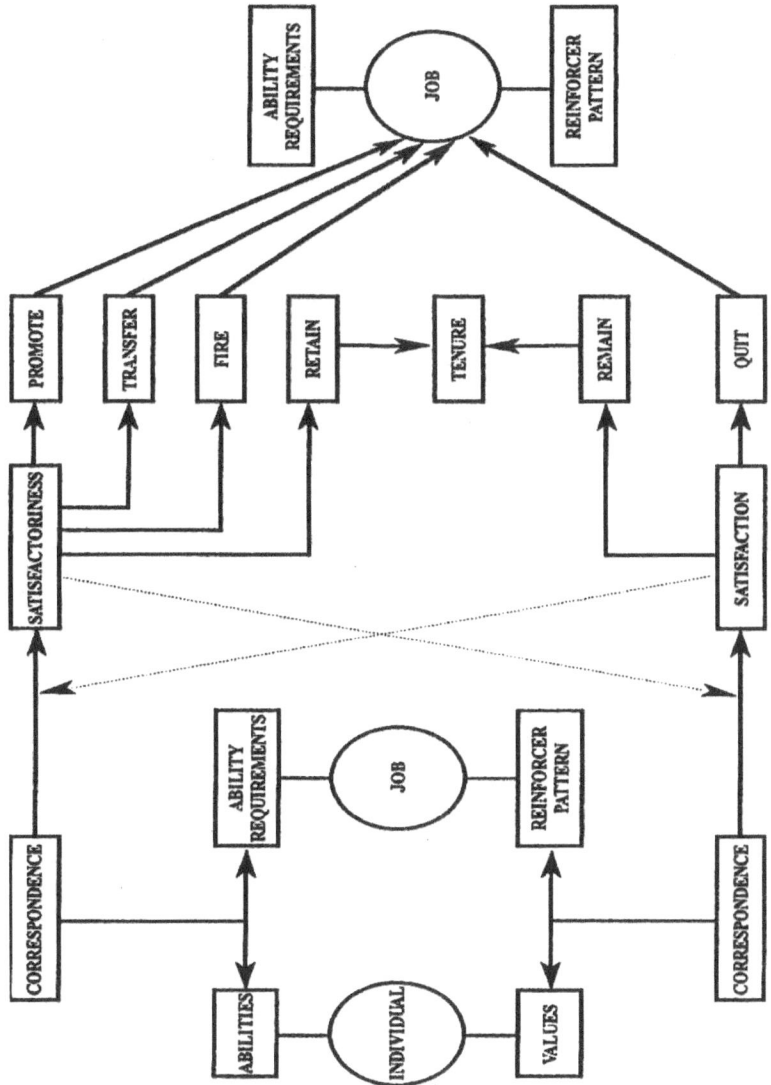

**Figure 5** A depiction of the Theory of Work Adjustment. (Adapted from Dawis and Lofquist, 1984). The dotted lines serve to illustrate how satisfaction and satisfactoriness function jointly to determine educational/career tenure. When an individual is not satisfactory, the environment is motivated to transfer or fire the individual, whereas if the individual is not satisfied, the person is motivated to leave.

Figure 5 highlights how mutually complementary people and their environments are when an individual is adjusted to work. Just as individuals have abilities and needs, so do environments. Environments can be described in terms of their response capabilities (to provide reinforcers attractive to individuals with correspondent needs) and in terms of their needs (or demands for individuals having correspondent abilities). School and work environments are, essentially, molecular ecologies defined by 1. their capability to reinforce and 2. the response requirements that they demand (Lubinski and Dawis, 1992; Lubinski and Thompson, 1986).

As noted above, gifted males compared to gifted females tend to have ability and preference profiles more congruent with optimal adjustment in math and science careers. As a result, one would expect more males and females in such careers, which is what we demonstrated above. The important message to take from this discussion is that, given the basic gender differences reviewed As noted above, gifted males compared to gifted females tend to have ability and preference profiles more congruent with optimal adjustment in math and above, to an appreciable degree males and females are most likely to thrive, disproportionately, in somewhat different occupational environments. To be sure, there will be overlap ; but disparate proportions are to be expected. Given that most vocational counselors underscore the importance of both abilities and expressed preferences throughout the educational and career decision making process, stressing the importance of vocational counseling is not likely to attenuate these differences. This basically is the main thrust of SMPY, to stress to gifted adolescents the personal significance of both satisfaction and satisfactoriness when choosing a college major or possible career, irrespective of whether male/female disproportion's ensue. If mathematically gifted females prefer to secure advanced degrees in biology, the humanities, law, or medicine (choices more congruent with their interests and values) and other disciplines for which they are likely to find more correspondent with their personal attributes, we see no problem with gender disparities. Here, our unit of analysis is the individual. Our goal is to facilitate individual development in ways that both the individual and the environments they choose find satisfying and satisfactory.

Yet, as a corollary to optimal intellectual development among the gifted, SMPY, because of the nature and scope of its data-collection operation, is often in a position to test more basic hypotheses and theoretical conjectures in psychological science. Some of these include postulated connections between intellectual precocity and underlying biological mechanisms. We turn next to our findings in this important area.

# Possible underlying reasons for the gender differences

In most treatments of causes for gender differences in abilities, interests, and values, socialization hypotheses have been emphasized (Halpern, 1992). This is perhaps due to the erroneous assumption that, if gender differences are environmentally determined, they are somehow more readily modifiable. Whether individual differences in a behavioral trait are pirmarily determined by biological or environmental factors is not what determines how responsive the differences will be to environmental intervention (Meehl, 1972). Nonetheless, SMPY and several other investigators have devoted considerable effort to identifying environmental determinants for gender differences in mathematical talent (Benbow, 1988). Although subtle effects of socialization could not be tested, the research conducted over the past 20 years has been unable to produce results consistent with an exclusively environmental explanation for the sex difference in SAT-M scores (Benbow, 1988).

Moreover, Lubinski and Benbow (1992) listed a number of findings that would appear curious if purported social influences are operating exclusively to attenuate in females the development of key attributes associated with satisfaction and satisfactoriness in engineering, mathematics, and the physical sciences. For example, females are superior to males on tests of arithmetic computation and they also (as a group) tend to get better grades in math courses. Some hypotheses attribue sex-role identification to gender differences in mathematical reasoning ability, but adolescents gifted in spatial and verbal abilities, like their mathematically gifted peers, are less gender stereotyped in nonacademic interests than the typical adolescent (cf. Lubinski and Humphreys, 1990b) ; and a recent meta-analytic review has called into question parents' differential socialization of boys and girls with respect to a number of abilities and social behaviors (Lytton and Romney, 1991). These factors led SMPY to begin exploring possible biological correlates of superior mathematical reasoning ability, hoping to stimulate subsequent and more sophisticated investigations into the underpinnings of precocity and the gender differences observed in several of its facets. This approach appeared fruitful, inasmuch as a genetic contribution to both abilities and preferences has been clearly documented (Benbow et al. 1983; Bouchard, 1991; Bouchard, et al., 1990; Lykken, 1982). SMPY's work in this area began with a neuropsychological investigation.

# Hemispheric specialization

The human brain is split into two parts, the right and left hemispheres, which are connected by the corpus callosum. The left hemisphere is specialized for language production, is analytical and sequential in processing of information, and is compartmentalized for various sensory modalities (Semrud-Clikeman and Hynd, 1990). The right hemisphere is specialized for  nonverbal abilities (e.g., spatial ability and judging emotions) and the distribution of attention across space (Kosslyn, 1987). It tends to be more holistic in the processing of information and integrates information across multiple modalities simultaneousy. SMPY's early work revealed that exceptionally precocious youth tend to be more frequently left-handed than their parents and siblings, average-ability students, and modestly gifted students (Benbow, 1986; Benbow and Benbow, 1984). Because the specialization of cognitive functions in the right and left hemispheres tend to be more diffuse in left than right handers, this finding had special significance for theoretical conjectures about brain organization (Bradsha and Nettleton, 1983). It led to a proposal that bilaterality or enhanced right hemispheric functioning may be associated with extreme intellectual precocity (Benbow, 1986; O'Boyle and Benbow, 1990). A series of studies has now provided support for this view.

Benbow and Benbow (1987) analyzed data from the visual modality. These date were obtained by tachistoscopically presenting stimuli (verbal and spatial) to each visual field and measuring reaction times. Results seemed to indicate that, indeed, the organization of skills within the two hemispheres was somewhat different for the intellectually gifted compared to typical students. O'Boyle and Benbow (1990) explored this idea further. They reported results of two experiments in which intellectually gifted and average-ability subjects (12 to 14 year-olds), all of whom were right handers, performed a verbal dichotic listening task and a free-vision chimeric face task. Typically, one would expect for right handers a right ear/left hemisphere advantage for the verbal dichotic listening task, while for the chimeric face task (a task involving the judging of emotions) a significant right hemisphere bias would be anticipated. For O'Boyle and Benbow's average ability control subjects, this was indeed the case. But the intellectually gifted subjects exhibited a quite different pattern. In the dichotic listening task, gifted subjects failed to show the usual left hemisphere advantage. Both hemispheres were equally effective in dealing with linguistic stimuli. For the chimeric face task the gifted, just like the average-ability subjects, also exhibited a right hemisphere advantage. This right-hemispheric bias for the gifted was, however, appreciably stronger by a magnitude of four than that revealed by the average-ability students.

O'Boyle and Benbow (1990) concluded from the above findings that the right hemisphere of the intellectually precocious is particularly engaged during cognitive processing. To lend further credence to this idea, more basic physiological data were collected. O'Boyle et al. (1991) conducted a preliminary electroencephalographic (EEG) investigation to determine if the pattern of hemispheric activation characterizing mathematically precocious males is different from that of average ability males. All subjects were right handed, and alpha activity at four brain sites was monitored. At baseline (looking at a blank slide) the left hemisphere of the precocious group compared to the average-ability group was found to be more active at all four sites. For the chimeric face task, the right hemisphere was markedly more active than the left, especially at the temporal lobe, while for the average ability students the left hemisphere was somewhat more active (see Figures 6 and 7). For the verbal task, the right hemisphere of the extremely precocious was somewhat more active with the opposite pattern for the average-ability subjects. A replication of this work, using both males and females as subjects, has now been completed (Alexander, 1992). The findings for males did replicate. Intellectually precocious males show enhanced right hemisphere

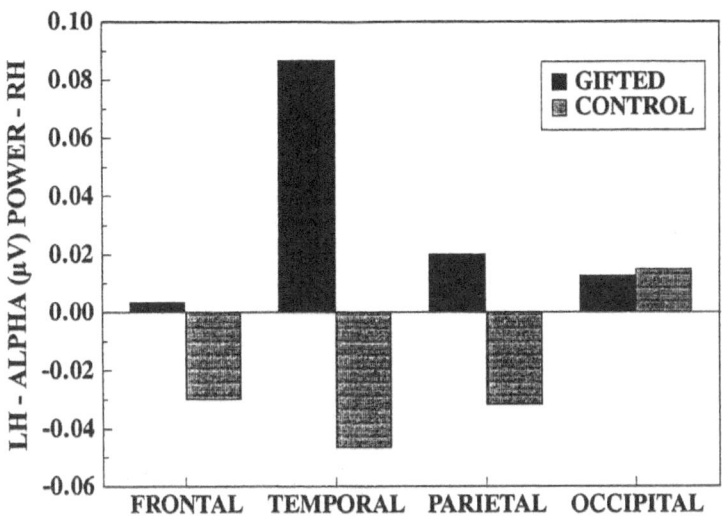

**Figure 6** Alpha power reduction (i.e., the reduction of alpha brain wave activity) (μV) for mathematically gifted and average ability control youths during the chimeric face task. (Adapted from O'Boyle et al., 1991).

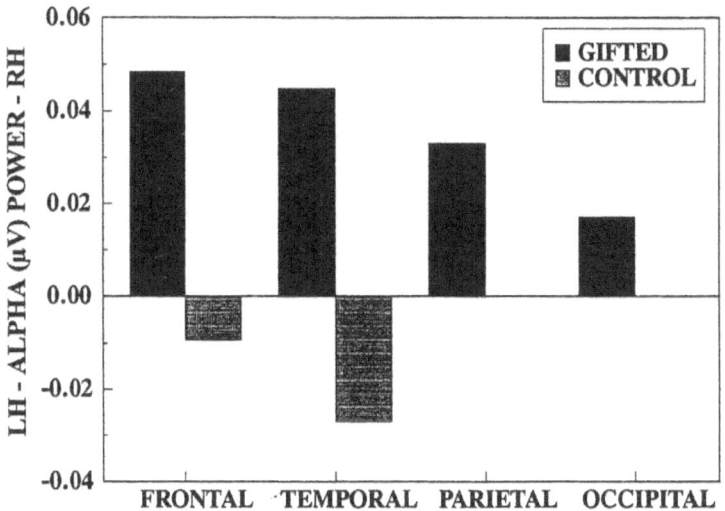

**Figure 7** Baseline alpha power (alpha brain wave activity) for mathematically gifted and average ability control youths. (Adapted from O'Boyle et al., 1991).

functioning, but the females did not. In sum, evidence is beginning to emerge indicating that the organization of cognitive functions within the left and right hemispheres in intellectually precocious males differs from that found for individuals with average abilities. These findings provide an especially attractive rationale for subsequent work involving recent advances in Positron Emission Topography (PET) technology.

Nonetheless, a question remains : why does enhanced right hemisphere functioning characterize males but not females?' We offer the following hypothesis : we suggest that it may have something to do with prenatal exposure to high levels of the hormone *testosterone* (Benbow, 1988). Further,we suggest a re-framing of the question, "Why do so few females possess exceptional levels of quantitative sophistication ?" The question might better be posed as : "Why is there an *overabundance* of mathematically gifted males" ?

Although purely speculative at this point, the excess of mathematically precocious males may be due to the more frequent exposure of males than females to high levels of fetal testosterone. Levy and Gur (1980) proposed that high levels of fetal sex hormones promote the maturational rate and cognitive capacity of the right hemisphere, and Gardner (1983) and Troup et al. (1983) reported that mathematical reasoning ability may be more directly under the influence of the right than left hemipshere. It may be that, just as there are continuous and taxonic avenues from which mental retardation can be traced (namely, simply systematic sources of individual differences at the low end or Mendelian inheritance, respectively), intellectual giftedness may stem from systematic sources of individual differences at the high end and, *possibly*, from underlying hormonal influences that function to produce discontinuities at the phenotypic level indicative of a taxonic phenomenon.

The work of Geschwind and Behan (1982) provides the theoretical basis for our speculations. Geschwind and Behan reported that left handers suffer more frequently from immune disorders, learning disabilities, and migraines than do right handers. The proposed explanation for this association involved prenatal exposure to testosterone. They suggested that if the developing fetus is exposed to high levels of testosterone or has an increased sensitivity to testosterone, at least two sequenced manifestations result. Testosterone affects the development of the thymus gland and, thereby, leads to increased susceptibility to immune disorders, such as allergies. Moreover, testosterone was predicted to enhance the development of the right hemisphere of the brain, which would lead to an increased likelihood of becoming lefhanded. Benbow (1986) and Benbow and Benbow (1987) presented data consistent with this hypothesis. Although, overall, intellectually precocious youth tend to be physically healthier than their normative peers (Lubinski and Humphreys, 1992), they also are more frequently left-handed, suffer more frequently from allergies (as well as other immune disorders), are more often first-born, and (quite curiously) tend to be born during a specified period of the year (February through July, with a peak in June), all findings that were predicted from the

Geschwind hormonal hypothesis and discussed in more detail by Benbow and Benbow (1987).

## Conclusion

Herein we have documented that gender differences among the giften have not diminished over the past 20 years in contrast to some recent reports that they may be disappearing in normative samples. Among the gifted there are gender differences at age 13, favoring males, in mathematical reasoning ability, that are accompanied by gender differences in spatial and mechanical reasoning abilities. (At the end of high school and college, there also are gender differences, favoring males, in mathematics and science achievement test scores). These differences at upper ability ranges are important and psychologically meaningful; even among SAT-M scores in the top 1 %, Benbow (1992) has demonstrated their predictive validity across 4-10 year temporal gaps for a host of academic achievement criteria.

In addition, there are differences in values and interests among the gifted at age 13 ; mathematically talented males are more theoretically oriented on the SOV and have primary interests in the investigative and realistic dimensions of Holland's Hexagon. In contrast, mathematically talented females are more socially and aesthetically oriented and have interests that are more evenly divided among investigative, social, and artistic pursuits. Thus, at age 13 more males than females possess ability and value profiles congruent with pursuing careers in the malth/sciences. This leads to gender disparities in educational attainment and in pursuing careers in math/science. These disparities become more intense at higher educational/professional levels, in part because males also demonstrate a stronger commitment to full-time work. Indeed, by drawing on longitudinal data available from SMPY on these students, we revealed that at age 23 more than twice as many males than females are pursuing advanced schooling and careers in the areas of mathematics, engineering, and physical science. The ability differences partially responsible for male/female disparities in physical science disciplines may have a biological basis. Mathematically talented males appear to possess enhanced right hemisphere functioning.

## Notes

[1] All subjects were identified by a talent search at age 13 and subsequently enrolled in a summer academic program for the gifted at Iowa State University (ISU). Students were qualified for this program if, as seventh graders, they earned scores of at least 500 on the mathematics SAT (SAT-M) or 430 on the verbal SAT (SAT-V). Only students with SAT-M > 350 (roughly the top 2% in mathematical reasoning ability) are included here. (Note that the group of students who took all of the tests is also included in the group who took at least one test). ISU's Talent Search is particularly noteworthy because it has the highest participation rate in the nation (more than 75% of all eligible students) and the highest ability scores. Students in these programs tend to be (personally) motivated and (family) supported : except for limited-income families, parents pay for them to attend.
Tests : College Board Scholastic Aptitude Test (mathematics = SAT-M; verbal = SAT-V; for participants beyond the seventh grade, SAT scores were adjusted downward 4 points/month); Raven's Progressive Matrices (Advanced), a nonverbal measure of general intelligence; Vandenberg Mechanical

Comprehension Test (Form AA), a test designed to assess inferences based on primitive kinds of physical mechanisms (gears, pulleys, springs etc.); Allport, Vernon and Lindzey (1970) Study of Values, a measure designed to assess the relative intensity of six "evaluative attitudes" used to approach life theoretical, aesthetic, social, economic, religious and political.

[2] The students in the sample were identified by a talent search requiring junior-high math achievement scores in the top 2% and had scores of at least 390 on the mathematics SAT or 370 on the verbal SAT when in seventh or eighth grade (years 1972-1974). The students were surveyed 10 years later (i.e. at age 23). The two bottom rows are rounded to the first whole number. The bracketed cells reveal the low rate at which mathematically gifted females pursue doctorates in mathematics or physical science. Samples defined at this level of mathematical reasoning have special significance for the math-science pippeline because these students earn degrees in math and science at 10 times the national rate. The all majors row includes low-frequency majors not reported in the above categories. (Adapted from Lubinski and Benbow, 1992)

# References

Aiken, L. (1986-1987). Sex differences in mathematical ability : a review of the literature. *Educ. Res. Quar.,* **10** : 25-35.

Albaum, G. (1976). Selecting specialized creators : the independent inventor. *Psych. Rep.,* **39** : 175-179.

Albaum, G. and Baker, K. (1977. Cross-validation of a creativity scale for the Adjective Checklist. *Educ. Psych. Meas.,* **37** : 1057-1061.

Alexander, J. E. (1992). *Behavioral and Electrophysiological Aspects of Hemispheric Functioning in Mathematically Precocious Males and Females,* Unpublished Doctoral Dissertation, Iowa State University.

Ailport, G. W., Vernon, P. E. and Lindzey, G. (1970). *Manual for the Study of Values,* Boston : Houghton-Mifflin.

Benbow, C. P. (1986). Physiological correlates of extreme intellectual precocity. *Neuropsychologia,* **24** : 719-725.

Benbow, C. P. (1988). Sex differences in mathematical reasoning ability among the intellectually talented : their characterization, consequences, and possible explanations. *Behav. Brain Sci.,* **11** : 169-232.

Benbow, C. P. and Benbow, R. M. (1984). Biological correlates of high mathematical reasoning ability. In : DeVries, J. G. et al. (Eds.), *Progress in Brain Research,* Amsterdam : Elsevier, **61** : 469-490.

Benbow, C. P. and Benbow, R. W. (1987). Extreme mathematical talent : a hormonally induced ability. In : Ottoson, D. (Ed.), *Duality and Unity of the Brain,* MacMillan, pp. 147-157.

Benbow, C. P. and Lubinski, D. (1992). *Gender Differences Among Intellectually-Gifted Adolescents : Implications for the Math/Science Pipeline,* Invited address at the annual convention of the American Psychological Society, San Diego.

Benbow, C. P. and Minor, L. L. (1986). Mathematically talented males and females and achievement in high school sciences. *Am. Educ. Res. J.,* **23** : 425-436.

Benbow, C. P. and Minor, L. L. (1990). Cognitive profiles of verbally and mathematically precocious students : implications for the identification of the gifted. *Gift. Child Quart.,* **34** : 21-26.

Benbow, C. P. and Stanley, J. C. (1982). Consequences in high school and college of sex differences in mathematical reasoning ability : a longitudinal perspective. *Am. Educ. Res. J.,* **19** : 598-622.

Benbow, C. P., Stanley, J. C., Zonderman, A. B. and Kirk, M. K. (1983). Structure of intelligence in intellectually precocious individuals and their parents. *Intell.,* **7** : 129-152.

Benbow, C. P., Zonderman, A. B. and Stanley, J.C. (1983). Assortative marriage and the familiality of cognitive abilities in families of extremely gifted students. *Intell.,* **7** : 153-161.

Bouchard, T. J. Jr. (1991). A twice-told tale : twins reared apart. In : Grove, W. M. and Cicchette, D. (Eds.), *Thinking Clearly About Psychology (vol. 2) : Personality and Psychopathology*, University of Minnesota Press : Minneapolis, pp. 188-215.

Bouchard, T. J., Jr. Lykken, D. T., McGue, M., Segal, N. L. and Tellegen, A. (1990). Sources of human psychological differences : the Minnesota study of twins reared apart. *Science,* **250** : 223-228.

Bradshaw, J. L. and Nettleton, N. C. (1983). *Human Cerebral Asymmetry*, Englewood Cliffs, NJ : Prentice-Hall.

Chambers, J. A. (1964). Relating personality and biographical factors to scientific creativity. *Psych. Monog.,* **78**, (Whole No. 584).

Cohn, S. J. (1991). Talent searches. In : Colangelo, N. and Davis, G.A. (Eds.), *Handbook of Gifted Education,* Boston : Allyn and Bacon, pp. 166-177.

Connell, R. W. (1987). *Gender and Power : Society, the Person and Sexual Politics,* Stanford, CA : Stanford University Press.

Dawis, R. V. and Lofquist, L. H. (1984). *A Psychological Theory of Work Adjustment : An Individual Differences Model and its Application,* Minneapolis, MN : University of Minnesota Press.

Feingold, A. (1988). Cognitive gender differences are disappearing. *Amer. Psych.,* **43** : 95-103.

Feingold, A. (1992). Sex differences in variability in intellectual abilities : a new look at an old controversy. *Rev. Educ. Res.,* **62** : 61-84.

Gardner, H. (1983). *Frames of Mind,* Basic Books.

Geschwind, N. and Behan, P. (1982). Left-handedness : associations with immune disease, migraine, and developmental learning disorders. *Proc. Natl. Acad. Sci.,* **79** : 5097-5100.

Halpern, D. F. (1982). *Sex Differences in Cognitive Abilities,* 2nd Edition, Hillsdale, NJ : Lawrence Erlbaum Associates.

Holland, J. C. (1985). *Making Vocational Choices : A Theory of Vocational Personalities and Work Environments* (2nd ed.), Englewood Cliffs, NJ : Prentice-Hall.

Humphreys, L. G., Lubinski, D. and Yao, G. (1992). Utility of predicting group membership : exemplified by the role of spatial visualization in becoming an engineer, physical scientist, or artist. *J. Appl. Psych.,* In press.

Hyde, J. S., Fennema, E., and Lamon, S. J. (1990). Gender differences in mathematics performance : a meta-analysis. *Psych. Bull.,* **107** : 139-155.

Keating, D. P. and Stanley, J. C. (1972). Extreme measures for the exceptionally gifted in mathematics and science. *Educ. Res.,* **1** : 3-7.

Kosslyn, S. H. (1987). Seeing and imaging in the cerebral hemispheres : a computational approach. *Psych. Rev.,* **94** : 148-175.

Levy, J. and Gur, R. C. (1980). Individual differences in psychoneurological organization. In : Herron, J. (Ed.), *Neuropsychology of Left-Handedeness,* Academic Press, pp. 199-210.

Lofquist, L. H., and Dawis, R. V (1991). *Essentials of Person-Environment-Correspondence Counseling,* Minneapolis, MN : University of Minnesota Press.

Lubinski, D., and Benbow, C. P. (1992). Gender differences in abilities and preferences among the gifted : implications for the math/science pipeline. *Cur. Dir. Psych. Sci.,* **1** : 61-66.

Lubinski, D., Benbow, C. P. and Sanders, C. E. (In press). Reconceptualizing gender differences in achievement among the gifted : an outcome of contrasting attributes for personal fulfillment in the world of work. In : Heller, K. A., Monks, F. J. and Passow, A. H. (Eds.), Oxford : Pergamon Press.

Lubinski, D. and Dawis, R. V. (1982). Aptitudes, skills, and proficiency. In : Dunnette, M. and Hough, L. M. (Eds.), *The Handbook Industrial/Organizational Psychology* (2nd ed.), Palo Alto, CA : Consulting Psychologists Press, pp. 3-59.

Lubinski, D. and Humphreys, L. G. (1990a). Assessing spurious "moderator effects" : illustrated substantively with the hypothesized ("synergistic") relationship between spatial and mathematical ability. *Psych. Bull.,* **107** : 385-393.

Lubinski, D. and Humphreys, L. G. (1990b). A broadly based analysis of mathematical giftedness. *Intell.,* **14** : 327-355.

Lubinski, D. and Humphreys, L. G. (1992). Some medical and bodily correlates of mathematical giftedness and commensurate levels of socioeconomic status. *Intell.,* **16** : 99-115.

Lubinski, D. and Thompson, T. (1986). Functional units of human behavior and their integration : a dispositional analysis. In : Thompson, T. and Zeiler, M. (Eds.), *Analysis and Integration of Behavioral Units,* Hillsdale, NJ : Erlbaum, pp. 275-314.

Lykken, D. T. (1982). Research with twins : the concept of emergenesis. *Psychophysiol.,* **19** : 361-373.

Lytton, H. and Romney, D. M. (1991). Parents' differential socialization of boys and girls : a meta-analysis. *Psych. Bull.,* **109** : 267-296.

MacKinnon, D. W. (1962). The nature and nurture of creative talent. *Amer. Psych.,* **17** : 484-495.

Marshall, S. P. and Smith, J. D. (1987). Sex differences in learning mathematics : a longitudinal study with item and error analyses. *J. Educ. Psych.,* **79** : 372-383.

Meehl, P. E. (1972). Specific genetic etiology, psychodynamics, and therapeutic nihilism. *Inter. J. Mental Health,* **1** : 10-27.

O'Boyle, M. W., Alexander, J. and Benbow, D. P. (1991). Enhanced right hemisphere activation in the mathematically precocious : a preliminary EEG investigation. *Brain and Cognition,* **17** : 138-153.

O'Boyle, M. W. and Benbow, C. P. (1990). Enhanced right hemisphere involvement during cognitive processing may relate to intellectual precocity. *Neuropsychologia,* **28** : 211-216.

Riger, S. (1992). Epistemological debates, feminist voices : science, social values, and the study of women. *Amer. Psych.,* **47** : 730-740.

Rosenthal, R. and Rubin, D. B. (1982). Further meta-analytic procedures for assessing cognitive gender differences. *J. Educ. Psych.,* **74** : 708-712.

Semrud-Clikeman, M. and Hynd, G. W. (1990). Right hemispheric dysfunction in nonverbal learning disabilities : social, academic, and adaptive functioning in adults and children. *Psych. Bull.,* **107** : 196-209.

Southern, M. L., and Plant, W. T. (1968). Personality characteristics of very bright adults. *J. Soc. Psych.,* **75** : 119-126.

Spranger, E. (1928). *Types of Men* (translated by P.J.W. Pigors), Halle : Niemeyer.

Stanley, J. C. (1977). Rationale of the Study of Mathematically Precocious Youth (SMPY) during its first five years of promoting educational acceleration. In : Stanly, J. D., George, W. D. and Solano, C. H. (Eds.), *The Gifted and the Creative : A Fifty-Year Perspective,* Baltimore MD : Johns Hopkins University Press, pp. 73-112.

Stanley, J. C. (1990). Leta Hollingworth's contributions to above-level testing of the gifted. *Rop. Rev.,* **12**, 166-171.

Stanley, J. C. and Benbow, C. P. (1986). Youths who reason exceptionally well mathematically. In : Sternberg, R. J., and Davidson, J. E. (Eds.), *Conceptions of Giftedness,* New York : Cambridge University Press, pp. 361-387.

Stanley, J. C., Benbow, C. P., Brody, L. E., Daubeer, S. and Lupkowski, A. (1992). Gender differences on eighty-six nationally standardized achievement and aptitude tests. In : Colangelo, N., Assouline, S. G. and Ambroson, D. L. (Eds.), *Talent Development,* Proceedings from the 1991 Henry B. and Jocelyn Wallace National Research Symposium on Talent Development, New York : Trillium Press, pp. 42-65.

Stanley, J. C., Keating, D. P. and Fox, L. H. (1974). *Mathematical Talent : Discovery Description and Development,* Baltimore : Johns Hopkins University Press.

Thorndike, E. L. (1911). *Individuality,* Cambridge, MA : Riverside Press.

Troup, G. A., Bradshaw, J. I. and Nettleton, N. D. (1983). The lateralization of arithmetic and number processing : a review. *Inter. J. Neurosci.,* **19** : 231-242.

# How and Why Sex Differences Evolve, with Spatial Ability as a Paradigm Example.

S. J. C. GAULIN

*Department of Anthropology, University of Pittsburgh, Pittsburgh, PA, USA*

## Why sex differences evolve

When articulated in genetic terms, Darwin's (1859) theory of evolution by natural selection is the most powerful tool we have for explaining why living things are as they are (Fisher, 1958; Dawkins, 1982). The theory is powerful because its prerequisite conditions are minimal and its implications ubiquitous. Natural selection will be at work anywhere entities make imperfect copies of themselves. For the kinds of organisms we know well, the imperfections of interest are mutations. These chance errors in gene copying create gene variants -alleles- at each chromosomal locus, alleles that are inevitably in competition with one another. An allele will win the competition, eventually replacing its competitors, if it has effects that cause it to be copied at a higher rate than any of its allelic alternatives. In this way genes that most favorably affect their own copying rates become common. The manifest traits of organisms are simply the allelic effects that led to maximal rates of gene copying.[1]

The theory of evolution by natural selection has many implications, one of which is that species tend to differ from one another. This is easy to explain: different species evolve divergent traits because a given genetic effect may lead to higher rates of gene copying in one environment and lower rates in another. In general, the members of a single species are similar because their genes have won the same sort of contest. They differ from other species because each species has its own unique environment and hence its own unique playing field of gene competition.

Thinking in terms of species differences highlights a problem. Why, within a sexual species, would females and males ever be different? They are by definition members of the same species, typically exploiting the same physical and biotic environments, eating the same foods, falling prey to the same predators and parasites. Beyond the primary reproductive organs, why should the sexes have been built differently by evolution?

Darwin (1871) asked himself this question and acknowledged that his theory of evolution by natural selection did not contain an answer. He recognized that one sex often exhibits structures or behaviors that seem to be useless (or even harmful) in dealing with the problems of surviving, finding food, avoiding

*M. Haug et al. (eds.), The Development of Sex Differences and Similarities in Behavior,* 111–130.

predators and the like. These traits - such as antlers, bright plumage or elaborate songs - were generally restricted to males. Why would such "ecologically useless" traits evolve at all, and why should they evolve in only one sex? Darwin realized that these traits were used extensively by males in a specific context, competing for and courting females. He argued, correctly we now believe, that traits conferring an advantage in this context would spread just as surely as traits that conferred an advantage in, say, disease resistance. He used the phrase "sexual selection" to refer to the spread of traits that are beneficial only in a mating context.[2] But this still does not explain why sexual selection has only affected males; why females lack antlers, bright plumage and elaborate songs.

Darwin's (1871) first answer was a skewed sex ratio. He suggested that if males were considerably more numerous than females, then from a male perspective females would be scarce, whereas from a female viewpoint males would be abundant. In such a world males would have more to gain from competing for mates than would females, who would already have more mates than they could use. Darwin was a committed empiricist and rapidly discovered that no such sex ratio imbalance existed; nevertheless his logic was sound and his idea captures the essence of contemporary sexual selection theory. Sexual reproduction requires equal genetic input from males and females. If members of one sex were especially numerous, they would find that partners were scarce.

The solution to Darwin's dilemma lies in recognizing that scarcity is only one cause of unavailability. Sometimes the sexes differ in their maximum reproductive rates, one sex requiring longer to complete a reproductive undertaking than the other. This will often be the case where one sex makes a greater commitment to rearing the offspring than does the other (Williams, 1966; Trivers, 1972). But regardless of what causes the difference in rate, members of the more slowly reproducing sex will generally find a good supply of potential mates, whereas members of the faster sex will often find few available partners due to the continuing commitment of these potential partners to some prior reproductive undertaking (Clutton-Brock and Vincent, 1991).

Consider a male and female engaged in a successful reproductive venture, i.e., one that eventually results in viable offspring. Their current success temporarily delays their future reproduction simply because success requires some irreducible temporal commitment. But this inevitable reproductive delay is not necessarily equivalent for females and males; in general, the delay is relatively long for females (for example, due to gestation and lactation in mammals) and relatively brief for males. In essence this situation allows males to reproduce more rapidly than females, or more precisely, it would allow males to reproduce more rapidly, if only they could find enough mates! Thus, sex differences in the length of the reproductive delay produce sex differences in (potential) reproductive rates and hence differences in the supply of reproductively available males and females. This situation can produce sexual selection just as intense as would a biased sex ratio. In fact its effects are identical. At any point in time there will be relatively few females who are available to begin a reproductive venture. In contrast, males return to the starting point of their reproductive cycle soon after copulation, so at any given time many males will be available and they will thus be forced to compete for the few available females. For males, fertilizable females will be genuinely scarce; for females, reproductively ready males will be abundant and eager.

Males generally can achieve higher reproductive rates than females, but this is not definitionally so. There are some species, which represent important test cases for sexual selection theory, where females have higher reproductive rates than males. This being the case, our discussion will be more precise if we ignore the words male and female for a while. Instead let us use the term "fast" to describe the sex that returns more quickly to reproductive condition (usually but not always males), and "slow" for the sex that has the lower reproductive rate.

Members of the fast sex could increase their reproductive output by increasing their copulatory frequency. Members of the "slow" sex require relatively few copulations to achieve their maximum reproductive rate. As a consequence of this difference, genes that augment copulatory success confer a significant evolutionary advantage in the fast sex but are of little evolutionary consequence for members of the slow sex. Generally speaking there are two categories of genetic effects that would tend to augment copulatory success: a gene could help the body in which it resides to defeat or intimidate other members of the fast sex, or alternatively it could help its body to charm any available members of the slow sex into mating. Thus traits that enhance same-sex competitiveness and traits that enhance cross-sex attractiveness are very common results of sexual selection. Of course these traits tend to be confined to the fast sex because only the fast sex benefits, in terms of total gene copying success, from the increased copulatory opportunities that such genetic effects provide.

This version of sexual selection theory is eminently testable and in fact does very well at predicting the cross-species distribution of "ecologically useless" traits used in fighting for and courting mates. These stigmata of sexual selection tend to be restricted to the fast sex (Clutton-Brock and Vincent, 1991). As Darwin noted, usually males are so marked but where females can reproduce more rapidly than males, they, not males, have been the principal targets of sexual selection.

A further implication of this theory should be explicitly stated. In some species the sexes do not differ in their maximum reproductive rates. This can result from strict monogamy, for example where the offspring are dependent for their survival on the attentions of both parents. In such cases, a male who deserted his partner to seek additional matings would doom his current offspring, and thus his own reproductive efforts, to failure. Under these conditions male and female reproductive rates are in lockstep; because neither sex benefits differentially from increases in copulatory frequency, sexual selection does not produce conspicuous sex differences.

In summary, sex differences in traits that are useful in competing for and courting mates will evolve in species where there are sex differences in reproductive rate; the fast sex alone will possess these traits. Such sex differences will be absent in species where the sexes have similar reproductive rates. This explains why sex differences evolve; we now turn to the question of how they evolve.

# How sex differences evolve, and what that tells us about how they develop

We saw how species differences evolve. A gene may have favorable effects on copying rates in one environment and unfavorable effects in another, thereby spreading in one population and being eliminated in the other. Thus, species differences evolve via genetic differentiation of the populations. But within any species males and females share most of their genes, so genetic differentiation is probably not the typical route by which sex differences evolve. This contrast between species and sexes is worth exploring in more detail.

Consider a pair of species, A and B. If a given allele has favorable effects in species A, it will spread in species A. If the allele has unfavorable effects in species B, it will be lost in B. The outcomes in species A and B are independent; they are not causally linked. Now, rather than thinking about a pair of species, think about the two sexes of a single species, and similarly imagine an allele with favorable effects on only one member of the pair. An example (in a species where males are the fast sex) would be an allele that helps a male to inseminate more than the average number of the females. By inseminating more females such a male will produce both more sons and more daughters than other males. In this way alleles with favorable effects on one sex are automatically spread to both sexes. If antlers, bright plumage or elaborate songs make successful fathers, fathers will in general pass the genes underlying these traits to both male and female progeny. This seems to produce a paradox. How can sex differences evolve if, every generation, successful fathers pass their genes to both sexes of offspring?

To begin to answer this question we need to consider the effects of these genes on sons and daughters. In species where females are the slow sex, daughters do not benefit by having antlers or any such copulation enhancing trait; in fact antlers, bright plumage and elaborate songs inevitably impose several types of costs on their bearers (Zahavi, 1975; Moller, 1989). For example, antlers must be built out of something. The necessary resources, over and above what would be necessary to build an antlerless body, must be harvested, processed and converted to antler tissue. The antlers have weight and therefore add to the metabolic costs of locomotion and could reduce the animal's top speed and stamina, making it more vulnerable to predators. Of course all traits have costs. But, for males, these costs may well be outweighed by a more-than-compensatory increase in copulatory frequency; in contrast females would suffer net costs because they reap minimal benefits from additional copulations.

Thus genes that, at some cost, increase copulatory frequency often produce different net effects depending on whether they are expressed in female or male bodies. There are many situations where such a gene will tend to spread as a result of the net benefits it confers on males, but will tend to be eliminated as a result of the net costs it imposes on females. Will sexual selection then end in a stalemate, where the characteristics of each sex are compromised for the benefit of the other? There may be a scrap of truth in this but sex differences are too pronounced for this to be the whole answer.

The evolutionary problem is to restrict the costs to the sex that can reap a net benefit by paying them (Lande, 1980). This could be accomplished if gene expression could be modulated according to sex. Some alleles are restricted to the heterogametic sex; for example, only male mammals can carry Y-chromosome genes. At least in humans the Y is known to be largely inert (Cavalli-Sforza and Bodmer, 1971), and there are strong theoretical reasons to expect that this is generally true (Hamilton, 1967). Since the Y is the only domain in which there could ever be genetic differentiation between the sexes in mammals, the inertness of the Y leads us to conclude that sex differences do not tend to evolve via genetic differentiation the way species differences do. But the Y nevertheless provides a wedge to begin to separate male and female ontogeny: despite its general inertness, the Y carries a gene called testes determining factor or TDF (Page, 1986; Vergnaud et al., 1986; Grumbach and Conte, 1992). What TDF does is activate autosomal genes (genes on chromosomes other than X and Y) whose products cause the fetal gonads to become testes. The testes then begin producing high levels of androgens that in turn influence the expression of many other autosomal genes. If TDF is absent, as in normal females, the fetal gonads become ovaries and a different hormonal regime washes the autosomes. Thus genes on the Y, genes that only one sex carries, are not in any direct sense responsible for sex differences. Instead, most sex differences result from the differential expression of autosomal genes, genes that, by definition, both sexes share. This differential expression is modulated by the best available cue about the sex of the body, sex hormones.

Here is another way of conceptualizing how sexual selection works at the level of the genes. Over the long haul of evolutionary time, the vast majority of genes spend about half of their careers in female bodies and the other half in male bodies. The sex of their next host body is in no way predictable from the sex of their current host body. Now consider two kinds of genes. The first kind produces fixed and definite effects. In species where there are differences in reproductive rate, some fixed effects will end up benefiting one sex of body but inflicting net costs on the other. The second kind of gene produces effects that are contingent on the sex of the body it is currently in; this latter kind somehow monitors the sex of its current host and adjusts its effects accordingly. It should be obvious that the latter type of gene will tend to win evolutionary competition in any species where there are sex differences in reproductive rate. Simply put, when sexual selection is operating, genes that have answers to the narrow problems "How do I make a fit female?" or "How do I make a fit male?" will eventually be replaced by genes than can solve both problems. Genes that can solve both problems need to be instructed about which problem they are solving this time around. They seem to receive that instruction from gonadal hormones. The result is that, by linking gene expression to hormone regimes, sexual selection designs sex-dependent ontogenetic programs: programs that foster the development of copulation enhancing traits in the fast sex, but repress these costly traits in the slow sex.

# Sexual selection for spatial ability

To illustrate my points I want to talk about sex differences in a particular behavioral domain. What I will emphasize is that the sex difference is not invariant: its presence or absence depends ultimately on the force of sexual selection and developmentally on gonadal hormones.

Sex differences in spatial performance are well described for humans (Harris, 1978; McGee, 1982; Rosenthal and Rubin, 1982; Linn and Petersen, 1985; Halpern, 1986) and laboratory rodents (Barrett and Ray, 1970; Joseph, 1979; Beatty 1984; Mishima et al., 1986). To begin to explain this sex difference in evolutionary terms, that is in terms of sexual selection, we must have some idea of how spatial ability might affect copulatory success. This part of the problem is not difficult.

The spatial organization of animal populations on the ground is known to depend on their mating system (Brown, 1966). In virtually all monogamous endotherms, mated pairs have isomorphic ranges (Figure 1), from which the

A Typical Monogamous Mammal

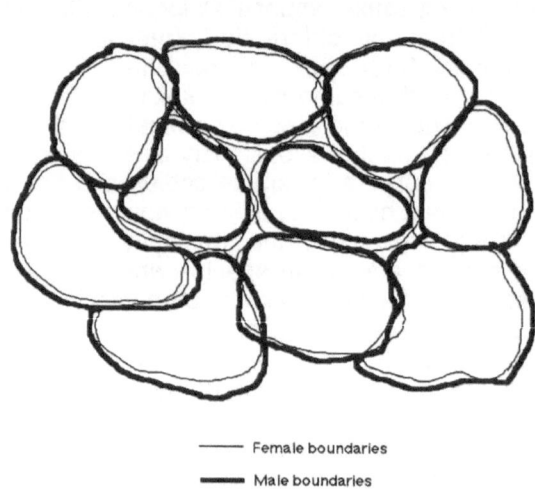

—— Female boundaries
━━ Male boundaries

**Figure 1** In monogamous species male and female partners tend to have isomorphic home ranges.

male and female exclude same-sex conspecifics, thereby enforcing the exclusivity of the mateship (Chivers, 1974; Kleiman, 1977). In many polygynous species the distribution of females may be quite similar to what it is under monogamy, each female occupying a relatively small, relatively exclusive range. However, because males can usually gain more than females from an increase in copulatory frequency, they may benefit differentially from increased exposure to potentially receptive partners. Hence, under polygyny, males who maximize the number of females they contact tend to leave more offspring than more sedentary males (Rodman, 1984; Kawata, 1988). Any genes that foster range expansion when they occur in male bodies will probably spread through the population, and sexually dimorphic ranging patterns will evolve (Figure 2).

A Typical Polygynous Mammal

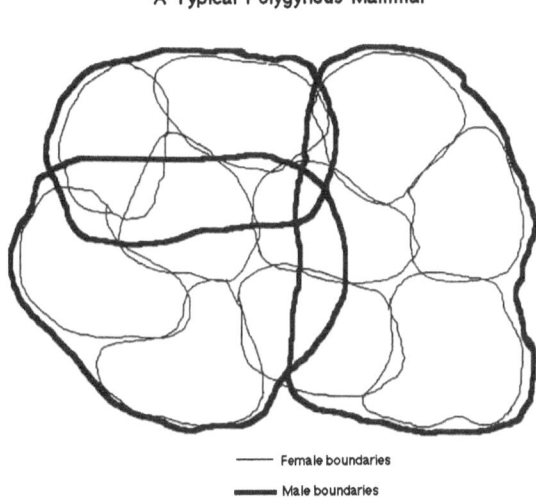

—— Female boundaries

▬▬ Male boundaries

**Figure 2** In many polygynous species male home ranges greatly exceed female home ranges.

Against this background, Figure 3 outlines a model to explain the evolution of sex differences in spatial ability. The assumptions of this model should be made explicit. First, what we call spatial ability is fundamentally a navigational adaptation. Animals will do best if they can acquire and manipulate accurate data on the distribution of rewards and risks in their environments. Within most species females and males exploit the environment in the same way and therefore confront very similar distributions of reward and risk: they will, to this extent, experience the same evolutionary demand for spatial ability. But when analysing a problem in terms of sexual selection, we also need to consider the impact of sex differences in reproductive rate. In non-monogamous species, males can usually reproduce more rapidly than females and they therefore experience a scarcity of females that is not reciprocal; data on the current location and reproductive status of females is much more relevant to male reproductive success than is parallel data on males to female reproductive success. Under these conditions, the ability to travel widely without disorientation has a greater impact on male than female fitness.

The second assumption involves cost: increases in range size and spatial ability are not free. There are energetic costs to patrolling a larger range and, under most assumptions about predator distribution, greater risks as well; increased spatial ability probably entails neural and metabolic costs. Of course costs do not invalidate a sexual selection explanation; they are part of it. If there were no costs, selection favoring a particular gene in one sex would simply drag the other sex along. In many species, a gene that buys a higher copulatory rate by inflicting costs will confer net benefits on males but net costs on females. Our

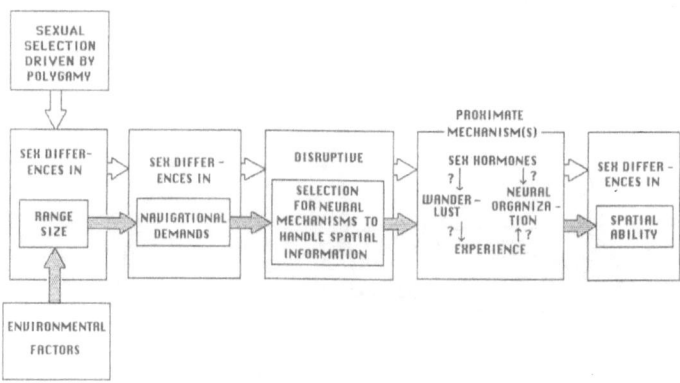

**Figure 3** Shaded arrows suggest how environmental factors, such as the spatial distribution of rewards and risks, might lead to the evolution of neural mechanisms for spatial processing. Open arrows emphasize that, in some polygamous mating systems, sexual selection could favor sexually dimorphic ranging behavior and thereby foster the evolution of sex differences in spatial skills.

theory tells us that these genes could have persisted only if they had a sex-limited expression.

To an evolutionist, the most obvious way to test this model is to examine its predictions about the distribution of the relevant sex differences. One of the most critical predictions is that sex differences in spatial ability and in ranging should covary. We have tested this prediction using the evolutionist's method of controlled comparison. Species that are distantly related to each other have typically evolved many different adaptations, whereas closely related species conserve many of the same adaptations from their recent common ancestor. Thus, if we expect that, for example, mating systems shape ranging patterns, it will be most informative if we examine closely related species which nevertheless differ in their mating systems.

In this research we have focused on wild rodents belonging to the genus Microtus, (commonly called voles) not because they are closely related to humans, but because there is an extraordinary amount of variation in the mating systems of its member species (Wolff, 1985). The model predicts that polygynous species will exhibit sex differences in ranging patterns and spatial ability. From the perspective of the psychological literature this is not a novel prediction because it is the baseline condition. Rats, mice and humans all exhibit the sex difference and all have a recent history of polygyny (Dewsbury, 1981; Murdock, 1986). Thus, the discovery of sex differences in spatial ability in another polygynous rodent could hardly be considered a strong validation of the model. The critical observations involve monogamous species.

We have studied two monogamous species, Microtus pinetorum (the pine vole) and M. ochrogaster (the prairie vole) and, as a control, one polygynous species, M. pennsylvanicus (the meadow vole). In the field, meadow voles shows marked sex differences in ranging, whereas the monogamous species (pine and prairie voles) reliably lack these sex differences, regardless of the time scale across which range sizes are computed (Table I). The situation in

**Table I**  Range sizes of breeding voles, by sex and species

| | N | 30–Day Range (m² ±se) | 48–Hour Range (m² ±se) | 24–Hour Range (m² ±se) |
|---|---|---|---|---|
| **Meadow Voles** | | | | |
| Males | 9 | | 623.3 ±163.7 | |
| Females | 12 | | 209.4 ±48.5 | |
| **Meadow Voles** | | | | |
| Males | 21 | 694.6 ±211.5 | | 198.6 ±41.9 |
| Females | 22 | 157.4 ±26.1 | | 64.0 ±10.4 |
| **Pine Voles** | | | | |
| Males | 10 | | 37.6 ±6.2 | |
| Females | 9 | | 40.8 ±4.5 | |
| **Prairie Voles** | | | | |
| Males | 21 | 277.6 ±63.7 | | 77.0 ±14.4 |
| Females | 26 | 183.2 ±24.0 | | 56.4 ±7.6 |

Data from Gaulin and FitzGerald (1986, 1989).

meadow voles is complicated and matches precisely what one would expect from a sexual selection perspective. In this polygynous species, there are no sex differences in range size prior to the attainment of sexual maturity (Table II)

**Table II**  Range sizes of meadow voles, by sex and reproductive status

| | N | Home Range (m² ±se) | Day Range (m² ±se) |
|---|---|---|---|
| **Males** | | | |
| Adults | 12 | 1124.8 ±321.1 | 310.6 ±53.8 |
| Subadults | 9 | 121.2 ±10.3 | 49.1 ±5.5 |
| **Females** | | | |
| Adults | 8 | 162.8 ±38.1 | 66.3 ±15.6 |
| Subadults | 14 | 154.3 ±35.7 | 62.7 ±14.0 |

Adults are reproductively active; subadults are not.  Data from Gaulin and FitzGerald (1989).

nor outside the breeding season; but during the breeding season, adult males have much larger ranges than do females (Figure 4). Augmented ranges are costly and should only occur when there is a compensatory benefit. Males derive no compensatory benefit in monogamous species and no compensatory benefit in polygynous species if they themselves are sexually immature or if local females are seasonally anestrus. These findings suggest that ranging patterns are indeed shaped by sexual selection. Have these ranging patterns generated sexual selection for spatial ability as outlined in Figure 3?

Using eight mazes of two different types, we have tested the spatial ability of voles under laboratory conditions. All three species have been examined; subjects were trapped from the same populations studied during our field work,

120

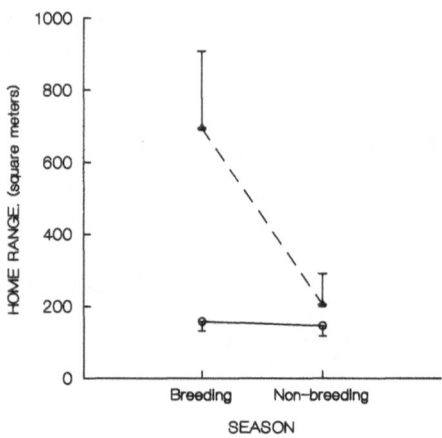

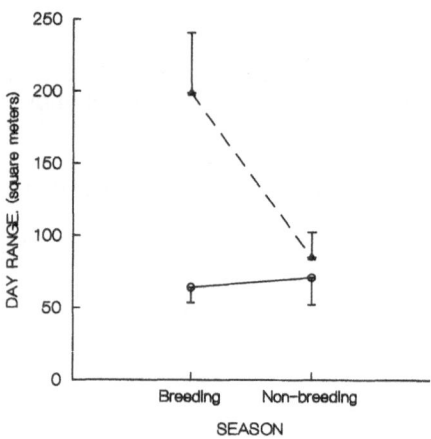

**Figure 4** Home and day ranges for meadow voles by sex and season. Male means are indicated by triangles, female means by circles. Data from Gaulin and FitzGerald (1989)

and in many cases were the very same individuals whose ranges had been measured in the wild. Pine and meadow voles were compared on a place-learning task in a sunburst maze (Table III); prairie and meadow voles were compared on a route-learning task in a series of seven symmetrical mazes (Figure 5). Our novel finding has been that the monogamous species do not show a sex difference, whereas their polygynous congeners, tested under identical conditions, do. Again the situation with meadow voles is complicated; the sex difference in maze performance is much more pronounced in animals trapped during the breeding season than in animals trapped during the non-breeding season (Figure 6). In meadow voles hormone regimes are known to

**Table III** Median ranks of voles in study 1 on the place-learning task, by sex, species

| | N | Median Rank | Mann–Whitney U-Test |
|---|---|---|---|
| **Meadow Voles** | | | |
| Males | 9 | 7.0 | p<.025 |
| Females | 11 | 15.0 | |
| **Pine Voles** | | | |
| Males | 8 | 10.5 | n.s. |
| Females | 13 | 11.0 | |

For each species, the U-test evaluates the significance of the
sex difference in rank. Data from Figure 3 of Gaulin and
FitzGerald (1986).

MEADOW VOLES

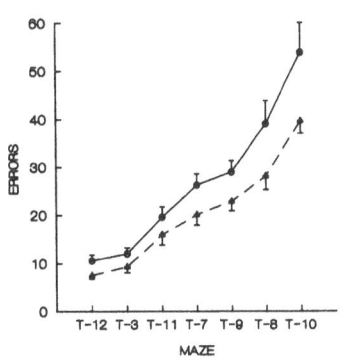

PRAIRIE VOLES

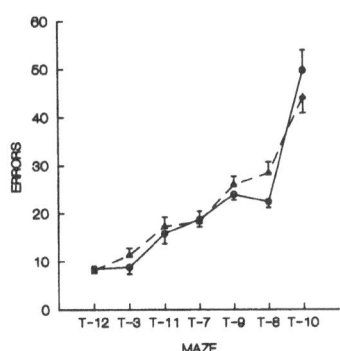

**Figure 5** Spatial performance by sex and species. Male means are indicated by triangles, female means by circles. Maze configurations (T-12, T-3, etc.) were drawn from Davenport et al. (1970). Data from Gaulin and FitzGerald (1989)

122

BREEDING SEASON

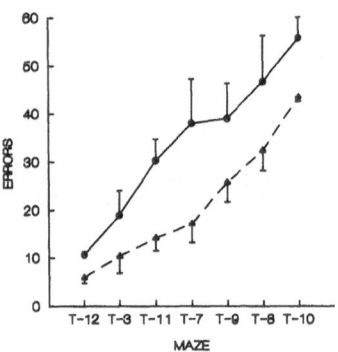

NON-BREEDING SEASON

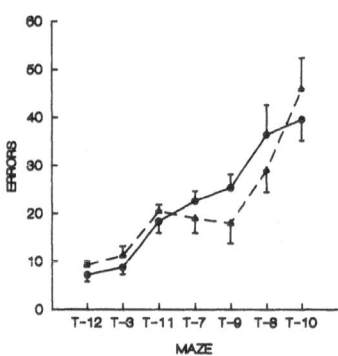

**Figure 6** Spatial performance of meadow voles by sex and season. Male means are indicated by triangles, female means by circles. Maze configurations (T-12, T-3, etc.) were drawn from Davenport et al. (1970). Figure presents a further partitioning of data from Gaulin and FitzGerald (1989).

differ between the breeding and nonbreeding seasons. Thus it is possible that hormones are responsible for the regression of sex differences in range size and maze performance among nonbreeding meadow voles.

Sex differences in spatial ability are sometimes attributed to sex differences in spatial experience. It is difficult to imagine how such an idea could have gained any credibility, given that laboratory rodents reliably exhibit the sex difference despite highly controlled rearing conditions. Nevertheless, we have evaluated this idea experimentally in voles. The essence of the experience hypothesis is that sex is irrelevant to "sex differences"; it posits that they are really experience differences. It follows that differences in spatial experience should produce differences in maze performance independent of sex. We have created spatially deprived groups of voles that differ greatly in experience from their wild-trapped counterparts without any perceptible deterioration of maze performance (Figure 7). The experience hypothesis should be laid to rest.

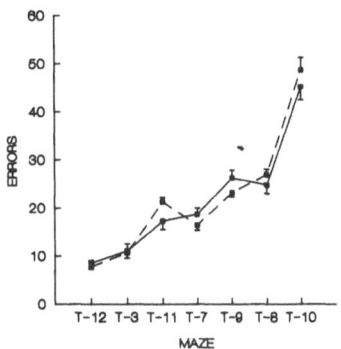

**Figure 7** Spatial performance of prairie voles by cohort. Means for spatially experienced wild-caught parents are open squares, means for spatially deprived lab-reared progeny are filled squares. Maze configurations (T-12, T-3, etc.) were drawn from Davenport et al. (1970). Data from Gaulin and Wartell (1990).

The sex differences we have observed in voles probably have a neuroanatomical basis (Jacobs et al., 1990). Anatomical, physiological and behavioral evidence from both birds and mammals (O'Keefe et al., 1975; Morris et al., 1982; O'Keefe and Speakman, 1987; Sherry and Vaccarino, 1989; Krebs et al., 1989; Sherry et al., 1989; Wehner et al., 1990) suggests that the hippocampus is critically involved in spatial processing (Sherry et al., in press). Voles present an interesting case in this regard precisely because some species show, and some species lack, sex differences in spatial ability. In meadow voles, males devote both absolutely and relatively more brain tissue to hippocampus than do females, while in pine voles there are no patterned sex differences (Table IV). A larger hippocampus is one of the several costs a male meadow vole pays in order to increase his copulatory frequency.

# Hormonal influences on spatial ability

Some other papers at this conference deal in greater depth with the ontogenetic mechanisms discussed below. My point is more general. I want to emphasize that the expectations of our evolutionary theory are bourne out: gonadal hormones do apparently shape the ontogeny of sex differences in spatial ability in a range of mammals. Both organizational and activational influences have been described.

**Table IV** Comparisons of hippocampal (HP) size, by sex, species

|  |  | HP Volume (mm³) | HP Volume x 100 / Brain Volume |
|---|---|---|---|
| Meadow Voles | | | |
| Males | 10 | 31.42 ±0.69 | 4.93 ±0.07 |
| Females | 10 | 28.22 ±0.89 | 4.50 ±0.12 |
| Pine Voles | | | |
| Males | 10 | 22.89 ±0.95 | 4.39 ±0.15 |
| Females | 10 | 22.42 ±0.74 | 4.57 ±0.23 |

Data from Figure 1 of Jacobs et al. (1990); in that original presentation, the two right-hand graphs are mislabeled on the y-axis: "x 100" should be deleted.

Experimental work with laboratory rodents suggests that the organizational effects are strong. Sex-specific patterns of maze performance can be completely reversed by early administration of appropriate hormones (e.g., Dawson et al., 1973, 1975; Stewart et al., 1975; Joseph et al., 1978; Williams et al., 1990). Most workers have examined the performance-enhancing effects of testosterone, on the logic that, if males normally perform better than females, male hormones must be responsible. But sexual differentiation of the rat brain is known to depend on the aromatization of certain androgens to estradiol within the central nervous system (e.g., McEwen et al., 1977); Williams has persuasively argued that sex differences in spatial ability are also largely a consequence in early CNS exposure to androgen-derived estradiol (Williams et al., 1990) and that the hippocampus is responsive to these estrogenic influences (Williams and Meck 1991).

No data exist on such organizational effects in wild rodents, although this would be fertile ground for research. If hormones organize the sex difference in spatial ability in meadow voles (as they appear to do in laboratory rodents), why do they not have similar effects in pine and prairie voles? It remains to be seen how these hormonal mechanisms have been modified by evolution so as to produce different results in these closely related species. The evidence we do have from wild rodents is indirect and bears more on activational effects. Significant variation in both range size and spatial performance is associated with hormonally mediated (Seabloom, 1985) changes in breeding status.

In humans, data on the relationship between gonadal steroids and spatial ability are clinical rather than experimental and derive from studies of patients with one of several rare hormonal syndromes. Among women there are both "masculinizing" and "feminizing" syndromes. In patients with Turner's Syndrome (46, XO) the fetal gonads do not differentiate and such individual are thus both androgen- and estrogen-deprived during fetal development. At the other extreme endocrine malfunction causes women with congenital adrenal hyperplasia (CAH) to be more androgenized than normal women. Among males there are also interesting contrasts; normal males can be compared with low-androgen, "hormonally feminized" males, such as those expressing Klinefelter's Syndrome and idiopathic hypogonadotropic hypogonadism.

Over the range of conditions discussed above, spatial skills are well correlated with early androgen dosage (Gaulin and Hoffman, 1988) - although this androgen may act primarily in an estrogenic aromatized form. Androgen-deficient females with Turner's Syndrome show a special deficit in spatial processing, that is their spatial ability is significantly lower than their verbal ability and significantly below the spatial ability of normal control females (Money, 1963; Alexander et al., 1964; Garron, 1977; Buchsbaum and Henkin, 1980; Gordon and Galatzer, 1980; Rovet and Netley, 1982), Of course Turner's women are estrogen-deficient as well, so they may not provide the best test case. Perhaps more telling is the case of CAH women; in CAH females only androgens are elevated above the normal female developmental baseline. Women with CAH score significantly above the mean of matched normal female controls on spatial tests (Perlman, 1973; Resnick, et al., 1986). Low-androgen males often have significantly depressed spatial ability relative to normal males (Bobrow et al., 1971; Buchsbaum and Henkin, 1980; Nyborg and Nielsen, 1981; Hier and Crowley, 1982). These results agree with the experimental data from laboratory rodents: early exposure to androgen (in some form) elevates subsequent spatial ability.

Among normal (i.e., non-feminized) males there is a range of androgenization in adulthood, and the most androgenized males seem to have lower spatial ability. This finding demonstrates an activational, not an organizational effect. Claims of a nonlinear relationship between androgen levels and spatial ability are restricted to males and based on current rather than fetal androgen exposure; among females higher current androgen levels are (like elevated fetal androgen levels) associated with higher scores on spatial tests (Shute et al., 1983; Gouchie and Kimura 1991). Estrogen (or other "female" hormones) may also have activational effects on spatial ability in that women perform better on spatial tasks during the menstrual phase of their ovulatory cycles (Hampson and Kimura 1988; Hampson 1990a, b). Data we have recently collected confirms this effect and shows that it is far from trivial (Table V).

**Table V**  Group differences on a spatial task

| Grouping Variable | Groups | (n) | 3-D Mental Rotation Mean (±se) | F | p |
|---|---|---|---|---|---|
| *Sex* | | | | | |
| | female | 108 | 8.22 ±0.66 | 29.44 | <.0001 |
| | male | 86 | 14.85 ±1.03 | | |
| (Females only) *Menstruating* | | | | | |
| | yes | 25 | 10.76 ±1.43 | 4.62 | .017 |
| | no | 83 | 7.45 ±0.73 | | |

# Summary and conclusions

In the study of sex differences, the nature/nurture issue has probably sparked more heat than light. While there are interesting questions here, much of the debate has been naive. For example, otherwise reasonable people have gone chasing after a sex-linked gene for spatial ability. At the other extreme, some environmentalists have drawn satisfaction from the fact the few sex differences seem directly traceable to genes on the X- or Y-chromosomes. An acquaintance with sexual selection would provide a good antidote to both kinds of confusion. To a great extent, evolution is constrained to build males and females out of the same genes. Those sex differences that have genuine biological bases are likely to be rooted in hormonally mediated gene expression rather than in gross allelic differences.

Beyond this, the evolutionary perspective explains the functional basis of sex differences, and by telling us what sex differences are for, it sheds light on many pragmatic questions. For example, if you know the adaptive significance of a particular sex difference you know where to look for it, which taxa are likely to exhibit the sex difference and which are not. Regardless of whether the topical concerns are endocrinological, neurobiological or psychological (to name a few), this is a powerful aid to research design because it tells us where to find natural controls. In addition, when sex differences are seen in the larger context of male and female reproductive strategies, it is apparent that some sets of sex differences are functionally linked, working together to maximize reproductive output in either a fast-sex or a slow-sex context. A reproductive strategy comprising a mix of male and female traits would probably be less successful than either coherent, pure strategy; thus, from an efficiency standpoint, we might expect functionally linked traits to be developmentally linked also. When we are studying the ontogenetic basis of sex differences, we are studying evolved developmental programs. These programs have an integral adaptive logic and thinking in terms of that logic will provide useful keys in unlocking their secrets.

## Notes

[1] Talking in terms of genes is the rigorous, but unfortunately not the most familiar, way to state evolutionary theory. More often the theory is argued in terms of competition among alternative traits (or, progressively worse, among alternative individuals or alternative populations). But there are many logical pitfalls on that path and it is best avoided. Traits do not spread directly; (much less so individuals) they spread because their genetic bases spread. To best understand a process, we should use an analytical model that matches the assumed mechanism as closely as possible. If it is more efficient to speak in terms of traits (or individuals), we must at least show occasionally that our arguments can be translated back in to the rigorous logic of genes.

[2] To many modern students of evolution Darwin's sharp distinction between sexual and natural distinction is unnecessary since in both processes a gene spreads due to its beneficial effects on its own copying rate. Because Darwin had emphasized the role of natural selection in adapting organisms to their environments he apparently felt obliged to distinguish a component of the evolutionary process that could actually degrade such environmental adaptation.

## References

Alexander, D., Walker, H. T. and Money, J. (1964). Studies in directional sense. *Arch. Gen. Psychiatry*, **10** : 337-339.

Barrett, R. J. and Ray, O. S. (1970). Behavior in the open field, Lashley III maze, shuttle box, and Sidman avoidance as a function of strain, sex, and age. *Dev. Psychol.*, **3** : 73-77.

Beatty, W. W. (1984). *Hormonal Organization of Sex Differences in Play Fighting and Spatial Behavior.* In : De Vries, G. J., De Bruin, J. P. C., Uylings, H. B. M. and Corner, M. A. (Eds.), *Sex Differences in the Brain, Prog. Brain Res. vol. 61,* Elsevier, Amsterdam, pp. 315-330.

Bobrow, A. A., Money, J. and Lewis, V. G. (1971). Delayed puberty, eroticism and sense of smell : a psychological study of hypogonadotropism, osmatic and anosmatic (Krallmann's syndrome). *Arch. Sex. Behav.*, **1** : 329-344.

Brown, L. E. (1966). Home range and movement in small mammals. *Symp. Zool. Soc. Lond.*, **18** : 111-142.

Buchsbaum, M. S. and Henkin, R. I. (1980). Perceptual abnormalities in patients with chromatin negative gonadal dysgenesis and hypogonadotropic hypogonadism. *Int. J. Neurosci.*, **11** : 201-209.

Cavalli-Sforza, L. L. and Bodmer, W. F. (1971). *The Genetics of Human Populations,* W. H.Freeman, San Francisco.

Chivers, D. J. (1974). *The Siamang in Malaya,* S. Karger, Basel.

Clutton-Brock, T. H. and Vincent, A. C. J. (1991). Sexual selection and the potential reproductive rates of males and females. *Nature,* **351** : 58-60.

Darwin, C. (1859). *On the Origin of Species,* John Murray, London.

Darwin, C. (1871). *The Descent of Man, and Selection in Relation to Sex,* John Murray, London.

Davenport, J. W., Hagquist, W. W. and Rankin, G. R. (1970). The symmetrical maze : an automated, closed-field test series for rats. *Behav. Res. Meth. Instr.*, **2** : 112-118.

Dawkins, R. (1982). *The Extended Phenotype,* Oxford University Press, Oxford.

Dawson, J. L. M., Cheung, Y. M. and Lau, R. T. S. (1973). Effects of neonatal sex hormones on sex-based cognitive abilities in the white rat. *Psychologia,* **16** : 17-24.

Dawson, J. L. M., Cheung, Y. M. and Lau, R. T. S. (1975). Developmental effects of neonatal sex hormones on spatial and activity skills in the white rat. *Biol. Psychol.*, **3** : 213-229.

Dewsbury, D. A. (1981). An exercise in the prediction of monogamy in the field from laboratory data on 42 species of muroid rodents. *The Biologist,* **63** : 138-162.

Fisher, R. A. (1958). *The Genetical Theory of Natural Selection,* Dover Publications, New York.

Garron, D. (1977). Intelligence among persons with Turner's syndrome. *Behav. Genet.*, **7** : 105-127.

Gaulin, S. J. C. and FitzGerald, R. W. (1986). Sex differences in spatial ability : an evolutionary hypothesis and test. *Amer. Nat.*, **127** : 74-88.

Gaulin, S. J. C. and FitzGerald, R. W. (1989). Sexual selection for spatial-learning ability. *Anim. Behav.*, **37** : 322-331.

Gaulin, S. J. C. and Hoffman, H. A. (1988). Evolution and development of sex differences in spatial ability. In : Betzig, L. L., Borgerhoff Mulder, M. and Turke, P. W. (Eds.), *Human Reproductive Behaviour : A Darwinian Perspective.* Cambridge University Press, Cambridge, pp. 129-152.

Gaulin, S. J. C. and Wartell, M. S. (1990). Effects of experience and motivation on symmetrical-maze performance in the prairie vole (Microtus ochrogaster). *J. Comp. Psychol.*, **104** : 183-189.

Gordon, H. W. and Galatzer A. (1980). Cerebral organization in patients with gonadal dysgenesis. *Psychoneuroendocrinol.*, **5** : 235-244.

Gouchie, C. and Kimura, D. (1991). The relationship between testosterone levels and cognitive ability patterns. *Psychoneuroendocrinol.*, **16** : 323-334.

Grumbach, M. M. and Conte, F. A. (1992). Disorders of sexual differentiation. In: Wilson, J. and Foster, D. (Eds.), *Williams Textbook of Endocrinology*, W.B. Saunders, Philadelphia, pp. 853-952.

Halpern, D. F. (1986). *Sex Differences in Cognitive Abilities*, Lawrence Erlbaum, Hillsdale, NJ.

Hamilton, W. D. (1967). Extraordinary sex ratios. *Science*, **156** : 477-488.

Hampson, E. (1990a). Variations in sex-related cognitive abilities across the menstrual cycle. *Brain and Cognition*, **14** : 26-43.

Hampson, E. (1990b). Estrogen related variations in human spatial and articulatory-motor skills. *Psychoneuroendocrinol.*, **15** : 97-111.

Hampson, E. and Kimura, D. (1988). Reciprocal effects of hormonal fluctuations on human motor and perceptual-spatial skills. *Behav. Neurosci.*, **102** : 456-459.

Harris, L. J. (1978). Sex differences in spatial ability : possible environmental, genetic, and neurological factors. In: Kinsbourne, M. (Ed.), *Asymmetrical Function of the Brain*, Cambridge University Press, New York, pp. 405-522.

Hier, D. B. and Crowley, W. F. (1982). Spatial ability in androgen deficient men. *New Engl. J. Med.*, **306** : 1202-1205.

Jacobs, L. F., Gaulin, S. J. C., Sherry, D. F. and Hoffman, G. E. (1990). Evolution of spatial cognition : sex-specific patterns of spatial behavior predict hippocampal size. *Proc. Natl. Acad. Sci. USA*, **87** : 6349-6352.

Joseph, R. (1979). Effects of rearing and sex on maze learning and competitive exploration in rats. *J. Psychol.*, **101** : 37-43.

Joseph, R., Hess, S. and Birecree, E. (1978). Effects of hormone manipulation and exploration on sex differences in maze learning. *Behav. Biol.*, **24** : 264-277.

Kawata, M. (1988). Mating success, spatial organization, and male characteristics in experimental field populations of the red-backed vole Clethrionomys rufocanus bedfordiae. *J. Anim. Ecol.*, **57** : 217-235.

Kleiman, D. G. (1977). Monogamy in mammals. *Quart. Rev. Biol.*, **52** : 39-69.

Krebs, J., Sherry, D. F., Healy, S. D., Perry, V. H. and Vaccarino, A. L. (1989). Hippocampal specialization of food-storing birds. *Proc. Natl. Acad. Sci. USA*, **86** : 1388-1392.

Lande, R. (1980). Sexual dimorphism, sexual selection, and adaptation in polygenic characters. *Evolution*, **34** : 292-305.

Linn, M. C. and Petersen, A. C. (1985). Emergence and characterization of sex differences in spatial ability : a meta-analysis. *Child Develop.*, **56** : 1479-1498.

McEwen, B. S., Lieberburg, I., Chaptal, C. Krey, L. C. (1977). Aromatization : important for sexual differentiation of the rat brain. *Horm. Behav.*, **9** : 249-263.

McGee, M. G. (1982). Spatial abilities : the influence of genetic factors. In: Potegal, M. (Ed.), *Spatial Abilities : Developmental and Physiological Foundations*, Academic Press, New York, pp. 199-222.

Mishima, N., Higashitani, F., Teraoka, K. and Yoshioka, R. (1986). Sex differences in appetitive learning of mice. *Physiol. Behav.*, **37** : 263-268.

Moller, A. P. (1989). Viability costs of tail ornaments in a swallow. *Nature*, **332** : 640-642.

Money, J. (1963). Cytogenic and psychosexual incongruities with a note on space-form blindness. *J. Psychiatry*, **119** : 820-827.

Morris, R. G. M., Garrud, P., Rawlins, J. N. P. and O'Keefe, J. (1982). Place navigation impaired in rats with hippocampal lesions. *Nature*, **297** : 681-683.

Murdock, G. P. (1986). *Ethnographic Atlas*, World Cultures 2 #4.

Nyborg, H. and Nielsen, J. (1981). Spatial ability of men with karyotype 47-XXY, 47-XYY, or normal controls. In: Schmid, W. and Nielsen, J. (Eds.), *Human Behavior and Genetics*, Elsevier/North Holland Biomedical Press, Amsterdam.

O'Keefe, J., Nadel, L., Keightly, S. and Kill, D. (1975). Fornix lesions selectively abolish place learning in the rat. *Exper. Neurol.*, **48** : 152-166.

O'Keefe, J. and Speakman, A. (1987). Single unit activity in the rat hippocampus during a spatial memory task. *Exper. Brain Res.*, **68** : 1-27.

Page, D. C. (1986). Sex reversal : deletion mapping of male-determining function of the human Y chromosome. *Cold Spring Harbor Symp. Quant. Biol.*, **51** : 229-235.

Perlman, S. M. (1973). Cognitive abilities of children with hormone abnormalities : screening by psycho-educational tests. *J. Learn. Disabil.*, **6** : 21-29.

Resnick, S. M., Berenbaum, S. A., Gottesman, I. I. and Bouchard, T. J. (1986). Early hormonal influences on cognitive functioning in congenital adrenal hyperplasia. *Develop. Psychol.*, **22** : 191-198.

Rodman, P. S. (1984). Foraging and social systems of orangutans and chimpanzees. In: Rodman, P. S. and Cant, J. G. H. (Eds.), *Adaptations for Foraging in Nonhuman Primates*. Columbia University Press, New York, pp. 134-160.

Rosenthal, R. and Rubin, D. B. (1982). Further meta-analytic procedures for assessing cognitive gender differences. *J. Educat. Psychol.*, **74** : 708-712.

Rovet, J. and Netley, C. (1982). Processing deficits in Turner's syndrome. *Develop. Psychol.*, **18** : 77-94.

Seabloom, F. (1985). Endocrinology. In: Tamarin, R. H. (Ed.), *Biology of New World Microtus*, American Society of Mammalogists Special Publications, pp 685-724.

Sherry, D. F., Jacobs, L. F. and Gaulin, S. J. C. (1992). Spatial memory and adaptive specialization of the hippocampus. *Trends Neurosci.*, **15** : 298-303.

Sherry, D. F. and Vaccarino, A. L. (1989). Hippocampus and memory for food caches in black-capped chickadees. *Behav. Neurosci.*, **103** : 308-318.

Sherry, D. F., Vaccarino, A. L., Buckenham, K. and Herz, R. (1989). The hippocampal complex of food-storing birds. *Brain Behav. Evol.*, **34** : 308-317.

Shute, V. J., Pellegrino, J. W., Hubert, L. and Reynolds, R. W. (1983). The relationship between androgen levels and human spatial abilities. *Bull. Psychon. Soc.*, **21** : 465-468.

130

Stewart, J., Skvarenina, A. and Pottier, J. (1975). Effects of neonatal androgens on open-field behavior and maze learning in the prepubescent and adult rat. *Physiol. Behav.*, **14** : 291-295.

Trivers, R. L. (1972). Parental investment and sexual selection. In: Campbell, B. G.(Ed.), *Sexual Selection and the Descent of Man : 1871-1971*, Aldine, Chicago, pp. 136-179.

Vergnaud, G., Page, D. C., Simmler, M. C., Brown, L., Rouyer, F., Noel, B., Botstein, D., de la Chapelle, A. and Weissenbach, J. (1986). A deletion map of the human Y chromosome based on DNA hybridization. *Amer. J. Hum. Genet.*, **38** : 109-124.

Wehner, J. M., Sleight, S. and Upchurch, M. (1990). Hippocampal protein kinase C activity is reduced in poor spatial learners. *Brain Res.*, **523** : 181-187.

Williams, C. L., Barnett, A. L. and Meck, W. H. (1990). Organizational effects of early gonadal secretions on sexual differentiation in spatial memory. *Behav. Neurosci.*, **104** : 84-97.

Williams, C. L. and Meck, W. H. (1991). The organizational effects of gonadal steroids on sexually dimorphic spatial ability. *Psychoneuroendocrin.*, **16** : 155-176.

Williams, G. C. (1966). *Adaptation and Natural Selection*, Princeton University Press, Princeton, NJ.

Wolff, J. O. (1985). Behavior. In: Tamarin, R. H. (Ed.), *Biology of New World Microtus*, American Society of Mammalogists Special Publications, pp. 340-372.

Zahavi, A. (1975). Mate selection -a selection for a handicap. *J. Theoret. Biol.*, **53** : 205-214.

# Hormonal and Neural Correlates of Sex-Typed Behavioral Development in Human Beings

## M. HINES

*Department of Psychiatry and Biobehavioral Sciences, 760 Westwood Plaza, School of Medicine, University of California, Los Angeles, CA, 90024-1759 USA*

It is well established that hormones have powerful and permanent influences on neural and behavioral development in experimental animals. (see, e.g., Goy and McEwen, 1980). In general, administering testosterone to genetic female animals prenatally or neonatally promotes development of male-typical characteristics and impairs development of female-typical characteristics. Similarly, removal of testosterone from developing males has the opposite effect. In addition, administering estrogen to developing females has many of the same effects as does testosterone administration, apparently because testosterone is converted to estradiol within the brain before exerting many of its neurobehavioral effects (McEwen et al., 1977a; McEwen et al., 1977b). Although these influences of androgens and estrogens were first demonstrated for reproductive behaviors, such as lordosis, mounting, intromission and ejaculation, they also apply to other behaviors that show sex differences, or are sex-typed, in the sense that they differ on the average for males and females of the species (Beatty, 1979). In addition, similar influences have been documented for brain regions that show sex differences. In these sexually differentiated areas, the early hormone environment influences basic processes of neural differentiation such as cell survival, anatomical connectivity, and neurochemical specification (Arnold and Gorski, 1984). Thus, it is thought that permanent hormone-induced changes in behavior result from hormone-induced changes in brain structure that occur during critical or sensitive periods of development.

The neural regions influenced by androgens or estrogens are those that have receptors for these steroid hormones, including subregions of the hypothalamus, such as the preoptic area, bed nucleus of the stria terminalis, and ventromedial hypothalamic nucleus, as well as portions of the amygdaloid nucleus and of the cerebral cortex (Stumpf and Grant, 1975). Although the location of steroid receptors in the developing brain has been studied most extensively in rodents (Pfaff and Keiner, 1973; Stumpf et al., 1975), receptor localization appears to be similar across a wide range of mammalian species including primates (Clark et al., 1988; Stumpf and Grant, 1975).

*M. Haug et al. (eds.), The Development of Sex Differences and Similarities in Behavior, 131–149.*
© 1993 *Kluwer Academic Publishers.*

In regard to non-reproductive behaviors that are influenced by androgens or estrogens during development, the majority of research has again focused on rodents, where social behaviors, such as aggression (Edwards and Herndon, 1970) and rough and tumble play (Meaney and Stewart, 1981), and cognitive traits, such as visuospatial abilities (Williams and Meck, 1991) and neural lateralization for vocal behavior (Holman and Hutchison, 1991), have been found to be sensitive to the same types of hormonal influences as are reproductive behaviors. Again, although there is less information on hormonal contributions to behavioral development in primates, the available data suggest that hormonal influences in rhesus macaques are similar to those demonstrated in rodents (Goy, 1978; Goy et al., 1988).

A major question regarding the importance and implications of this research area is its relevance to understanding human development. In this chapter I will describe research related to the possibility that gonadal hormones influence human neural and behavioral development in a manner similar to that documented in other species. First, studies examining sex-typed behaviors in human beings exposed to unusual hormone milieus during development will be summarized. Second, research reporting sex differences in human brain structure will be reviewed. Finally, recent data correlating neural sex differences with behavioral sex differences will be described.

# Gonadal hormones and human behavioral development

In experimental animals, critical periods for the influences of gonadal hormones on neurobehavioral development correspond to times when androgen levels differ in developing males versus females. In humans, androgen levels are higher in males than in females prenatally from approximately week 8 of gestation to approximately week 24, and then again neonatally from about the first to the sixth month of life (Smail et al., 1981). Thus, these times could be critical periods for gonadal hormone influences on human development.

Because it is not ethical to administer hormones to developing human beings for experimental purposes, research investigating gonadal hormone influences on the development of human behavior has focused on "experiments of nature" in which people developed in unusual hormone milieus because of genetic problems or because their mothers were prescribed hormones during pregnancy. Populations available for study include: 1. girls and women with Congenital Adrenal Hyperplasia (CAH), a disorder in which the adrenal gland overproduces androgens, beginning prenatally; 2. girls and women with Turner Syndrome, who experience ovarian regression and consequently reduced levels of androgens and estrogens (usually beginning prenatally); 3. boys and men who have idiopathic hypogonadotrophic hypogonadism (IHH) and who are consequently exposed to lower than normal levels of androgens and estrogens during neonatal life; 4. girls and women whose mothers were prescribed the synthetic estrogen, diethylstilbestrol (DES), during pregnancy; and 5. individuals whose mothers were prescribed progesterone or synthetic progestins during development. These progestational compounds are of interest because some mimic the actions of androgens (androgenic progestins), and others interfere with the actions of androgens (anti-androgenic progestins).

Because experimental animal research indicates that behaviors that show sex differences are influenced by manipulations of androgens or estrogens during development, behaviors that show sex differences in human beings might be hypothesized to relate to the early hormone environment. The question of which human behaviors show sex differences or are sex-typed, even in the simple sense of differing on the average for males and females, has been disputed. However, since the late 1970's there has been general agreement that at least a small group of behaviors, including physical aggression, certain cognitive functions (e.g., visuospatial abilities, verbal fluency and language lateralization), childhood play patterns (e.g., toy preferences and rough and tumble play), and sexual orientation show sex differences (Halpern, 1987; Hines and Green, 1991; Maccoby and Jacklin, 1974; McGlone, 1980). The differences between males and females are not absolute. In regard to each of the behaviors there is overlap between the sexes. Nevertheless, when groups of males and females are tested, differences are seen reliably. The size of most of these behavioral sex differences is approximately one-sixth to one-half the size of the sex difference in height (for review see Hines, 1990). The exception is sexual orientation, for which the sex difference is larger. For example, it is estimated that about 90% of men have a primary erotic attraction to women, whereas this is the case for only about 5% of women. Similarly, although about 95% of women have a primary erotic attraction to men, only about 10% of men have a primary erotic attraction of this sort (Hyde, 1990; King et al., 1991; Kinsey et al., 1948; Kinsey et al., 1953).

Studies of the behavior of individuals exposed to unusual hormone environments during development ("experiments of nature") are relevant to determining if biology plays a role in the development of these behaviors that show sex differences. As described below, there is some evidence supporting a hormonal contribution to human variability in each category of sex-related behavior.

## Sex-typed play patterns

As early as the age of 12 months, sex differences can be measured in the play of boys and girls (Snow et al., 1983). Beginning at that age and continuing through childhood, boys tend to prefer vehicles and building toys for their play activities, whereas girls tend to prefer dolls (Fagot, 1978; Sutton-Smith et al., 1963). Boys also spend more time than girls do in rough and tumble play, particularly involving play fighting and overall body contact (DiPietro, 1981). Early reports on girls exposed to high levels of androgens prenatally, because they have CAH or because their mothers were prescribed androgenic progestins during pregnancy, suggested they were "tomboys" (Ehrhardt and Baker, 1974; Ehrhardt et al., 1968; Ehrhardt and Money, 1967). These results were reported for androgenized girls compared to matched controls (Ehrhardt et al., 1968), as well as to unaffected sisters of children with CAH (Ehrhardt and Baker, 1974). The results were derived from interviews with the girls and their mothers in which the girls were described as prefering boys' activities, boys as playmates, boys' clothes, and rough, active outdoor play usually considered more characteristic of boys than of girls.

Girls with CAH are often born with some degree of virilization of the external genitalia. Typically, parents are instructed to raise the child as a girl and the genital virilization is corrected early in life. However, it has been argued that interview-based reports of behavioral masculinization in girls with CAH reflect faulty parental perceptions of behavioral virilization based on the girls' early physical virilization, or result from changes in the way that parents treat CAH girls, again based on genital virilization at birth (Quadagno et al., 1977). Recently we conducted a study relevant to the validity of these arguments (Berenbaum and Hines, 1992). In the study, we observed the behavior of girls with CAH directly, rather than infering behavioral changes from interview data, and found that at least some aspects of sex-typed play in girls with CAH are masculinized. Videotapes were made of 3 to 8 year old girls and boys with CAH and of their unaffected 3 to 8 year old male and female relatives playing individually in a playroom. Toys available in the playroom included some typically prefered by boys (e.g., cars, trucks, Lincoln Logs), some typically prefered by girls (e.g., a Barbie doll, dishes, an infant doll) and some typically prefered equally by boys and girls (e.g., books and board games). The videotapes were coded by raters who did not know which children had CAH and which did not. The results indicated that the control children showed the predicted sex differences in toy choices. The unaffected boys spent more time than did the unaffected girls with the boy-prefered toys, and the unaffected girls spent more time than did the unaffected boys with the girl-prefered toys. In addition, the girls with CAH showed a masculine-typical pattern of behavior. In comparison to unaffected female relatives, they spent more time with the boy-prefered toys and less time with the girl-prefered toys. No differences were seen between any of the groups in preferences for the neutral toys, suggesting that the behavioral changes in the girls with CAH were specific to sex-typed behaviors.

As mentioned above, criticisms of research on girls with CAH are two-fold. First, it has been suggested that the girls do not show altered behavior, but rather that their parents perceive their behavior as more masculine because they recall their genital virilization at birth. The data just described argue against this possibility. However, they do not address the second part of the criticism--that parental knowledge of virilization at birth causes differences in childrearing that lead to behavioral masculinization. This possibility seems unlikely, since parents are instructed to raise girls with CAH as girls and might be expected to combat rather than promote masculine inclinations. Nevertheless, to provide information relevant to this possibility, we obtained medical records and assessed the degree of virilization at birth for each CAH girl. We then correlated the degree of physical virilization with the amount of behavioral masculinization. These correlations were not significant (Berenbaum and Hines, 1992). In fact, some girls who were most severely virilized physically showed relatively low preferences for toys normally prefered by boys and some who were least virilized showed strong preferences for the boy-prefered toys. Thus, the suggestion that behavioral masculinization in CAH girls is caused by their genital virilization was not supported by our data.

## Physical aggression

Across the life-span and in disparate cultures human males show more physical aggression than human females (Maccoby and Jacklin, 1974). Although no direct observations of aggression in hormone-exposed groups have been reported, data from two studies using indirect measures suggest a role for the early hormone environment in propensities to physical aggression. In the first study, children exposed prenatally to androgenic progestins were found to self-report higher levels of physical aggression in response to provocation when compared to a control group of their unexposed siblings (Reinisch, 1981). Importantly, the progestin-exposed girls in this study were not physically virilized, ruling out this mechanism for the behavioral difference. In the second study, females androgenized prenatally because of CAH scored higher on the aggression subscale of a personality inventory than did their unaffected sisters and female first cousins (Resnick, 1982).

## Cognitive traits

Although men and women are similar in overall intelligence, as measured by IQ tests, they differ in regard to some specific intellectual functions (Halpern, 1987; Hines, 1990; Linn and Petersen, 1985; Maccoby and Jacklin, 1974). Notably, on the average, men perform better than women on measures of visuospatial abilities, particularly those involving mental rotation of three-dimensional figures and, to a lesser extent, those involving disembedding of simple patterns from complex backgrounds. In contrast, on the average, women outperform men on measures of verbal fluency, such as tests requiring the production of words or sentences that meet certain constraints of meaning or form. Men and women also differ in language lateralization, or the organization of the two cerebral hemispheres for processing or producing language (McGlone, 1980). On the average, in comparison to women, men show more language lateralization, or a greater reliance on a single hemisphere for verbal tasks.

Studies of individuals exposed during early development to abnormal hormone milieus suggest that these cognitive sex differences may have an endocrine component. For instance, postpubescent girls and women exposed to high levels of androgens during development, because of CAH, have been reported to have enhanced visuospatial abilities compared to unaffected sisters and female first cousins of CAH patients (Resnick et al., 1986). In addition, men exposed to lower than normal levels of androgens from early life, because they have IHH, have been reported to show reduced visuospatial abilities compared to healthy controls, as well as to men whose hypogonadism began after puberty (Hier and Crowley, 1982). Also, women exposed to DES prenatally, because their mothers were prescribed this hormone during pregnancy, have been reported to show increased language lateralization compared to their unexposed sisters (Hines and Shipley, 1984). Finally, many studies have found that girls and women exposed to lower than normal levels of gonadal hormones prenatally, because of ovarian regression associated with Turner Syndrome, show reduced visuospatial ability and reduced language lateralization in comparison to matched controls (Gordon and Galatzer, 1980; Money, 1973; Rovet and Netley, 1982).

## Sexual orientation

Several studies suggest alteration in sexual orientation associated with prenatal exposure to androgens or estrogens. One study reported that women exposed to high levels of androgens during development, because of CAH, are more likely than women with other endocrine disorders to self-report a bisexual or homosexual orientation (Money et al., 1984). A second study found similar results for a sample of German women with CAH (Dittman et al., 1992). Finally, a recent study of a third group of women with CAH found them to indicate reduced sexual experience (heterosexual or homosexual) compared to their sisters without CAH (Zucker et al., 1992). One possible interpretation of the data from the last study is that women with CAH show diminished sexual interest in general, both heterosexual and homosexual. However, it is also possible that the women have homosexual interest, but that they do not feel free to express this interest, because of social constraints, and so express no sexual interest at all. Further research is needed to distinguish between these possibilities.

Data on sexual interest and behavior in women with CAH are problematic because of their genital virilization at birth, and because the surgery to correct virilization does not always produce genitalia identical with those of normal females. In fact, in some cases, characteristics of the genital repair are such that heterosexual intercourse can be painful. Therefore, data on women exposed to hormones that influence the development of sex-linked characteristics in experimental animals, but who are born with normal external genitalia, are of interest. Such data have come from women exposed prenatally to DES, a hormone that produces masculine-typical brain structure and sexual behavior in female rodents exposed during critical developmental periods, without producing genital virilization (Döhler et al., 1984; Hines et al., 1987; Hines and Goy, 1985). Similarly, female human beings exposed to DES prenatally are not virilized physically. However, two studies suggest that DES-exposed women are more likely than matched controls, and than their unexposed sisters, to have a bisexual or homosexual orientation (Ehrhardt et al., 1985; Ehrhardt et al., 1987). In these studies, approximately 30 to 40% of the DES-exposed women versus 0 to 10% of the controls were bisexual or homosexual.

The above section described a number of studies that reported predicted relationships between the early hormone environment and human behavior. There are also studies that failed to find such relationships for cognitive function (Baker and Ehrhardt, 1974; Kester et al., 1980; McGuire et al., 1975; Reinisch and Karow, 1977; Yalom et al., 1973), aggression (Ehrhardt and Baker, 1974; Money and Schwartz, 1976), childhood play behavior (McGuire et al., 1975) or sexual orientation (Ehrhardt et al., 1968; Lev-Ran, 1974). Methodological aspects of these studies may have limited their ability to detect hormone-behavior relationships. For instance, the studies generally used smaller samples than those reporting positive results and in some cases did not include comparison groups. In many cases, they also used measures that show small sex differences or included substantial numbers of prepubertal individuals who would not be expected to show reliable sex differences on some measures of sex-typed behavior (for example, measures related to sexual orientation and some of the commonly employed measures of visuospatial ability and language lateralization). Some studies also focused on hormone-exposed males, for whom reliable changes in sex-typed behaviors would not be predicted from animal models, or analyzed data for males and females combined, despite evidence from animal models of different predictions for the two sexes. Thus, a lack of experimental power may have precluded seeing hormone-behavior relationships in these studies. (See Hines and Green, 1991; Hines and Shipley, 1984; Resnick et al., 1986 for further discussion of these issues).

Nevertheless, although several studies suggest hormonal influences on sex-typed behavior in humans, the overall pattern of results suggests that these relationships are complex. For instance, although DES-exposed women and women with CAH indicate more bisexual or homosexual experience than do controls, many hormone-exposed women indicate a heterosexual orientation (Ehrhardt et al., 1985; Ehrhardt et al., 1987; Money et al., 1984). Thus, it appears that factors other than hormones contribute to a person's sexual orientation, and that, in at least some cases, these other factors are dominant. Another complexity involves the ability of hormones to affect some sex-typed behaviors without affecting others. For instance, although DES-exposed women have been found to show increased bisexuality or homosexuality (Ehrhardt et al., 1985; Ehrhardt et al., 1987) and increased language lateralization (Hines and Shipley, 1984), they show no changes in visuospatial abilities (Hines and Shipley, 1984). In contrast, individuals with other hormone syndromes, involving changes in androgens as well as estrogens, do show alterations in visuospatial abilities (Hier and Crowley, 1982; Money, 1973; Resnick et al., 1986). In animal models, although estrogen and androgen have similar influences on a large number of neurobehavioral characteristics, some characteristics are sensitive only to androgen during development (Arnold and Gorski, 1984; Meaney and Stewart, 1981). Thus, some differences in the consequences of androgen versus estrogen might be expected for human neurobehavioral development as well. Similarly, in experimental animal models, the timing of hormone exposure within the overall critical period determines specific behavioral outcomes. If a hormone perturbation is brief, some sex-linked behaviors will be influenced whereas others will not be (Christensen and Gorski, 1978; Goy et al., 1988). Thus, human offspring exposed to hormones at different times during prenatal or neonatal development might show different behavioral outcomes.

# Sex differences in human brain structure

In animals, hormone-induced changes in behavioral development are thought to result from hormone-induced alteration in the differentiation of specific neural regions that show sex differences. Thus, a question related to possible hormone influences on human behavioral development is whether or not there are portions of the human brain that differ for males and females.

## The anterior hypothalamic/preoptic area (AH/POA)

The AH/POA has been of particular interest in the search for structural sex differences in the brain, because it is known to contain a high density of receptors for sex steroids and because lesion and stimulation studies indicate its importance for several sex-linked functions, including gonadotropin regulation, maternal behavior and male sexual behavior (for reviews see Allen et al., 1989; Arnold and Gorski, 1984; Goy and McEwen, 1980). In 1978 a sex difference was described in a subregion of the preoptic area of the rat brain, and was named the sexually dimorphic nucleus of the preoptic area (SDN-POA) (Gorski et al., 1978; Gorski et al., 1980). The SDN-POA shows a dramatic sex difference, being several fold larger in the brains of male rats compared to females. Subsequently, similar volumetric sex differences were observed in subregions of the preoptic area in other mammalian species, including gerbils, guinea pigs and ferrets (Commins and Yahr, 1984; Hines et al., 1985; Tobet et al., 1986) Also, additional sex differences, some favoring females and some favoring males, were reported in other subregions of the rodent preoptic area. All the evidence to date suggests that these sex differences in brain structure are determined by the actions of androgens and estrogens during critical periods of development (see Arnold and Gorski, 1984 for a review).

Several research groups have searched for similar sex differences in the human brain. An early report claimed that the human SDN-POA had been found (Swaab and Fliers, 1985). However, two subsequent studies failed to find a sex difference in this nucleus (Allen et al., 1989; LeVay, 1991). It is possible that the original report actually reflected an age difference rather than a sex difference. The volume of the nucleus that was called the human SDN-POA declines dramatically with age (Allen et al., 1989), and the women studied in the report finding what appeared to be a sex difference were approximately 10 years older on average than the men (see Allen et al., 1989 for further discussion). Alternatively, the nucleus may show a small sex difference or, because of differences in the timing of age-related neural changes in men and women (Gur et al., 1991), may appear to show a sex difference in some age ranges.

What's in a name? Attachment of the name "human SDN" or "sexually dimorphic nucleus" to a brain region that does not show a reliable sex difference has produced confusion. For instance, a subsequent study failed to find a sex difference in the nucleus in the brains of children (Swaab and Hofman, 1988). Based on the lack of a sex difference in "the human SDN" in children it was concluded that sexual differentiation of the human brain occurs after childhood, and thus can not relate to the prenatal hormone environment. However, if the nucleus named the "human SDN" does not show a reliable sex difference, no conclusions can be drawn about the ontogeny of sexual differentiation by failing to observe a sex difference in the nucleus in children. Similarly, a report that the "human SDN" is similar in size in heterosexual and homosexual men (Swaab and Hofman, 1988) does not allow conclusions regarding the ontogeny or neural basis of human sexual orientation. If the nucleus does not show a sex difference, it would not be expected to relate to sex-linked characteristics.

Subsequent reports of sex differences in the human preoptic area may prove to be more reliable. For instance, in a study of four nuclei in the human preoptic area, named the interstitial nuclei of the anterior hypothalamus (INAH) numbers 1, 2, 3 and 4, we found two of the nuclei (INAH 2 and INAH 3) to be larger in men than in women (Allen et al., 1989). Pending additional information on these nuclei, such as neurochemical characterization and localization of steroid receptors, it is not possible to say if either is a human equivalent of the rodent SDN-POA. However, the sex difference in one of the nuclei (INAH 3) has been replicated (LeVay, 1991). Thus, it may provide a useful marker for studying processes involved in human sexual differentiation.

## The corpus callosum

The corpus callosum is the main fiber tract connecting the two hemispheres of the cerebral cortex. It has been estimated to contain two million neuronal fibers (Tomasch, 1954), and its importance to human cognition has been demonstrated by evidence of behavioral abnormalities following abnormal callosal development or callosal damage (Chiarello, 1980; Sparks and Geschwind, 1968; Sperry, 1982). In 1982, the posterior fifth of the callosum, or splenium, was reported to be greater in area, wider, and more bulbous, in women than in men, the difference being particularly marked when splenial area was considered as a function of total brain size (de Lacoste-Utamsing and Holloway, 1982). Subsequently, it was reported that other callosal subregions also show sex differences. The genu, or anterior portion of the callosum, was reported to be larger in men than in women (Reinarz et al., 1988; Witelson, 1989) and, among right-handed individuals, the isthmus, or posterior third minus fifth, was reported to be larger in women than in men (Witelson, 1989).

The corpus callosum can be visualized relatively easily and there have been many attempts to replicate the sex differences, particularly those in the splenium. Some attempts have been successful (Clarke et al., 1989; Reinarz et al., 1988), whereas others have not (Byne et al., 1988). Methodological problems limit the validity of many of the attempted replications (see, e.g., Hines, 1990 for a discussion). In addition, the sex difference may be small or present only in certain subgoups of the population. Related to this possibility is evidence from animal models that experience can influence cortical and hippocampal sex differences (Juraska, 1991). Specifically, in the splenium, patterns of sex differences have been found to relate to the environment in which male and female rats are raised (Juraska and Kopcik, 1988). Sex differences in the number and size of splenial fibres differ in rats raised post-weaning in environmental complexity (group cages with objects available) versus environmental isolation (single housing without objects). In complex environments, female rats have more myelinated axons than do males, whereas the sex difference is reversed for animals raised in isolation. Similarly, the diameter of myelinated axons is greater in males than in females raised in complex environments, but there is no sex difference in animals raised in isolated conditions. In addition to suggesting that environment and experience may be important in development of the splenium and its relationship to sex, these results may help explain the variability in results of studies of sex differences in the human corpus callosum. Specifically, it may be necessary to control for individual differences in developmental history in order to understand patterns of sex differences completely. However, even without extensive data on developmental history, the available data on sex differences in the human corpus callosum suggest that posterior callosal regions tend to be larger in females, while anterior regions may be larger in males, particularly when considered as a function of overall brain size (See Hines, 1990 for further discussion).

Several other regions of the human brain have also been reported to show sex differences, including the massa intermedia (Allen and Gorski, 1987; Morel, 1948; Rabl, 1958), the bed nucleus of the stria terminalis (Allen and Gorski, 1990), the planum temporale (Wada et al., 1975) and the anterior commissure (Allen and Gorski, 1992; Demeter et al., 1988). These reports reinforce the conclusion that sex differences in brain structure are not limited to infrahuman animals, but are characteristic of human beings as well.

# Brain/behavior relationships

One purpose in describing sex differences in human brain structure is the hope of identifying regions of the brain that are involved in regulation of behaviors that show sex differences. Thus far, attempts have been made to relate individual differences in sexually dimorphic brain structures to individual differences in sexually dimorphic behaviors.

## Sexual orientation and the brain

In 1991, it was reported that INAH-3, a nucleus in the human AH/POA that had previously been found to be larger in men than in women (Allen et al., 1989), also varied with sexual orientation among men. The nucleus was found to be larger in heterosexual men than in those who were homosexual or bisexual (LeVay, 1991). In fact, in the homosexual and bisexual men, INAH-3 was similar in volume to the mean for a control group of women. This report generated an extraordinary amount of media attention, and was widely interpreted to indicate that INAH-3 was directly involved in male sexual orientation in human beings. However, although the AH/POA in general has been related to aspects of male sexual behavior, such as mounting, intromission and ejaculation, in experimental animals (Oomura et al., 1983;

Robinson and Mishkin, 1966), INAH-3 is a very small subregion of the AH/POA, and is unlikely, in and of itself, to regulate these behaviors. In addition, even in rodents, where rigorous experiments can be conducted, it is not clear that regions of the AH/POA that show the most dramatic sex differences are those that relate causally to male sexual behavior. For instance, in the rat at least, dorsal POA lesions, but not SDN-POA lesions themselves, have been found to impair male sexual behavior (Arendash and Gorski, 1983). Finally, it is not clear that rodent behaviors such as mounting, intromission and ejaculation are similar conceptually to human sexual orientation.

What then is the cause of a correlation between sexual orientation and the size of INAH-3? One possibility is that whatever factors, including hormonal factors, determine a person's sexual orientation also leave their imprint on the brain. Thus, one might predict that many, or even all, neural regions that show dramatic structural sex differences would differ in individuals differing in the most dramatically sex-typed of human behaviors, sexual orientation. In keeping with this hypothesis, we have found that the size of the splenial region of the corpus callosum, which as described above has been reported to be larger in women than in men, may relate to sexual orientation in women. This result was obtained in the course of a study designed primarily to examine relationships between cognitive sex differences and subregions of the corpus callosum (a study that will be described in detail below). Although sexual orientation was not a major focus of the study, a subset of women in the study completed a questionnaire concerning same-sexed versus opposite-sexed sexual experience. Because the sample was small, conclusions must be tentative. However, our results were consistent with predictions based on the direction of sex differences reported in the splenium and in sexual orientation. Women with a history of some homosexual experience had significantly smaller midsagittal splenial areas than those whose sexual experience involved men only (Hines et al., 1990). Similarly, a recent report suggests that the anterior commissure, another structure with no apparent relationship to sexual or reproductive behavior, shows a sex difference and varies with sexual orientation in men (Allen and Gorski, 1992). The anterior commissure was found to be larger in heterosexual men than in women, and, as was the case for the prior report on INAH-3, homosexual men resembled women in regard to the size of this structure. Interpretation of these data is complicated by a separate report that the anterior commissure shows a sex difference in the opposite direction (i.e., larger in men than in women, see e.g. Demeter et al., 1988). Nevertheless, taken as a whole, the data suggest that many neural regions that vary with sex may vary with sexual orientation as well.

## Sex-typed cognitive function and the brain

The first report of a sex difference in the human corpus callosum suggested that this neural sex differences might relate to cognitive sex differences (de Lacoste-Utamsing and Holloway, 1982). Recent data from my laboratory support this prediction (Hines et al., 1992). We studied a group of normal, healthy women, in whom the corpus callosum was visualized in mid-sagittal section using magnetic resonance imaging (MRI). On a separate occasion, the same group of women completed measures of cognitive traits that show sex differences. Results indicated that the cross sectional surface area of posterior regions of the callosum, particularly the splenium, related positively to verbal fluency and negatively to language lateralization. These data were consistent with predictions based on patterns of sex differences in the callosum and in cognitive traits. Specifically, the data suggest that women with more "female-typical" brain structure also have more "female-typical" cognitive patterns, at least in regard to the verbal characteristics measured. The data are also consistent with information from other areas of inquiry. For instance, human language abilities depend extensively on temporal-parietal-occipital (TPO) association cortex (Penfield and Roberts, 1974), and the interhemispheric fibers connecting left and right TPO association cortices course through the isthmus and splenium of the corpus callosum (de Lacoste et al., 1985; Pandya and Rosene, 1985). In addition, these fibers are more likely to traverse through the splenium in humans than in non-human primates (de Lacoste et al., 1985; Pandya and Rosene, 1985), suggesting that the splenium may be particularly important for interhemispheric transfer of language related information.

As noted above, the splenium was also found to relate to sexual orientation in a subset of this group of women, and it may be that relationships between sex differences in brain structure and sex differences in behavior are non-specific. That is, a common set of factors may determine the range of brain structures that show sex differences as well as the range of behaviors that show sex differences. In this respect, it is important to note that the relationship observed between the splenium and sex-linked verbal traits showed some specificity. Measures of visuospatial abilities that show sex differences were not found to relate to splenial area (Hines et al., 1992). In addition, significant relationships were not observed between other callosal subregions that have been reported to show sex differences (the genu and isthmus) and the sex-related cognitive traits.

# Summary

In experimental animals, administration of androgens or estrogens during critical periods of development causes permanent changes in behaviors that show sex differences. The same hormonal manipulations that alter behavior produce sex-related differences in brain structure and the behavioral changes are thought to result from hormone-induced alterations in basic processes of neural differentiation. Studies of human beings exposed to unusual hormone milieus during development suggest that androgens and estrogens also influence the development of human behaviors that show sex differences. In addition, there are sex differences in human brain structure similar to those described in experimental animals.

Patterns of sex differences in human brain and behavior may help us understand sources of variability in human behaviors that show sex differences. For instance, both sexual orientation and language lateralization have been found to be altered in individuals exposed prenatally to atypical hormone environments (Hines and Green, 1991). In addition, variability in sexual orientation has been found to relate to the size of a sexually dimorphic region in the AH/POA (LeVay, 1991) and variability in verbal fluency and language lateralization has been found to relate to the size of a sexually dimorphic region in the corpus callosum (Hines et al., 1992). It is possible that the hormone-related behavioral differences result in part from hormone-induced changes in brain structure in human beings, as appears to be the case in other species.

The role of experience in development of neural as well as behavioral sex differences can not be discounted, however. For example, although there is an association between the early hormone environment and sexual orientation, this relationship is not one to one. In addition, there is evidence from experimental animal models that patterns of neural sex differences in cortical and hippocampal regions differ depending on the rearing environment of animals. Therefore, although the existence of sex differences in brain structure might at first appear to suggest inherent or immutable sex differences in behavior, alteration and even reversal of these sex differences by post-weaning experience, as well as by the prenatal and neonatal hormonal milieu, suggests neurobehavioral systems that are subject to modification at many points in the lifespan and by many types of factors. The neural sex differences might be viewed most appropriately as "final common pathways" regulating the expression of sex-linked behaviors and reflecting the myriad factors that contribute to their development. Thus, although one value of identifying sex differences in brain structure is their potential for elucidating the neural basis and underlying causes of individual variation in behaviors that show sex differences, it is unlikely that any single approach will provide final answers in this complex domain.

# References

Allen, L. S. and Gorski, R. A. (1987). Sex differences in the human massa intermedia. *Soc. Neurosci. Abstr.,* 13.

Allen, L. S. and Gorski, R. A. (1990). Sex difference in the bed nucleus of the stria terminalis of the human brain. *J. Comp. Neurol.,* **302** : 697-706.

Allen, L. S. and Gorski, R. A. (1992). Sexual orientation and the size of the anterior commissure in the human brain. *Proc. Natl. Acad. Sci. USA.,* **89** : 7199-7202.

Allen, L. S., Hines, M., Shryne, J. E. and Gorski, R. A. (1989). Two sexually dimorphic cell groups in the human brain. *J. Neurosci.,* 9 : 497-506.

Arendash, G. W. and Gorski, R. A. (1983). Effects of discrete lesions of the sexually dimorphic nucleus of the preoptic area or other medial preoptic regions on the sexual behavior of male rats. *Brain Res. Bull.,* **10** : 147-154.

Arnold, A. P. and Gorski, R. A. (1984). Gonadal steroid induction of structural sex differences in the central nervous system. *Ann. Rev. Neurosci.,* 7 : 413-442.

Baker, S. W. and Ehrhardt, A. A. (1974). Prenatal androgen, intelligence and cognitive sex differences. In : Friedman, R. C.,Richart, R. N. and Vande Wiele, R. L. (Ed.), *Sex Differences in Behavior,* Wiley, New York, pp. 53-76.

144

Beatty, W. W. (1979). Gonadal hormones and sex differences in nonreproductive behaviors in rodents : organizational and activational influences. *Horm. Behav.,* **12** : 112-163.

Berenbaum, S. A. and Hines, M. (1992). Early androgens are related to childhood sex-typed toy preferences. *Psychol. Sci.,* **3** : 203-206.

Byne, W., Bleier, R. and Houston, L. (1988). Variations in human corpus callosum do not predict gender : a study using magnetic resonance imaging. *Behav. Neurosci.,* **102** : 222-227.

Chiarello, C. (1980). A house divided? Cognitive functioning with callosal agenesis. *Brain and Language,* **11** : 128-158.

Christensen, L. W. and Gorski, R. A. (1978). Independent masculinization of neuroendocrine systems by intracerebral implants of testosterone or estradiol in the neonatal female rat. *Brain Res.,* **146** : 325-340.

Clark, A. S., MacLusky, N. J. and Goldman-Rakij, P. S. (1988). Androgen binding and metabolism in the cerebral cortex of the developing rhesus monkey.*Endocrinol.,* **123** : 932-940.

Clarke, S., Kraftsik, R., van der Loos, H. and Innocenti, G. M. (1989). Forms and measures of adult and developing human corpus callosum : is there sexual dimorphism? *J. Comp. Neurol.,* **280** : 213-220.

Commins, D. and Yahr, P. (1984). Adult testosterone levels influence the morphology of a sexually dimorphic area in the mongolian gerbil brain. *J. Comp. Neurol.,* **224** : 132-140.

de Lacoste, M. C., Kirkpatrick, J. B. and Ross, E. D. (1985). Topography of the human corpus callosum. *J. Neuropathol. Exper. Neurol.,* **44** : 578-591.

de Lacoste-Utamsing, C. and Holloway, R. L. (1982). Sexual dimorphism in the human corpus callosum. *Science.,* **216** : 1431-1432.

Demeter, S., Ringo, J. L. and Doty, R. W. (1988). Morphometric analysis of the human corpus callosum and anterior commissure. *Human Neurobiol.,* **6** : 219-226.

DiPietro, J. A. (1981). Rough and tumble play : a function of gender. *Develop. Psychol.,* **17** : 50-58.

Dittman, R. W., Kappes, M. E. and Kappes, M. H. (1992). Sexual behavior in adolescent and adult females with congenital adrenal hyperplasia. *Psychoneuroendocrinol.,* **17** : 1-18.

Döhler, K. D., Coquelin, A., Davis, F., Hines, M., Shryne, J. E. and Gorski, R. A. (1984). Pre- and postnatal influence of testosterone propionate and diethylstilbestrol on differentiation of the sexually dimorphic nucleus of the preoptic area in male and female rats. *Brain Res.,* **302** : 291-295.

Edwards, D. A. and Herndon, J. (1970). Neonatal estrogen stimulation and aggressive behavior in female mice. *Physiol. Behav.,* **5** : 993-995.

Ehrhardt, A. A. and Baker, S. W. (1974). Fetal androgens, human central nervous system differentiation, and behavior sex differences. In : Friedman, R. C.,Richart, R. M. and van de Wiele, R. L. (Eds.), *Sex Differences in Behavior,* Wiley, New York, pp. 33-52.

Ehrhardt, A. A., Epstein, R. and Money, J. (1968). Fetal androgens and female gender identity in the early-treated adrenogenital syndrome. *Johns Hopkins Med. J.,* **122** : 165-167.

hrhardt, A. A., Meyer-Bahlburg, H. F. L., Rosen, L. R., Feldman, J. F., Veridiano, N. P., Zimmerman, I. and McEwen, B. S. (1985). Sexual orientation after prenatal exposure to exogenous estrogen. *Arch. Sex. Behav.,* **14** : 57-77.

hrhardt, A. A., Meyer-Bahlburg, H. F. L. and Veridiano, N. P. (1987). Women with a history of prenatal exposure to diethylstilbestrol (DES): sexual functioning and reproductive concerns. In: *Proceedings of the Workshop on Psychosexual and Reproductive Issues Affecting Patients with Cancer,* American Cancer Society, New York, pp. 54-57.

hrhardt, A. A. and Money, J. (1967). Progestin-induced hermaphroditism : IQ and psychosexual identity in a study of ten girls. *J. Sex Res.,* **3** : 83-100.

agot, B. I. (1978). The influence of sex of child on parental reactions to toddler children. *Child Develop.,* **49** : 459-465.

ordon, J. W. and Galatzer, A. (1980). Cerebral organizations in patients with gonadal dysgenesis. *Psychoneuroendocrinol.,* **5** : 235-244.

orski, R. A., Gordon, J. H., Shryne, J. E. and Southam, A. M. (1978). Evidence for a morphological sex difference within the medial preoptic area of the rat brain. *Brain Res.,* **148** : 333-346.

orski, R. A., Harlan, R. E., Jacobson, C. D., Shryne, J. E. and Southam, A. M. (1980). Evidence for the existence of a sexually dimorphic nucleus in the preoptic area of the rat. *J. Comp. Neurol.,* **193** : 529-539.

oy, R. W. (1978). Development of play and mounting behaviour in female rhesus virilized prenatally with esters of testosterone or dihydrotestosterone. In : Chivers, D. J. and Herbert, J. (Eds.), *Recent Advances in Primatology,* Academic Press, New York, pp. 449-462.

oy, R. W., Bercovitch, F. B. and McBrair, M. C. (1988). Behavioral masculinization is independent of genital masculinization in prenatally androgenized female rhesus macagues. *Horm. Behav.,* **22** : 552-571.

oy, R. W. and McEwen, B. S. (1980). *Sexual Differentiation of the Brain.* MIT Press, Cambridge, Massachusetts.

ur, R. C., Mozley, P. D., Resnick, S. M., Gottlieb, G. L., Kohn, M., Zimmerman, R., Herman, G., Atlas, S., Grossman, R., Berretta, D., Erwin, R. and Gur, R. E. (1991). Gender differences in age effect on brain atrophy measured by magnetic resonance imaging. *Proc. Natl. Adac. Sci. USA.,* **88** : 2845-2849.

alpern, D. F. (1987). *Sex Differences in Cognitive Abilities,* Erlbaum, Hillsdale, N.J.

ier, D. B. and Crowley, W. F. (1982). Spatial ability in androgen-deficient men. *N. Engl. J. Med.,* **306** : 1202-1205.

ines, M. (1990). Gonadal hormones and human cognitive development. In : Balthazart, J. (Ed.), *Hormones, Brain and Behaviour in Vertebrates. 1. Sexual Differentiation, Neuroanatomical Aspects, Neurotransmitters and Neuropeptides.,* Karger, Basel, pp. 51-63.

ines, M., Alsum, P., Roy, M., Gorski, R. A. and Goy, R. W. (1987). Estrogenic contributions to sexual differentiation in the female guinea pig : influences of diethylstilbestrol and tamoxifen on neural, behavioral and ovarian development. *Horm. Behav.,* **21** : 402-417.

Hines, M., Chiu, L., McAdams, L. A., Bentler, P. M. and Lipcamon, J. (1992). Cognition and the corpus callosum : verbal fluency, visuospatial ability and language lateralization related to midsagittal surface areas of callosal subregions. *Behav. Neurosci.,* **106** : 3-14.

Hines, M., Davis, F. C., Coquelin, A., Goy, R. W. and Gorski, R. A. (1985). Sexually dimorphic regions in the medial preoptic area and the bed nucleus of the stria terminalis of the guinea pig brain : a description and an investigation of their relationship to gonadal steroids in adulthood. *J. Neurosci.,* **5** : 40-47.

Hines, M. and Goy, R. W. (1985). Estrogens before birth and development of sex-related reproductive traits in the female guinea pig. *Horm. Behav.,* **19** : 331-347.

Hines, M. and Green, R. (1991). Human hormonal and neural correlates of sex-typed behaviors. *Rev. Psychiat.,* **10** : 536-555.

Hines, M., Green, R., Chiu, L. and Lipcamon, J. (1990). Corpus callosum shape and sexual orientation in women. (submitted for publication).

Hines, M. and Shipley, C. (1984). Prenatal exposure to diethylstilbestrol (DES) and the development of sexually dimorphic cognitive abilities and cerebral lateralization. *Develop. Psychol.,* **20** : 81-94.

Holman, S. D. and Hutchison, J. B. (1991). Lateralized action of androgen on development of behavior and brain sex differences. *Brain Res. Bull.,* **27** : 261-265.

Hyde, J. S. (1990). *Understanding Human Sexuality,* McGraw Hill, New York.

Juraska, J. M. (1991). Sex differences in "cognitive" regions of the rat brain. *Psychoneuroendocrinol.,* **16** : 105-119.

Juraska, J. M. and Kopcik, J. R. (1988). Sex and environmental influences on the size and ultrastructure of the rat corpus callosum. *Brain Res.,* **450** : 1-8.

Kester, P., R., G., Finch, S. J. and Williams, K. (1980). Prenatal 'female hormone' administration and psychosexual development in human males. *Psychoneuroendocrinol.,* **5** : 269-285.

King, B. M., Camp, C. J. and Downey, A. M. (1991). *Human Sexuality Today,* Prentice Hall, Englewood Cliffs, New Jersey.

Kinsey, A., Pomeroy, W. and Martin, C. (1948). *Sexual Behavior in the Human Male,* Saunders, Philadelphia.

Kinsey, A., Pomeroy, W. and Martin, C. (1953). *Sexual Behavior in the Human Female,* Saunders, Philadelphia.

Lev-Ran, A. (1974). Sexuality and educational levels of women with the late-treated adrenogenital syndrome. *Arch. Sex. Behav.,* **3** : 27-32.

LeVay, S. (1991). A difference in hypothalamic structure between heterosexual and homosexual men. *Science.,* **253** : 1034-1037.

Linn, M. C. and Petersen, A. C. (1985). Emergence and characterization of sex differences in spatial ability : a meta-analysis. *Child Develop.,* **56** : 1479-1498.

Maccoby, E. E. and Jacklin, C. N. (1974). *The Psychology of Sex Differences,* Stanford University Press, Stanford, CA.

McEwen, B. S., Lieberburg, I., Chaptal, C. and Krey, L. C. (1977a). Aromatization : important for sexual differentiation of the neonatal rat brain. *Horm. Behav.,* **9** : 249-263.

McEwen, B. S., Lieberburg, I., MacLusky, N. and Plapinger, L. (1977b). Do estrogen receptors play a role in the sexual differentiation of the rat brain? *J. Steroid Biochem.,* **8** : 593-598.

McGlone, J. (1980). Sex differences in human brain asymmetry : a critical survey. *Behav. Brain Sci.,* **3** : 215-263.

McGuire, L. S., Ryan, K. O. and Omenn, G. S. (1975). Congenital adrenal hyperplasia II : cognitive and behavioral studies. *Behav. Genet.,* **5** : 175-188.

Meaney, M. J. and Stewart, J. (1981). Neonatal androgens influence the social play of prepubescent rats. *Horm. Behav.,* **15** : 197-213.

Money, J. (1973). Turner's syndrome and parietal lobe functions. *Cortex,* **9** : 387-393.

Money, J. and Schwartz, M. (1976). Fetal androgens in the early treated adrenogenital syndrome of 46XX hermaphroditism : influence on assertive and aggressive types of behavior. *Aggres. Behav.,* **2** : 19-30.

Money, J., Schwartz, M. and Lewis, V. (1984). Adult erotosexual status and fetal hormonal masculinization and demasculinization : 46 XX congenital virilizing adrenal hyperplasia and 46 XY androgen-insensitivity syndrome compared. *Psychoneuroendocrinol.,* **9** : 405-414.

Morel, R. (1948). La massa intermedia ou commissure grise. *Acta Anat.,* **4** : 203-207.

Oomura, Y., Yoshimatsu, H. and Aou, S. (1983). Medial preoptic and hypothalamic neuronal activity during sexual behavior of the male monkey. *Brain Res.,* **266** : 340-343.

Pandya, D. N. and Rosene, D. L. (1985). Some observations on trajectories and topography of commissural fibers. In : Reeves, A. G. (Ed.). *Epilepsy and the Corpus Callosum,* Plenum, New York, pp. 21-39.

Penfield, W. and Roberts, L. (1974). *Speech and Brain Mechanisms,* Athenum, New York.

Pfaff, D. W. and Keiner, M. (1973). Atlas of estradiol-concentrating cells in the central nervous system of the female rat. *J. Comp. Neurol.,* **151** : 121-158.

Quadagno, D. M., Briscoe, R. and Quadagno, J. S. (1977). Effects of perinatal gonadal hormones on selected nonsexual behavior patterns: a critical assessment of the nonhuman and human literature. *Psychol. Bull.,* **84** : 62-80.

Rabl, R. (1958). Strukturstudien an der massa intermedia des thalamus opticus. *J. Hirnf.,* **4** : 78-112.

Reinarz, S. J., Coffman, C. E., Smoker, W. R. K. and Godersky, F. C. (1988). MR imaging of the corpus callosum : normal and pathologic findings and correlation with CT. *Amer. J. Radiol.,* **151** : 791-798.

Reinisch, J. M. (1981). Prenatal exposure to synthetic progestins increases potential for aggression in humans. *Science.,* **211** : 1171-1173.

Reinisch, J. M. and Karow, W. G. (1977). Prenatal exposure to synthetic progestins and estrogens : effects on human development. *Arch. Sex. Behav.,* **6** : 257-288.

148

Resnick, S. M. (1982). *Psychological Functioning in Individuals with Congenital Adrenal Hyperplasia : Early Hormonal Influences on Cognition and Personality,* Doctoral dissertation, University of Minnesota.

Resnick, S. M., Berenbaum, S. A., Gottesman, I. I. and Bouchard, T. (1986). Early hormonal influences on cognitive functioning in congenital adrenal hyperplasia. *Develop. Psychol.,* **22** : 191-198.

Robinson, B. W. and Mishkin, M. (1966). Ejaculation evoked by stimulation of the preoptic area in monkeys. *Physiol. Behav.,* **1** : 269-272.

Rovet, J. and Netley, C. (1982). Processing deficits in Turner's syndrome. *Develop. Psychol.,* **18** : 77-94.

Smail, P. J., Reyes, F. I., Winter, J. S. D. and Faiman, C. (1981). The fetal hormone environment and its effect on the morphogenesis of the genital system. In : Kogan, S. J. and Hafez, E. S. E. (Eds.), *Pediatric Andrology,* Martinus Nijhoff, The Hague, pp. 9-20.

Snow, M. E., Jacklin, C. N. and Maccoby, E. E. (1983). Sex of child differences in father-child interaction at one year of age. *Child Develop.,* **54** : 227-232.

Sparks, R. and Geschwind, N. (1968). Dichotic listening in man after section of neocortical commissures. *Cortex.,* **4** : 3-16.

Sperry, R. (1982). Some effects of disconnecting the cerebral hemispheres. *Science.,* **217** : 1223-1226.

Stumpf, W. E. and Grant, C. D. (1975). *Anatomical Neuroendocrinology,* Basel : Karger.

Stumpf, W. E., Sar, M. and Keefer, D. A. (1975). Atlas of estrogen target cells in rat brain. In : Stumpf, W. E. and Grant, C. D. (Eds.), *Anatomical Neuroendocrinology,* Karger, Basel, pp. 104-119.

Sutton-Smith, B., Rosenberg, B. G. and Morgan, E. F. Jr. (1963). Development of sex differences in play choices during preadolescence. *Child Develop.,* **34** : 119-126.

Swaab, D. and Hofman, M. (1988). Sexual differentiation of the human hypothalamus : ontogeny of the sexually dimorphic nucleus of the preoptic area. *Develop. Brain Res.,* **44** : 314-318.

Swaab, D. F. and Fliers, E. (1985). A sexually dimorphic nucleus in the human brain. *Science.,* **228** : 1112-1115.

Tobet, S. A., Zahniser, D. J. and Baum, M. J. (1986). Sexual dimorphism in the preoptic/anterior hypothalamic area of ferrets : effects of adult exposure to sex steroids. *Brain Res.,* **364** : 249-257.

Tomasch, J. (1954). Size, distribution, and number of fibres in the human corpus callosum. *Anat. Rec.,* **119** : 119-135.

Wada, J. A., Clarke, R. and Hamm, A. (1975). Cerebral hemispheric asymmetry in humans. *Arch. Neurol.,* **32** : 239-246.

Williams, C. L. and Meck, W. H. (1991). The organizational effects of gonadal steroids on sexually dimorphic spatial ability. *Psychoneuroendocrinol.,* **16** : 155-176.

Witelson, W. F. (1989). Hand and sex differences in the isthmus and genu of the human corpus callosum : a postmortem morphological study. *Brain,* **112** : 799-835.

Yalom, I. D., Green, R. and Fisk, N. (1973). Prenatal exposure to female hormones : effect on psychosexual development in boys. *Arch. Gen. Psychiat.,* **28** : 554-561.

Zucker, K. J., Bradley, S. J., Loiver, G., Hood, J. E., Blake, J. and Fleming, S. (1992). Psychosexual assessment of women with congenital adrenal hyperplasia : preliminary analyses. *Abstracts : International Academy of Sex Research,* Prague.

# Are Sex or Gender Relevant Categories to Language Performance ? A Critical Review

M. KAIL

Laboratoire de Psychologie Expérimentale, Université René Descartes, URA CNRS 316, 28 rue Serpente 75006 Paris, France

The study of sex differences (or similarities) in language is clearly an integral part of the wider investigative frame of interactions between social and biological processes. The seminal work on this subject, Maccoby and Jacklin's"The Psychology of Sex Differences"(1974), covers a broad range of studies on this topic and discusses the state of the art of that time. The first distinguishing feature of this volume is that it presents an exhaustive critical overview of the literature on this topic published between 1965 and 1973, and cites more than 1400 studies on samples ranging in age from 1 day to adulthood. Its second feature is that it demonstrates that this area of research is particularly prone to bias, as Sherman and Denmark (1978) point out. This bias arises from an unchallenged position that sex differences have an impact, from a belief that sex differences exist.

Among these biases, which can arise from choice of experimental techniques (data generation) as well as from the dissemination of information, in particular pressure to publish, the major ones include:
- stressing differences, regardless of how minimal they are, and inflating their impact, while dismissing similarities which have less chance of being published
- viewing sex as a causal factor, and not taking other sources of variation into account.

Maccoby and Jacklin suggest classifying the most widely shared beliefs about sex differences into three categories: beliefs which are unfounded, beliefs which have received a fair amount of support (girls are superior to boys in verbal ability, boys are superior to girls in visuo-spatial tasks and in mathematics, and boys are more aggressive) and beliefs where there is not enough empirical data (tactile sensitivity, anxiety, level of activity and competitiveness). One of the major criticisms of the Maccoby and Jacklin book was formulated by Block (1976) who argued that contrary to the Maccoby and Jacklin contention, boys and girls are socialized differently as of birth, which makes it practically impossible to segregate out biological factors from

M. Haug et al. (eds.), The Development of Sex Differences and Similarities in Behavior, 151–174.
© 1993 Kluwer Academic Publishers.

environmental ones. In addition, the available data are not as unequivocal as Maccoby and Jacklin claim. Some of the cognitive differences they consider to be founded are not as firmly established as they assume, in particular as regards to verbal abilities, as will be shown below. Furthermore, as Fairweather (1976) points out, Maccoby and Jacklin appear to consider that any genuine psychological difference has a biological foundation. The best example is that of brain lateralization, which implies the notion of an innate determinism, built into the anatomical substrate and the neurophysiological functions.

## Sex differences in the lateralization of language: controversial and inconclusive evidence

The main kinds of information which are currently considered to be evidence for sex differences in language-related cognition relate in one way or another to differences in lateralization or hemispheric differentiation of language processing.

The left cerebral hemisphere has been found to be more involved in the processing of linguistic information, whereas the right hemisphere has been found to be more involved in the processing of nonlinguistic stimuli. For example, stimuli such as faces, complex designs, environmental sounds and melodies have been shown to be more efficiently processed by the right hemisphere, and stimuli such as printed or spoken words are more efficiently processed by the left hemisphere.

Nevertheless, on the basis of commissurotomized patients, it has been suggested that the left hemisphere may be more specialized for analytic processing and the right for gestalt processing (Levy and Trevarthen, 1977; Nebes, 1971, 1972, 1973, 1974). In a study on hemispheric specialization for serial and parallel processing, Cohen (1973) reported a tendency for the left hemisphere to process letter stimuli serially and for the right hemisphere to do so in parallel or holistically, but a tendency for both hemispheres to process unnameable shapes holistically. Patterson and Bradshaw (1975) used schematic faces with a same-different matching paradigm and found that the left hemisphere tended to operate analytically and the right by gestalt matching. Similarly, a study by Martin (1979) using the Stroop test to investigate hemispheric specialization in right handed adults, showed that the processing of local aspects of a linguistic stimulus is more efficient in the left hemisphere, whereas global processing does not appear to be strongly lateralized.

Investigations of the correlation beween sex and brain organization have a long history, but have received considerably more attention in the last twenty years. The importance of works on sex differences in brain lateralization (primarily published in Neuropsychologia, Cortex, Brain and Language) is that these studies draw direct connections between cognitive differences and structural differences in the brain or in brain functioning. In 1980, McGlone published a critical overview in Behavioral and Brain Sciences which has become a reference in the field of sex differences and brain assymmetry. McGlone argues that evidence from brain-damaged patients shows that men's and women's speech is impaired differently when there is trauma to the same areas. Women present less impairment of speech than men overall when the left hemisphere is traumatized, suggesting greater involvement of both hemispheres in language processing and less hemispheric specialization of cognitive functions than for men.

Aside from this overview, McGlone's article contains commentaries of thirty three well known researchers in the field and her own responses to their commentaries. The value of McGlone's work, who is convinced that men's brains are more asymmetrical than women's, is her careful analysis of all the studies she reviews, including works whose theses run counter her own. She reviews fourteen studies on verbal ability in men and women which use the classic experimental technique in the area, namely dichotic listening. Dichotic listening has proved to be a reliable behavioral measure of hemispheric specialization of the processing of auditory stimuli. In a dichotic listening task, different stimuli are presented simultaneously to each ear, via earphones. The validity of this paradigm is based on the assumption that stimuli presented to each ear are processed more efficiently by the contralateral hemisphere. When the stimuli presented are verbal or analytic in nature, such as spoken syllables or words, there is a right ear (left hemisphere) advantage in correctly reporting the stimuli. When the stimuli are non-speech or more holistic in nature such as melodies, there is a left ear (right hemisphere) advantage in correctly reporting the stimuli.

Nine of the fourteen studies cited in the McGlone article report no relationship between subject gender and degree of superiority of the right ear. Four report superiority of the right ear in men (corroborational finding) and one reports superiority of the right ear in women.

McKeever (1987) presents an overview of work using tachistoscopic tasks which have been shown to be a reliable measure of hemispheric specialization of the processing of visual stimuli. This task involves rapid simultaneous visual presentations of different stimuli, one to each visual field (right and left of a central fixation point). Stimuli in each visual field are processed in the contralateral hemisphere. The hemisphere that is specialized for the visual material presented processes the stimuli more efficiently. The typical finding is that verbal or analytic material presented visually (i.e. words) are processed more efficiently in the right visual field (left hemisphere) and non linguistic or more holistic visually presented stimuli (faces or nonsense designs) are processed more efficiently in the left visual field (right hemisphere). Out of about twenty visual laterality task studies, only five found a sex difference, and one of these (MacKeever and Van Deventer, 1977) found females more lateralized than males. The results in general are not supportive of the hypothesis of greater verbal function laterality in females since about 12% of the dichotic and 27% of the tachistoscopic study results found females to be less lateralized. Similarly, in a review of sex differences in visual laterality, Fairweather (1982) showed that five out of forty nine studies that reported males to be more lateralized, two studies indicated females to be more lateralized and forty two studies found no sex differences whatsoever.

Piazza (1980) points out that many studies that have assessed the effect of sex or lateralization of function have neglected the potential effect of handedness. Piazza found that handedness, familial sinistrality and sex all affect hemispheric specialization. However the effects of these factors differ as a function of the task. In general, left handedness (and familial sinistrality) is associated with atypical or bilateral hemispheric specialization. Sex interacts with handedness and familial sinistrality in the lateralization of the auditory tasks used, but sex does not influence processing of visually presented stimuli (words and faces) in this study. Similarly, McKeever and Hoff (1982), McKeever et al. (1983) stress that the relationship between cerebral organization and sex is interesting but complex. They present evidence that sex is a factor, if it is considered relative to familial sinistrality. In a tachistoscopic task, females lacking familial sinistrality and males with familial sinistrality have smaller right visual field superiority than females with familial sinistrality and males who do not.

More recently, investigators have attempted to relate the cerebral specialization of brain function to changes in electrophysiological measures (EEG and evoked potential) recorded from the surface of the scalp in normal individuals. What differentiates evoked potential from the more traditional EEG measure is that the event-related potential (ERP) is a portion of the ongoing EEG activity of the brain; i.e. it is time-locked (Molfese, 1990) to the onset of some event in the subject's environment.

Electrophysiological investigations tend to support those using other techniques showing differential functioning between the two hemispheres. Studies on adults (Morrell and Salamy, 1971; Molfese et al.,1975) found that auditory evoked potentials produced by speech sounds were significantly higher in amplitude in the left temporal area than the right. However, other studies (Tanguy, 1976; Gevins et al., 1980, 1981) failed to obtain a differential effect of this type.

As regards the relationship between sex and visual event related potentials (ERPs), Friedman et al., (1985) found effects of sex on P550 and slow Wave (SW) components of ERPs in response to continuous performance. Females presented larger P550 activity for non target than for target stimuli whereas males did not exhibit this difference. Picton et al., (1984) also reported sex differences on the visual P3 for target stimuli which are significantly larger in females than in males.

Regardless of method of investigation, the inconsistency of the findings is based on the underestimation of certain variables such as the nature of the task. Bradshaw and Gates (1978) attempted to account for possible differential involvement of the left hemisphere as a function of type of task. They showed that a manual response in a lexical decision task tends to produce consistent right field advantages in males but not in females. Yet, when an oral report of the same kind of stimuli is required, both sexes appeared to be more equally lateralized. The findings may imply that females may be more consistently lateralized to the left hemisphere for a language task that is more productive in nature such as oral reporting, and less lateralized for a language discrimination task such as lexical decision.

What emerges clearly is that task requirement is an important variable to take into account in studies of sex differences in laterality. Attentional biases have been shown to interact with performance on visual laterality tasks (Kinsbourne, 1973, 1975). In their experiment, Healy et al., (1985) used different linguistic tasks - discrimination vs production and control of attention. The findings show that for language discrimination, the sexes were fairly equally lateralized whereas on production tasks, females showed greater laterality differences. The attempt to control for attention resulted in higher field differences in particular for females. These findings suggest that females, rather than being less lateralized for language functions, may be lateralized in a somewhat different way, a conclusion which has also been reached by Inglis et al., (1982).

As a theoretical rationale, it has been argued (Geschwind and Galaburda, 1985) that cerebral dominance is based in most instances on asymmetries of structure. The authors assume that language lateralization depends to a great extent on the size of the planum temporale, which is larger on the left side in about 65% of all brains (Geschwind and Levitsky, 1968). In adult women, the planum temporale shows increased development on the right side as compared to that of males (Kelly, 1981; Wada et al., 1975 ; Wittelson and Pallie, 1973). This difference is not found in infancy.

The apparent change in structure with age is consistent with the proposals put forward by Lenneberg (1966, 1967) and Zangwill (1960) that a critical period of neurological development responsible for the observed differences in language development occurs between the ages of 2 and 12 years. According to Waber, (1976, 1977) rapid maturation leads to increased bilateral language representation in the brain. Waber suggested that sex differences arise from the relatively faster rate of physical development seen in girls as compared to boys. The slower maturation rate in males is thought to allow for increased lateralization of language: available cortical areas of the nondominant hemisphere are then dedicated to visual spatial function an area in which males usually demonstrate superior performance.

Commenting on the Weber theory, Fairweather (1976) writes:

*"A recent speculation in terms of maturation rate is embarassed factually by a failure to find a sex difference. And logically by a miscued syllogism: early maturers differ, cognitively from late maturers; girls mature earlier than boys, therefore sex differences in cognition are a function of maturation rate. The first "premise" awaits substantial replication; the second awaits verification for psychologically relevant indices, and the conclusion is not possible since it contains more information than the premises,i.e. that there are sex differences, a statement which as we have seen, requires considerable qualification"*

Another theory put forward by Geschwind and Galaburda (1985) postulates that left hemisphere language dominance and right handedness reflect the normal differential rates of growth of the cerebral hemispheres during fetal life.

According to their view, the normal differential rates can be influenced by exposure of the fetus to excessive testosterone. They suggested that such fetal exposure or unusual sensitivity to testosterone could slow the growth of the left hemisphere and that this retardation could allow the right hemisphere to compete more effectively for control of mechanisms for which the left hemisphere would normally have been dominant. In a more recent version, Galaburda et al., (1987) suggested that excessive fetal testosterone exposure accelerates the development of right hemisphere, rather than slowing down the growth of the left hemisphere. But, as stressed by Rich and McKeever, (1990) this *"does not alter the postulated final effect of a weakening of preprogrammed left hemisphere dominance"*.

Finally, it has been hypothesized that the corpus callosum could play an important role in hemispheric integration and possibly in hemispheric specialization (Wittelson, 1985). Larger parts of this interhemispheric tract found in females (De Lacoste-Utamsing and Holloway, 1982) and left handers may imply larger numbers of fibers which possibly provide the anatomical basis for a greater connectivity between the hemispheres. This may be associated with greater functional bilateralization. Recently, Hassler (1990) found that the relationship between lateral dominance and cognitive variables was influenced by sex and musical talents and the ability to paint. Her results seem to support the assumption that left hemisphere and right hemisphere functions contributing to processes associated with verbal processing are more effectively integrated in musicians than in non musicians, as in females and left-handers.

As a conclusion to this section devoted to sex differences and lateralization, several comments are in order. First of all, methodological caution is a necessity, as pointed out by Alper (1985) in an excellent paper entitled "Sex differences in Brain Asymmetry, a critical analysis". The main methodological flaws are the following: - selection of a sample of subjects which is generally too small, in clinical studies of brain asymmetry no sampling is done at all, and in experimental studies, subjects are students. In both cases, studies are not justified in assuming that sex differences observed in the study exist in the general population. Secondly the choice of cognitive tasks raises a number of problems, because there is no theory which explains which tests of cognitive function are relevant to the study of brain function. Thirdly, Alper presents different instances where there is a confounding of purely biological variables and environmental variables. For example, the different environments women and men experience could be responsible for differences in brain structure and function which in turn could lead to cognitive differences. A hypothesis of this type has been put forward suggesting that the brains of Japanese and Western children develop differently over the course of their learning very different types of languages (Shibatani, 1980).

Even in interactive models where genetic and environmental differences act in concert to produce cognitive differences, confounding biological variables have been reported and discussed by the commentators of McGlone's review (1980). For example, Martin (1980) notes that *"normal differences in cerebral vascularization between men and women, as well as consistent differences in the locus and extent of vascular accidents between the sexes may account completely for the differences in testing results".* Similarly, Mc Guiness (1980) found that men are more right eared than women and that this difference rather than brain differences is responsible for the sex differences found in dichotic listening tests. Finally, Alper discusses how behavioral differences are evaluated.

Statistical tests determine whether a difference is significant. Alper shows that intra-group variation is generally greater than inter-group variation, which in most cases is extremely small and the distributions overlap. (A detailed analysis by Hurtig and Pichevin (1991a) on various areas of differential psychology of sex differences reaches the same conclusions). He concludes that sex as a factor has low predictive value. Furthermore, small differences which are found to be statistically significant are not necessarily meaningful, in particular because there are no theoretical restrictions on the number of variables available to investigation: anatomical features, electrophysiological indicators, etc...

Alper's conclusion is that modern theories of sex differences in brain structure and function are based on the presumption that the sexes are characterized by innate differences in cognitive abilities.

Given the fact that intragroup variation is so much larger than intergroup variation, why is there so much interest in intergroup differences? McGlone herself (1980) provides one answer: *"One must not overlook perhaps the most obvious conclusion, which is that basic patterns of male and female brain asymmetry seem to be more similar than they are different. Nevertheless, it is only by focusing on those differences that our knowledge of brain function will expand".*

Alper (1985) fails to be convinced by this argument: *"The research field exists because sex is an interesting and important category in our culture, not because it has proved to have any particular relevance for an understanding of brain function".* I will return later to this issue.

My final theoretical comment is related to the generalization to language in reports of findings on highly specific tasks. Language is a complex phenomenon with multiple facets and no firm conclusions should be drawn before a detailed analysis of the different features of language - lexicon, syntax, semantic, and pragmatic features - has been carried out. This holds for both clinical and experimental studies. Labelling studies as well as verbal identification studies in dichotic listening tasks are only one extremely restricted area of linguistic competence.

# Sex differences in language acquisition: equally controversial and inconclusive evidence

Maccoby and Jacklin (1974) state in their extensive survey that *"female superiority on verbal tasks has been one of the more solidly established generalizations in the field of sex differences and recent research continues to* support the generalization to a degree". Merz (1979) states that " everybody is convinced that girls and women do speak better than men and boys. Empirical investigations confirm this general stereotype".

The analysis below is restricted to the developmental psycholinguistic aspects of this general stereotype. The issue is the following: in what way, if any, does the sex of a child influence his or her language acquisition? The data reviewed here rely heavily on an overview by Klann-Delius (1981). I focus on empirical studies dealing with the beginnings of language acquisition, phonological development, the development of syntax and semantics, and studies focusing on the acquisition of pragmatic rules and general communicative abilities.

## The beginnings of language acquisition

It has been reported that girls not only start speaking earlier but also talk more than boys. Some researchers have found that preverbal girls vocalize more frequently than boys, but others have failed to replicate this difference. What kind of significance this different preverbal behavior may have on the development of language is however another question.

Studies on the onset of speech as measured by age at use of the first words also show a slight tendency for girls to be earlier, but the trends are not statistically significant. Mean length of utterance (MLU) has also been shown to correlate at early stages with the complexity of a child's grammar. However, measures of MLU at times favor girls and at other times, boys.

## Phonological development

Empirical studies have shown that during the first year of life boys and girls do not differ for the acoustic qualities of their utterances (Murry et al. 1975; Murry et al., 1977). Strikingly, however, from the age of three on the voices of boys and girls differ to the extent that the gender of a child can be guessed correctly on the basis of voice alone (Edwards, 1979).

Learning to read seems to be less difficult for girls than for boys. Pathological retardation in language development and speech impediments such as stuttering occur more often in boys than in girls (Eme, 1979; Fairweather, 1976). Analyses of phonetic and phonological development indicate that there are sex differences in articulatory style between boys and girls.

## Development of syntax and semantics

Empirical research on the first phases of syntax development rarely relates to sex differences. Ramer (1976) found that girls were faster than boys in progressing from their first two word utterances to the use of syntactically more advanced subject-verb complement constructions. Whether girls are faster than boys in later acquisition of syntactic categories and relatives is controversial. No consistent sex differences have been reported for vocabulary or lexicon structure.

# The development of communicative competence

Up to the age of one and a half to two, girls are reported to have more sustained and frequent exchanges with their mothers (or caretakers). There are however few systematic studies. A contrast has been reported in communicative attitudes (girls tending towards relationships with others, boys tending to privilege object relationships) but there is no clearcut evidence for differences in competence: both boys and girls at roughly age four are able to adjust their utterances to the situation (Shatz and Gelman, 1973; Sachs and Devin, 1976). At about age 7, they are both able to take role into account (mother, father, children; see Andersen, 1978), and later, at about age 11 realize that certain features of language are associated with gender roles in a stereotyped fashion (Edelsky, 1976).

These studies stress that one of the determinants of language acquistion is the type of social environment, which is known to differ for boys and girls. Overall, these studies indicate that girls are the subjects of more linguistic stimulation in the first years of life but that once school starts the reverse is true: teachers tend to talk more with boys than with girls, because boys are harder to discipline and have a harder time adapting to school norms, in particular as regards language (Cherry, 1975; Dittmann, 1977; Maccoby and Jacklin, 1974).

It is obvious that these studies are influenced by representations of child socialization. Those which stress the effect of motherese (Snow, 1972; Ringler, 1973) - the impact of the mother's specific language behavior on the development of the child's communicative competence - show almost no differences as regards gender.

Recently Gleason (1987) reported on a series of studies on sex differences in the language of two to five year old American middle class children and their caretakers. An explicit effort is made to draw connections between the language produced by the children and the inputs to them. Gleason argues that language input to children is linked to sex in two ways: as a function of target and as a function of the source of the message. The language variables analyzed are lexical selection and politeness (politeness routines, interruptions, and directness of directives). On some variables, Gleason found differences in input language tied to the sex of the parent as speaker, but not to the sex of children as addressee. For example, she reports that fathers used more sophisticated vocabulary items than mothers to their children of both sexes. This provocative result needs further confirmation. Similarly, with respect to other variables (directives and imperatives) Gleason found differences in language use tied to the sex of both source and target. Fathers interrupt children more than mothers. Parents of both sexes interrupt girls more than boys. Fathers use more direct imperatives than mothers, in particular to boys.

On the theoretical level, the mechanisms of transmission remain difficult to disentangle. The socializing effect of motherese seems to be relevant to language development only insofar as it meets the development-specific concepts of language structure the child has formed him or herself in a way which is relatively autonomous of the linguistic surroundings (Newport et al., 1977). This effect appears to be limited to cognitive procedures of assimilation and analysis of information, both of which are presumably not sex-related.

In contrast, socialization concepts which derive from the theory of identification predict differences: the main claim is that the child acquires features of his or her environment in a way that is directly proportional to the extent that these features correspond to traits or expectations conveyed by the person who is the object of the child's libidinal investment. Changes are expected to take place over the course of development as a function of changes in the libidinal object, and differences in parental language behavior are assumed to be reflected in the child's language.

There is no doubt that a child's interactions with the social environment - which vehicles sex-role differentiation - need to be incorporated in any theory of language development. Nevertheless, the level of theorization remains weak and empirical work in this area reflects this conceptual fuzziness. However, it is worth noting that the concept of difference in terms of absence has been discarded, and that there have been efforts in particular in the area of social interaction theory to define those areas of behavior where differences in the semantico-pragmatic features of language can be expected (see Klann-Delius, 1981).

Nevertheless, the issue of the relationship between sex and language acquisition cannot be resolved solely on the basis of empirical studies. The findings are contradictory and above all flawed by conceptual and methodological weaknesses. Aside from the obstacles mentioned formerly (in particular intra/intergroup variations and low statistical validity) there are other problems with the specific area of analysis of language behavior. The first problem is related to choice of linguistic reference model and differences in the ways models segment language activities (i.e. word, sentence, utterance, or longer discourse strings). Isolated linguistic items which are relevant on one level of analysis may not be qualitatively or quantitively relevant on others. For example, children are able to express completely different intentions in utterances of the same length (Lieven, 1978). Thus the relevance of unit of analysis can vary as a function of level of development. For example, as a function of developmental level, a child may choose to give the maximum amount of information, and thus to produce longer utterances, or in contrast to adapt to the situation and only produce ellipses (Wells, 1978). Thus the validity of MLU as a measure is entirely relative.

This latter example points indirectly the particularly thorny problem of the relationship between the implicit and the explicit which arises almost immediately when dealing with the development of pragmatic skills and communicative competence. Here again, choice of linguistic reference model is critical, and empirical studies on sex differences in this area have themselves been regrettably implicit as to their options.

Lastly, there are virtually no longitudinal studies on sex differences. Most works are cross sectional, and only deal with specific areas of language development, and hence provide extrapolated starting points which are uninformative as to the central issue of those mechanisms of language acquisition which are specifically sex-linked, and changes over the course of development. Exploring this issue calls for empirical grounding in a theoretical model of the relationships between gender and language. Without a model of this type, language acquistion data will remain fuzzy, contradictory, non-replicable and unexploitable in terms of a better understanding of language processing and sex differences.

Two overall conclusions can be drawn from these studies. The first is that the existence of biological differences in the structure of brain organization and function is open to question. The second is that language acquisition data provides no support for the contention that the sexes differ for either acquisition mechanisms or language development. On the contrary, similarities appear to dominate. Clearly, as Steele (1987) points out *"the link between the two kinds of work is more abstract".* In fact even though the neurophysiological literature suggests that there are systematic differences between males and females, these differences do not touch on the basic cognitive capacities involved in the language acquisition process. There is no reason to believe that eventual differences discussed at one level are the basis for the differences assumed to exist at another level.

## Sex revisited: some new perspectives

The issues and comments developed here in deal with sex as a locus of real theoretical upheaval in both Psychology and Linguistics. New theories have arisen from doubt as regards the sex variable. Sex has emerged as a constructed variable, and as such contrasts with the commonly held view that sex is a *sui generis* variable, a given.

In their discussion of the status of the sex variable in psychology, Hurtig and Pichevin (1985) show that in the vast majority of studies, the sex variable has been ignored, marginalized or masked (Maccoby and Jacklin, 1974; Grady, 1979; Unger, 1979 a,b). General psychology is "blind" to the sex of its subjects.When the sex variable is not ignored, it is however not defined. Sex is generally construed as a given, beyond the scope of scientific investigation, or more precisely as a given with a preestablished scientific value.

Sex is considered to be a biological given which dichotomizes homo- sapiens into two clearly distinct categories, whose psychological and social attributes devolve "naturally" from the biological difference. These attributes are themselves dichotomized to define the masculine and feminine spheres. This allows the data to adhere to naive common sense, and to form a postulate that escapes scientific inquiry.

Biological sex has thus been elevated to the status of explanatory principle. The sex principle has been posited in the majority of cases without even the most elementary precautions to account for differences that are seen as the links between the biological and the social. Practically all the studies cited in the first section of this chapter fall into this category: language differences are expected to exist as a function of sex and are accounted for in terms of sex.

This leads to an implicit theory of sex differences based on illusory beliefs, which in turn however create a set of norms and ideals individuals invoke to justify their behavior (Grady, 1977, 1981).

This concept of sex does not totally skirt the problem of the relationship between the sexes. However the issue is restricted to a relationship of "natural" complementarity, since it is linked to reproduction. As Star (1979) Hubbard and Lowe (1979), Hubbard et al., (1979) have contended, there are no innate sex differences which are not directly linked to reproduction.

In classic studies on sex differences, the sex variable is identified as the genetic, chromosomal sex. However sex is a composite, multidimensional reality and, as a function of level of description, can be broken down into various components such as genetic sex, gonadic sex, endocrinian sex, anatomical sex, sex determination at birth, psychological sex, etc. Works by Money and Ehrhardt (1972) on individuals with discordancies between these different chromosomal, hormonal and morphological sex components suggest that the strength of the correlation between these components is likely to be lower than formerly believed. Studies on transexualism (Stoller, 1968) corroborate this contention, and stress the flexibility and malleability of the genetic system, including dimorphic sex programming which is not as absolute as was thought in the past (Eisenberg, 1978).

The issue of the genetic determinism of sex itself has undergone constant revision. After having shown that the Y chromosome could not be the sole factor in sexual differentiation, the HY antigen was the most promising factor in the 1980s. More recently, researchers have opted for ZFY genes (Page, 1986) which have currently been supplanted by SRY genes. However, as Peyre et al., (1991) point out, the search for the "sex" gene, which would corroborate the idea that there is a watertight boundary between the sexes, is incompatible with the notion that sexual differentiation is the result of a conglomerate of features acting in a coordinated fashion and by interregulation. This notion challenges the theoretical groundwork for sexual dimorphism itself, which is the necessary foundation for psychological and behavioral dimorphism.

The data obtained in recent years in a whole host of studies in different fields have exposed the ideological dimension of a presumed causal tie between human modes of functioning and the biological difference between the sexes.

*"It has become clear that dichotomizing homo-sapiens into two distinct and discontinuous classes, men and women, is only possible through successive reductions which restrict the definition of the two classes to one (or a small number) of indicators, which furthermore vary as a function of context. These are thus constructed, rather than bona fide classes" (Hurtig et al., 1991).*

This recasting of the processes of differentiation has led to clarifications and the development of more operational concepts that are better equipped to account for the heterogeneity of reality, in particular the concept of gender. In what has become a watershed publication, Unger (1979b), after having distinguished sex as "a subject variable" from sex as "a stimulus variable" uggests that the term gender *"may be used to describe those non-physiological components of sex that are culturally regarded as appropriate to males or to females. Gender may be used for those traits for which sex acts as a stimulus variable, independently of whether those traits have their origin within the subject or not".*

When gender is taken as a variable, it can be a better predictor of behavior han biological sex (Unger, 1979a and1979b). A similar attempt to analyze sex categorization and its modes of functioning in human cognitive organization prompted Bem (1981, 1983) to put forward the concept of gender schema. The gender schema is a cognitive mechanism which can process information, structure experiences and regulate behavior. It is a bipolar schema elaborated out of designations of the two sexes and is structured around male and female prototypes. A number of studies on children and adults have shown how this schema, which is characterized by its salience and early emergence, operates n perceptual (Deaux and Major, 1987) and mnemonic activities (Jennings, 1975; Bem, 1981).

However, as Hurtig and Pichevin (1985, 1986) stress, these gender concepts do not come to grips with the social hierarchy of the sexes. Bern's gender schema for example is structurally symmetrical. Hurtig and Pichevin on the contrary argue that this sociocognitive schema is intrinsically asymmetrical since the social hierarchy between the sexes implies the existence of male dominance over women and has structural implications on the psychological evel.

*"The representation of sex is an asymmetrical structure, in other words the role and function of the two sexes is not equivalent; male/female sex asymmetry, which is concommitant with social status, is a determinant of the structure and mode of functioning of the representation of sex".*

The gender schema thus vehicles the social hierarchy between the sexes. The gender schema has strong implications for the study of language in that language actualizes and reinforces the bicategorization of the sexes through the presence of a specific linguistic marker system: gender.

# Gender: a linguistic category unlike others

Although markers of gender are characteristic of Indoeuropean languages (with a few notable exceptions) they are not universal. In most languages gender is plurifunctional and gender markers are integrated into case and number. Gender is classically defined as a system of classification and although the male/female (and neutral) opposition is a major one, other oppositions such as animate/inanimate and human/non human also affect the definition of gender (Douay-Soublin, 1985). Languages differ greatly in the way they mark gender. In Indoeuropean languages, formal markers of gender apply to:
- the range of categorization: there are languages with 4 genders (masculine, feminine, common, and neuter), languages with three genders (masculine, feminine, neuter) such as German and Greek, and languages with two genders

such the Romance languages. This variability is even greater in non-indoeuropean languages. Finno-hungarian languages do not have a gender distinction, even in those areas such as personal pronouns where it is seen elsewhere as fundamental. In contrast, in the Bantu group of African languages, gender distinctions incorporate the state of matter (liquid/solid, big/small, continuous/discontinuous, etc).
- the variety of sectors of the language which are marked by gender: nouns, articles, adjectives, pronouns, verb inflections
- the range of levels on which different phonetic, morphological, semantic rules apply and their scope in a given language.

The issue of the origin and the evolution of grammatical gender raises a series of thorny problems for the language sciences on a number of levels (methodological, theoretical, ideological). These questions were not really approached until the 19th century. Theories of gender have tended to be speculative and can be classified into two categories (Fodor, 1959) as a function of the type of explanation they put forward.

In group 1, extralinguistic factors are cited to account for the emergence of this system of classification. In the second group, the evolution of grammatical gender and languages in general is thought to arise from internal constraints on the system (phonological changes for example).

In Wundt's theory ( see Fodor, 1959) for example, which is representative of the first group, grammatical gender is rooted in the bicategorization of the sexes. According to Wundt, the system of classification of nouns operates according to a differentiation principle based on object valence. The male/female distinction, according to Wundt is coded in language via this principle andthe encoding of sex differences is the prime determinant for the emergence of grammatical gender.

In contrast, Paul (see Fodor, 1959) views grammatical agreement as the fundamental cause for the emergence of gender in indoeuropean languages.

As regards the neuter, Meillet (1921) suggested that the neuter arose because emergence of the three genders was not simultaneous. Because of the preponderance of the animate/inanimate distribution, nouns were first split into animate nouns and inanimate nouns (neuter). Animate nouns were then divided into two groups, masculine and feminine, without a clearcut motivation for this division. Meillet stresses that *"grammatical gender is one of the least logical grammatical categories and one of the most unexpected"*, and the masculine/feminine distinction is *"totally meaningless"*.

In gender languages, there is a tendency for the feminine to be absorbed or neutralized (Michard, 1986; Douay-Soublin, 1985; Violi, 1987), and the dissymmetry between the masculine and the feminine can be seen on all the structural levels of language.

Meillet (1921) was not mistaken when he commented *"if we want to account for the fact that in languages which make a distinction between the masculine and the feminine, the feminine is always derived from the masculine, never from the root form, we cannot do so without recalling the respective social*

*tuation of man and woman at the time at which these grammatical forms came
to being".*
Without going into a critical assessment of these theories, what emerges is
at they run the gamut from a totally motivated concept to a totally arbitrary
oncept of gender. Nevertheless, all share a naturalistic view of gender which
kes the sex of the referents as a given, and hence appear to justify the
xistence of a level of language - natural gender - which is directly tied to an
nchallenged extra-linguistic dichotomy. These views were not really subjected
 criticism before the advent of feminist research (Kail,1989). This is
articularly true for the postulate of a fundamental transparency of language
nd its neutrality. The greatest amount of work on relationships between
inguage and biological sex and socio-conceptual gender variables has been
one in the USA (see Michard and Viollet, 1991).
Although most studies point clearly to the fallaciousness of the concept of
atural gender, in particular because it suggests there is a symmetry between
emantic features (male and female) represented as the direct linguistic
anslation of a physical property of referents in the extra-linguistic universe,
ere are a variety of interpretations as to "sex differences" in language.
The first interpretation places primary emphasis on symbolic and imaginary
eterminations. In a recent study on the origins of grammatical gender, Violi
1987) shows that grammatical gender is neither unmotivated nor arbitrary and
at language reflects basic dimensions of our experience, one of which being
ex differences. Sex difference is seen as one of the categories upon which our
erception and representation of the world is based, a feature which most
nguistic theories attempt to cloak.

*As a categorial schema of our existence, the sex opposition is embodied in
anguage structure in the form of grammatical gender. But this embodiment is
either neutral or contingent, and reflects the position of the feminine in the
ymbolic universe".*

Violi indirectly suggests that the semantic role of gender could be made
ymmetrical and that the "natural opposition" could be handled symbolically in
ther ways.
The second view stresses social and ideological determinants and sees
nguistic gender as *"the linguistic materialization of dominance relationships"*
Michard, 1991).
Michard (1988a,b) argues for a restructuring of the gender category in
nguistics, based on a sociological approach which conceptualizes the
ategorial system of sex in terms of relationships between the
lominant/dominated group (Guillaumin, 1978a,b, 1992). On the basis of
heoretical and empirical works which challenge the classic idea of a neutral
emantic level, Michard hypothesizes that there is a dissymmetrical
tructuration of the properties of sex in homo-sapiens: the dominant sex "has a
ex" whereas the dominated sex "is a sex". This type of hypothesis leads to the
onclusion that gender traits are human vs female (rather than male/female),

and gender is the model for a system which excludes women from the human while maintaining women in a specific, "feminine" gender. Gender becomes a fundamental semantic category based on the dissymmetry which is its precondition for existence.

The gender issue is linked to problems in cognitive psychology explored by Hurtig and Pichevin (1990, 1991a,b) on the role of sex categorization in the perception of others. One of the major contributions of these works is to have shown that one and the same categorization process can generate different cognitive spaces as a function of the category of sex involved. The sex category is thought to have a greater information organization capacity for the feminine than for the masculin sex. The members of the dominated group - women - define people, who define themselves and are defined by their category membership. The members of the dominant group - men - tend to be described by distinctive individual features. Thus sex is only an identity marker for women.

Although it has often been pointed out that there is a referential asymmetry within the group of animate nouns - where masculine gender is associated with referents having female sex but not the reverse - there are practically no studies on the impact of this asymmetry, except for anglosaxon feminist works dealing mainly with generics and prounouns, the generic "he" for example ( MacKay, 1980; Mac Kay and Toshi Konishi, 1980; Martyna, 1978, 1980a,b; Moulton, 1981).

The findings obtained in these experiments on the interpretation of male generics (man) or undifferentiated generics (person, adult) are extremely convergent. Subjects of both sexes choose masculine referents more frequently for terms with undifferentiated meanings. Nevertheless, women tend to interpret "man" and "person" more frequently as meaning a human being, and thus make more undifferentiated interpretations. Work by Martyna on pronouns shows that women prefer to use "her or she" or "they" instead of "he". In addition, women interpret "he" as an undifferentiated generic more frequently than men, without however identifying with this undifferentiated semantic value: seven times as many men as women state they imagine themselves in neutral sentences.

These works as well as others show the need to promote genuine generics (in other words forms which explicitly include both sexes or neutral forms such as chair-person for example).

The rare studies in developmental psycholinguistics on the construction of gender have focused on the issue of how young children learn the conceptual and semantic traits that underlie the gender system and the relationships between phonological, morphological, lexical and syntactic variables that are specific to the native language. In a volume devoted to reference, Karmiloff-Smith (1979) studied the production of gender by young French-speaking children. The ingenious experimental design used by Karmiloff-Smith consisted of presenting children two identical drawings of an imaginary object in two different colors, to which a fictitous name had been associated (for example maudrier, bicron, plichette, fascine, etc.) One of objects then undergoes a transformation which the child is asked to describe ("you turned e grey maudrier over"). In this situation, the experimenter provides no idications as to the gender of the noun, and the child must assign one through hoice of article and inflected adjective. This experiment was carried out with hildren aged 3 to 11. The findings show that as of age three, children are esponsive to the regularity of markers of gender in French. Strikingly, armiloff-Smith notes that at age nine and over, there is a tendency to assign lasculine gender to all unknown words,including those with feminine endings, hich she interprets as the use of the masculine as a "neuter". In another study armiloff-Smith creates a conflict between the sex of the person in the drawing after having made sure that the children had identified the sex correctly) and le noun which appeared without an article. For example: here are two ictures. Are they girls or boys? It's just two girls. They are two plichons. Then le transformation takes place. The findings examine conflict by comparing lese cases to cases of compatibility between sex and phonological ending. he comparisons show that up to the age of ten, children use the phonological idicator to generate the article, whether the picture depicts a girl or a boy.

To sum up, assignment of gender to fictitious nouns by young children ppears to be dominated in French by the phonological markers of nouns ather than by semantic factors ("natural gender" or syntactic markers agreement of the article). Karmiloff-Smith argues that the regularity of honological patterns accounts for this trend.

In a series of cross-linguistic studies on the acquisition of personal pronouns l German and English three and four year olds, Mills (1984, 1986) shows that ierman children show earlier mastery and argues that it is not the semantic imensions (conceptualized in terms of natural gender) which condition the cquisition of gender but rather the structural properties of the language system lat are specific to the target language. These studies on ontogenesis are ertinent because they appear to indicate that the hypothesis that natural ender is the precondition for the acquisition of grammatical gender should be econsidered. However, as I have pointed out above, it is the concept of natural lender itself which should be abandoned, since it masks the perception of eferential asymmetry and its consequences as regards assignment of rammatical gender.

## Concluding comments

n conclusion, advances in technology in the area exploring  brain asymmetry lnd language differences between men and women have led to the voicing of certain number of criticisms of previous findings. There have been calls for :ontrol groups, larger samples, and the need to take the sex variable into lccount along with other variables in a multivariation approach.

Appeals for conceptual clarification in particular as regards the distinction )etween sex and gender have prompted use of the term gender in )ublications. Unfortunately, gender has become somewhat a buzz word which las simply replaced sex and has rendered it meaningless. Choice of term is merely a concession that introduces no changes in the explanatory system itself.

In the field of language acquisition, the sex variable tends to be seen as a given. As I have pointed out elsewhere (Kail, 1984) its predictive value is virtually zero.

Nevertheless, under the joint influence of the Women's Movement and certain schools of thought in Psychology, sex has been the object of new theorizations, which view it as a biosocial variable in Unger's terms (1979b).

*"A biosocial variable - not one that is the result of biological and social causes, but one that produces effects because of generalized sociocultural assumptions about universal biological processes".*

Analyses which view sex into a constructed, structurally asymmetric variable are comparable to those found in certain areas of linguistics, in particular those areas which conceptualize gender as a socio-cognitive variable.

This theoretical convergence should be a promising point of departure for sorely needed new empirical research. The preconditions for taking the sexuated dimension of the individual into account in the processing and appropriation of language have now been met. Research is now equipped to overcome a scientific deadend, and escape the myth of *"the pleasant difference between the sexes".*

# References

Alper, J. S. (1985) Sex differences in brain asymmetry: A critical analysis. *Feminist Studies.*, **11** : 7-37.

Andersen, E. (1978). Will you please don't snore ? Directives in young children's role-play speech. *Papers and Reports on Child Language Develop..*, **14** : 140-150.

Bem, S. L. (1981). Gender schema theory: a cognitive account of sex typing. *Psychol. Bull.*, **88** : 354-364.

Bem, S. L. (1983). Gender schema theory and its implications for child development: raising gender-aschematic children in a gender-schematic society. *Signs.*, **8** : 598-616.

Block, J. H. (1976). Issues, problems and pitfalls in assessing sex differences : a critical review of"The Psychology of Sex Differences". *Merrill-Palmer Quart.*, **22** : 283-308.

Bradshow, J. L. and Gates, E. A. (1978). Visual field difference in verbal tasks: effects of task familiarity and sex of subject. *Brain Language,* **5** : 166-187.

Cherry, L. (1975). The preschool teacher-child dyad: sex differences in verbal interaction.*Child. Develop.*, **46** : 532-535.

Cohen, G. (1973). Hemispheric differences in serial versus parallel processing. *J. Exp. Psychol.*, **97** : 349-356.

Deaux, K. and Major, B. (1987). Putting gender into context: an interactive model of gender-related behavior. *Psychol. Rev.*, **94** : 369-389.

De Lacoste-Utamsing, C. and Holloway, R. I. (1982). Sexual dimorphism of the human corpus callosum. *Science.*, **216** : 1431-1432.

ittmann, A. T. (1977). Development of conversational behavior. In :Freedmann, N. and Grand, S. (Eds.),*Communicative Structures and Psychic Sructures,* Plenum Press, New York, pp. 133-147.

ouay-Soublin, F. (1985). Fonctionnements linguistiques de la catégorisation de sexe. *Bief.,* **17** :103-109 and 116-123.

delsky, C. (1976). The acquisition of communicative competence: recognition of linguistic correlates of sex roles. *Merrill-Palmer Quart.,* **22** : 47-59.

dwards, J. R. (1979). Social class differences and the identification of sex in children's speech. *J. Child. Lang.,* **6** : 121-127.

isenberg, L. (1978). La répartition différentielle des troubles psychiatriques selon le sexe. In: Sullerot, E. (Ed.), *Le Fait Féminin,* Fayard, Paris, pp.313-335.

me, R. F. (1979). Sex differences in childhood psychopathology. *Psychol. Bull.,* **86** : 574-595.

airweather, H. (1976). Sex differences in cognition. *Cognition,* **4** : 231-280.

airweather, H. (1982). Sex differences : little reason for females to play midfield. In : Beaumont, J. H. (Ed.), *Divided Visual Field Studies of Cerebral Organization,* Academic Press, New York, pp. 192-207.

odor, I.(1959).The origin of grammatical gender. *Lingua.,* **8** : 1-41 and 186-214.

riedman, D., Boltri, J., Vaughan, H., Erlenmeyer-Kimling, L. (1985). Effects of age and sex on the endogenous brain potential components during two continuous performance tasks. *Psychophysiol.,* **2** : 440-452.

ialaburda, A. M., Corsiglia, J., Rosen, G. D. and Sherman, G. F. (1987). Planum temporale asymmetry reappraisal since Geschwind and Levitsky. *Neuropsychologia,* **25** : 853-868.

ieschwind, N. and Galaburda, A. M. (1985). Cerebral lateralization: biological mechanisms associations and pathology: a hypothesis and program for research, *Arch. Neurol.,* **42** : (I). 428-459 ; (II). 521-552 ; (III). 634-654.

ieschwind, N. and Levitsky, W. (1968). Human brain: left-right asymmetries in the temporal speech region. *Science,* **161** : 186-187.

ievins, A. J., Doyle, J. C., Schaffer, R. E., Callaway, E. and Yeager,C. L. (1980). Lateralized cognitive processes and the electroencephalogram. *Science,* **207** : 1006-1007.

ievins, A. J., Doyle, J. C., Cutillo, B. A., Schaffer, R. E., Tannehill, R. S., Ghannam, J. H., Gilcrease,V. A. and Yeager, C. L. (1981). Electrical potentials in human brain during cognition: new method reveals dynamic patterns of correlation. *Science,* **213** : 918-922.

ileason, J. B. (1987). Sex differences in parent-child interaction. In : Philips, S. V., Steele, S. and Tanz, C.(Eds), *Language, Gender and Sex in Comparative Perspective.,* Cambridge University Press, Cambridge, pp. 189-200.

irady, K. E. (1977). *Sex as a Social Label: The Illusion of Sex Differences,* PhD Thesis, City University of New-York.

irady, K. E. (1979). Androgyny reconsidered. In : Williams, J. H. (Ed.), *Psychology of Women: Selected Readings.,* Norton, New-York, pp. 172-177.

Grady, K. E. (1981). Sex bias in research design. *Psychol. Women Quart.*, **5**: 628-636.

Guillaumin, C. (1978a). Pratique du pouvoir et idée de Nature : (1) L'appropriation des femmes. *Questions Féministes,* **2** : 5-30.

Guillaumin, C. (1978b). Pratique du pouvoir et idée de Nature : (2) Le discours de la Nature. *Questions Féministes,* **3** : 5-28.

Guillaumin, C. (1992). *Sexe, Race et Pratique du Pouvoir*, Editions Côté Femmes, Paris.

Hassler, M. (1990). Functional cerebral asymmetries and cognitive abilities in musicians, painters and controls. *Brain Cognition,* **13** : 1-17.

Hubbard, R. and Lowe, M. (Eds). (1979). *Genes and Gender II: Pitfalls in Research on Sex and Gender,* Gordian Press, New York.

Hubbard, R. , Henifin, M. S. and Fried, B. (1982). *Biological Woman: The Convenient Myth,* Schenkman, Cambridge.

Hurtig, M. C. and Pichevin, M. F. (1985). La variable sexe en psychologie : donné ou construct ?, *Cahiers Psychol.Cogni.,* **5** : 187-228.

Hurtig, M. C. and Pichevin, M. F. (1986). Conclusions. In : Hurtig, M. C. and Pichevin, M. F. (Eds). *La Différence des Sexes,* Questions de Psychologie, Editions Tierce, Paris, pp. 321-331

Hurtig, M. C. and Pichevin, M. F. (1990). Salience of the sex category system in person perception: contextual variations. *Sex Roles,* **22** : 369-395

Hurtig, M. C. and Pichevin, M. F. (1991a). Sex Typicality and Sex conformity. In: Haug, M., Brain, P. F. and Aron, C. (Eds.), *Heterotypical Behaviour in Man and Animals*, Chapman and Hall, London, pp. 16-41.

Hurtig, M. C. and Pichevin, M. F. (1991b). Catégorisation de sexe et perception d'autrui. In : Hurtig, M. C., Kail, M. and Rouch, H. (Eds.), *Sexe et Genre*, Editions du CNRS, Paris, pp. 169-180.

Hurtig, M. C., Kail, M. and Rouch, H. (1991). Introduction. In : Hurtig, M. C., Kail, M. and Rouch, H. (Eds.), *Sexe et Genre*, Editions du CNRS, Paris, pp.11-21.

Inglis, J., Ruckman, M., Lawson, J. S., Maclean, A. W. and Monga, T. N. (1982). Sex differences in the cognitive effects of unilateral brain damage. *Cortex,* **18** : 257-276.

Jennings, S. A. (1975). Effects of sex typing in children's stories on preference and recall. *Child Develop.,* **46** : 220-223.

Kail, M. (1984). Le sexe parle-t-il ? In : *Femmes, Féminisme et Recherches*, Editions AFER, Toulouse, pp. 790-800.

Kail, M. (1989). Aspects du fonctionnement langagier du genre. In : Daune-Richard, A. M. Hurtig, M. C. and Pichevin, M. C. (Eds.), *Catégorisation de Sexe et Constructions Scientifiques*, Editions CEFUP, Aix en Provence, pp. 51-62.

Karmiloff-Smith, A. (1979). *A Functional Approach to Child Language : A Study of Determiners and Reference*, Cambridge University Press, Cambridge.

Kelly, D. D. (1981). Sexual differentiation of the nervous system. In : Kandel, E. R. and Schartz, J. H. (Eds.), *Principles of Neural Science*, Elsevier / North Holland, Amsterdam, pp. 771-783.

insbourne, M. (1973). The control of attention by interaction between the cerebral hemispheres, In : *Attention and Performance IV*, Academic Press, New York, pp. 239-253.

insbourne, M. (1975). The mechanism of hemispheric control of the lateral gradient of attention. In : *Attention and Performance V*, Academic Press, New York, pp. 81-95.

lann-Delius, G. (1981). Sex and language acquisition: is there any influence?. *J. Pragmatics*, **5** : 1-25.

enneberg, F. (1966). *Speech development: its anatomic and physiologic concomitants. Brain Function.* University of California Press, Stanford.

enneberg, F. (1967). *Biological Foundations of Language*, Wiley, New York.

evy, J. and Trevarthen, C. (1977). Perceptual, semantic and phonetic aspects of elementary language processes in split-brain patients. *Brain*, **100** : 105-118.

ieven E. (1978). Conversations between mothers and young children: Individual differences and their implications for the study of language learning. In: Waterson, N. and Snow, S. (Eds.), *The Development of Communication*, Wiley, New York, pp.173-187.

Maccoby, E. E. and Jacklin, C. N. (1974).*The Psychology of Sex Differences*, Stanford University Press, Stanford.

MacKay, D. G. (1980). Psychology, prescriptive grammar and the pronoun problem. *Amer. Psychol.*, **35** : 444-449.

MacKay, D. G.and Toshi K. (1980). Personification and the pronoun problem. *Women's Studies Int. Quart.*, **3** : 149-163.

McGlone, J. and Commentators. (1980). Sex differences in human brain asymmetry: a critical survey. *Behav. Brain Sci.*, **3** : 215-263.

McGuiness, D. (1980). Comments. In: McGlone, J. and Commentators. Sex differences in human brain asymmetry: a critical survey. *Behav. Brain Sci.*, **3** : 215-263.

McKeever W. F. (1987). Cerebral organization and sex: interesting but complex. In: Philips, S. V., Steele, S. and Tanz, C. (Eds.), *Language, Gender and Sex in Comparative Perspective*, Cambridge University Press, Cambridge, pp. 268-278.

McKeever, W. F. and Hoff, A. L. (1982). Familial sinistrality, sex and laterality differences in naming and lexical decision latencies of righhanders, *Brain Language*, **7** : 175-190.

McKeever, W. F., Seitz, K. S., Hoff, A. L., Diehl, J. A. and Marino, M. F. (1983). Interactive sex and familial sinistrality characteristics influence both language lateralization and spatial ability in right handers. *Neuropsychologia*, **21** :661-668.

McKeever, W. F. and Van Deventer, A. D. (1977). Visual and auditory language processing asymmetries: influences of handedness, familial sinistrality and sex. *Cortex*, **13** : 225-241.

Martin, M. (1979). Hemispheric specialization for local and global processing. *Neuropsychologia*, **17** : 33-40.

Martin, E. J. (1980). Comments. In: MacGlone, J. and Commentators. Sex differences in human brain asymmetry : a critical survey. *Behav. Brain Sci.*, **3** : 215-263.

Martyna, W. (1978). What does he mean ?. *J. Commun.*, **28** : 131-138.

Martyna, W. (1980a). Beyond the he/man approach - The case for language change. *Signs.*, **5** : 482-493.

Martyna, W. (1980b). The psychology of the generic masculine. In: McConnel-Ginet, S. (Ed.), *Linguistics and the Feminist Challenge*, Praeger, New York, pp. 69-78.

Meillet, A. (1921). *Linguistique Historique et Linguistique Générale*, Champion, Paris.

Merz, F. (1979). *Geschlechtunterschiede und Ihre*. Entwicklung. Hogrefe, Göttingen.

Michard, C. (1986). *Le Genre en Français Contemporain. Matérialisations Linguistiques de la Catégorie Socio-Conceptuelle de Sexe*, Rapport ATP CNRS , Paris.

Michard, C. (1988a). Some socio-enunciative characteristics of scientific texts concerning the sexes. In: Seidel, G. (Ed.), *The Nature of the Right*, Benjamins, Amsterdam, pp.27-59.

Michard, C. (1988b). Les valeurs sémantiques humain et humain mâle : univocité, ambiguïté ou ambivalence ? In: Fuchs, C. (Ed.), *L'ambiguïté et la Paraphrase*, Centre de Publications de l'Université de Caen, Caen, pp. 135-138.

Michard, C. (1991). Approche matérialiste de la sémantique du genre. In: Hurtig, M. C., Kail, M. and Rouch, (Eds.). *Sexe et Genre*, Editions du CNRS, Paris, pp. 147-157.

Michard, C. and Viollet, C. (1991). Sex and gender in linguistics: fifteen years of feminist research in the United States and in West Germany. *Feminist Issues*, **11** : 1. 53-88.

Mills, A. (1984). *The Acquisition of Gender in English and German*. Habilitationschift. University of Tubingen.

Mills, A. (1986). The acquisition of gender in English and German. *York-Springer Series in Language and Communication*, **20**.

Molfese, D. L. (1990). Auditory evoked responses recorded from 16 month-old human infants to words they did and did not know. *Brain Language*, **38** : 345-363

Molfese, D. L., Freeman, R. and Palermo, D. (1975). The ontogeny of brain lateralization for speech and nonspeech stimuli. *Brain Language, 2* : 356-368.

Money, J. and Ehrhardt A. A. (1972). *Man and Woman, Boy and Girl,* John Hopkins University Press, Baltimore.

Morrel, L. and Salamy, J. (1971). Hemispheric asymmetry of electrocortical responses to speech stimuli. *Science*, **174** : 164-166.

Moulton, J. (1981). The myth of the neutral man. In: Vetterling-Braggin (Ed.), *Sexist Language,* Adams and Co, Littlefield, pp. 100-115.

lurry, T., Amundson, P. and Hollien, H. (1977). Acoustical characteristics of infant cries: fundamental frequency. *J. Child Language,* **4** : 321-328.

lurry, T., Hollien, H. and Muller, E. (1975). Perceptual responses to infant crying: maternal recognition and sex judgments. *Quart. Rep.,* **13** : 27-34.

ebes, R. D. (1971). Superiority of the minor hemisphere in commissurotomized man for the perception of part-whole relations. *Cortex,* **7** : 333-347.

ebes, R. D. (1972). Dominance of the minor hemisphere in commissurotomized man in a test of figural unification. *Brain,* **95** : 633-638.

ebes, R. D. (1973). Perception of dot patterns by the disconnected right and left hemispheres in man. *Neuropsychologia,* **11** : 285-290

ebes, R. D. (1974). Hemispheric specialization in commissurotomized man. *Psychol. Bull.,* **81** : 1-14.

ewport, E. L., Gleitman, H. and Gleitman, L. R. (1977). Mother I'd rather do myself: some effects and non effects of material speech. In: Snow, C. and Ferguson, C. (Eds.), *Talking to Children,* Cambridge University Press, New York, pp. 109-149.

age, D. (1986). Sex reversal: delition mapping the male determining function of the human Y chromosome, Cold Spring Harbor Symposia on Quantitative Biology, Ll, pp. 229-235.

atterson, K. and Bradshaw, J. L. (1975). Differential hemispheric mediation of non verbal visual stimuli. *J. Exp. Psychol.,* 246-252.

eyre, E., Wiels, J. and Fonton, M. (1991). Sexe biologique et sexe social. In: Hurtig, M. C., Kail, M. and Rouch, H.(Eds.), *Sexe et Genre,* Editions du CNRS, Paris, pp. 27-50.

iazza, D. M. (1980). The influence of sex and handedness in the hemispheric specialization of verbal and non verbal tasks. *Neuropsychologia,* **18** : 163-176.

icton,T. W., Stuss, D. T., Champagne, S. C. and Nelson, R. F. (1984). The effects of age on human even-related potentials. *Psychophysiol.,* **21** : 312-325.

amer, A. L. H. (1976). Syntactic styles in emerging language. *J. Child Language,* **3** : 49-62.

lich, D. A. and McKeever W. F. (1990). An investigation of immune system disorder as a marker for anomalous dominance. *Brain Cognition,* **12** : 55-72.

lingler, N. (1973). *Mother's Language to Their Young Children and to Adults Over Time,* Doctoral dissertation, Case Western Reserve University.

achs, J. and Devin, J. (1976). Young children's knowledge of age appropriate speech styles. *J. Child. Lang.,* **3** : 81-98.

hatz, M. and Gelman, R. (1973). The development of communicative skills, modifications in the speech of young children as a function of listener. *Mon. Soc. Res. Child. Develop.,* **38** :

herman, J. A. and Denmark, F. L. (Eds.). (1978). *The Psychology of Women: Future Directions of Research,* Psychological Dimensions, New York.

hibatani, A.(1980). The japanese brain. *Science,* **6** : 24-26.

Snow, C. (1972). Mother's speech to children learning language. *Child Develop.*, **43** : 549-565.

Star, S. L. (1979). Sex differences and the dichotomization of the brain: methods, limits and problems in research on consciousness. In: Hubbard, R. and Lowe, M. (Eds.), *Genes and Gender II: Pitfalls in Research on Sex and Gender*, Gordian Press, New York, pp.62-74.

Stoller, R. J. (1968). *Sex and Gender*. Science House Edition, New York, 1968. Traduction Française : *Recherches sur l'Identité Sexuelle*, Gallimard, Paris, 1978.

Tanguay P., Tanb, J., Doubleday, Y. and C., Clarkson, D. (1977). An interhemispheric comparison of auditory evoked responses to consonant vowel stimuli. *Neuropsychologia*, **15** : 123-131

Unger, R. K. (1979a). *Female and Male: Psychological Perspectives*, Harper and Row, New York.

Unger, R. K. (1979b). Toward a redefinition of sex and gender. *Amer. Psychol.*, **34** : 1085-1094

Unger, R. K. (1981). Sex as a social reality: field and laboratory research. *Psychol. Women Quart.*, **5** : 645-653.

Violi, L. (1987). Les origines du genre grammatical. In: Irigaray, L. (Ed.), *Le Sexe Linguistique*, Langages, **85** : 15-34.

Waber, D. P. (1976). Sex differences in cognition: a function of maturation rate ?. *Science*, **193** : 572-574.

Waber, D. P. (1977). Biological substrates of field dependence: implications of the sex difference. *Psychol. Bull.*, **84** : 1076-1087.

Wada, J. A., Clarke, R., and Hamm, A. (1975). Cerebral hemispheric asymmetry in humans. *Arch. Neurol.*, **32** : 239-246.

Wells, G. (1978). What makes for successful language development. In: Campbell, P. and Smith, R. (Eds.), *Recent Advances in the Psychology of Language*, Plenum Press, New York, pp.449-469.

Witelson, S. F. (1985). The brain connections: the corpus callosum is larger in left handers. *Science*, **229** : 665-668.

Witelson, S. F. and Pallie, F. (1973). Left hemisphere specialization for language in the newborn: neuroanatomical evidence of asymmetry. *Brain*, **96** : 641-646.

Zangwill, O. (1960). *Cerebral Dominance and its Relation to Psychological Function*, IL, Thomas, Springfield.

# Organizational Effects of Gonadal Hormones Induce Qualitative Differences in Visuospatial Navigation

## C. L. WILLIAMS[1] and W. H. MECK[2]

[1]Department of Psychology, Barnard College of Columbia University, New York, New York 10027, USA

[2]Department of Psychology, Columbia University, New York, New York 10027, USA

Since the pioneering work of Phoenix, Goy, Gerall, and Young in 1959, considerable evidence has demonstrated that gonadal hormones, which are secreted in high quantities by the neonatal male mammal and which act at specific neural receptor sites in the brain, are the proximate cause of a number of neuroanatomical and behavioral differences between male and females. Hormone-dependent structural dimorphisms have been described in a number of brain regions including: hypothalamus, preoptic area, cerebral cortex, hippocampus, habenula and spinal cord (for review see Arnold and Gorski, l984; Toran-Allerand, 1984), and hormone-induced sexual dimorphisms occur in a variety of reproductive (see Goy and McEwen, 1980) and nonreproductive behaviors (see Beatty, 1992). However, with the possible exception of the frog and songbird vocal control centers (see DeVoogd, 1984; Kelley, 1987), the sexually dimorphic spinal nucleus of the bulbo-cavernosus, which innervates the penile musculature for erection (see Fishman and Breedlove, 1988), and the medial and lateral sexually dimorphic area of the gerbil hypothalamus which appears to be essential for masculine sexual behavior (Yahr, this volume) the precise sexually dimorphic functions subserved by these neuroanatomical differences or even subserved by the regional localization of these differences is largely unknown. These sexually dimorphic systems in which brain and behavior can be related rely on behaviors which are present in the male, but are absent or not frequently displayed by the female. The central control appears to be equally dimorphic. For example, the adult male rat possesses a spinal motor nucleus for the bulbo-cavernosus muscle, while the adult female rat does not. In song birds, the nuclei along the song pathway are dramatically larger in males, and one nucleus, Area X, is not even distinguishable in the female zebra finch. These quantitative differences

175

M. Haug et al. (eds.), The Development of Sex Differences and Similarities in Behavior, 175–189.
© 1993 Kluwer Academic Publishers. Printed in the Netherlands.

between males and females in brain regions and behaviors related to reproduction have served as models for how hormones regulate sexually dimorphic function, and have greatly influenced the questions that we ask about sexually dimorphic behavior.

One class of sexually dimorphic behavior that does not fit this standard model is visuospatial ability. Unlike birdsong or male sexual behavior in which one sex normally displays the behavior and the other does not, both males and females readily solve visuospatial problems and use visuospatial cues to navigate. In quantitative analyses of visuospatial skills in both human and nonhuman animals, there is overwhelming evidence that males outperform females (e.g., Dawson et al., 1975; Beatty, 1979, 1984; Halpern, 1992; Gaulin and Fitzgerald, 1986; Linn and Petersen, 1985), but the differences are small (compared to sex differences in birdsong or sex behavior), often disappear when the task is well-learned (Burstein et al., 1980; Beatty, 1984; Roof and Havens, 1992), and rarely can be detected if the task is too simple (see Williams and Meck, 1991 for discussion). Furthermore, initial findings (MacLusky et al., 1979) revealed that telencephalic areas thought to be involved in cognitive function were relatively devoid of steroid receptors early in development. Together, these findings have fueled the controversy about whether sexually dimorphic visuospatial ability is caused by hormones acting to organize brain regions involved with spatial ability, by hormones acting indirectly on other behavioral characteristics (e.g., motivation, exploration, activity), by nonhormonal experiential factors (see Beatty, 1992; Halpern, 1992), or whether the differences exist at all.

In the last 4-5 years there has been increasing evidence that sexually dimorphic visuospatial ability is caused by hormonal mechanisms similar to those described for sexually dimorphic reproductive behavior. One reason for this change of view is that new behavioral analyses have allowed us to see that performance differences between the sexes are likely due to qualitative differences in the cognitive and/or behavioral processes used to solve a spatial task, rather than the degree to which either sex possesses basic visuospatial skills. A second reason is that receptors for steroid hormones have now been detected in brain regions likely to control visuospatial ability. Thus, the standard model for the hormonal induction of sexually dimorphic function that relies on quantitative differences in brain and behavior may need to be expanded to include sex differences in cognitive function. This qualitative sexual dimorphism and its hormonal control are the focus of this chapter.

Work from our laboratory (Williams et al.,1990a; Williams and Meck, 1991; Williams et al., 1990b; Williams et al., 1992) has carefully examined the behavioral differences between male and female rats when they solve a visuospatial task, and has begun to determine the hormonal control of this sex difference. In our studies, we have utilized the radial-arm maze procedure (Olton and Samuelson, 1976), a laboratory version of a foraging task. This maze has a central circular platform from which long arms radiate at equal angles. In the standard training procedure, food is placed in a small well at the end of each arm at the start of each day's trial, and the rat is left on the maze until it visits every arm and finds all the food. After each choice, the rat must return to the central platform to choose another arm. We have used a modification of this task, in which only a subset of arms (8 of 12) is baited with food, and the pattern of baited and unbaited arms remains the same from day to day. This task is more difficult for the rat, because it discourages the use of a motor bias, or response strategy and encourages a greater reliance on memory strategies (see Williams and Meck, 1991 for further discussion of this issue). In this chapter, evidence will be presented to show that: 1. sex differences in visuospatial memory of rats develop through exposure to the organizational influence of aromatizable androgens during perinatal life; and 2. differences between the sexes in maze performance are not due to quantitative differences in memory but rather to qualitative differences in the use of visuospatial cues that guide spatial navigation.

## Hormonal organization of sex differences in visuospatial memory

Although there is little argument that sex differences in visuospatial ability exist in both human and non human species (see Linn and Petersen, 1986; Williams and Meck, 1991), the issue of what causes these differences has been largely unexplored. To date most evidence supports the view that behavioral differences between the sexes are due to perinatal exposure to gonadal hormones. For example, administration of testosterone to neonatal female rats improves their performance on maze tasks (Lashley III, Hebb-Williams, water maze, radial-arm maze), while neonatal castration disrupts male performance to varying degrees (Dawson et al., 1975; Joseph et al., 1978; Roof and Havens, 1992; Stewart et al., 1975). Despite these repeated demonstrations, reviewers of the literature do not all agree that early hormonal exposure causes sex differences in visuospatial memory. Beatty (1992), for example, argues that the interpretation of these studies is complicated by the fact that in some maze tasks exploratory activity is inversely correlated with maze performance, so hormones may indirectly alter performance by influencing activity (Stewart et al., 1975). However, recent work demonstrates that sex differences in maze performance can be found that are not correlated with activity levels (Gaulin et al., 1990). A second concern is that subjects in these studies were not always gonadectomized as adults. Therefore, it is not clear whether postpubertal differences in circulating hormones, in perinatal hormone exposure, or both is the proximate cause of the dimorphism in behavior. Third, these studies did not address the issue of whether testosterone is acting via its intracellular conversion to estradiol, as it appears to do for the organization of other sexually dimorphic behaviors (e.g., Christensen and Gorski, 1978; Clemens and Gladue, 1978; Whalen et al., 1986) or whether it is acting directly via androgen receptors. Work from our laboratory has addressed these latter two issues.

We have recently reported (Williams et al., l990a; Williams and Meck, 1991) that early organizational effects of gonadal secretions influence visuospatial memory, and that the active hormone for this process may be estradiol. Neonatally gonadectomized male rats, and females showed the least accurate choice performance during acquisition of a radial-arm maze task with 8 baited and 4 unbaited arms (the first 9-10 days of training), while females which had received injections of estradiol benzoate (EB) during the first 10 days of life (500 μg total) and normal males showed the most accurate choice performance. At asymptotic performance these differences disappear but they can be reinstated by various manipulations of the test environment (see discussion below). More recently, we have provided direct evidence that aromatization of testosterone to estradiol plays a significant role in the sexual differentiation of spatial ability in male rats (Williams et al., 1992). The aromatase inhibitor, androst-1,4,6-triene-3,17-dione (ATD) was administered to newborn male rats in subcutaneously implanted Silastic capsules during the first 10 days of life, and the spatial memory of these rats and their control male littermates was assessed in adulthood on a 12-arm radial maze with 8 baited and 4 unbaited arms. In this study control rats outperformed their ATD-treated littermates when they were trained as adults. ATD-treatment caused accuracy of choice performance of male subjects during acquisition of the task to decrease to the level normally shown by control females. The effectiveness of ATD-treatment was further assessed by giving all subjects tests for female sexual behavior after priming with EB and progesterone. Control males showed lordosis on less than 20% of trials, while the ATD-treated male rats showed lordosis on more than 60% of trials.

In both these studies adult rats were gonadectomized at 60 days of age to remove the confounding influence of adult gonadal secretions on radial-arm maze performance. Thus, the differences in visuospatial ability are due to organizational effects of estradiol on the developing brain. Activational effects of steroid hormones do not appear to be required for the expression of this sexually dimorphic behavior. This does not rule out the possibility that circulating hormones in adult animals might modulate visuospatial memory function (e.g., Hampson and Kimura, 1988). Together, these two lines of research suggest that aromatization of testosterone into estradiol plays a significant role in the sexual differentiation of spatial ability during the first postnatal week in the Sprague-Dawley rat.

Until recently, the hypothesis that aromatized androgen acted on telencephalic regions involved in cognitive function met with skepticism; there was no evidence that estrogen biosynthetic ability occurred in the telencephalon. New techniques, however, have demonstrated low levels of estrogen biosynthesis from hippocampus and cortex in mouse and rat brain (MacLusky et al., 1986; MacLusky et al.,1987; MacLusky and Toran-Allerand, 1989). These brain regions also contain estrogen receptors (MacLusky et al., 1979; Maggi and Bettini, 1990; Shughrue et al., 1990). Telencephalic estrogen receptors appear just before birth, increase to very high levels during the first week of life and then decline to lower adult levels (O'Keefe and Handa, 1990; Shughrue et al., 1990). In the mouse brain, receptors appear first in the deep cortex. By postnatal day 8 estrogen target cells are strongly concentrated in the cingulate/paracingulate and suprarhinal cortex. In 12-day-old mice, estrogen target cells are mainly in laminae II and III, and by day 25, cell numbers decline, and most cells appear in superficial layers (Shughrue et al., 1990). This ontogenetic profile is different from that seen in the hypothalamus, where levels of estrogen target cells rise during the first week of life and remain high in the adult (MacLusky et al., 1979). These data parallel the behavioral findings that hypothalamically-controlled reproductive behavior requires hormonal activation for its expression, while it appears that sexually dimorphic visuospatial ability does not require adult hormone priming. Recently, O'Keefe and Handa (1990) have found that treating week-old rats with the synthetic estrogen, diethylstilbestrol (DES), increases the levels of estrogen receptors in the hippocampal nuclear extract. The fact that DES causes the induction of estrogen receptors strongly supports the view that the hippocampus is a potential substrate for estrogen-mediated organizational actions.

Neuropsychological investigations of the frontal cortex and hippocampus implicate these brain regions in the control of working and reference memory, respectively (e.g., Kesner et al., l987; Meck et al., 1987; Meck et al., 1989). Because these brain regions possess estrogen receptors and aromatase activity early in development we have investigated the effect of estradiol placed directly into these brain areas in neonatally castrated male rats (Williams et al., 1990b). As a first attempt to relate hormonally-induced changes in telencephalic structures to hormonally-induced changes in a behavior modulated by that system, we have completed a study in which we examined the radial-arm maze performance of neonatally castrated male rats which received bilateral implants of estradiol (approximately 10 ng) aimed at either the frontal cortex, the medial hippocampus, or the ventromedial hypothalamus, or which received no implant, and compared their performance to male rats castrated at puberty (Controls). At 60 days of age, the rats were trained on our radial-arm maze task. After the rats' choice performance reached steady-state in the first test room (Room A), rats were transferred to a novel training environment (Room B) for two days of reacquisition. Rats were then returned to Room A for one week until steady-state performance was reattained. Rats were then transferred to a second novel environment (Room C) for two more days of reacquisition. These transfer tests were designed to reveal sex differences that are more evident early in training. These design of the experiment are shown in Figure 1.

During acquisition of the task in Room A (Figure 2) , control males and neonatally castrated males with implants aimed at either the hippocampus or cortex were significantly more accurate in choice performance than either the castrated males that received no implants or the neonatally castrated males with implants aimed at the hypothalamus. These differences disappeared at steady-state. During the transfer tests, control males and neonatally castrated males with implants aimed at the hippocampus were more accurate in their choice performance than neonatally castrated rats with no implants or with implants aimed at the hypothalamus. The choice performance of rats with implants aimed at the frontal cortex did not differ significantly from the rats with hypothalamic implants but their choice performance was significantly more accurate than the performance of the neonatal castrates with no implants. These data provide preliminary evidence implicating the hippocampus and

180

perhaps the frontal cortex as sites of estradiol action for the organization of sexually dimorphic visuospatial ability.

### Experimental Design for Behavioral Training

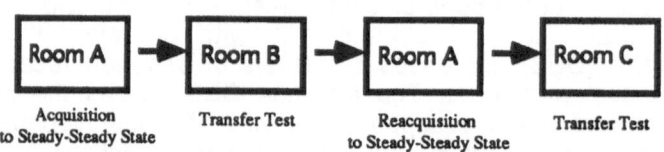

**Figure 1** Rats were trained for 30 days in Room A, transferred to Room B (a room with different geometry and landmark cues from Room A) for 2 days of training, returned to Room A for a week of retraining, and then transferred to Room C (a room with different geometry and landmark cues from Rooms A and B) for 2 days of training.

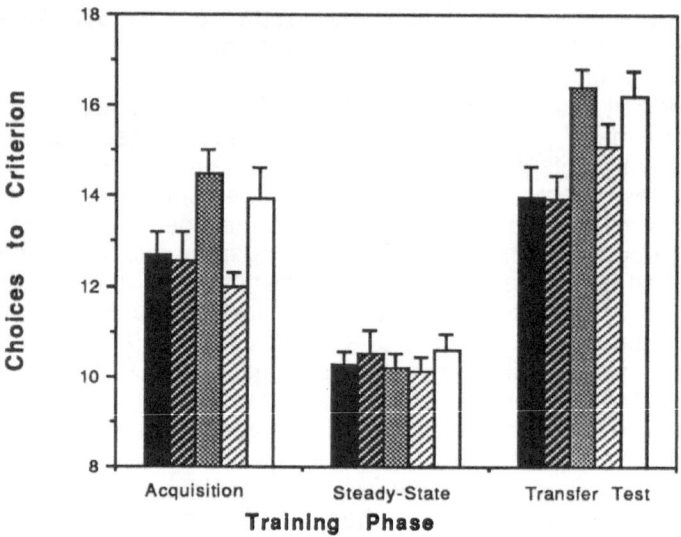

**Figure 2** Mean number of number of choices to locate all 8 baited arms ± S.E.M. during Acquisition (Room A acquisition training), Steady State (Room A asymptotic performance), and Transfer (Training in novel Rooms A and B), for CON (male rats castrated at 60 days of age), CAS (male rats castrated within 6 hrs of birth), HIP (male rats castrated within 6 hrs of birth and bilaterally implanted with 10 ng estradiol benzoate-EB aimed at the medial hippocampus); HYP (male rats castrated within 6 hrs of birth and bilaterally implanted with 10 ng estradiol benzoate-EB aimed at the ventromedial hypothalamus), and COR (male rats castrated within 6 hrs of birth and bilaterally implanted with 10 ng estradiol benzoate-EB aimed at the frontal cortex).

Further work to demonstrate site specificity of this estrogen effect, and to examine the neural consequences of estradiol action in the developing hippocampus and cortex are ongoing in our laboratory. Additional support for the contention that the hippocampus is a target for the early organizational effects of gonadal steroids on visuospatial memory comes from a recent report (Roof and Havens, 1992) showing that when tested as adults, females rats treated with testosterone propionate during the first week of life (total 300 μg) and control males locate a hidden escape platform significantly faster during the acquisition of a distal cue water maze task than do untreated females. Maze performance correlated with the width of the dentate gyrus granule cell layer across all groups. Thus, while cause and effect between anatomy and behavior cannot be established by these studies, these data support the hypothesis that hormonally-induced sex differences in hippocampus may underlie sex differences in visuospatial memory.

# Behavioral processes responsible for sex differences in spatial ability

Although it is possible to assess sex differences in visuospatial ability by comparing performance on a variety of maze-type tasks, these studies do not address the issue of what underlying behavioral mechanism is involved. Based on our current understanding of sexually dimorphic reproductive behavior, the implicit assumption has been that because males outperform females on visuospatial tasks they must have bigger or better spatial memory and perhaps more brain space devoted to this function. There is increasing evidence, however, that performance differences between the sexes on a variety of visuospatial tasks are more qualitative than quantitative. Males and females may use different problem solving strategies (Sherman, 1978; Blough and Slavin, 1987), may be differentially dependent upon response biases and spatial memory (Williams and Meck, 1991), and may employ different visuospatial cues (Ward et al., 1986; Williams et al., 1990a; Bever, 1992). These differences often translate into quantitative differences in maze performance. As described above, one difficulty with this type of assessment is that sex differences are often masked at steady state performance because males and females can both solve visuospatial problems and remember spatial locations. Once rats have reached steady state and sex differences are no longer apparent, we have effectively utilized several probe tests that place added demands on rats' spatial memory which cause differences to reemerge. Data from these probe tests have revealed that males and females use spatial information differently. It appears that males simplify the task by utilizing a single type of distal cue - the shape or global geometry of the test room. Females, in contrast, appear to rely on multiple cues; unlike males they make use of landmarks - large objects in the environment - as well as other distal cues. Three examples that demonstrate this differential cue use by male and female rats are described below.

As described above, females rats that were injected with 10 mg EB on postnatal days 1, 3, 5, 7, 9 (FNE) and control males (MC) make fewer errors during acquisition of a radial-arm maze task than oil-treated females (FC) and neonatal male castrates (MNC) (Williams et al., 1990a). After rats reached steady state-performance, and no sex differences in choice behavior were detectable, we manipulated the visual cues in the room which we believed the rats might be using to navigate. Our assumption was that if we altered the cues used to navigate, rats' choice performance would be dramatically disrupted, as if the rats had been moved to an unfamiliar room. Specifically, we evaluated rats for their use of geometry (shape of the room) and landmark (movable objects in the room) cues. Geometry was either: 1. maintained as in original training or 2. modified by enclosing the maze within a circular arena thus eliminating the possibility that rats could determine the locations of food caches by the correct alignments of angles and distances obtained from the shape of the enclosure. At the same time, the arrangement of landmarks was either: 1. unmodified, 2. modified by unsystematic rearrangement of landmarks, or 3. modified by removal of the most salient landmarks. These conditions were evaluated by the use of a 2 x 3 factorial design.

Rats exposed to neonatal hormones (MC and FNE groups) were disrupted in their performance in conditions in which room geometry was modified, regardless of the landmark location. In contrast, rats exposed to no or low levels of gonadal steroids neonatally (FC and MNC groups) were disrupted only if both the landmarks and geometry were removed. If either the landmarks or the geometry alone were removed, they were not significantly disrupted in their performance. These rats were also disrupted if the landmarks were rearranged but the geometry was unmodified. These design and results of this experiment can be seen in Figure 3 and 4.

This pattern of results suggests that males attend to a single feature of the environment - room geometry - perhaps one to which they were biologically "prepared" to attend. Males' performance is never disrupted by the removal or rearrangement of landmarks, only by changes in room shape. Females appear to use two or more features from different dimensions (e.g., landmarks and geometry) in order to locate a target. Thus, either type of cue alone, can guide female navigation. However, if landmarks are rearranged within the same geometric frame, female performance is disrupted, suggesting that when multiple cues are present females use them in combination. Therefore, group differences in the acquisition of the radial-arm maze task might be due to differences in the number and/or type of cues used to locate food caches. Use of a single cue may act to simplify the task, and thereby improve performance under the circumstances which happen to be common in the rats' natural habitat and in the usual design of spatial navigation tasks employed in the laboratory. Males also simplify the task early in training by relying more on response biases and less on spatial memory (see Williams and Meck 1991).

A second study that we have recently run in our laboratory, also points to differential cue use in male and female rats. Adult male and female Sprague Dawley rats that were gonadectomized at 60 days of age were trained for 30 days on our version of the radial-arm maze procedure (Figure 5). During the last block of 3 days of training, there were no significant differences between male and female performance. On day 31 of training, all large movable objects in the room were removed, and instead of illuminating the room with 2 banks of fluorescent ceiling lights, the room was lit by a single dim red light bulb hung

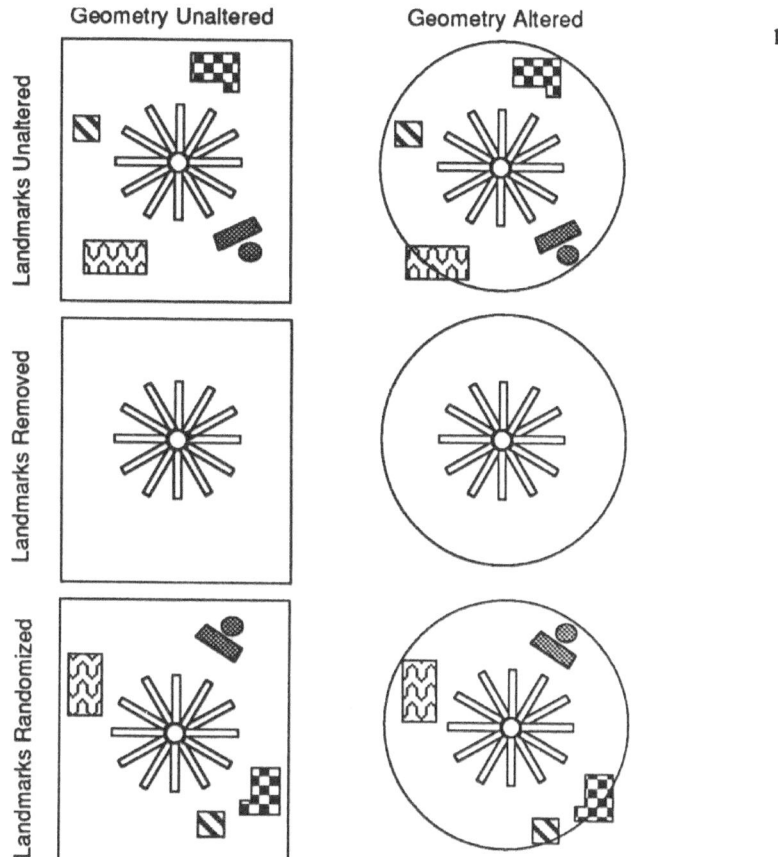

**Figure 3** Schematic diagram to represent the 2 by 3 design used in this experiment. Geometry (room shape) was either unaltered or altered by hanging a circular curtain around the maze. Landmarks (large movable objects in the room) were either unaltered, removed, or unsystematically randomized.

from the center of the room, directly over the maze. Under these conditions, the geometric frame, or shape of the room was still visible; however, the landmarks in the room were removed and the configuration of large objects in the ceiling and on the walls were obscured. As can be seen in Figure 6, when training was conducted under the dim lighting conditions, female rats were significantly more disrupted in their choice performance than were male rats. When the original cues were returned to the room and rats were re-tested under the original conditions, choice performance returned to levels seen prior to the probe test and there were no significant differences. Again, these data suggest that males are more reliant on cues about angles and distances that come from the Euclidian properties of the room shape. Females are disrupted if the large objects in the room are removed or obscured by a change in lighting. An alternate explanation of these data may be that both males and females

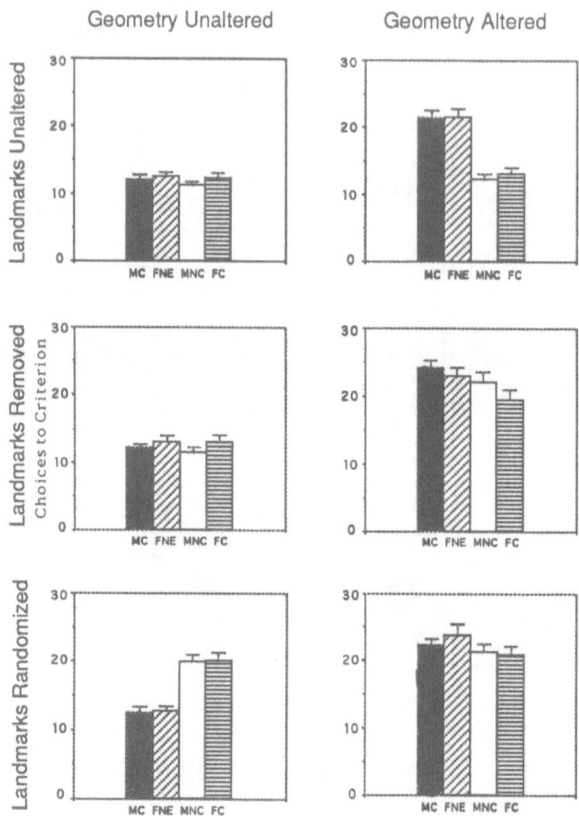

**Figure 4** Mean choices to locate all 8 baited arms ± S.E.M. for MC (male control), FNE (females treated with 10 μg EB on postnatal days 1, 3, 5, 7, and 9 of life), MNC (males castrated within 24 hrs of birth) and FC (female control) in each of the 6 cue configurations depicted in the left panel.

behave as if they were in a new room (e.g., see the description of the transfer test in Figure 1), because males are more accurate in their choice performance early in training. This may be due to the males' greater reliance on response biases (see Williams and Meck, 1991).

Recent work by Bever (1992) using both rats and humans has also revealed differential cue use by males and females. In his studies subjects are trained in enclosed hallways (college students) or in a maze with high walls (rats) so that only cues within the hallways/maze can easily be used to navigate. This differs from the procedures described above in which rats use extramaze cues to navigate. The hallway and maze were shaped like a symmetrical figure 8 with corners at 90° angles. Subjects were required to go from a start point at the top of the figure to a goal area at the bottom of the figure, and to avoid making a wrong turn down the center cross-over. Hidden barricades marked wrong turns.

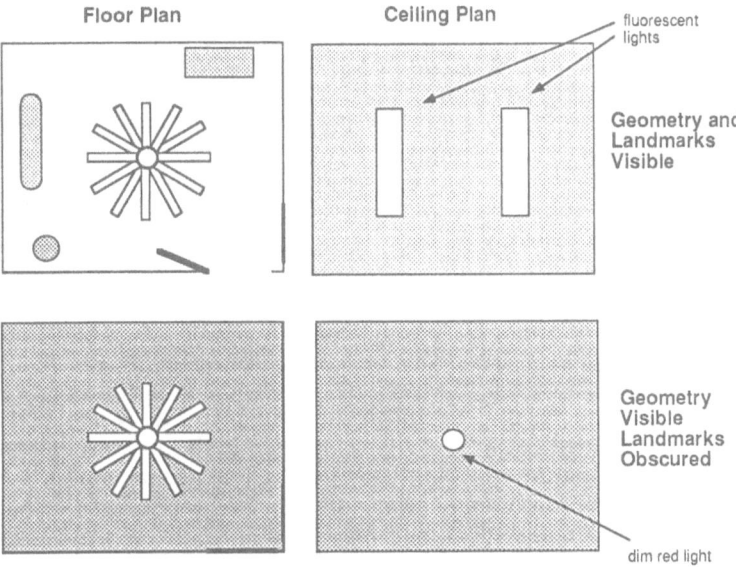

**Figure 5** Schematic diagram to represent the 2 cue conditions used in this experiment. Geometry (room shape) and Landmarks (large movable objects and objects and lighting on the walls and ceiling) were either visible or the Geometry was visible but the Landmarks were removed (movable objects on the floor) or obscured (by using only a single dim red light centered directly over the maze platform.

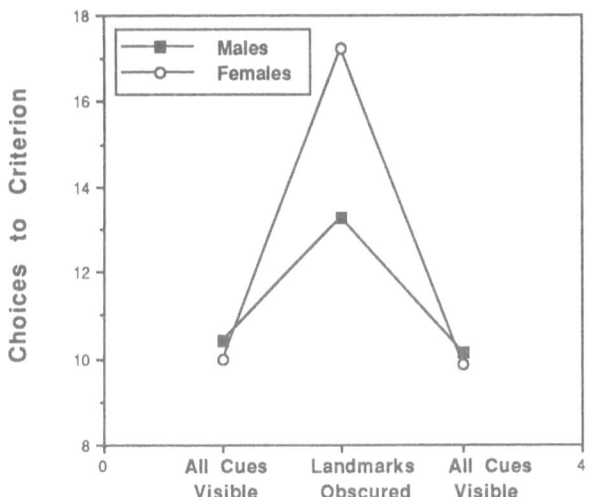

**Figure 6** Mean choices to locate all 8 baited arms for male and female rats when geometry and Landmarks were visible, and when landmarks were removed or obscured.

186

When males and females were trained by always starting at the same location (one-way training), no differences between the sexes were found. However, if the start and goal areas were reversed on each trial (two-way training), males outperformed females. One interpretation of these data is that in the two-way condition each landmark (objects or markings within the hallways or maze) has two opposite meanings depending on one's running direction, however, since the maze is symmetrical, reliance on angles and distances would be the same regardless of direction of training. Thus, males outperform females because reliance on angles and distances overshadows use of landmarks. Interestingly, using a task where adult male and female subjects were required to learn a specified route from a novel map, Galea and Kimura (1991) demonstrated that males outperformed females in their rate of acquisition, overall accuracy and knowledge of Euclidian properties. While there was a clear female superiority in remembering landmarks on and off the route (beyond that which could be accounted for by their advantage in visual item recall), both females and males appeared to be using the same geometrically-based (versus landmark based) spatial strategy for solving this task. Again, females appear to utilize multiple cues to navigate, while the male advantage may be due to task simplification.

## Summary and conclusion

The evidence presented in this chapter suggests that the current model of sexual differentiation of brain and behavior that has been developed from studies of the origins of sex differences in reproductive behavior can be usefully applied to the study of sex differences in visuospatial ability of rats. It appears that androgens secreted by the neonatal male are aromatized intracellularly to estradiol in hippocampus, and perhaps frontal cortex, to masculinize visuospatial processing. Activational influences of circulating androgens and estrogens are not needed to reveal sexual dimorphic adult visuospatial abilities. However, the model must be expanded to consider behavioral differences that are qualitative in nature rather than quantitative. Unlike sex differences in birdsong, rough and tumble play, or male or female sexual behavior in which one sex performs the behavior and the other sex rarely or never shows the behavior, cognitive processing of visuospatial information is effectively accomplished by both male and female animals. An examination of the behavioral processes underlying visuospatial navigation points to a qualitative sex difference in the content of spatial memory. In particular, males make almost exclusive use of cues based on the angles and distances (geometric information), while female utilize multiple cues, including landmark-based navigation. The exact neuroanatomical and neurophysiological basis for such differences awaits further research. Preliminary work, however, points to the hippocampus and regions of the cortex as potential sites for the action of estradiol on the organizational of visuospatial function.

# References

Arnold, A. P. and Gorski, R. A. (I984). Gonadal steroid induction of structural sex differences in the central nervous system. *An. Rev. Neurosci.,* **7** : 413-442.

Beatty, W. W. (1979). Gonadal hormones and sex differences in non-reproductive behaviors in rodents: organizational and activational influences.*Horm. Behav.,* **12** : 112-163.

Beatty, W. W. (1984). Hormonal organization of sex differences in play fighting and spatial behavior. *Prog. Brain Res.,* **6** : 320-324.

Beatty, W. W. (1992). Gonadal hormones and sex differences in nonreproductive behaviors. In: Gerall, A. A., Moltz, H. and Ward, I. L. (Eds.),*Handbook of Behavioral Neurobiology, Sexual Differentiation,* **11**, Plenum, New York and London, pp. 85-128.

Bever, T. (1992). The logical and extrinsic sources of modularity. In: Gunnar, M. and Maratsos, N. (Eds.), *Modularity and Constrains in Language,* Minnesota Symposia on Child Psychology, 25, Lawrence Erlbaum, Hillsdale, N.J., pp. 179-211.

Blough, P. M. and Slavin, L. K. (1987). Reaction time assessments of gender differences in visual-spatial performance. *Percep. Psychophys.,* **41**: 276-281.

Burstein, B., Bank, L. and Jarvik, L. (1980). Sex differences in cognitive functioning: evidence, determinants, implications. *Hum. Devel.,* **23** : 289-313.

Christensen L. W. and Gorski, R. A. (I978). Independent masculinization of neuroendocrine systems by intracerebral implants of testosterone or estradiol in the neonatal rat. *Brain Res.,* **146** : 325-340.

Clemens, L. G. and Gladue, B. A. (I978). Feminine sexual behavior in rats enhanced by prenatal inhibition of androgen aromatization. *Horm. Behav.,* **11** : 190-201.

Dawson, J. L. M., Cheung, Y. M. and Lau, R. T. S. (1975). Developmental effects of neonatal sex hormones on spatial and activity skills in the white rat. *Biol. Psychol.,* **3** : 213-229.

DeVoogd, T. (1984). The avian song system: relating sex differences in behavior to dimorphism in the central nervous system. *Prog. Brain Res.: Sex Diff. Brain.,* **6** : 171-184.

Fishman, R. B. and Breedlove, S. M. (1988). Sexual dimorphism in the developing nervous system. In: Meisami, E. and Timiras, P. S. (Eds.), *Handbook of Human Growth and Developmental Biology,* CRC Press, Boca Raton, FL., pp. 45-57.

Galea, L. and Kimura, D. (1991). *Sex Differences in Route Learning,* University of Western Ontario Publications.

Gaulin, S. J. C. and Fitzgerald, R. W. (I986). Sex differences in spatial ability: an evolutionary hypothesis and test. *Amer. Natur.,* **I27** : 74-88.

Gaulin, S. J. C., FitzGerald, R. W. and Wartell, M. S. (1990). Sex differences in spatial ability and activity in two vole species (Microtus ochrogaster and M. pennsylvanicus). *J. Comp. Psychol.,* **104** : 88-93.

Goy R. W. and McEwen, B. S. (1980). *Sexual Differentiation of the Brain,* The MIT Press, Cambridge.

Halpern, D. F. (1992). *Sex Differences in Cognitive Abilities,* Lawrence Erlbaum Associates, Hillsdale, N.J.

Hampson, E. and Kimura, D. (1988). Reciprocal effects of hormonal fluctuation on human motor and perceptual-spatial skills. *Behav. Neurosci.,* **102** : 456-459.

Joseph, R., Hess, S. and Birecree, E. (1978). Effects of hormone manipulations and exploration on sex differences in maze learning. *Behav. Biol.,* **24** : 364-377.

Kelley, D. (1987). The genesis of male and female brains. *Trends Neurosci.,* **9** : 499-502.

Kesner, R. P., DiMattia, B. V. and Crutcher, K. A. (1987). Evidence for neocortical involvement in reference memory. *Behav. Neur. Biol.,* **47** : 40-53.

Linn, M. C. and Petersen, A. C. (1985). Emergence and characterization of sex differences in spatial ability: a meta-analysis. *Child Devel.,* **56** : 1479-1498.

MacLusky, N. J., Clark, A. S. and Toran-Allerand,C.D. (1986). Aromatase activity in explant cultures of the developing mouse brain: is the rodent cerebral cortex a target for locally-synthesized estrogen? *Soc. Neurosci. Abstr.,* **12** : 1217.

MacLusky, N. J., Lieberburg, I. and McEwen, B. S. (1979). The development of estrogen receptor systems in the rat brain: perinatal development. *Brain Res.,* **178** : 129-142.

MacLusky, N. J. and Toran-Allerand, C. D. (1989). Estrogen biosynthesis in the developing rat brain: regional and temporal aspects. *Soc. Neurosci. Abstr.,* **15** : 88.

MacLusky, N. J., Clark, A. S., Naftolin, F. and Goldman-Rakic, P. S. (1987). Estrogen formation in the mammalian brain: possible role of aromatase in sexual differentiation of the hippocampus and neocortex. *Steroids,* **50** : 459-463.

Maggi, A. and Bettini, E. (1990). Estrogen receptor gene expression in the rat hippocampus. *Soc. Neurosci. Abstr.,* **16** : 1311.

Meck, W. H., Church, R. M., Wenk, G. L. and Olton, D. S. (1987). Nucleus basalis magnocellularis and medial septal area lesions differentially impair temporal memory. *J. Neurosci.,* **7** : 3505-3511.

Meck, W. G., Smith, R. A. and Williams, C. L. (1989). Organizational changes in cholinergic activity and enhanced visuospatial memory as a function of choline administered prenatally, postnatally, or both. *Behav. Neurosci.,* **103** : 118-146.

McEwen, B. S., Lieberburg, I., Chaptal, C. and Krey, L. C. (1977). Aromatization: important for sexual differentiation of the neonatal rat brain. *Horm. Behav.,* **9** : 249-263.

O'Keefe, J. A. and Handa, R. J. (1990). Transient elevation of estrogen receptors in the neonatal rat hippocampus. *Dev. Brain Res.,* **57** : 119-127.

Olton D. S. and Samuelson, R. J. (1976). Remembrance of places past: spatial memory in rats. *J. Exp. Psychol.: Anim. Behav. Proc.,* **2** : 97-116.

Phoenix, C. H., Goy, R. W., Gerall, A. A. and Young, W. C. (1959). Organizing action of prenatally administered testosterone propionate on the tissues mediating mating behavior in the guinea pig. *Endocrinology*, **65** : 369-382.

Roof, R. L. and Havens, M. D. (1992). Testosterone improves maze performance and induces development of a male hippocampus in females. *Brain. Res.*, **572** : 3130-313.

Sherman, J. (1978). *Sex-Related Cognitive Differences: an Essay on Theory and Evidence*, Thomas, Springfield, IL.

Shughrue, P. J., Stumpf,W. E., MacLusky, N .J., Zielinski, J. E. and Hochberg, R. B. (1990). Developmental changes in estrogen receptors between birth and postweaning: studied by autoradiography with 11β-methoxy-16α-[125I]Iodoestradiol. *Endocrinology*, **126** : 1112-1125.

Stewart, J., Skvarenina, A. and Pottier, J. (1975). Effects of neonatal androgens on open-field behavior and maze learning in the prepubescent and adult rat. *Physiol. Behav.*, **14** : 291-295.

Toran-Allerand, C. D. (1984). On the genesis of sexual differentiation of the central nervous system. In: De Vries, G. J., De Bruin, J. P. C., Uylings, H. B. M. and Corner , M. A. (Eds.), *Progress in Brain Research: Sex Differences in the Brain*, Elsevier, Amsterdam, pp. 63-98.

Ward, S. L., Newcombe, N. and Overton, W. F. (1986). Turn left at the church, or three miles north. A study of direction giving and sex differences. *Envir. Behav.*, **18** : 192-213.

Whalen, R. E., Gladue, B. A. and Olsen, K. L. (1986). Lordotic behavior in male rats: genetic and hormonal regulation of sexual differentiation. *Horm. Behav.*, **20** : 73-82.

Williams, C. L., Barnett, A. M. and Meck, W. H. (1990a). Organizational effects of early gonadal secretions on sexual differentiation in spatial memory. *Behav. Neurosci.*, **104** : 84-97.

Williams, C. L., Benedict, G. S., Williams, J. F. and Meck, W. H. (1992). Masculinization of spatial memory and defeminization of sexual behavior are blocked by postnatal inhibition of androgen aromatization. *Behav. Neurosci.*, under review.

Williams, C. L., Cohen, R. and Meck, W. H. (1990b). Development of sexually dimorphic spatial ability: neural sites of estradiol action. *Soc. Neurosci. Abstr.*, **16** : 472.

Williams, C. L. and Meck, W. H (1991). Organizational effects of gonadal steroids produce sexually dimorphic spatial ability. *Psychoneuroendocrinology*, **16** : 157-177.

# Intraspecific Aggression in Mice (Mus Domesticus): Male and Female Strategies

P. PALANZA, P. F. BRAIN[1] and S. PARMIGIANI

*Dipartimento di Biologia e Fisiologia Generali, Università di Parma, 43100 Parma, Italy*

*[1]University College of Swansea, School of Biological Sciences, Swansea, SA28PP, Wales, U K*

Aggression is used to compete for resources (like space, mates, food) and in any situations where the selfish interests of individuals conflict (Wittenberger, 1981). Indeed, agonistic interactions resulting in death (e.g. infanticide), dispersion or inhibition of reproductive functions may play a major role in shaping social structure and spatial distribution of rodents.

The house mouse provides an experimental model for understanding the relationships between individual aggressiveness, competitive strategies and spatial distribution. Indeed, this species is amongst the most versatile of mammals, having colonised an enormous range of habitats, either living commensally with man or under feral conditions (Berry, 1981). House mice populations may assume a variety of social organizations (ranging from exclusive male territoriality to hierarchical groups) depending on different socio-ecological conditions. The actual social organization employed seems to reflect variations in the degrees of male and female aggressiveness (Busser et al., 1974; Parmigiani et al., 1989a; Brain and Parmigiani, 1990).

This chapter describes a series of laboratory experiments on domesticated and wild stocks of mice analyzing different forms of male and female aggression, in an attempt to elucidate the proximal and ultimate causes of competitive strategies in this species.

## The male

Aggressive behavior towards (generally same sex) conspecifics in male mice mostly occurs in the context of territory establishment and defence. Successful reproduction seems to be a prerogative of dominant or exclusively territorial males (Reimer and Petras, 1967; Wolff, 1985; Hurst, 1987). Levels of male aggressiveness vary within and between laboratory strains or wild populations; indeed, males with differing potentials for intermale aggression and sociability may predispose populations to assume varied social structures (Brown, 1975; Busser et al., 1974; Brain and Parmigiani, 1990). It follows that all factors affecting the development of a male's aggressive behavior towards other males

*M. Haug et al. (eds.), The Development of Sex Differences and Similarities in Behavior, 191–203.*
© 1993 Kluwer Academic Publishers.

are of paramount importance in determining his reproductive fitness and shaping social structures.

Although it has been assumed that variations in aggressiveness are primarily due to genetic differences between individuals or groups, *in utero* exposure to steroid hormones and previous social experiences have potent effects on behavioural phenotypes in mice. Aggressive responses are also strongly influenced by the type of eliciting stimulus (i.e. type of opponent) and socio-environmental context (Brain, 1981).

Intrauterine position can influence many aspects of a rodent's anatomy, physiology and behavior (vom Saal, 1984a, for a review), but the majority of studies on this phenomenon have been limited to a single stock of mice. The impact of this variable was consequently studied on subsequent social responses of adult males in both outbred Swiss and inbred BALB/c mice (Yousif et al., 1990). Males from known intrauterine positions were produced by time-mating females, and delivering fetuses by Caesarean section a few hours prior normal parturition. Males which developed between two sisters (0M), between one sister and one brother (1M) and between two brothers (2M) were raised by foster mothers and, as adults, confronted standard opponents in a resident/intruder test. Males rendered anosmic by nasal lavage with a 4% zinc sulphate solution were used as standard intruders. A significant strain effect was recorded, with the Swiss albino line showing more offense (e.g. attack, threat) and defence (e.g. avoidance, submission) and less non social activity than the BALB/c. Intrauterine position influenced many behavioral parameters in adult male mice (Figure 1).

2M males displayed the highest levels of both offense and defence and showed less social investigation but more non social activities, than 1M and 0M counterparts (see Figure 1). What emerges from these data is that, during social encounters, 2M males are more aggressive and generally more active than 1M and 2M counterparts; conversely, 1M and 0M animals are likely to be more sociable. Exposure to androgens during intrauterine life may, indeed, exert a sensitizing effect on the neural substrates mediating intermale aggression in adulthood (vom Saal, 1984a). As the impact of intrauterine position is more marked on a range of social behaviors in the outbred Swiss albino mice than in inbred BALB/c subjects, the relative importance of this phenomenon may depend on the gene pool of a particular mouse population. The phenotypically variable mice generated by exposure to different titers of sex steroids may be suited to different ecologies or phases of the population cycle. The behavioral features facilitating reproductive success in mice may depend on the various phases of the population cycle (van Oortmersen and Busser, 1989). The enhanced levels of agonistic and non social activities shown by 2M males may predispose such animals to become territorial and intolerant towards same sex conspecifics. Conversely, 0M males could be mainly suited to situations where group living rather than potentially damaging and energetically wasteful territorial defence would be advantageous, e.g. immediately prior the migratory phases. Thus, changes due to the intrauterine position may be beneficial to a "r" reproductive strategist.

Male competitive strategies are not limited to direct interactions with adult conspecifics but they can also include interactions with their offspring. A high proportion of sexually naive male mice will attack and cannibalize young conspecifics, although with variations due to strain differences. As in other mammalian species, one of the commonest natural circumstances in which male mice kill unrelated young is when taking over a reproductive area to gain access to mates (Hrdy, 1979; vom Saal and Howard, 1982). This behavior seems to have evolved via sexual selection as a form of postmating competition among males (Hrdy, 1979; vom Saal and Howard, 1982). In fact, the infanticidal male eliminates a competitor's offspring and accelerates the females' return to estrus, thus advancing his mating opportunities and increasing reproductive success (vom Saal 1984b). Infanticide may thus be considered a unique form of intraspecific aggression (leading to the death of interacting animals) rather than intraspecific predation (cannibalism). This suggestion was assessed by giving the serotonergic agonist fluprazine to groups of males pre-selected for respectively showing intermale fighting, infanticide or predatory attack on a beetle larva similar in size and ability to move to a newborn mouse pup. The hypothesis that similar neuro-chemical substrates underlie male social aggression and infanticide was confirmed, as fluprazine inhibited infanticide and intermale attack at the same doses and to the same degree, but did not significantly alter predatory attack. This finding supports the Hrdy's view that this

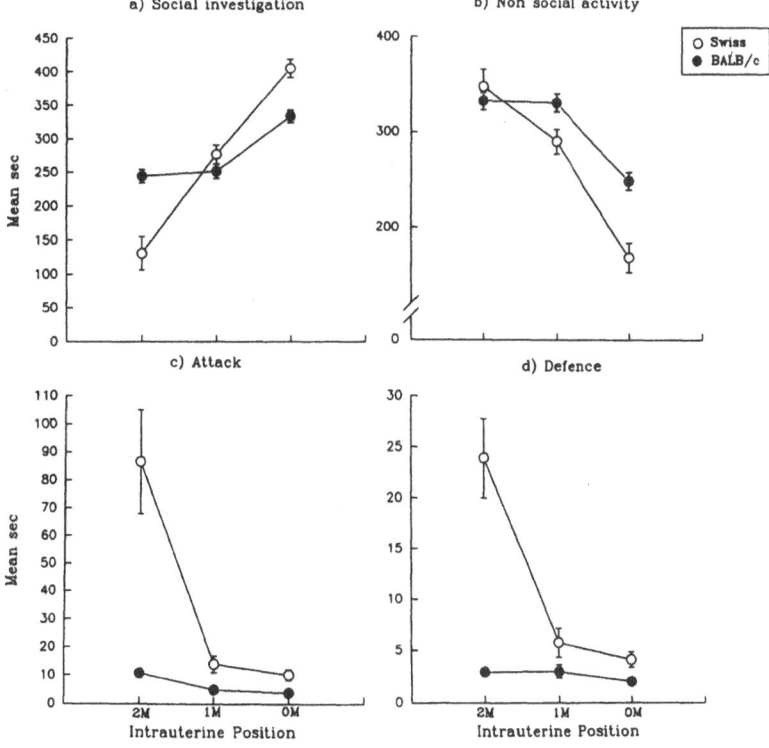

**Figure 1** Mean of times (sec.) allocated to different categories of behavior by Swiss and BALB/c males from different intrauterine position.

kind of infanticide is a competitive strategy, providing an indirect prove that infanticide is a form of intraspecific aggression as far as the neural domain is concerned (Parmigiani and Palanza, 1991).

The adaptiveness of "sexually selected" infanticide assumes the existence of mechanisms inhibiting infanticidal males from killing their own offspring. Indeed, male mice do not harm their own pups even if when infanticidal prior to mating. Although multiple mechanisms mediating the inhibition of infanticide can coexist within a mouse population (Palanza and Parmigiani, 1991), several studies suggest that male socio-sexual interactions with females play a crucial role in this phenomenon (Huck et al., 1982; vom Saal and Howard, 1982; Elwood and Ostermeyer, 1984; Jakubowsky and Terkel, 1982; Palanza and Parmigiani, 1991). The behavioral polymorphism in the factors mediating the transition from killing to caring for pups among (and within) domesticated and wild lines of mice might be due to varied reproductive strategies in response to different selection pressures (Palanza and Parmigiani, 1991). After mating and cohabitation with the pregnant mate, males do not kill related (their own) or unrelated young, either in the presence or in absence of the familiar lactating female (Parmigiani, 1989). Thus suppression of infant killing occurs at time when there is a strong probability that a male will encounter his own offspring. In fact, once a male has established a territory and achieved dominance, he is likely to sire the majority of the litters within that area (Reimer and Petras, 1967). Consequently, the preferential survival of related infants appears a by-product of the typical social structure of the mouse. This mechanism resulting in kin selection does not necessitate the animals having to show kin recognition.

# The female

The stereotype of the female mouse is that of a "non aggressive" and "passive" animal in response to conspecifics (Mackintosh, 1981). This view was partially due to the fact that isolation (a procedure that increases social aggression in males) failed to enhance aggressiveness in laboratory female mice, thus suggesting a non-territorial nature of this gender (Valzelli, 1974). It was implied that aggression was under the control of male androgens, and because females lack the Y chromosome and have lower circulating levels of androgens, they do not ordinarily have the biological substrates for the exhibition of aggression (Edwards, 1968). It was traditionally maintained that female mice become aggressive only during pregnancy and lactation in order to defend their parental investment (Ostermeyer, 1983; Svare, 1989). Several current observations suggest that female aggression is not restricted to pup's protection and can play an important role in social dynamics (e.g. Yasukawa et al., 1985).

Even so-called "maternal aggression" in mice is a complex and heterogeneous phenomenon subserving a variety of functions according context and characteristics of conspecific intruders (Parmigiani, 1986; Parmigiani et al., 1988). For instance, lactating females may use aggression in competing with same sex conspecifics to establish a social hierachy, to space rivals and in defence of the litter from infanticidal conspecifics (Parmigiani et al., 1989b). In this view, maternal aggression toward males (the more infanticidal gender) has been interpreted as a counterstrategy to infanticide. However, in laboratory studies, maternal attack rarely prevents male infanticide. A recent study[1] investigating the effects of confronting lactating females with sexually naive male intruders of differing potentials for infanticide and intermale aggression, suggests that the female's response as well as the possibility of successfully protecting her young is modulated by the aggressive tendency (fighting ability) of the intruder male, rather than by the potential risk for the young (Parmigiani et al., 1993).

One may speculate on the ultimate causation of maternal aggression towards male intruders. Females whose litters are destroyed quickly come back into estrus and can be inseminated by the intruder male. Consequently, female attack might also assess the fighting ability and indirectly the genetic quality, in terms of Resources Holding Potential (RHP) [see Parker, 1974 and Maynard-Smith, 1982] of the interloper male, that is likely to become her future mate and the father of her next litter. Indeed, when the stud male is absent (i.e. the territory is vacant), the cost of defending the previous parental investment may be outweighed by the gain of a new mate characterized by good RHP. In this scenario, maternal aggression prevents reproduction with males of low aggressive potential. Indeed, lactating females do not engage in costly fights (i.e. in terms of energy expenditure) with the interloper males when her mate (i.e. the father of the litter) is not aggressive and submissive to the intruder (Parmigiani et al., 1993). Moreover, social status of males modulates sexual preferences and subsequent mating in mice and courtship in this species resembles an agonistic interaction with the male subduing the female prior the copulation (Parmigiani et al., 1982; Hurst, 1986). Aggression by lactating females towards males may thus serve as a counterstrategy defending the parental investment but also could be involved in intersexual selection by females for males with "good genes" (Krebs and Davies, 1981; Trivers, 1985).

The presence of a territorial male plays a crucial role in modulating interfemale competition. Female laboratory mice may become aggressive towards same sex conspecifics after 24 hours of cohabitation with a male (Parmigiani et al., 1989a). How does the male alter the aggressive behavior of the female? Since olfactory cues are important in the regulation of aggressive behavior in mice (Bronson 1983), the effects of exposure to male urinary odors on female aggressive responses were evaluated. Swiss albino virgin females were individually housed for 24 hours in cages containing clean sawdust or previously inhabited by a male, for 48 hours. The twenty females in each category, confronted an unfamiliar same sex intruder for 30 minutes. After a 10 minute break, they confronted an adult sexually naive male. In both experimental conditions, about 50 % of Swiss resident female displayed agonistic behaviors, like aggressive grooming and mounting-like behavior, but exposure to male bedding increased the proportion of resident females that attacked ($X^2 = 6.5$, P < 0.01) a female intruder, compared to counterparts isolated in clean cages. The attack recorded is similar to that observed during male-male encounters. No females showed aggressive responses towards male intruders. Similar results have been obtained in wild mice (unpublished observation). These findings suggest that females compete among themselves not for space (i.e. territory) but for a male who has taken possession of an area. Since male odors are known to induce estrus (the so-called Whitten effect c.f.

196

Whitten, 1958), the increased female aggressiveness could facilitate a successful mating by dispersing same sex rivals that could interfere with reproduction.

Female mice spend a significant portion of their adult life span pregnant or lactating and these reproductive periods are associated with rapid neuroendocrine changes and significant maternal investment in the successful rearing of the young. These factors, along with the associated risk of infanticide by males, intuitively suggest that sexually, and therefore reproductively, active female mice are more likely to exhibit aggressive behavior than non reproductive (e.g. virgin) animals (Svare, 1989). The relation of interfemale competition to reproductive activity is confirmed to some degree by the variation of infanticidal behavior in relation to the reproductive cycle (McCarthy and vom Saal, 1985).

In Swiss females, the frequency of infanticide varies with their reproductive state and the age of the alien pup (Parmigiani et al., 1993). While virgin females are generally parental both towards newborn pups and preweaning young, pregnant females kill pups and attack preweaning young in 50% of cases. Lactating females behave parentally towards strangers of the same age of their own offspring but vigorously attack older pups. There appears to be an age-dependent discrimination of unfamiliar pups by lactating females and that this phenomenon is modulated by the stage of lactation and the age difference between the pup and the female's own offspring. The parental behavior of resident lactating mice towards alien young of the same age as their litters could reduce the risk of killing related pups since, in a deme, females (which are often genetically related) generally synchronize estrus and pup delivery (Crowcroft and Rowe, 1963; Pennycuik et al., 1986). Alien pups which are older than a female's own pups are likely to be immigrants and thus genetically unrelated competitors of the resident lactating females own young, and should be attacked. This falls under Hrdy's definition of resource competition infanticide (Hrdy, 1979). When resident females are lactating, the territory holding male is generally inhibited in his attack and killing of young (see previous section). Consequently, the female's intolerance towards alien young whilst reproducing may prevent immigration of juveniles which would compete for resources with her offspring.

# Roles of male and female aggression

In order to understand male and female competitive strategies, and their roles in shaping social structure, a longitudinal study in artificial territories was carried out. All mice used in this study were originally derived from a population of wild house mice captured near Capalbio (Central Italy) and had been bred in the laboratory of the University of Parma for about five generations. The experimental apparatus consisted of 8 artificial territories, each consisting of 12 transparent plastic cages, of different sizes (40x25x15 cm and 23x18x14 cm.), connected by blockable tunnels of wire netting, 5 cm in diameter. The total area covered by each territory was approximately 2 meters square, including the tunnels. Experimental subjects were virgin mice (8 males and 8 females) 90 days old. The experimental procedure followed four main stages:

-Stage 0: establishment of a pair, in which one male and one female were allowed to colonize an enclosure (these were the resident animals). Intruder tests were carried out at different stages of the reproductive cycle.
-Stage 1: intruder test before breeding (48 h. after colony establishment).
-Stage 2: intruder test during pregnancy (after 18 days).
-Stage 3: intruder test during lactation, when resident female was nursing pups (two days after delivery).
In each stage, a virgin female, a virgin male and two pups were separately introduced into the enclosure, 24 hours separating each introduction. Whenever a new individual was introduced into a territory, observation was made continually for the first hour and then continued for 6 hours whenever further activity occurred. Pups were removed after first recorded attack. After 24 hours, tolerance of intruders was checked and the intruders were left in the enclosure throughout the study in stage 1 or removed in stages 2 and 3. In any stage, subjects becoming injured or cornered and continually attacked were removed from the territory.

Male and female residents mainly attacked like-sexed intruders (Figure 2). Male residents were always highly aggressive toward male intruders but did not attack female intruder in the first stage, usually showing a sexually related

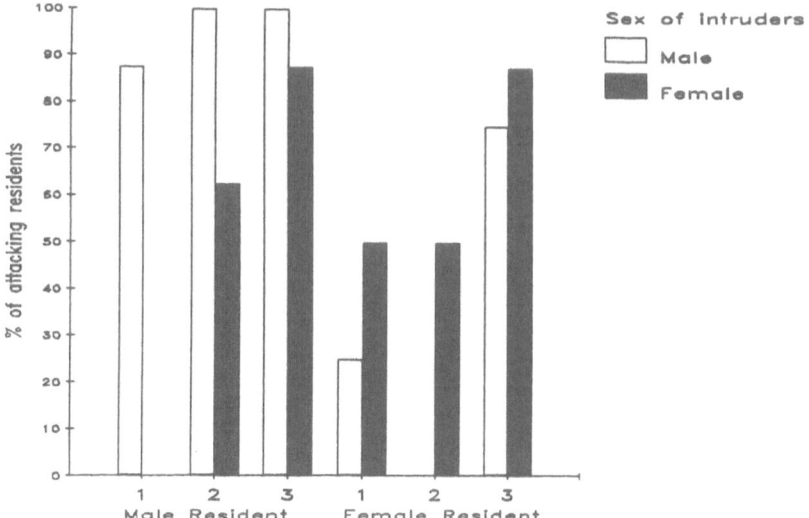

**Figure 2** Percentages of male and female residents attacking male and female intruders during different reproductive stages: 1-before breeding; 2-pregnancy; 3-lactation.

aggression on female intruders in stages 2 and 3 (with low intensity of attack and no viscious bites and mounting attempts). In two cases in stage 3 female intruders were strongly attacked by male residents.

In the first two stages (immediately after colony formation and during pregnancy) 50% of resident females attacked preferentially (or rather exclusively) same sex intruders. In the following hours, virtually all females attacked. In the third stage, resident lactating females attacked both male and female intruders, though attacks on males were less intense.

Male intruders were never tolerated inside the territory in any stage. Conversely, during the first stage, female intruders were tolerated in five out eight territories. Tolerance of females progressively decreased, with 3 and 1 female intruders tolerated in stage 2 and 3, respectively. Male and female residents appear intolerant of same sex intruders. There was a significant increase in the intensity of attack by both male and female residents on same sex intruders between stage 1 and stages 2 and 3, when the resident female is pregnant or lactating. Since in this stock of mice virtually all males (92%) and most of females (67%) exhibited infanticide as virgins, the increased rate of aggression displayed by both sex residents during peri-parturition phases seems related to the protection of parental investment.

The majority of resident males killed the intruder pups in stage one and two, but all displayed parental behavior (retrieving the pup) during the stage three, when their own litters were present into the enclosures (Figure 3).

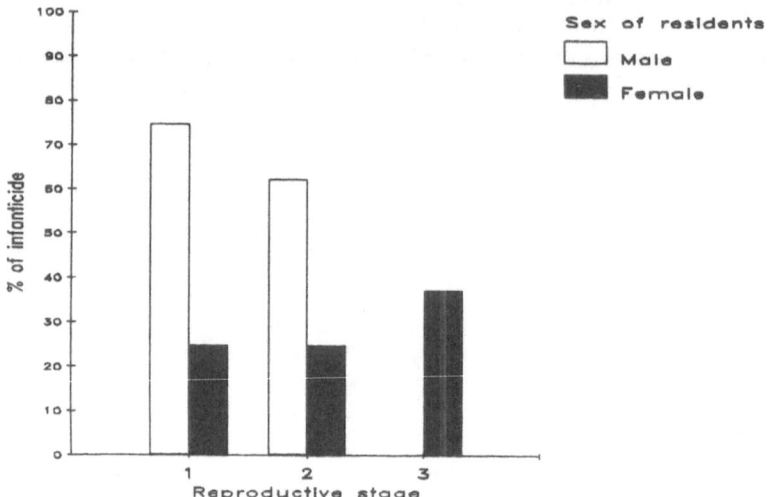

**Figure 3** Percentages of infanticide toward strange pups by male and female residents at different reproductive stages.

This finding substantially confirms previous data on infanticide inhibition in Swiss mice (see earlier). Since it was usually the male that found the intruder pups first, data on infanticide by females are limited. It is however interesting that three lactating residents attacked strange pups of the same age as their own, in stage three (see Figure 3).

When two females were present into a territory, the resident female was largely responsible of aggression towards intruders. In this situation, only one female reproduced successfully: in three territories only the resident became pregnant and delivered pups successfully. This suggests that the two females established a hierachycal polarity and only the dominant female in the pair was able to ovulate and mate. In the remaining two territories, both the females were pregnant and delivered their litters a few day apart, but only the offspring of the second female to deliver survived. As previously mentioned, during the last part of pregnancy, the proportion of female mice exhibiting infanticide increases (see Mc Carthy and vom Saal, 1986 for wild mice). The second female to deliver may have killed the first litter, although infanticide was not directly observed. These findings suggest that, as is true for males, females of this stock compete among themselves for the opportunity to reproduce. They can be exclusively territorial or form a dominance hierarchy which determines reproductive success (see also Franks et al., 1993). This can strongly affect social structure. Indeed, female aggression toward same sex adult conspecifics may limit the reproductive output of the dominant male in a deme. Thus, although house mice tend to be polygynous, interfemale aggression as well as infanticide by females could prevent males from acquiring additional mates, thus leading to forced monogamy for males in this stock.

# Conclusion

Male and female mice can both be aggressive but can show differences in the display and the timing of aggression toward adult and young conspecifics. Males are competitive only among each others for establishing and holding a territory and/or establishing social rank, in order to mate with females. Since reproduction is largely confined to dominant or exclusively territorial male (Wolff, 1985; Hurst, 1986), intermale aggression can limit reproductive potential of same sex conspecifics and facilitate dispersion and colonisation. Females become aggressive only when they become associated with a male holding a territory; suggesting that interfemale competition arises in relation to reproductive activity.

Situational determinants and reproductive status strongly affect the behavioral responses of male and female adult mice towards unrelated young. Males are most likely to show infanticide when they are sexually naive and when taking over of a reproductive area, whereas females exhibit the highest propensity of killing unrelated young when they are near parturition and/or lactating and the stud territorial male is not infanticidal. In male mice, infanticide involves intraspecific competition for mates, whereas, in females, it appears to be a resource competition strategy increasing the probability of access to food and survival of their offspring. The killing of unrelated young by females may serve the function of territorial defence against juvenile immigrants.

The presence of a territorial male seems a key-factor in controlling social organization, since impregnation or just stimuli coming from a male holding an area are necessary to induce female aggression. However, females seem to be largely responsible of the regulation of the reproductive potential of a deme unit throughout intrasexual aggression (intolerance towards other females), inhibition of subordinate reproduction and killing of unrelated young.

The sex differences in the display and timing of competitive strategies can generate conflict of interests (like the limitation of male reproductive output due to interfemale competition or female's parental defence against male infanticide) but may also maximize both male and female reproductive success when they form a demic unit (i.e. preventing immigration of strange conspecifics which would compete for resources and mates). In this respect, if the reproductive fitness of a male depends on his ability to acquire and defend a territory or social status, then the most successful strategy for females seems to become associated (to mate) with a male with a good fighting ability and thus capable to defend territory. The resident male provides indeed a necessary defender of the pups when the intruder is a male, as maternal aggression *per se* can not prevent male infanticide. The spatial and temporal stability of demes seems indeed a crucial factor in determining the reproductive success of both male and female residents.

# Note

[1] In order to examine the functions of maternal aggression, we investigated the effects of Four categories of previously selected males were used as intruders : 1. infanticidal and aggressive (IA; N = 12); 2. infanticidal and non-aggressive (INA, N = 10); 3. non-infanticidal aggressive (NIA, N = 4); 4. non-infanticidal non-aggressive (NINA, N = 10). Detailed behavioral recording lasted 10 minutes, but occurrence of infanticide was subsequentely checked in the following hours. The male was removed after first recorded attack on any pup. Lactating females attacked all categories of males to similar degrees, but exhibited shorter latencies to attack toward infanticidal aggressive males than toward INA and NINA counterparts. In the initial ten minutes, the majority of Infanticidal Aggressive males and a few males in the other categories of intruders started to attack the female and her pups; over the next 12 hours, all IA and the majority of INA attacked the pups, whereas the other categories showed no further augmentation. These findings suggest that attack by lactating females prevented or delayed pup killing only in weakly aggressive males.

# References

Berry, R. J. (1981). The biology of the house mouse. *Symposium of the Zoological Society of London* , Academic Press, New York.

Bradford, L. D., Olivier, B., van Dalen, D. and Schipper, J. (1984). Serenics: the pharmacology of fluprazine and DU 28412. In: MiczeK, K., Kruk, M. and Olivier, B. (Eds.), *Ethopharmacological Aggression Research*, Alan R. Liss Inc., New York, pp. 191-207.

Brain, P. F. (1981). Differentiating types of attack and defence in rodents. In: Brain, P. F. and Benton, D. (Eds.), *Multidisciplinary Approaches to Aggression Research*, Elsevier/North-Holland, Amsterdam, pp.53-78.

Brain, P. F. and Parmigiani, S. (1990). Variation in aggressiveness in house mouse populations. *Biol. J. Linnean Soc.*, **41** : 257-269

Bronson, F. H. (1983). Chemical communication in house mice and deer mice: functional roles in reproduction of wild populations. In: Eisenberg, J. F. and Kleiman, D. G. (Eds.), *Advances in the Study of Mammalian Behavior,* Special Publication N.7, The American Society of Mammalogists, pp. 198-238.

Brown, J. L. (1975). *The Evolution of Behavior*, W. Norton, New York.

Busser, J., Zweep, A. and van Oortmerssen, G. A. (1974). Variability in the aggressive behavior of *Mus domesticus*, its possible role in population structure. In: Abeleen J. H. F. (Ed.), *The Genetics of Behaviour*, North-Holland Publishing Co., Amsterdam, pp.185-199.

owcroft, P. and Rowe, F. P. (1963) Social organization and territorial behavior n the wild house mouse (*Mus musculus L.*). *Proc. Zool. Soc. London*, **140** : 517-531.

Jwards, D. A. (1968). Mice : Fighting by neonatally androgenized females. *Science*, **161** : 1027-1028.

wood, R. W. and Ostermayer, M. C. (1984). Does copulation inhibit infanticide n male rodents? *Anim. Behav.*, **32** : 293-305.

anks, P., Parmigiani, S. and vom Saal, F. S. (1993). Nest defence and survival of offspring in highly aggressive canadian female house mice. In press.

rdy, S. B. (1979). Infanticide among animals : a review, classification, and examinations of the implications for the reproductive strategies of females. *Ethol. Sociobiol.*, **1** : 13-40.

uck, U. W., Soltis, R. L. and Coopersmith, C. B. (1982). Infanticide in male laboratory mice : effects of social status, prior sexual experience, and bases for discriminating between related and unrelated young. *Anim. Behav.*, **30** : 1158-1165.

urst, J. L. (1986). Mating in free living wild house mice *(Mus domesticus Rutty)*. *J. Zool.*, **210** : 623-628.

urst, J. L. (1987). Behavioural variation in wild house mice *(Mus domesticus Rutty)* : a quantitative assessment of female social organization. *Anim. Behav.*, **35** : 1864-1857.

akubowsky, M. and Terkel, J. (1982). Infanticide and caretaking in non lactating *Mus musculus* : influence of genotype, family group and sex. *Anim. Behav.*, **30** : 1029-1035.

rebs, C. B. and Davies, N. B. (1981). *An Introduction to Behavioral Ecology*, Blackwell Scientific Publication, Oxford.

lackintosh, J. H. (1981). Behaviour of the House Mouse. *Symposium of the Zoological Society of London*, **47** : 337-335.

laynard-Smith, J. (1982). *Evolution and the Theory of Games*, Cambridge University Press, Cambridge.

lcCarthy, M. M. and vom Saal, F. S. (1985). The influence of reproductive state on infanticide by wild female house mice *(Mus musculus)*. *Physiol. Behav.*, **35** : 843-849.

)stermeyer, M. (1983). Maternal aggression. In : Elwood, R. (Ed.), *Parental Behavior in Rodents*, Wiley and Sons, Chirchester, pp.151-179.

'alanza, P. and Parmigiani, S. (1991). Inhibition of infanticide in male Swiss mice : behavioral polimorphism in response to multiple mediating factors. *Physiol. Behav.*, **49** : 797-802.

'arker, G. A. (1974). Assessment strategy and the evolution of fighting behavior. *J. Theoret. Biol.*, **47** : 223-243.

'armigiani, S. (1986). Rank order in pairs of communally nursing female mice and maternal aggression towards conspecific intruders of differing sex. *Aggres. Behav.*, **12** : 377-386.

'armigiani, S. (1989). Inhibition of infanticide in male house mouse *(Mus domesticus)* : is kin recognition involved? *Ethol. Ecol. Evol.*, **1** : 93-98.

'armigiani, S. and Palanza, P. (1991). Fluprazine inhibits intermale attack and infanticide, but not predation, in male mice. *Neurosci. Biobehav. Rev.*, **15** : 511-513.

Parmigiani, S., Brain, P. F. and Palanza, P. (1989a). Ethoexperimental analysis of different forms of intraspecific aggression in the house mouse *(Mus domesticus)*. In : Blanchard, R., Brain, P. F., Blanchard, D. C. and Parmigiani, S. (Eds.), *Ethoexperimental Approaches to the Study of Behavior*, Klüwer Academic, Dordrecht, pp. 418-431.

Parmigiani, S., Brunoni, V. and Pasquali, A. (1982). Behavioral influences of dominant, isolated and subordinated male mice on female socio-sexual preferences. *Boll. Zool.*, **49** : 73-78.

Parmigiani, S., Palanza, P. and Brain, P. F. (1989b). Intraspecific maternal aggression in the house mouse *(Mus domesticus)* : a counterstrategy to infanticide by male? *Ethol. Ecol. Evol.*, **1** : 341-352.

Parmigiani, S., Palanza, P., Brain, P. F. and Mainardi, D. (1993). Infanticide and protection of young in house mouse *(Mus domesticus)* : female and male strategies. In : Parmigiani S., Svare B. and vom Saal F. (Eds.), *Infanticide and Parental Care in Animals and Man*, Harwood Academic Publishers, Chur (in press).

Pennycuik, P. R., Johnston, P. G., Westwood, N. H. and Reisner, A. H. (1986). Variation in numbers in a house mouse population housed in a large outdoor enclosure : seasonal fluctuations. *J. Anim. Ecol.*, **55** : 371-391.

Reimer, J. and Petras, M. L. (1967). Breeding structure of the house mouse *(Mus musculus)* in a population cage. *J. Mammal.*, **48** : 88-99.

Svare, B. (1989). Recent advances in the study of female aggressive behaviour in mice. In : Brain, P.F., Mainardi, D., and Parmigiani, S. (Eds.), *House Mouse Aggression : A Model for Understanding the Evolution of Social Behaviour.* Harwood Academic Press, Chur, pp. 135-159.

Trivers, R. L. (1985). *Social Evolution*, The Benjamin/Cumming Co, Manlo Park.

Valzelli, L. (1974). Aggressiveness by isolation in rodents. In : de Wit, J. and Hartup, W. W. (Eds.), *Determinants and Origins of Aggressive Behavior*, Mouton, The Hague, pp. 299-308.

van Oortmerssen, G. A. and Busser, J. (1989). Studies on wild house mice: distruptive selection of aggression as a possible force in evolution. In : Brain, P. F., Mainardi, D. and Parmigiani, S. (Eds.), *House Mouse Aggression.* Harwood Academic Publ. Chur, pp.87-118.

vom Saal, F. S. (1984a). The intrauterine position phenomenon : effects on physiology, aggressive behavior, and population dynamics in house mice. In : Flanelly, K. J., Blanchard, R. J. and Blanchard,D. C. (Eds), *Biological Perspectives on Aggression*, Alan R. Liss Inc., New York, pp.135-180.

vom Saal, F. S. (1984b). Proximate and ultimate causes of infanticide in parental behavior in male house mice. In : Husfater, G. and Hrdy, S. B. (Eds.), *Infanticide : Comparative and Evolutionary Perspectives*, Aldine Publishing Co., New York, pp. 401-425.

vom Saal, F. S. and Howard, L. S. (1982). The regulation of infanticide and parental behavior : implication for reproductive success in male mice. *Science*, **215** : 1270-1272.

Whitten, W. K. (1958). Modification of the estrus cycle of the mouse by external stimuli associated with the male. *J. Endocr.*, **13** : 339.

Wittenberger, J. F. (1981). *Animal Social Behavior*, Duxbury Press, Boston.

Iolff, J. O. (1985). Maternal aggression as a deterrent to infanticide in *Peromyscus leucopus* and *P. maniculatus*. *Anim. Behav.*, **33** : 117-123.

asukawa, N. J., Harvey, M., Leff, F. L. and Christian, J. J. (1985). Role of female behavior in controlling population growth in mice. *Aggres. Behav.*, **11** : 49-64.

ousif, Y, Palanza, P, Parmigiani, S., Mainardi, M. and Brain, P. F. (1991). Effects of genotype and intrauterine position on behavior of male mice during social encounters. *Boll. Zool.*, **58** : 119-124.

# A Comparison of Drug Responses by Male and Female Rats During Aggression Tests

**J. MOS[1] and B. OLIVIER[1,2]**

[1]*Department of CNS-Pharmacology, Solvay Duphar B.V., P.O. Box 900, 1380 DA Weesp, The Netherlands*

[2]*Department of Psycho-pharmacology, Faculty of Pharmacy, State University of Utrecht, The Netherlands*

The scope of this chapter is to compare the differences and similarities of the neuropharmacology of male and female aggression in rats. Unfortunately such a task is far from easy because aggression research in the realm of neuropharmacology has mainly focussed on males, notably in rodents. The reasons for this choice are obvious and valid. With some exceptions, under many circumstances males are more aggressive than females. However, the generality of our conclusions and our knowledge on brain-behavior relationships is severely limited by this bias to study male aggression. In contrast to the more etho-ecologically oriented studies, in most psycho-pharmacological experiments there is no emphasis on the function of the observed behavior, which may profoundly differ in males and females. Indeed the adaptive or survival value of aggression in rodents housed under laboratory conditions can only be extrapolated from their feral counterparts. However, to study the neuro-pharmacological organization under more ecologically relevant conditions is not very practical, not to say impossible. We therefore have to rely on extrapolations from the laboratory situation to more naturalistic situations and *vice versa*.

A comparison of the neuropharmacology of male and female aggression is interesting for different reasons. First, it is important to understand the regulation of aggression within different genders of the same species where internal and external factors evoking aggression may differ profoundly. Is the basic neuropharmacology similar despite the diversity in the other regulatory mechanisms? Second, it is of interest to know whether drugs that modulate aggression in males are equally effective and selective in both sexes. Our work was to a large extent governed by the latter interest. Since we have discovered and developed drugs that exert unique anti-aggressive actions in animals, we wanted to know whether these drugs could be equally useful for treating (pathological) aggression in males and females.

*M. Haug et al. (eds.), The Development of Sex Differences and Similarities in Behavior, 205–225.*
© 1993 *Kluwer Academic Publishers.*

In this chapter we describe studies comparing male and female aggression in rats. We mainly focussed our own work on resident-intruder aggression test as a valid, ethologically relevant aggression model in male rats. Female aggression can readily be evoked under laboratory conditions by the introduction of an intruder during the post-partum period of a female rat (Erskine et al., 1978a,b). Although these two models are by no means suggested to be representative of all forms of male and female aggression in rats, let alone in other species, the present set of data provides a within-laboratory comparison of a wide range of different psychoactive compounds. First, the choice for resident-intruder and maternal aggression will be discussed. Subsequently a selected number of compounds including those affecting serotonergic and dopaminergic neurotransmission will be compared in males and females. Finally these data are compared to available literature and a synopsis of the conclusions will be given.

# The choice for maternal aggression and resident-intruder aggression

Several reasons underlie the emphasis that has previously been placed on male agonistic behavior. There is a widely held belief that females are less aggressive than males and selective citation is an easy tool to support this notion. However, already in the early days of aggression research in the laboratory rat, the bias of the investigators was clearly present as evident from the following statement:

*"The chief difference between the social interactions of males and those of females can be most succinctly, if not objectively, described by saying that the females were less concerned with the problem of status ..... Fights occurred among females but with less decisive effect on their subsequent reactions (Seward, 1945a,b,c)".*

It is evident that Seward was not primarily interested in the occurrence of aggressive acts in a situation of competition, but rather in the establishment of clearcut dominance-subordinance relationships. And although females displayed aggressive acts at the same levels as males, they failed to establish dominance (Seward, 1945a, page 189).

For many years the study of aggression in the laboratory was guided by 'dominance' type of studies often employing round robin techniques pairing different individuals repeatedly. Females were often neglected in these studies.

The psychopharmacological studies that started to develop at the end of the fifties used isolation induced aggression in mice. The emergence of isolation-induced aggression in mice as a valuable tool for studying the psychopharmacological control of aggression occurred at the same time when the procedures for shock-induced fighting and "predatory aggression", both in rats and mice were developed. But neither in shock-induced fighting, nor in "predatory aggression" investigators have paid much attention to comparative studies on the neuropharmacological mechanisms in males and females (Olivier et al., 1989c).

Rather recently, aggression research has moved to the stage where ethopharmacologial approaches play an important role (see Krsiak, 1991). The studies on colony formation and intruder attack in rats (Luciano and Lore, 1975; Blanchard and Blanchard, 1977) and the subsequent modification of these paradigms to more simple resident-intruder (RI) paradigms (Thor and Flannelly, 1976a,b; Olivier, 1977; Lehman and Adams, 1977; Miczek, 1979; Lore et al., 1984) has been paralleled by much more sophisticated methods in the recording of aggression. In fact, not only aggressive elements were recorded using computer-assisted scoring systems, but also other behavioral categories like exploration, social interest, self-care, inactivity, defence and avoidance were more routinely scored. Thus the emphasis changed from scoring limited (often single) parameters indicative for aggression to a complete analysis of the behavioral repertoire of the animal in the context of an aggression test.

Simultaneously, the distinction between offense and defense in rat aggression models led to a re-appraisal of the animal models (Blanchard et al., 1977; Adams, 1979). Nowadays the more naturalistic models of offensive aggression like resident-intruder aggression, isolation-induced aggression, colony aggression and maternal aggression are preferred to predatory aggression, chemically- or lesion-induced aggression and footshock or withdrawal aggression. Although 'dominance studies', especially competitive studies over food, water, sucrose etc. are still used, their application in psychopharmacology has still been limited.

As a model for female aggression we chose maternal or postpartum aggression. In retrospect it is not easy to establish the precise reasons why we have not focussed our attention on the female in analogy to the resident-intruder model in rats. Although several studies (Brain et al., 1980; DeBold and Miczek, 1981) have suggested that female residents are quite capable of attacking female intruders, we were impressed by the fierce attacks produced by lactating female rats and mice towards an intruder as well as the striking differences in the neurobiological organization of maternal aggression compared with resident-intruder aggression (see Svare and Gandelman, 1973; Svare et al., 1981; Mos et al., 1989a). Earlier studies (Olivier et al., 1985; Olivier and Mos, 1986; Yohismura, 1987) showed the potential use of studying maternal aggression in psychopharmacology and finally we chose to compare several reference drugs in males and lactating females.

# Drug studies in resident-intruder and maternal aggression in rats

The effects of various drugs from different classes is summarized in the Figures 1 to 5, in which the mean duration scores of behavioral categories are expressed as percentage of vehicle treatment. For inactivity, which increased after drug treatment, the highest dose was set at 100% as this results in better graphical presentation. Grouping the different behavioral elements into broader behavioral categories does mask some more subtle effects, but it is easier to visualize the significance of the main findings.

The mixed serotonergic 1A/1B receptor agonist eltoprazine reduced aggression dose-dependently in males and females (Figure 1), although the dose response curve appeared somewhat steeper for males. Social interest was not affected and inactivity slightly increased at the highest dose. The only major difference was the fact that males reacted with increased exploration after eltoprazine whereas such effects were absent in females.

(±)-Propranolol, a ß-adrenoceptor antagonist with significant serotonin 1A/1B receptor affinity reduced aggression in male rats, but at the highest dose also reduced social interest and inactivity. Exploration was increased at the middle doses. By contrast (±)-propranolol treatment failed to change any of the behaviors of lactating females (Figure 1).

In maternal aggression the full 5-HT1A agonist 8-OH-DPAT (Figure 2) reduced aggression rather abruptly at a dose of 0.1 mg/kg and doubling the dose resulted in a decrease in social interest and an increase in inactivity. An almost identical profile of drug-induced changes was seen in residential males. Thus for 8-OH-DPAT there appears to be a good correspondence between maternal aggression and RI aggression, both quantitatively and qualitatively.

Figure 2 also shows that DOI, a 5-HT1C/2 receptor agonist with hallucinogenic properties, induced qualitatively similar effects on aggression and inactivity in male and female rats, but the dose response curve seems shifted towards the right for maternal aggression.

Fluvoxamine, a specific 5-HT reuptake inhibitor reduced aggression quite specifically in females, i.e. the decrease in aggression was not caused by overt signs of sedation, nor was social interest disrupted (Figure 3). However, in RI aggression, fluvoxamine reduced aggression only at higher doses and the profile of changes differed from that of females. Residential males showed reduced social interest and increased inactivity.

The benzodiazepine agonist oxazepam had biphasic effects on aggression: it increased aggression at the lower doses both in males and females (Figure 3), but at the highest dose aggression had returned to baseline levels again, without notable sedation. Both compounds reduced exploration at all doses, but did not affect social interest. This decrease is probably not similar to effects observed with sedating doses, because social interest and inactivity were not affected.

Haloperidol (Figure 4) reduced aggression in males at all doses, therefore in females a lower range of doses was selected. Unfortunately the drop in aggression in females did not reach statistical significance. In males the general sedatory effects of haloperidol are evidenced by the reductions of time spent on social interest and exploration, concomitant with a massive increase in inactivity. Females only suffered from an increase in inactivity at doses where social interest and exploration had not significantly been affected.

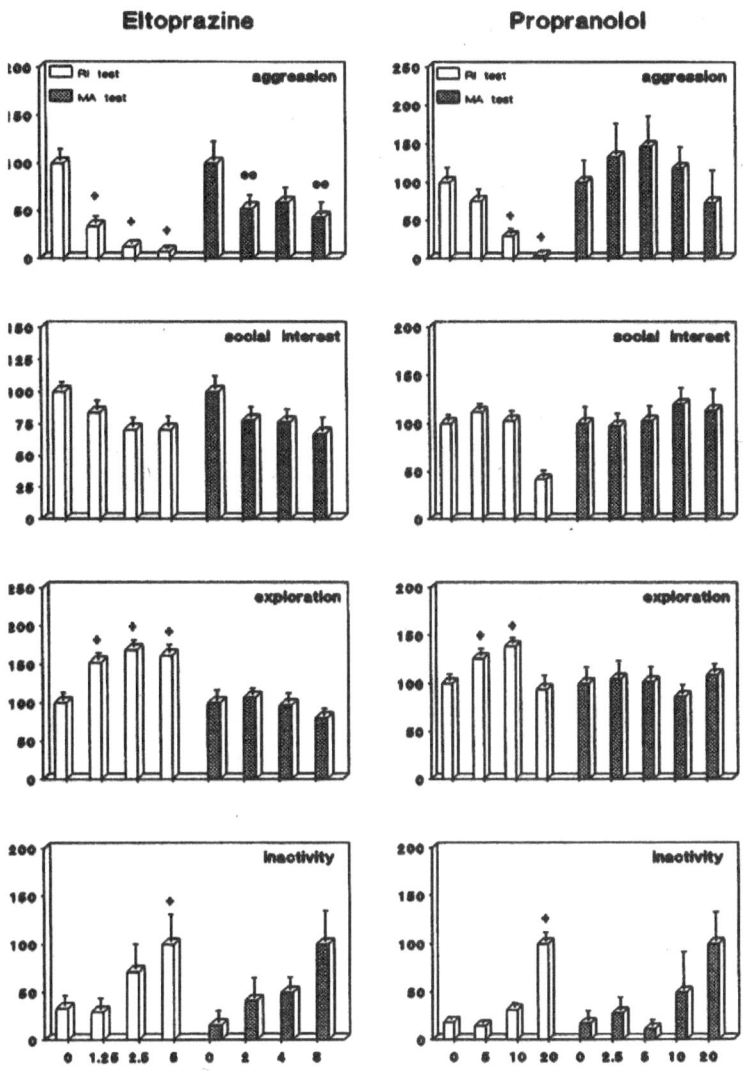

**Figure 1** Effects of eltoprazine and ± propranolol on four behavioural categories. Eltoprazine was given orally 60 minutes before the test to males and females. ± Propranolol was given i. p. 30 minutes before testing to the females and p.o. 60 minutes before testing to the males. + or o significant from vehicle.

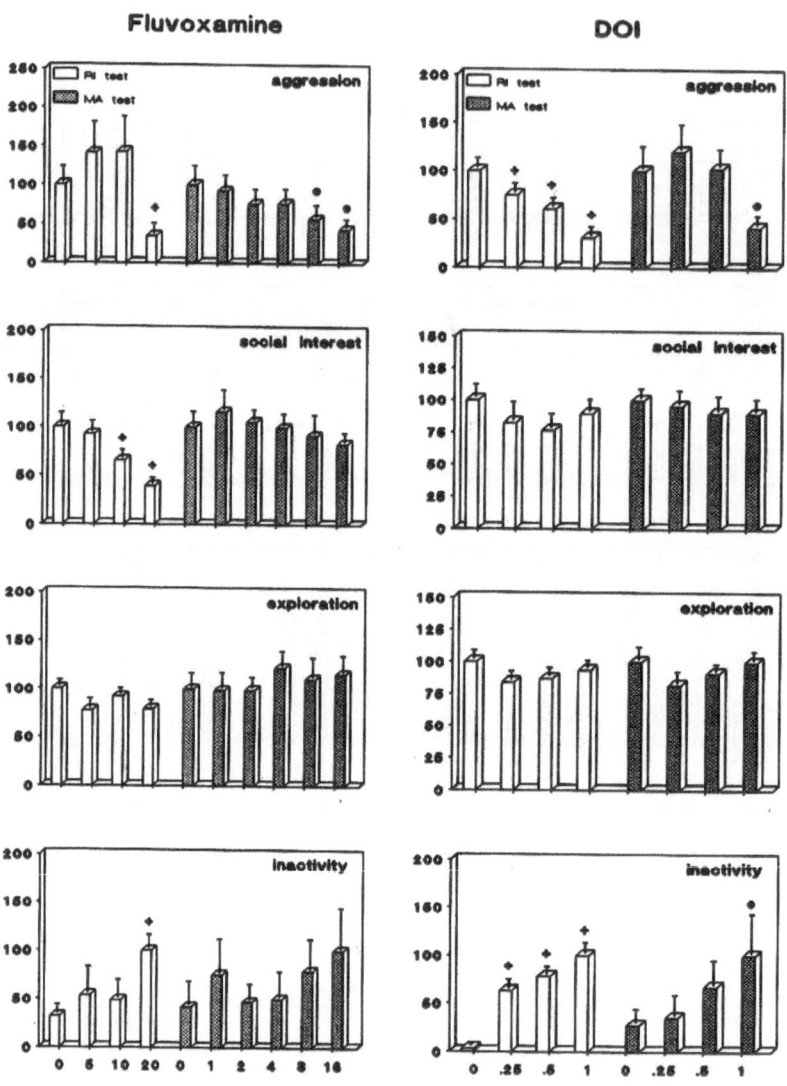

**Figure 2** Effects of fluvoxamine and DOI on four behavioral categories. 8-OH-DPAT was given subcutaneously 30 minutes before the test. DOI was given i. p. 30 minutes before testing. + or o significant from vehicle.

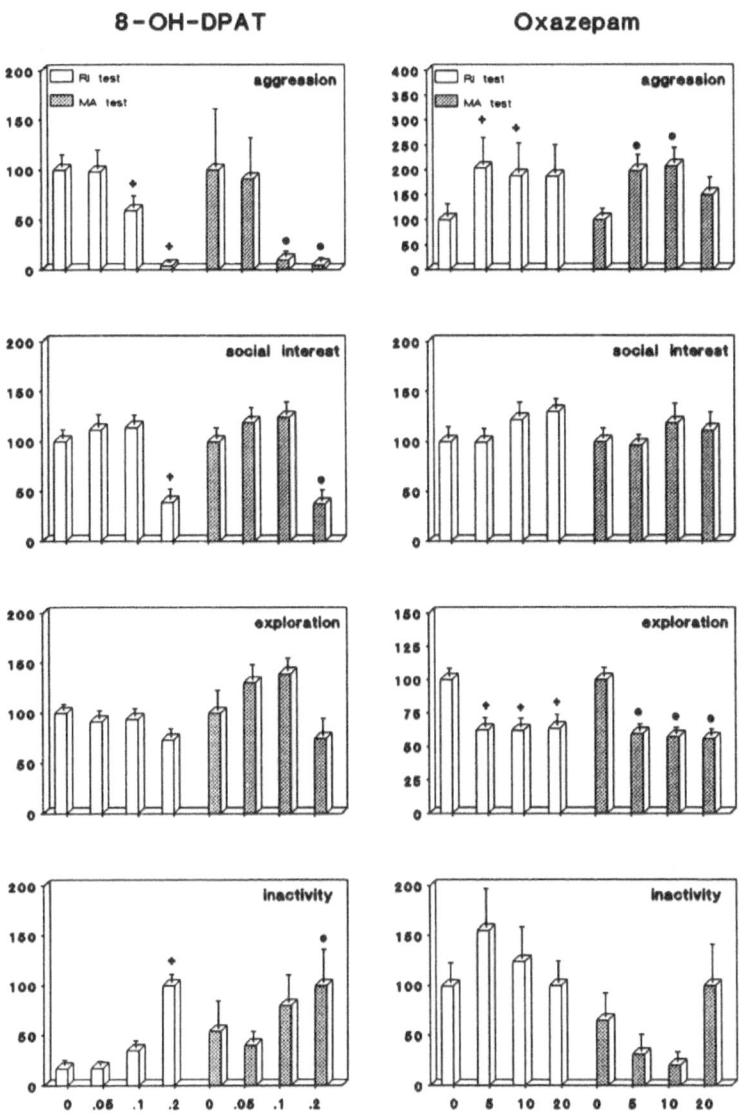

**Figure 3** Effects of 8-OH-DPAT and oxazepam on four behavioral categories. Fluvoxamine was given i. p. 30 minutes before the test. Oxazepam was given 30 minutes before testing (i. p.). + or o significant from vehicle.

For d-amphetamine (Figure 4) the females were again less sensitive, because even at the highest dose of 2 mg/kg, the reduction of aggression by 40% had not yet reached statistical significance. Exploration was increased at 0.5 and 1 mg/kg, which is more in line with the effects observed in males. While at all doses aggression was reduced in residential males, the detrimental effects of amphetamine on social interest were only evident at 1 mg/kg.

Scopolamine (Figure 5) reduced aggression in males and females and increased exploration. In males the decrease in social interest was evident at all doses, whereas in females no reduction was found, but rather an increase at the highest dose, although this was of modest size. In the males inactivity was unexpectedly high under control conditions and this was subsequently reduced by scopolamine treatment. Such effects were absent in females, but they showed no inactivity in this experiment under control conditions.

Neither in males nor in females did ethanol produce any significant change in aggressive behavior. The other behaviors displayed in the context of this aggression test were neither affected (Figure 5).

# Comparison with other data/literature

It is more or less a matter of taste, a choice based on personal preference, whether the differences or the similarities of these drug studies are emphasized. Although there are sometimes qualitative differences in the profile of behavioral changes, these are not consistently pointing to a certain direction. It should be noted that the experiments described form a dataset which was gathered over many years. Since there was no a priori goal to precisely compare male and female aggression, we sometimes used other doses. In view of the variance that thus inevitably entered conservatively.

By contrast, a more general finding is that the sensitivity of females to drug effects is usually less, i.e. the dose-response curves are somewhat shifted to the right.

By and large we are more impressed by the similarities of drug effects in the male resident-intruder and maternal aggression paradigms, than by the differences. Such similarities in drug sensitivity strongly suggest that, notwithstanding the large differences in the factors governing aggression in males and females, the basic organization of the neural substrates of aggressive behavior in both genders is largely identical.

Our findings on a number of reference drugs as shown in this article can be compared to those of others. d-Amphetamine, a psychostimulant, had no clear anti-aggressive action in females (this study; Olivier and Mos, 1986; Mos et al., 1990) but a clear anti-aggressive action in residential males (Olivier et al., 1984). The contradicting effects of d-amphetamine on aggression are well-known (Miczek, 1987), which may be caused by different factors like prevalent pattern of aggressive behavior, the dose administered, the baseline level of aggression, the behavioral history of the drug recipient (Haney et al., 1990) and the drug state of the victim of aggression (Miczek, 1987; Mos et al., 1987c).

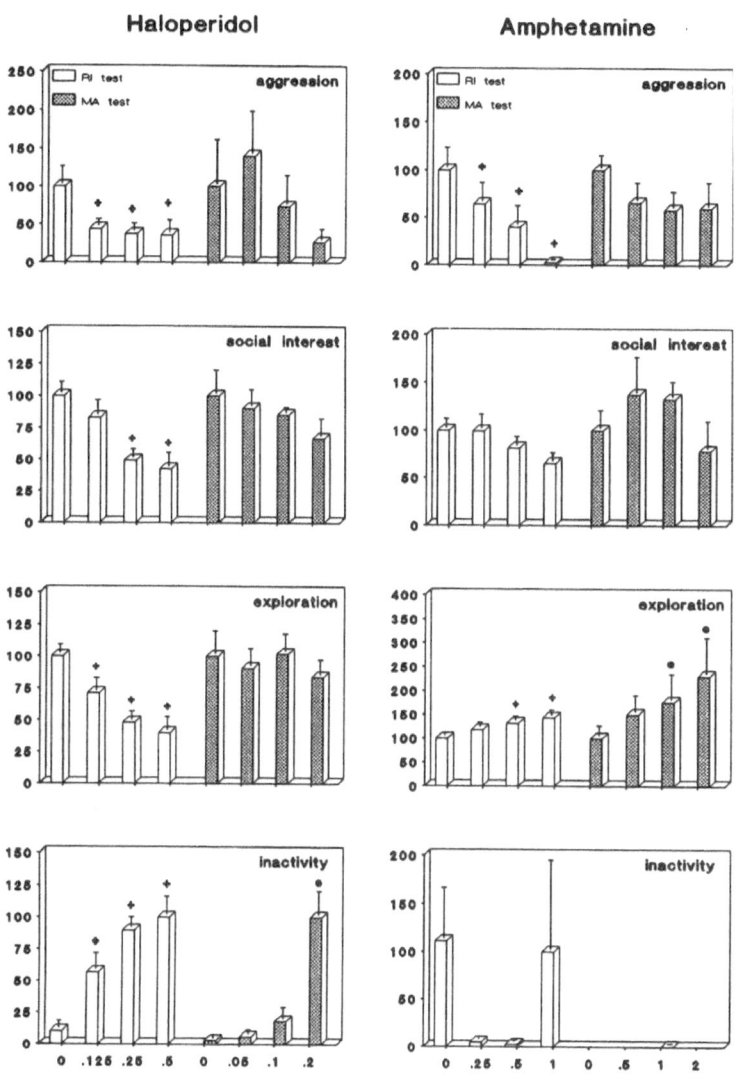

**Figure 4** Effects of haloperidol and d-amphetamine on four behavioral categories. Haloperidol was given i. p. 30 minutes before the test. d-amphetamine was given 30 minutes before testing (i. p.). + or o significant from vehicle.

214

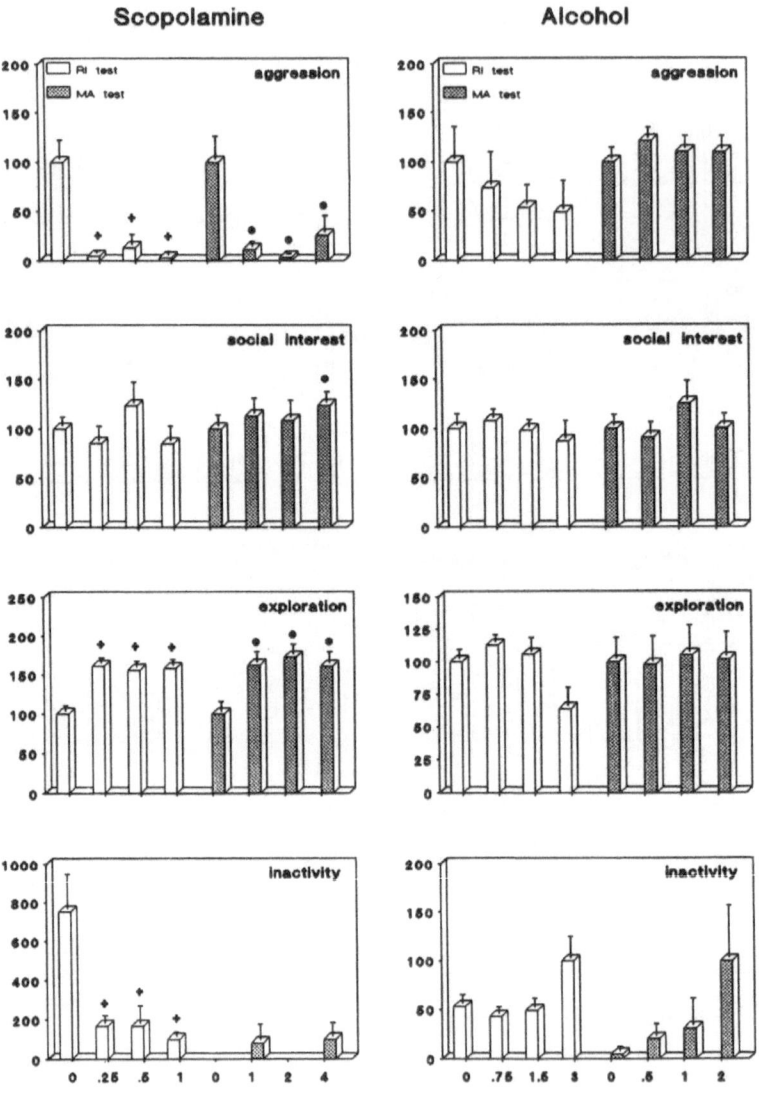

**Figure 5** Effects of scopolamine and alcohol on four behavioral categories. Scopolamine was given i. p. 30 minutes before the test. Alcohol was given orally 60 minutes before testing. + or o significant from vehicle.

Several lines of evidence (Miczek, 1983; Olivier et al., 1984; Poshivalov and Khodko, 1984; Schmidt, 1984) suggest that d-amphetamine disorganizes complex sequences and patterns of social interactions. This indirect influence of d-amphetamine can be deduced from brain-stimulation-induced (hypothalamic) aggression (Kruk et al., 1987; Kruk, 1991; own unpublished results) in which d-amphetamine, up to the high dose of 2 mg/kg had no effect on aggression, although locomotion was enhanced.

Haloperidol, a dopamine D2 receptor antagonist, reduced aggression and enhanced inactivity in residents, but less so in females, probably due to the lower doses used. A similar profile as in males would probably become manifest with higher doses as evidenced in the already significantly enhanced inactivity in maternal aggression. Such a profile, a highly nonspecific anti-aggressive effect, is seen before in RI - aggression in rats (Olivier et al., 1984), in hypothalamically-induced aggression in rats (Olivier et al., 1986), in resident-intruder aggression in mice (Miczek and DeBold, 1983; Olivier and van Dalen, 1982; Yoshimura, 1987) and in maternal aggression in mice (Yoshimura and Ogawa, 1989). The patterns after haloperidol in male and female aggression paradigms are largely similar, i.e., a strongly sedative profile.

Alcohol, over a broad dose range, was without effect on maternal aggression, thereby confirming several other studies we and others have performed in male rats (Kruk et al., 1987; Kruk, 1991; Mos and Olivier, 1988a; Olivier and Mos, 1986). However, several studies indicate that under special circumstances low doses of alcohol actually may enhance maternal aggression (Blanchard and Blanchard, 1987; Blanchard et al., 1987), particularly when small intruders were used. On the other hand, these authors could not find such an effect in male rats, independent from the level of fear imposed on the dominant animals. Other authors have found more convincing aggression-enhancing effects of low doses of alcohol, e.g., in mice, rats, and squirrel monkeys (Krsiak, 1975, 1976; Miczek and Barry, 1977; Winslow et al., 1987; Yoshimura and Ogawa, 1983). Miczek (1987) gives an extensive review on the relationship between alcohol and aggression, and suggests that one of the key phenomena of aggression enhancement lies in the presence of high levels of testosterone in the blood (Winslow et al., 1987), a finding observed both in monkeys and mice. Miczek (1987) suggests that alcohol's aggression-modulating effects may be mediated by alcohol's action on an androgen-sensitive neural mechanism. The question then is whether it is possible to observe aggression-enhancing effects of alcohol in females. We did not find an increase, but Blanchard and Blanchard (1987) reported enhanced aggression. In a colony situation with dominant (high androgen level) and subordinate (lower androgen level) male rats, we were not able to see aggression-enhancing effects in either of the two kinds of males (Mos and Olivier, 1988a). This strongly indicates that, besides testosterone, several other factors may play a role in alcohol effects on aggression.

Scopolamine strongly reduced aggressive behavior, which is replaced by stereotyped behavior, especially sniffing. A similar pattern has been observed in a resident-intruder paradigm (unpublished observations; Kruk et al., 1987; Kruk, 1991). Remarkably, scopolamine did not reduce aggression in hypothalamically induced aggression, although it showed a stimulatory (enhanced locomotion) pattern (Kruk et al., 1987; Kruk, 1991). These data suggest that the anti-aggressive activity is most likely due to the stereotypies induced by scopolamine. Anti-aggressive effects of scopolamine have been found by others: in mice (Donat and Krsiak, 1982; Yoshimura and Ogawa, 1982), in rats (Van der Poel and Remmelts,, 1971), and in juvenile rats (Thor and Hollaway, 1983). Our data suggest a similar profile of scopolamine in aggressive behavior of males and females.

ß-Adrenergic blockers have been suggested effective anti-aggressive drugs in the management of violent behavior in patients (e. g. Ratey et al., 1986; 1987). Originally it was thought that the anti-aggressive action was due to blockade of the ß-adrenoceptors, but several of these agents have fairly high affinities for 5-HT1A and 1B receptors. It is quite possible that the latter activity may explain their anti-aggressive profile. (±)-propranolol had an anti-aggressive profile in the RI-test, but remarkably, had no effect in maternal aggression. In fact, this is the compound showing a significant difference between both paradigms. Several studies have reported anti-aggressive effects of ß-blockers (mainly propranolol) in aggression paradigms, suggesting the (-) or (I) enantiomer as the active isomer of the racemic-propranolol (e. g. Yoshimura, 1987; Yoshimura et al., 1987). The 5-HT1 receptor affinity of these ß-blockers is apparently also located in the (-) enantiomer, thereby reinforcing the hypothesis that the anti-aggressive activity might be due to the serotonin involvement. Much more work is needed to really exclude the ß-adrenoceptor involvement although we found (unpublished results) that timolol, a potent ß-blocker without significant serotonergic affinity, was inactive in the resident-intruder paradigm, up to very high doses. It could therefore be possible that the 5-HT1A receptor antagonistic activity of certain ß-adrenoceptor antagonists might be responsible for the rather specific anti-aggressive effects. Why (±)-propranolol was virtually without such an effect in maternal females remains to be elucidated. Whether this may be due to the "tone" in the serotonergic system, which may determine whether a partial receptor agonist becomes an antagonist or an agonist, remains to be investigated. Alternatively, these ß-blockers may possess 5-HT1B (partial) receptor agonistic activity, as deduced from drug discrimination studies (Ybema et al., 1992). 5-HT1B receptor agonists have an anti-aggressive profile in various paradigms and genders (Olivier et al., 1991).

Oxazepam, a benzodiazepine receptor agonist, enhanced aggressive behavior in RI- and MA-tests at low drug doses. At higher doses aggression returned to control levels and at much higher doses (not shown in the present studies) aggression is decreased presumably caused by the severe muscle relaxing and hypnotic effects. Such biphasic, inverted U-shaped dose response curves have been observed for other BDZ receptor agonists like chlordiazepoxide, diazepam and alprazolam (Mos et al., 1990; Olivier et al., 1991; Mos and Olivier, 1987) both for male and female aggression paradigms. However, the pro-aggressive actions of BDZ are not invariably found. In hypothalamically-induced aggression no such effects could be detected (Kruk et al., 1987; Kruk, 1991), whereas chlordiazepoxide in a number of different strains of mice was also not able to evoke enhanced aggression at low doses (Everill et al., 1991). It was found that the baseline level of aggression is a critical determinant of the aggression-enhancing effect of BDZ receptor agonists (Miczek and Krsiak, 1979; Mos et al., 1987a,b), whereas also the size of the opponent may be important (Mos et al., 1987c). It was hypothetized that BDZ receptor agonists increase aggressive behavior in all these situations when this behavior is strongly reduced by internal or external factors, e. g. by anxiety or fear. Whether the anxiolytic effects of BDZ are reflected in their aggression-enhancing effects is however far from settled, because another putative class of anxiolytics, the 5-HT1A receptor agonists, do not exert such a pro-aggressive effect. In contrast, they rather show a monotonic "anti-aggressive" profile, although these drugs may have disinhibitory properties, like e. g. in feeding and sexual behavior (Dourish et al., 1985; Ahlenius and Larsson, 1984).

In the present study a systematic comparison was made between the effects of various serotonergic drugs on two forms of aggressive behavior in male and female rats, and it is especially interesting to further evaluate these results. These drugs differentially affect serotonergic transmission and 5-HT receptor subtypes. Although certain subtypes of receptors are more selectively affected than after lesions or dietary manipulations, the conclusions about the role of serotonin in aggression are still limited by the specificity of the 'tools' available. All 5-HT receptor agonistic drugs described here reduce aggression, irrespective of their neurochemical mode of action. Thus we seem to confirm the general inhibitory role of serotonin for male and female aggression in rats, however the drugs differ with respect to the specificity of the effects.

The reduction in aggressive behaviors by male and female rats after treatment with the selected serotonergic drugs can be compared with effects of some of these drugs in other animal models and species. In mice isolation-induced aggression is blocked by 5-HT1A receptor agonists like buspirone, ipsapirone and 8-OH-DPAT (McMillen et al., 1987, 1988b; Olivier et al., 1989b). Mouse-killing by rats has been reported to be unaffected (McMillen et al., 1988a; Olivier et al., 1987) or to be inhibited (Molina et al., 1987). Our own previous studies with TFMPP, RU 24969 and eltoprazine in mice and rats suggest specific reductions of attacks in isolation-induced aggression in mice, as well as in (intermale) aggression in mice and mouse-killing in rats (Olivier et al., 1987, 1989a).

Fluvoxamine has been demonstrated to be weakly active in inhibiting muricidal behavior and intraspecific aggression in mice (Mos and Olivier, 1988b). For other 5-HT reuptake blockers like fluoxetine and zimeldine reductions in mouse-killing have also been described. While for DOI as far as we know no anti-aggressive properties have been published, quipazine has repeatedly been shown to inhibit various forms of aggression. Resident-intruder aggression in mice (Lindgren and Kantak, 1987), muricide and shock-induced fighting in rats (Pucilowski et al., 1985) were decreased, although not always without reductions in locomotion. In vervet monkeys up to 1 mg/kg, quipazine had no effects on aggression displayed either by the dominant or the subordinate males of a colony (Raleigh et al., 1985).

By and large, these data confirm that serotonergic drugs may be effective to reduce aggressive behavior. However, many of these studies were too limited to deduct the role of specific 5-HT receptor subtypes in aggressive behavior. 5-HT1A receptor agonists like 8-OH-DPAT, buspirone and ipsapirone reduce aggression at doses which are similar or close to those resulting in non-specific behavioral interference, e.g. caused by sedation. For ipsapirone these results are at variance with the data reported by Glaser (1988) who presented data of more specific suppression of male aggression in rats. Apart from trivial strain differences there is no satisfactory explanation for this discrepancy. Mixed 5-HT1A/B receptor agonists like eltoprazine and RU24969 suppress aggression specifically, i.e. no sedation is found, but rather an increase in exploration, most notably for RU 24969 and eltoprazine where exploration is increased in maternal and resident intruder aggression. TFMPP, a somewhat more specific 5-HT1B receptor agonist (but by far not so specific as e.g. the 5-HT1A ligands) has a similar profile as RU 24969 in RI, but resulted in more inactivity in MA. Since at these doses social interest and exploration were not decreased these effects were not of a general sedatory nature.

The role for the 5-HT1C receptor remains to be established, but specific receptor agonists and antagonists are as yet scarce. The fact that eltoprazine is a 5-HT1C receptor antagonist and TFMPP an agonist suggests that the 5-HT1C site is not primarily involved in the regulation of aggression. Preliminary experiments in our laboratory have also indicated that specific (partial) 5-HT1C receptor agonists do not exert a specific profile of anti-aggressive action (unpublished results). The 5-HT2/5-HT1C receptor antagonist ritanserine did not significantly affect maternal aggression (Mos and Olivier, 1986), neither did the 5-HT3 receptor antagonists ondansetron nor MDL72222 change maternal aggression (Mos et al., 1990). These substances, however, have not yet been tested in the RI model.

While the effects of 5-HT1-like receptor agonists on aggression are quite similar in male and female rats, more discrepancies were found when the 5-HT reuptake blocker fluvoxamine was used. Females reacted with a specific, dose-dependent decrease in aggression, whereas male rats were non-specifically inhibited at the highest dose. Also after quipazine treatment male and female rats reacted differentially. Exploration was decreased in male rats, whereas females showed increased activity in exploring their homecage. Although this might be explained by a different sensitivity to drug doses, the behavioral effects on aggression were quite similar in dose range. Similarly, the wet dog shaking supposed to result from 5-HT2 activation followed a similar dose response curve in males and females. No sex differences were found after DOI, neither on the dose-response curve for wet dog shakes, nor on exploration. The quipazine experiment with maternal aggression therefore remains elusive.

As mentioned earlier, the specificity of the serotonergic tools for the various receptor subtypes is far from convincing. Therefore conclusions about the role of receptor subtypes must remain tentative. However, the behavioral profile of mixed 5-HT1A/B and 5-HT1B receptor agonists is the most specific one. Aggression is dose-dependently reduced, but this is not caused by sedatory actions of the drug. Social interest and exploration remains intact (or are even increased). Since the complete behavior of the animal is scored reductions in time spent of aggression must 'necessarily' be compensated by increases in other behaviors.

# Conclusions

It is not easy to objectively evaluate and compare male and female aggression, including the neuropharmacological basis underlying these behaviors. A description of the neurobiology of maternal aggression reveals marked differences in causation, morphology and (neuro)hormonal factors in females as compared to males (Svare and Gandelman, 1973; Svare et al., 1981; Mos et al., 1989a). However, a number of features also shows resemblance to male aggression. Although the context and causation of maternal aggression differs, it can be argued that the neural substrates subserving aggression is quite comparable to that of males. In this paper we particularly investigated the neuropharmacological basis for aggression by modulation of specific neurotransmitter systems. On the one hand this study revealed that males and females react by and large in the same way to those drugs, i.e. although the sensitivity might differ somewhat and the degree of specificity of the anti-aggressive effects did vary, no systematic evidence was obtained suggesting a different neuropharmacological organization. Of course this conclusion only holds for what we have investigated, since other than mice and rats we have little data on male and female aggression and its modulation by drugs.

From our point of view - the interest in developing drugs to treat pathological aggression or destructive behavior - it is important to know that male and female rats react more or less similar. Although no systematic data exist on a comparison of human male and female pathological aggression, it is by no means justified to limit aggression problems exclusively to males. Thus a first hint that serotonergic drugs might be useful in the treatment of both male and female aggression does arise from these studies.

From a behavioral point of view it is interesting to compare male and female aggression and to speculate upon the organization of aggressive behavior in the brain. Contrary to sexual behavior in which male and female behavioral elements are strikingly different, aggressive behavior is more similar. By and large male and female rats use the same aggressive elements although the frequency and intensity may vary. Even though the context and the function of aggression in males and females differ, they tend to use 'the same motor apparatus'. This does not imply, however, that drugs act at this output system and that therefore the similarities of drug effects are also consistent. Drug actions can also be targeted at the level of motivation and perception.

Since we do not know at which sites of the brain the drugs act, it remains unclear whether sexually dimorphic brain regions are involved. Neither is much attention given to compare drug effects on aggression of 'masculinized' females or 'feminized' males. Thus many questions on brain organization and similarities and differences in aggression remain unsolved. From a pharmacological perspective the endpoint, i.e. the neuropharmacological control of aggression, the similarities in males and females are more striking than the differences.

## Acknowledgements

The technical support and the highly skilled contributions of Hans van Aken and Ruud van Oorschot in obtaining the data are gratefully acknowledged. Marijke Mulder assisted in the preparation of the manuscript.

## References

Adams, D. B. (1979). Brain mechanisms for offense, defense, and submission. Behav. *Brain Res., 2* : 201-241.

Ahlenius, S. and Larsson, K. (1984). Lisuride, LY-141865, and 8-OH-DPAT facilitate male sexual behavior via a non-dopaminergic mechanism. *Psychopharmacology,* **83** : 330-334.

Blanchard, R. J. and Blanchard, D. C. (1977). Aggressive behavior in the rat. *Behav. Biol.,* **21** : 197-224.

Blanchard, R. J., Takahashi, L. K. and Blanchard, D. C. (1977). The development of intruder attack in colonies of laboratory rats. *Anim. Learn. Behav.,* **5** : 365-369.

Blanchard, R. J. and Blanchard, D. C. (1987). The relationship between ethanol and aggression: studies using ethological models. In: Olivier, B., Mos, J. and Brain, P. F. (Eds), *Ethopharmacology of Agonistic Behavior in Animals and Humans,* Martinus Nijhoff, Dordrecht, pp. 145-161.

Blanchard, D. C., Flannelly, K., Hori, K. and Blanchard, R. J. (1987). Ethanol effects on female aggression vary with opponent size and time within session. *Pharmacol. Biochem. Behav.,* **27** : 645-648.

Brain, P. F., Benton, D., Howell, P. A. and Jones, S. E. (1980). Resident rats' aggression toward intruders. *Anim. Learn. Behav.,* **8** : 331-335.

DeBold, J. F. and Miczek, K. A. (1981). Sexual dimorphism in the hormonal control of aggressive behavior of rats. *Pharmacol. Biochem. Behav.,* **14** : 89-93.

Donat, P. and Krsiak, M. (1982). Effects of scopolamine on agonistic behavior of aggressive and non-aggressive mice. *Act. Nerv. Sup.,* **24** : 278-279.

Dourish, C. T., Hutson, P. H. and Curzon, G. (1985). Characteristics of feeding induced by the serotonin agonist 8-hydroxy-2-(Di-n-propylamino) Tetralin (8-OH-DPAT). *Brain Res. Bull.,* **15** : 377-384.

Erskine, M. S., Barfield, R. J. and Goldman, B. D. (1978a). Intraspecific fighting during late pregnancy in rats and effects of litter removal. *Behav. Biol.,* **23** : 206-218.

Erskine, M. S., Denenberg, V. H. and Goldman, B. D. (1978b). Aggression in the lactating rat: effects of intruder age and test arena. *Behav. Biol.,* **23** : 52-66.

Everill, B., Brain, P. F., Rustana, A., Mos, J. and Olivier, B. (1991). Ethoexperimental analysis of the impact of chlordiazepoxide (CDP) on social interactions in three strains of mice. *Behav. Process.,* **25** : 55-67.

Glaser, T. (1988). Ipsapirone, a potent and selective 5-HT1A receptor ligand with anxiolytic and antidepressant properties. *Drugs of the Future*, **13** : 429-439.

Haney, M., Noda, K., Kream, R. and Miczek, K. A. (1990). Regional serotonin and dopamine activity: sensitivity to amphetamine and aggressive behavior in mice. *Aggr. Behav.*, **16**, 259-270.

Krsiak, M. (1975). Timid singly-housed mice: their value in prediction of psychotropic activity of drugs. *Br. J. Pharmacol.*, **55** : 141-150.

Krsiak, M. (1976). Effect of ethanol on aggression and timidity in mice. *Psychopharmacology*, **51** : 75-80.

Krsiak, M. (1991). Ethopharmacology: a historical perspective. *Neurosci. Biobehav. Rev.*, **15** : 439-445.

Kruk, M. R., Van Der Poel, A. M., Lammers, J. H. C. M., Hagg, T., De Hey, A. M. D. M., Oostwegel, S. (1987). Ethopharmacology of hypothalamic aggression in the rat. In: Olivier, B., Mos, J. and Brain, P. F. (Eds.), *Ethopharmacology of Agonistic Behavior in Animals and Humans,* Martinus Nijhoff, Dordrecht, pp. 35-45.

Kruk, M. R. (1991). Ethology and pharmacology of hypothalamic aggression in the rat. *Neurosci. Biobehav. Rev.*, **15** : 527-538.

Lehman, M. N. and Adams, D. B. (1977). A statistical and motivational analysis of the social behaviors of the male laboratory rat. *Behaviour*, **61** : 238-275.

Lindgren, T. and Kantak, K. M. (1987). Effects of serotonin receptor agonists and antagonists on offensive aggression in mice. *Aggr. Behav.*, **13** : 87-96.

Lore, R. K., Nikoletsas, M. and Takahashi, L. (1984). Colony aggression in laboratory rats: a review and some recommendations. *Aggr. Behav.*, **10** : 59-71.

Luciano, D. and Lore, R. K. (1975). Aggression and social experience in domesticated rats. *J. Comp. Physiol. Psychol.*, **88** : 917-923.

McMillen, B. A., Chamberlain, J. K. and DaVanzo, J. P. (1988a). Effects of housing and muricidal behavior on serotonergic receptors and interactions with novel anxiolytic drugs. *J. Neur. Transm.*, **71** : 123-132.

McMillen, B. A., DaVanzo, E. A., Scott, S. M. and Song, A. H. (1988b). N-Alkyl-substituted aryl-piperazine drugs: relationship between affinity for serotonin receptors and inhibition of aggression. *Drug Devlp. Res.*, **12** : 53-62.

McMillen, B. A., Scott, S. M., Williams, H. L. and Sanghera, M. K. (1987). Effects of gepirone, an aryl-piperazine anxiolytic drug, on aggressive behavior and brain monoaminergic neurotransmission. *Naunyn Schmiedeberg's Arch. Pharmacol.*, **335** : 454-464.

Miczek, K. A. A new test for aggression in rats without aversive stimulation: differential effects of d-amphetamine and cocaine. *Psychopharmacology*, **60** : 253-259.

Miczek, K. A. and Barry, H. III (1977). Effects of alcohol on attack and defensive-submissive reactions in rats. *Psychopharmacology*, **52** : 231-237.

Miczek, K. A. (1983). Ethologic analysis of drug action on aggression, defense and defeat. In: Spigelstein, M. Y. and Levy, A. (Eds.), *Behavioral Models and the Analysis of Drug Action,* Elsevier, Amsterdam, pp. 225-239.

Miczek, K. A. (1987). The psychopharmacology of aggression. In: Iversen, L. L., Iversen, S. D. and Snyder, S. H. (Eds.), *Handbook of Psychopharmacology: Behavioural Pharmacology,* Plenum Press, New York, vol. 19, pp. 183-328.

Miczek, K. A. and DeBold, J. F. (1983). Hormone-drug interactions and their influences on aggressive behavior. In: Svare, B. B. (Ed.), *Hormones and Aggressive Behavior,* Plenum Press, New York and London, pp. 313-347.

Miczek, K. A. and Krsiak, M. (1979). Drug effects on agonistic behavior. In: Thompson, T. and Dews, P. B. (Eds.), *Advances in Behavioral Pharmacology,* Academic Press, New York, vol 2, pp. 87-162.

Molina, V., Ciesielski, L., Gobaille, S., Isel, F. and Mandel, P. (1987). Inhibition of mouse killing behavior by serotonin-mimetic drugs: effects of partial alterations of serotonin neurotransmission. *Pharmacol. Biochem. Behav.,* **27** : 123-131.

Mos, J. and Olivier, B. (1987). Pro-aggressive action of benzodiazepines. In: Olivier, B., Mos, J. and Brain, P. F. (Eds.), *Ethopharmacology of Agonistic Behavior in Animals and Humans,* Martinus Nijhoff, Dordrecht, pp. 187-206.

Mos, J. and Olivier, B. (1988a). Differential effects of selected psychoactive drugs on dominant and subordinate male rats housed in a colony. *Neurosci. Res. Comm.,* **2** : 29-36.

Mos, J. and Olivier, B. (1988b). Fluvoxamine and aggression in rats and mice. In: Olivier, B. and Mos, J. (Eds.), *Depression, Anxiety and Aggression : Preclinical and Clinical Interfaces,* Medidact, Houten, pp. 103-120.

Mos, J., Olivier, B. and Van der Poel, A. M. (1987a). Modulatory actions of benzodiazepine receptor ligands on agonistic behavior. *Physiol. Behav.,* **41** : 265-278.

Mos, J., Olivier, B., Lammers, J. H. C. M. C., van der Poel, A. M., Kruk, M. R. and Zethof, T. (1987b). Postpartum aggression in rats does not influence threshold currents for EBS-induced aggression. *Brain Res.,* **404** : 263-266.

Mos, J., Olivier, B. and van Oorschot, R. (1987c). Maternal aggression towards different sized male opponents: effect of chlordiazepoxide treatment of the mothers and d-amphetamine treatment of the intruders. *Pharmacol. Biochem. Behav.,* **26** : 577-584.

Mos, J., Olivier, B., van Oorschot, R., van Aken, H. and Zethof, T. (1989a). Experimental and ethological aspects of maternal aggression in rats. Five years of observations. In: Blanchard, R. J., Brain, P. F., Blanchard, D. C. and Parmigiani, S. (Eds.), *Etho-experimental Approaches to the Study of Behavior,* Klüwer Academic Publishers, Dordrecht, pp. 385-398.

Mos, J. Olivier, B. and van Oorschot, R. (1990). Behavioral and neuropharmacological aspects of maternal aggression in rodents. *Aggr. Behav.,* **16** : 145-163.

Olivier, B. (1977). The ventromedial hypothalamus and aggressive behavior in rats. *Aggr. Behav.,* **3** : 47-66.

Olivier, B., Mos, J. and van Oorschot, R. (1985). Maternal aggression in rats: effects of chlordiazepoxide and fluprazine. *Psychopharmacology,* **86** : 68-76.

Olivier, B. and Mos, J. (1986). A female aggression paradigm for use in psychopharmacology: maternal agonistic behavior in rats. In: Brain, P. F. and

Ramirez, J. M. (Eds), *Cross-Disciplinary Studies on Aggression*, Sevilla University Press, Seville, pp. 73-111.

Olivier, B. and Van Dalen, D. (1982). Social behavior in rats and mice: An ethologically based model for differentiating psychoactive drug. *Aggr. Behav.*, **8** : 163-168.

Olivier, B., van Aken, H., Jaarsma, I., van Oorschot, R., Zethof, T. and Bradford, D. (1984). Behavioral effects of psychoactive drugs on agonistic behavior of male territorial rats (resident-intruder model). In: Miczek, K. A., Kruk, M. R. and Olivier, B. (Eds.), *Ethopharmacological Aggression Research,* Alan R. Liss Inc, New York, pp. 137-156.

Olivier, B., Van Dalen, D. and Hartog, J. (1986). A new class of psychoactive drugs : serenics. *Drugs of the Future,* **11** : 473-499.

Olivier, B., Mos, J., Van der Heyden, J. A. M., Schipper, J., Tulp, M., Berkelmans, B. and Bevan, P. (1987). Serotonergic modulation of agonistic behavior. In: Olivier, B., Mos, J. and Brain, P. F. (Eds.), *Ethopharmacology of Aggression in Animals and Humans,* Martinus Nijhoff, Dordrecht, pp. 162-186.

Olivier, B., Mos, J., Tulp, M., Schipper, J. and Bevan, P. (1989a). Modulatory action of serotonin in aggressive behavior. In: Bevan, P., Cools, A. R. and Archer, T. (Eds.), *Behavioral Pharmacology of 5-HT,* Lawrence Erlbaum, New Jersey, pp. 91-117.

Olivier, B., Mos, J., Van der Heyden, J. and Hartog, J. (1989b). Serotonergic modulation of social interactions in isolated male mice. *Psychopharmacology,* **97** : 154-156.

Olivier, B., Mos, J. and Van Oorschot, R. (1989c). Etho-experimental studies of similarities and differences in male and female agonistic behavior. In: Blanchard, R. J., Brain, P. F., Blanchard, D. C. and Parmigiani, S. (Eds.), *Ethoexperimental Approaches to the Study of Behavior,* Klüwer Academic Publishers, Dordrecht, pp. 494-507.

Olivier, B., Tulp, M. Th. M. and Mos, J. (1991). Serotonergic receptors in anxiety and aggression: evidence from animal pharmacology. *Hum. Psychopharm. Clin. Exptl.,* **6** : S73-S78.

Olivier, B. and Wiepkema, P. R. (1974). Behavior changes in mice following electrolytic lesions in the median hypothalamus. *Brain Res.,* **65** : 521-524.

Poshivalov, V. P. and Khodko, S. T. (1984). Mathematical description and experimental pharmaco-ethological analysis of animal intraspecific agonistic behavior. In: Miczek, K. A., Kruk, M. R. and Olivier, B. (Eds.), *Ethopharmacological Aggression Research,* Alan R. Liss Inc, New York, pp. 59-80.

Pucilowski, P., Plaznik, A. and Kostowski, W. (1985). Aggressive behavior inhibition by serotonin and quipazine injected into the amygdala in the rat. *Behav. Neural Biol.,* **43** : 58-68.

Raleigh, M. J., Brammer, G. L., McGuire, M. T. and Yuwiler, A. (1985). Dominant social status facilitates the behavioral effects of serotonergic agonists. *Brain Res.,* **348** : 274-282.

Ratey, J. J., Mikkelsen, E. J., Smith, G. B., Upadhyaya, A., Zuckerman, H. S., Martell, D., Sorgi, P., Pokaloff, S. and Bemporad, J. (1986) Beta-blockers in

224

the severely and profoundly mentally retarded. *J. Clin. Psychopharmacol.,* 6 : 103-107.

Ratey, J. J., Mikkelsen, E. J., Sorgi, P., Zuckerman, H. S., Pokaloff, S., Bemporad, J., Bick, P. and Kadish, W. (1987). Autism: the treatment of aggressive behaviors. *J. Clin. Psychopharmacol.,* 7 : 35-41.

Schmidt, W. J. (1984). Involvement of dopaminergic neurotransmission in the control of goal-directed movements. *Psychopharmacololgy,* 80 : 360-364.

Seward, J. P. (1945a). Aggressive behavior in the rat. I. General characteristics, age and sex differences. *J. Comp. Psychol.,* 38 : 175-197.

Seward, J. P. (1945b). Aggressive behavior in the rat. II. An attempt to establish a dominance hierarchy. *J. Comp. Psychol.,* 38 : 213-224.

Seward, J. P. (1945c). Aggressive behavior in the rat. III. The role of frustration. *J. Comp. Psychol.,* 38 : 225-238.

Svare, B. and Gandelman, R. (1973). Postpartum aggression in mice : experiential and environmental factors. *Horm. Behav.,* 4 : 323-334.

Svare, B. and Betteridge, C., Katz, D. and Samuels, O. (1981). Some situational and experiential determinants of maternal aggression in mice. *Physiol. Behav.,* 26 : 253-258.

Thor, D. H. and Flannelly, K. J. (1976a). Age of intruder and territorial-elicited aggression in male Long-Evans rats. *Behav. Biol.,* 17 : 237-241.

Thor, D. H. and Flannelly, K. J. (1976b). Intruder gonadectomy and elicitation of territorial aggression in the rat. *Physiol. Behav.,* 17 : 725-727.

Thor, D. H. and Hollaway, W. R. Jr. (1983). Scopolamine blocks play fighting behavior in juvenile rats. *Physiol. Behav.,* 30 : 545-549.

Van Der Poel, A. M. and Remmelts, M. (1971). The effect of anticholinergics on the behavior of the rat in a solitary and in a social situation. *Arch. Int. Pharmacodyn.,* 189 : 394-396.

Winslow, J. T., DeBold, J. F. and Miczek, K. A. (1987). Alcohol effects on the aggressive behavior of squirrel monkeys and mice are modulated by testosterone. In: Olivier, B., Mos, J. and Brain, P. F. (Eds.), *Ethopharmacology of Agonistic Behavior in Animals and Humans,* Martinus Nijhoff, Dordrecht, pp. 223-244.

Ybema, C. E., Slangen, J. L., Olivier, B. and Mos, J. (1992). Discriminative stimulus properties of the serotonergic compound eltoprazine. *J. Pharmacol. Exp. Therap.,* 260 : 1045-1051.

Yoshimura, H. (1987). Studies contrasting drug effects on reproduction induced agonistic behavior in male and female mice. In: Olivier, B., Mos, J. and Brain, P. F. (Eds.), *Ethopharmacology of Aggression in Animals and Humans,* Martinus Nijhoff, Dordrecht, pp. 94-109.

Yoshimura, H. and Ogawa, N. (1982). Pharmaco-ethological analysis of agonistic behavior between resident and intruder mice: effect of anticholinergic drugs. *Jap. J. Pharmacol.,* 32 : 1111-1116.

Yoshimura, H. and Ogawa, N. (1983). Pharmaco-ethological analysis of agonistic behavior between resident and intruder mice: effects of ethylalcohol. *Folia Pharm. Jap.,* 81 : 135-141.

'oshimura, H. and Ogawa, N. (1989). Acute and chronic effects of psychotropic drugs on maternal aggression in mice. *Psychopharmacology*, **97** : 339-342.

'oshimura, H., Kihara, V. and Ogawa, N. (1987). Psychotropic effects of adrenergic ß-blockers on agonistic behavior between resident and intruder mice. *Psychopharmacology*, **91** : 445-450.

# Sex Differences in Primate Social Behavior

## E. B. KEVERNE

*Sub-Department of Animal Behaviour, University of Cambridge, Madingley, Cambridge CB3 8AA, U K*

The behavior of monkeys is strongly influenced by their social organisation. This influence is all pervasive, starting early in life when the infant monkey knows and is concerned with only a very small part of its group, namely the mother, kin and peers. At this early stage, influence is brought to bear on that infant through these close family members and peer relationships. Hence the daughters of high ranking mothers are themselves more likely to achieve high ranking status (Simpson and Simpson, 1982). Interactions with peers are essential to the development of normal adult sexual behavior, and monkeys raised with only a mother show little play or sexual behavior when adult (Harlow and Harlow, 1969; Suomi et al., 1970). Social environments which are restricted to unisexual interactions also influence the development of sexual behavior. Rearing infants in mother-infant groups with play contact restricted to the same sex, reduce the male-typical mounting of males, but increase this behavior in isosexually reared females relative to heterosexually reared females (Goldfoot and Wallen, 1978). The behavior of primates develops, therefore, in a very complex manner, involving factors that shape and organise their society and determine an individuals role within that society.

## Social rank and socio-sexual strategies

The effects of social rank on reproductive success in monkeys is similar for males and females in that reproduction is less successful among subordinates. Studies from a number of primate populations (reviewed in Harcourt, 1987) has revealed that high ranking females are more likely to conceive, and have higher reproductive rates than low ranking females. There has been a long-standing disagreement as to whether or not high dominance rank also confers high mating success and paternity in male primates. A recent comprehensive and detailed analysis of this work shows fairly conclusively that there is a general relationship between a male's rank and his ability to gain access to females around the time of ovulation (Cowlishaw and Dunbar, 1991). More direct studies of paternity using DNA fingerprinting provide unequivocal evidence of dominance and reproductive success, at least for one group of feral macaques (de Ruiter et al., 1992). Hence, the biological consequences of

*M. Haug et al. (eds.), The Development of Sex Differences and Similarities in Behavior, 227–240.*
© *1993 Kluwer Academic Publishers. Printed in the Netherlands.*

rank is similar for both males and females in that reproduction is less successful in subordinates. However, the kind of behavioral strategies by which this is achieved are remarkably different in males and females, and this has been studied in some detail in the Talapoin monkey in groups of different sociosexual composition (Keverne, 1985).

In the isosexual group, male Talapoin monkeys show high levels of overt aggressive behavior compared with isosexual groups of females. In males, attacks and threats occur at approximately 10 times the frequency seen in females. Mild aggression, in the form of displacements involving non-contact aggression to occupy a cage position held by another monkey is however, no more frequent in males than females. Affiliative behavior, in the form of huddling and grooming (Figure 1) is the prerogative of females with relatively little of this behavior being observed among males. Indeed, female rank is linearly correlated with grooming, highest ranking females receiving most of the affiliative behavior, while among males it is the aggressive behavior which determines individual rank.

In marked contrast, aggressive interactions among females decreased when they moved into the heterosexual group, while their affiliative behavior remained high. A sequence analysis of the behavioral interactions reveals further differences in the behavioral strategies adopted by males and females during heterosexual interactions. Within 30 seconds of a female approaching a male, the most likely behavior to follow is mounting if the encounter is with a dominant male, and aggression from other males, or withdrawal, if the male is subordinate. Among females, those of high rank solicit males more frequently, but low ranking females are no more likely to receive aggression from others than are high ranking females. However, when low ranking females solicit males, the most likely behavior to follow is male solicitation from higher ranking females. Hence, females in contrast to males do not show overt suppression of their own sex, but compete for male attention, while males aggressively attack subordinates when they show interest in females.

As a result of such differing behavioral strategies, there are no long term consequences for the sexual behavior of subordinate females and in the absence of other females, subordinates immediately show high levels of sexual interactions. Subordinate males do not, in contrast to females, show high levels of sexual activity for some time after dominant males are removed (Eberhart et al., 1985). Although there is an indication of increased arousal with increases in testosterone in subordinates, no sexual activity was observed in the first three weeks following removal of high ranking males. Since levels of plasma cortisol in subordinate males also increase under these conditions, this would imply that these males found interactions with females stressful. Those subordinate males which had been tested with females prior to group formation, and hence before the experience of chronic subordination, had shown perfectly normal levels of sexual behavior (Yodyingyuad et al., 1982). This would suggest that subordination in males and the aggression they receive in the context of female approaches, produces a kind of learned suppression of their sexual activity.

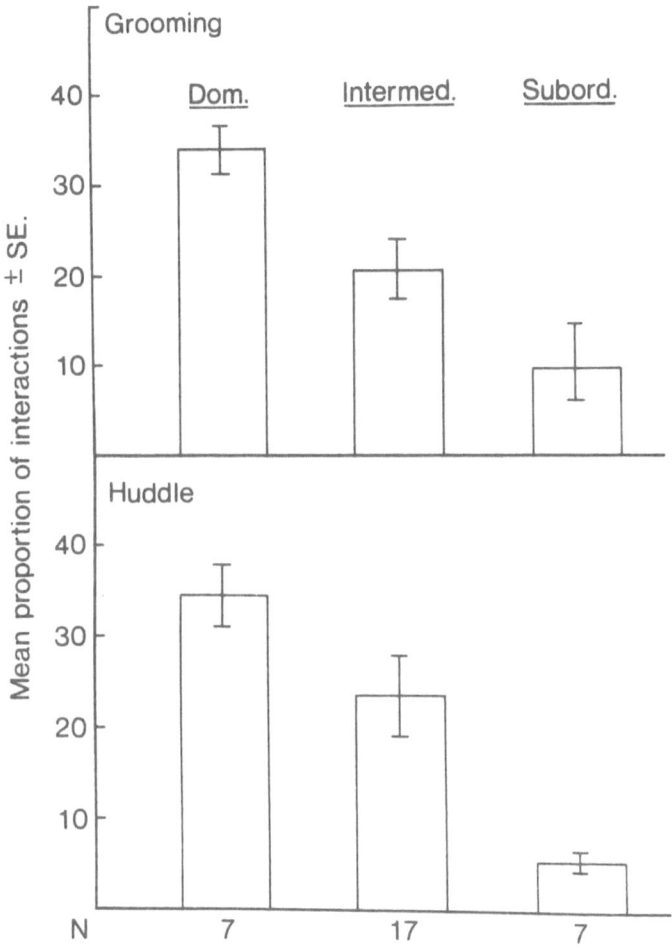

**Figure 1** Affiliative behavior in seven groups of monkeys (females.
Affiliate behavior (grooming and huddling) is high in females and is related to the hierarchy with highest ranking females receiving most attention from others. Based on 7 groups of monkeys observed daily over a five week period.

# Behavioral emancipation from gonadal hormones

It is often the case that observers of free ranging monkeys note that sexual behavior is restricted to certain seasons of the year and to periods in the menstrual cycle associated with ovulation (Lancaster and Lee, 1965). This has led to usage of the term "estrus" in order to contrast the monkey's menstrual cycle with that of women, and thereby more closely associate the primate behavioral cycle with that of other mammals. Likewise a widely cited distinction made by anthropologists between human sexuality and that of other primates is the apparent loss of estrus in the human female associated with copulation at times other than when fertilisation occurs (Alexander and Noonan, 1979). The implications of such reports bring primates in line with other mammals and make clear distinctions between them and the human condition. Superficially this evidence is compelling, but is not sustained by a critical appraisal of published findings which take into account laboratory studies. In reviewing the findings from studies of 20 species of both wild and captive simian primates, (Martin, 1992) concluded that most exhibit copulation at times when fertilisation seems unlikely. Others have questioned the usage of estrus as an appropriate term in describing simian sexual behavior (Keverne, 1981). Laboratory studies have shown that sexual interactions occur at all times of the menstrual cycle (Keverne, 1976) and have further revealed a role for ovarian hormones in determining these interactions (Keverne, 1985). Perhaps the most significant effects of ovarian hormones is to influence female attractiveness. This is brought about by a somatic action of hormones on the swelling and colouration of the perineal area and by changing vaginal and urinary odors which serve as powerful cues in the attraction of males (Keverne, 1976). Ovarian hormones have little effect on receptive or proceptive behavior and this has led to the view that the simian brain has become emancipated from fluctuations in gonadal hormones. This does not imply that female monkeys are permanently receptive any more than women are, but it does provide for neural mechanisms determining sexual behavior to be free from gonadal control, and thereby more amenable to social influences and higher order processing for integration of past experiences and partner preferences.

Studies of sexual behavior in male simian primates have languished somewhat, perhaps because of the investment in the time required to find any significant effects of castration. Sexual behavior will persist in castrated adult monkeys for at least a year in the laboratory, while castrate males released into free ranging groups have been observed mounting females some seven years following their release. Castration does, however, impair sexual performance, particularly intromission (Michael and Wilson, 1973). In those individuals where mounting stops, it is therefore difficult to determine the relative contribution of adverse learning experiences during their impaired performance. Hence, a male monkey can be induced to continue sexual behavior for longer periods after castration by simply changing the female partner. On the other hand, the male will stop sexual interactions sooner if other males are introduced that compete for the female partner. Indeed, the social environment imposes hierarchies which influence many aspects of male reproductive behavior.

In the case of talapoin monkeys, all aspects of male sexual behavior (inspects, looks, approaches to female, mounts and ejaculations) are related to the hierarchy, and while the appetitive behaviors (looks, approaches, inspects) are seen in all males, overt sexual consummatory behavior resulting in ejaculation is the prerogative of the highest ranking males (Keverne et al., 1978). Correlated with this is the increase in levels of testosterone measured in dominant males on moving into the heterosexual group, raising the question as o whether or not these changes are causatively linked to reproductive success Eberhart et al., 1980). To address this issue, males have been castrated in heir respective groups and given testosterone replacement at maintenance Joses similar in all animals. Among dominant males, castration never :ompletely eliminated their sexual interest in females, while subordinates failed o be sexually active even with very high doses of testosterone administration. Fhis finding together with the finding of phase shifts in the circadian rhythm of estosterone secretion in subordinate males following heterosexual interactions Martensz et al., 1987), suggests that testosterone secretion is influenced by Jehavioral interactions with respect to rank, rather than having a determining ?ffect on sexual behavior or rank.

Hence, the socio-sexual behavior of monkeys is best characterised by the ligh level of dependence on social influences and the low level of dependence Jn endocrine influences. Although largely independent of hormonal secretions rom the gonads, behavioral interactions within the social group do have major :onsequences for these and other endocrine systems.

# Endogenous opioids and the socio-sexual strategies of males and females

t is axiomatic that social structure determines primate behavior, but a question Jf some importance concerns the neural mechanisms that sustain social nteractions, and how such mechanisms may have evolved. In simian primates, social behavior may itself be considered a motivational force, but one that is 1evertheless intimately interlinked with sexual, aggressive and parental Jehavior. All these categories of behavior also have a common link with the brains endorphin system. Blockade of endogenous opiates impairs sexual and maternal behavior, while aggressive behavior may increase the release of opiates, producing an acute analgesia. It can therefore be hypothesised that the role of the endorphin system in sustaining the bond seen in the consort and mother-infant relationships has expanded to encompass social interactions in the broader context of the group as a whole. The evolutionary development of the underlying neural mechanisms has been aided by the emancipation from strict gonadal control of the component behaviors (sexual, aggressive and parental) important in social interactions.

Considerable attention has been given by sociobiologists to the advantages that have accrued among primates from living socially. These include finding food more efficiently (Clutton-Brock and Harvey, 1977), reducing the costs of predation (Bertram, 1978; van Schaik, 1983), and forming alliances to compete for access to feeding and sleeping sites (Wrangham, 1983). The advantages of social grouping may be different for each sex (Wrangham and Smuts, 1980); females rarely lack mates, whereas males often do, and food getting is an important social strategy for females, which means they often form more permanent alliances than males. Many primate societies are therefore referred to as being "female-bonded" (Wrangham, 1980).

Advantages such as these have formed the ultimate factors in the evolution of sociality. Although attempts have been made to describe proximate factors

(Hinde, 1983), with particular emphasis on grooming (Seyfarth, 1983), little has been published on the underlying physiological mechanisms of social reward in primates. Several studies have pointed to the involvement of endogenous opioids as underlying social emotion and social attachment (Panksepp, 1986), and it has been suggested that the positive affect arising from the mother-infant relationship is mediated by cerebral endorphin-containing systems (Panksepp et al., 1978). This hypothesis was based on findings of opiate alleviation of the stress arising from mother/infant separation in guinea pigs and puppies. Other studies have reported that opiate receptor blockade interferes with maternal behavior and disrupts pup-retrieval in dogs (Panksepp, 1986). In sheep, the onset of maternal behavior is impaired by central administration of an opiate receptor blocker (Kendrick and Keverne, 1989) while central morphine administration potentiates the selective bonding of a non-parturient ewe with a lamb (Keverne and Kendrick, 1991).

The rhesus monkey mother-infant relationship is characterised by high levels of social grooming in the early post-natal period (Hinde et al., 1964). The infant is attractive to other females in the group, and the mother normally restricts their grooming and attention to a minimum by restraining her infant from moving away (Hinde and Spencer-Booth, 1967). Treatment of the mother with low doses of the opiate receptor blocker at this time produce a dramatic effect on the mother's social behavior towards her infant (Martel et al., in press). Mothers both groom and restrain their infants less, and permit more infant grooming interactions by other females. This changed relationship with their infants is progressive with the continued naloxone treatment in contrast to the mothers grooming relationships with other females, which declined soon after the start of treatment (Figure 2).

There were no overall effects on activity, feeding, or the time infants were permitted on the nipple. Hence, in the early post-partum period when the mothers social interactions are predominantly with her infant, opiate receptor blockade impairs the security of this relationship.

Among adult primates, the ß-endorphin system is activated by social grooming and opiate activity relates to the motivation to be groomed and to groom, (Keverne et al., 1989). Blockade of opiate receptors (Figure 3) with either naloxone or naltrexone results in monkeys increasing their need to be groomed (invitations) and their grooming of others, which is a behavioral strategy to initiate reciprocal grooming (Fabre-Nys et al., 1982).

There are no effects on self-grooming or scratching. Because grooming is known to release central ß-endorphin (Keverne et al., 1989), it seems likely that the increased grooming that a monkey requests in this pharmacological paradigm is an attempt to compensate for loss of endogenous opiates induced by receptor blockade.

Increased grooming and grooming invitations normally occur in pair bonding of primates during and following copulation (Michael et al., 1966), in cementing social relationships (Seyfarth et al., 1978), particularly between mothers and

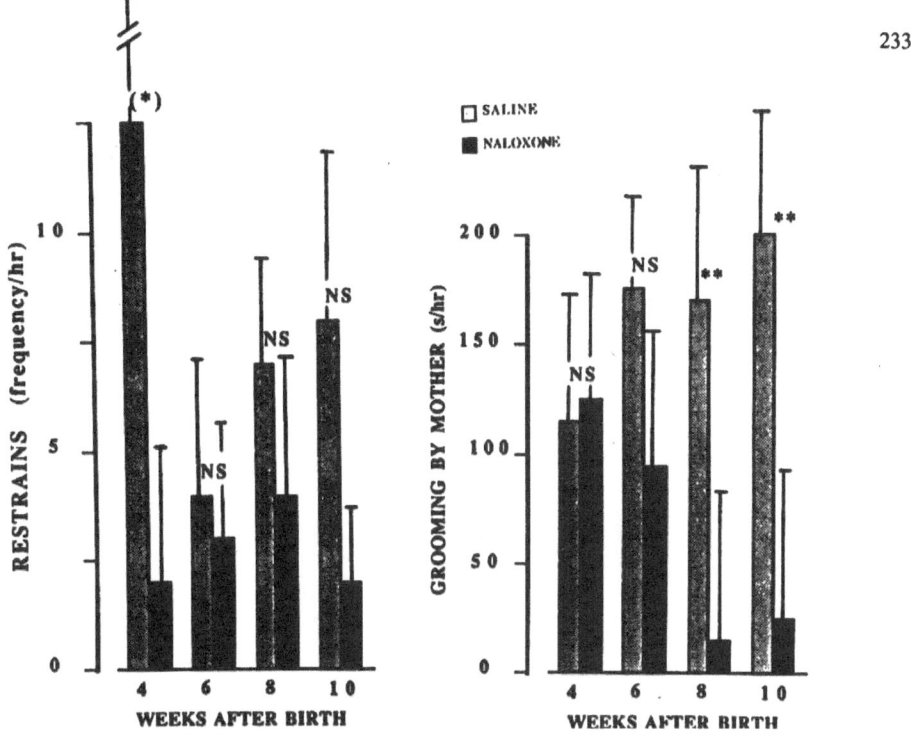

**Figure 2** Effects of opiate receptor blockade on mothers grooming their infants and restraining their interactions with others. ( *  P< 0.05 ; ** P< 0.01).

infants (Lee, 1983), in maintaining peace and cohesion in primate societies (Simpson, 1973), and following aggressive outbursts (Kummer, 1981). Grooming interactions form a predominant part of the females behavioral repertoire, occurring in different social situations and having in common the provision of bonding and comfort to the participants rather than being purely hygienic (Dunbar, 1989). It therefore appears that grooming is a significant proximate factor in social bonding and is accompanied by a rapid increase in ß-endorphin in cerebral spinal fluid (CSF) contingent on receiving grooming. Hence, at the neural level the brain's endorphin system may provide the basis for a common bonding mechanism, but the nature of the relationships bonded clearly differ (mother/infant; consortships; peers). Nevertheless, it is surely no coincidence that in female primates all of these relationships share a strong mutual grooming component.

Aggressive behavior is a predominant feature of male social interactions, resulting in the establishment of clear-cut hierarchies. Within such a hierarchy, subordinate male talapoin monkeys have approximately three times higher intra-cerebral CSF levels of ß-endorphin than do dominant animals (Martensz et al., 1986).

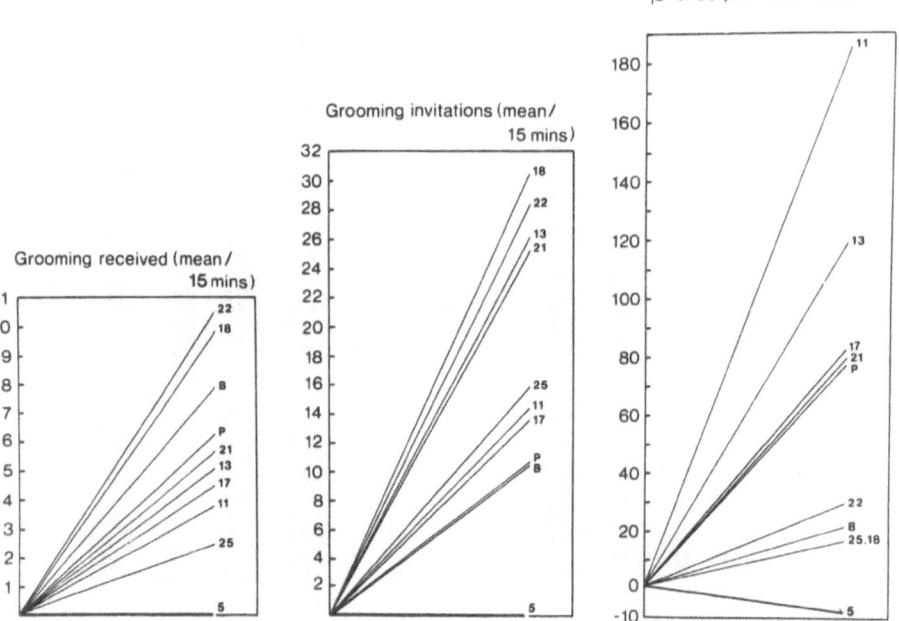

**Figure 3**   Changes in grooming behavior and CSF endorphin levels in monkeys re-united for 15 min. after 24 h. of social isolation. 11-25 and B, P represent individual animals.

This finding and the behavioral and neuroendocrine profile of subordinate monkeys (Figure 4) suggests a heightened activity in the ß-endorphin neurones. This correlates with their low level of sexual behavior and depressed gonadal function when compared with dominant males. This is also consistent with the observation that acute treatment of dominant males with the μ-receptor agonist (morphine) in low doses (2 μg/kg$^{-1}$) inhibits their sexual behavior, decreases testosterone secretion, and increases cortisol and prolactin, giving them an endocrine as well as behavioral profile similar to that of subordinates.

Monkeys of different rank can also be distinguished by the reactivity to opiate blockade of the neuroendocrine system controlling LH secretion. Dominant males release significant amounts of LH in response to doses of naloxone as low as .25 mg/kg, whereas doses 20 times this concentration (5 mg/kg) are ineffective in subordinate monkeys (Martensz et al., 1986). This represents an apparent inconsistency between the differential effects of opiate blockade with naloxone and postulated levels of activity or cerebral ß-endorphin in these monkeys. However, chronically high levels of ß-endorphin in subordinates may have down-regulated receptors to such an extent that they no longer respond to the acute administration of the antagonist. Though the exact interpretation of these results is not yet clear, they reinforce the conclusion that chronic subordination is associated with altered opiate activity, and this may be part of

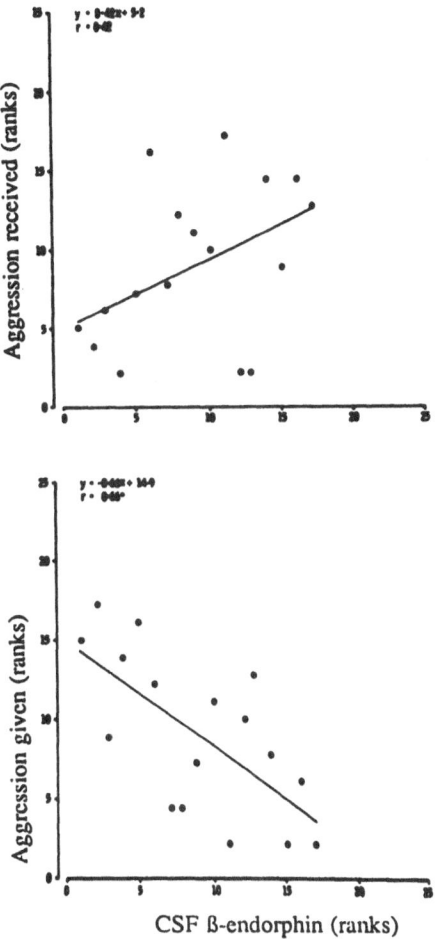

**Figure 4** CSF ß-endorphin and aggression in males. Receipt of high aggression leads to high levels of ß-endorphin, whilst the giving of aggression does not increase CSF ß-endorphin.

the neuroendocrine machinery of reproductive suppression characteristic of this condition.

A further paradox stems from the way in which opiate antagonists influence behavior in the social group. High-ranking males treated chronically with the opiate antagonist naltrexone show a significant reduction in sexual behavior, a deficit that does not recover rapidly after withdrawal of the drug (Meller et al., 1980). The data we have so far collected from monkeys living socially suggest that subordinate monkeys have much in common at the behavioral, neuroendocrine, and neural levels with dominant monkeys treated with the opiate receptor blockers naloxone or naltrexone. In other words, chronic subordination would seem to result in a failure of the monkey's brain to respond to its own endogenous opiates.

# Conclusions

In considering the evolution of group social structure and the distinct roles of males and females within this, ecological influences have played a key role. Wrangham (1987) suggests that since food is a significant limiting factor in female reproduction, the females' interaction with their environment has adaptive priority. Female reproductive success is rarely constrained by a shortage of males, but food availability, predation and other ecological factors (parasites, sleeping sites) have powerful effects on female fitness. In many primate societies, females are the permanent members of the group and form extensive kinship alliances with other females, often based on grooming relationships. Such social groups are referred to as being "female-bonded". However, the advantages and consequences of social living may be different for each sex, since the reproduction of males and females is constrained in different ways (Wrangham, 1983). Male reproductive success is primarily limited by their access to receptive females, and males are attracted to groups of females. Nevertheless, male strategies add complexity to the social structure : males compete and suppress the sexual behavior of some males and occasionally form alliances with others; they develop long-term and short-term affiliative bonds with females (Smuts, 1983) and threaten infanticide of infants not fathered by themselves (Hrdy and Hausfatr, 1984). Sexual competition is an important factor in male relationships and males frequently leave their natal group to breed because of the restricted mating opportunities within their established social group.

It would seem, therefore, that an understanding of the mechanisms which influence female social relationships is pertinent to understanding social structure, and the different behavioral predispositions of males and females within this structure. This chapter has outlined how the behavioral strategies of male and female monkeys differ, and the consequences of these differing strategies on the brain's endogenous opiate system. Affiliative behavior brings about acute increases in CSF endorphins and since this behavior is the prerogative of females, it may represent a mechanism important to "female-bonded" societies. Parental care is also the prerogative of female monkeys and is also in part dependent on opiate mechanisms. The female investment in the post-natal relationship ultimately leads to the development of extended family alliances. Following puberty, males may leave the natal group but females remain and the status of their matriline has marked influences on the development of their own status. High ranking mothers tend to produce high ranking daughters. This may also be related to the social attention they receive, since grooming is strongly correlated with rank.

Field primatologists never refer to social groups as being "male bonded". On the contrary, the behavioral strategies of males are constructed around competition, and sexual exclusion of young males results in male mobility being a common feature of many primate societies. This often produces solitary males that remain peripheral to the social group for extended periods. Even the groupings of male chimpanzees are thought to have evolved from a

ypothetical solitary male system (Wrangham, 1987), arising from the
ulnerability of young chimpanzees to attack (Goodall, 1986). It is therefore not
urprising to find that the functional activation of endogenous opiate release in
males is driven primarily in the context of aggression (Figure 4). This may lead
o the highest levels of CSF ß-endorphin being found in subordinate males, but
aradoxically their brain responds as if the system were totally inactive,
robably because of a down regulation of receptors. One consequence of this
s a neuroendocrine cascade which renders subordinates psychologically
astrated and incapable of performing with females even when the opportunity
s available. Hence, although similar neural mechanisms are available to
males and females, the way in which these are employed is very different.
Evolution has shaped the sexual strategies of males and females in ways that
ptimise the benefits to individuals of a given sex, rather than to the group as a
vhole.

# References

Alexander, R. and Noonan, K. M. (1979). Concealment of ovulation, parental
care, and human social evolution. In : Chagnon, N. A., Irons, W. G. (Eds.),
*Evolutionary Biology and Human Social Organisation*, Duxburg Press,
Chicago, pp. 436-453.

Bertram, B. C. R. (1978). Living in groups : predators and prey. In : Davies, N. B.
and Krebs, J. R. (Eds.), *Behavioral Ecology : An Evolutionary Approach*,
Blackwell, Oxford, pp. 269-285.

Clutton-Brock, T. H. and Harvey, P. H. (1977). Primate ecology and social
organisation. *J. Zool.*, **183** : 1-39.

Cowlishaw, G. and Dunbar, R. J. M. (1991). Dominance rank and mating
success in male primates. *Anim. Behav.*, **41** : 1045-1056.

de Ruiter, J. R., Scheffrahn, W., Trommelen, G. J J. M., Uitterlinden, A. G.,
Martin, R. D. and van Hoof, J. A. R. A. M. (1992). Male social rank and
reproductive success in wild long-tailed Macaques. In : Martin, R. D., Dixson,
A. F. and Wickings, E. J. (Eds.), *Paternity in Primates : Genetic Tests and
Theories*, Karger, Basel, pp. 175-191.

Dunbar, R. (1989). Functional significance of social grooming in primates. *Folia
Primat.*, **49** : 1-23.

Eberhart, J., Yodyinyuad, U. and Keverne, E. B. (1985). Subordination in male
Talapoin monkeys lowers sexual behaviour in the absence of dominants.
*Physiol. Behav.*, **35** : 673-678.

Eberhart, J. A., Keverne, E. B. and Meller, R. E. (1980). Social influences on
plasma testosterone levels in male talapoin monkeys. *Horm. Behav.*, **14** :
247-266.

Fabre-Nys, C., Meller, R. E. and Keverne, E. B. (1982). Opiate antagonists
stimulate affiliation behaviour in monkeys. *Pharmacol. Biochem. Behav.*, **16** :
653-659.

Goldfoot, D. A. and Wallen, K. (1978). Development of gender role behaviours
in heterosexual and isosexual groups of infant monkeys. In : Chivers, D. and
Herbert, J. (Eds.), *Recent Advances in Primatology*, Academic Press, London,

pp. 155-160.

Goodall, J. (1986). *The Chimpanzees of Gombe : Patterns of Behaviour.*, Harvard University Press, Cambridge.

Harcourt, A. H. (1987). Dominance and fertility among female primates. *J. Zool. Lond.*, **213** : 471-487.

Harlow, H. F. and Harlow, M. K. (1969). Effects of various mother infant relationships on rhesus monkey behaviour. In : Foss, B. M. (Ed.), *Determinants of Infant Behaviour, Vol.4*, Metheun, London, pp. 15-36.

Hinde, R. A. (1983). Description of the proximate factors influencing social structure. In : Hinde, R. A. (Ed.), *Primate Social Relationships*, Blackwell, Oxford, pp. 176-181.

Hinde, R. A. and Spencer-Booth, Y. (1967). The behaviour of socially living rhesus monkeys in their first two and a half years. *Anim. Behav.*, **15** : 169-196.

Hinde, R. A., Rowell, T. E. and Spencer-Booth, Y. (1964). Behaviour of socially living rhesus monkeys in their first six months. *Proc. Zool. Soc. Lond.*, **143** : 609-649.

Hrdy, S. B. and Hausfater, G. (1984). Comparative and evolutionary perspectives on infanticide : an introduction and overview. In : Hausfater, G. and Hrdy, S. B., (Eds.), *Infanticide : Comparative and Evolutionary Perspectives*, Hawthorne, New York.

Kendrick, K. and Keverne, E. B. (1989). Intracerebroventricular infusions of naltrexone and phentolamine on central and peripheral oxytocin release and on maternal behaviour induced by vaginocervical stimulation in the ewe. *Brain Res.*, **505** : 329-332.

Keverne, E. B. (1976). Sexual receptivity and attractiveness in the female monkey. *Adv. Study. Behav.*, **7** : 155-200.

Keverne, E. B. (1981). Do old world primates have oestrus? *Malays. Appl. Biol.* : 119-126.

Keverne, E. B. (1985). Hormones and the sexual behaviour of monkeys. In : Gilles, R. and Balthazar, J. (Eds.), *Neurobiology and Behaviour*, Springer Verlag, Berlin, pp. 37-47.

Keverne, E. B. and Kendrick, K. (1991) Morphine and CRF potentiate maternal acceptance in multiparous ewes after vaginocervical stimulation. *Brain Res.*, **540** : 55-62.

Keverne, E. B., Eberhart, J. A., Yodyinyuad, U. and Abbott, D. A. (1985). Social influences on sex-differences in the behaviour and endocrine state of talapoin monkeys. *Progr. Brain Res.*, **61** : 331-347.

Keverne, E. B., Martensz, N. D. and Tuite, B. (1989). ß-endorphin concentrations in CSF of monkeys are influenced by grooming relationships. *Psychoneuroendocrinol.*, **14** : 155-161.

Keverne, E. B., Meller, R. E. and Martinez-Arias, A. M. (1978). Dominance, aggression and sexual behaviour in social groups of talapoin monkeys. In : Chivers, D. J. and Herbert, J. (Eds.), *Recent Advances in Primatology, Vol. 1*, Academic Press, New York, pp. 533-548.

Kummer, H. (1981). *Primate Societies*, Aldine-Atherton, Chicago, Illinois.

Lancaster, J. B. and Lee, R. B. (1965). The annual reproductive cycle in monkeys and apes. In : DeVore, I. (Ed.), *Primate Behaviour*, Holt, Rinehart and

Winston, New York, pp. 486-513.

Lee, P. C. (1983). Caretaking of infants and mother-infant relationships. In : Hinde, R. A. (Ed.), *Primate Social Relationships*, Blackwell, Oxford, pp. 146-151.

Martel, F. L., Nevison, C. M., Rayment, D., Simpson, M. and Keverne, E. B. (1992). Opiate receptor blockade reduces maternal affect in rhesus monkeys. *Psychoneuroendocrinol.*, (in press).

Martensz, N. D., Vellucci, S. V., Fuller, L. M., Everitt, B. J., Keverne, E. B. and Herbert, J. (1987). Relationship between aggressive behaviour and circadian rhythms in cortisol and testosterone in social groups of talapoin monkeys. *J. Endocrinol.*, **115** : 107-120.

Martensz, N. D., Vellucci, S. V., Keverne, E. B. and Herbert, J. (1986). ß-endorphin levels in the cerebrospinal fluid of male talapoin monkeys in social groups related to dominance status and luteinizing hormone response to naloxone. *Neuroscience*, **18** : 651-658.

Martin, R. D. (1992). Female cycles in relation to paternity in primate societies. In : Martin, R. D., Dixson, A. F. and Wickings, E. J., (Eds.), *Paternity in Primates : Genetic Tests and Theories*, Karger, Basel, pp. 238-274.

Meller, R. E., Herbert, J. and Keverne, E. B. (1980). Behavioural and endocrine effects of naltrexone in male talapoin monkeys. *Pharmacol. Biochem. Behav.*, **13** : 663-672.

Michael, R. P. and Wilson, M. I. (1973). Effects of castration and hormone replacement in fully adult male rhesus monkeys. *Endocrinol.*, **95** : 150-159.

Michael, R. P., Herbert, J. and Welegalla, J. (1966). Ovarian hormones and grooming behaviour in the rhesus monkey (Macaca mulatta) in the laboratory. *J. Endocrinol.*, **36** : 263-279.

Panksepp., J. (1986). The psychobiology of prosocial behaviours : separation distress, play and altruism. In : Zahn-Waxler, C., Cummings, E. M. and Jannotti, R., (Eds.), *Altruism and Aggression : Biological and Social Origins*, Cambridge University Press, Cambridge, pp. 19-57.

Panksepp., J., Herman, B. H., Connor, R., Bishop, P. and Scott, J. P. (1978). The biology of social attachment : opiates alleviate separation distress. *Biol. Psychiat.*, **13** : 607-618.

Seyfarth, R. M. (1983). Grooming and social competition in primates. In : Hinde, R.A. (Ed.), *Primate Social Relationships*, Blackwell, Oxford, pp. 182-189.

Simpson, M. J. A. (1973). The social grooming of male chimpanzees. In : Michael, R. P. and Crook, J. H. (Eds.), *The Comparative Ecology of Behaviour of Primates*, Academic Press, New York, pp. 411-506.

Simpson, M. S. and Simpson, A. E. (1982). Birth sex ratios and social rank in rhesus monkey mothers. *Nature*, **300** : 440-441.

Smuts, B. B. (1983). Special relationships between adult male and female olive baboons : selective advantages. In : Hinde, R. A. (Ed.), *Primate Social Relationships*, Blackwell, Oxford, pp. 262-266.

Suomi, S. J., Harlow, H. F. and Domek, C. J. (1970). Effect of repetitive infant separation of young monkeys. *J. Abnorm. Psychol.*, **76** : 161-172.

van Schaik, C. P. (1983). Why are diurnal primates living in groups? *Behaviour*, **87** : 120-144.

Wrangham, R. W. (1980). An ecological model of female bonded groups. *Behaviour*, **75** : 262-300.

Wrangham, R. W. (1983). Ultimate factors determining social structure. In : Hinde, R. A. (Ed.), *Primate Social Relationships*, Blackwell, Oxford, pp. 255-261.

Wrangham, R. W. (1987). Evolution and social structure. In : Smuts, B. B., Cheney, D. L., Seyfarth, R. M., Wrangham, R. W. and Struhsaker, T. T. (Eds.), *Primate Societies*, Univ. Chicago Press, Chicago, pp. 282-296.

Wrangham, R. W. and Smuts, B. B. (1980). Sex differences in the behavioural ecology of chimpanzees in Gombe National Park, Tanzania. *J. Reprod. Fert.*, **28** : 1-20

Yodyingyuad, U., Eberhart, J. A. and Keverne, E. B. (1982). Effects of rank and novel females on behaviour and hormones in male talapoin monkeys. *Physiol. Behav.*, **28** : 995-1005.

# What, How, and Why of Gender Differences from an Evolutionary Perspective

L. PETRINOVICH

*Department of Psychology, University of California Riverside, CA 92521, USA*

will discuss some issues and concepts regarding evolutionary models adequate to deal with reproduction, with a special focus on issues related to gender. I hope to introduce those of you who do not track current trends in evolutionary theory to some of the basic concepts and controversies rather than present a review of basic principles involved in evolutionary processes. From an evolutionary perspective one would expect to find gender differences in relation to general intra- and inter-sexual relationships, specific courtship patterns, mating behaviors, patterns of parental care, and life-history strategies. I want to stress a few things I think are important to keep in focus when considering issues related to gender. Steve Gaulin (this volume) very clearly covered some of the pertinent issues regarding sexual selection, and male and female reproductive strategies, and I will avoid repetition of that material. All of the concerns I will raise here will involve questions in human evolutionary psychology, and will be driven by a construal of the ultimate questions in evolution, where the currency is differential reproductive success. At the end of this paper I will discuss my first steps toward constructing a human moral ethogram. First, a message from our basic evolutionary sponsor, which will set the stage for talking about the evolution of human nature.

## Some basic evolutionary concepts

It is important to emphasize that evolutionary theory operates at two distinct levels: at the proximate level where the concern is with how processes work, and the ultimate level where the currency is differential reproductive success. Evolutionary explanations are not complete unless they address both levels, and a consideration of each can lead to insights regarding the nature of the other.

*M. Haug et al. (eds.), The Development of Sex Differences and Similarities in Behavior, 241–253.*
© 1993 *Kluwer Academic Publishers.*

## Fitness

Fitness is an important concept which has been defined in terms of differential survival and reproductive success. Some philosophers have argued that there is a danger of circularity in this simple form of the concept because fitness differences cannot be used to explain differential survival and reproductive success without creating a tautology. The problem of circularity can be avoided by identifying the multiple factors that determine the values of the theoretical term "fitness". When the task of identifying the physiological and ecological factors that influence fitness levels is undertaken, the theoretical term "fitness" acquires value as a theoretical principle.

In the long run, fitness will have a relationship to the outcome variables of survival and differential reproduction. The outcome currency is not at the level of individual survival, fertility, and fecundity (which are at the proximate level), but at the ultimate level, at least counting as far as of the number of grandoffspring produced. It matters not that a healthy and fertile offspring is produced if it, in turn, is unable, for any of a variety of reasons, to raise its own offspring. It is entirely possible that, due to chance occurrences, a very fit organism will perish while a less fit one will survive; however, this fact does not lessen the power of the concept of fitness when it is viewed from a probabilistic perspective.

## Selection

For evolution to occur the process of natural selection must be operative. This process acts on the variation presented by different organisms in the population and it acts to destroy that variation through a process which favors some genes (and their organismic carriers) at the expense of others. The characteristics of individual organisms are stable throughout a lifespan, but through selection the gene frequencies, or combinations, in the gene pool will change.

Especially when considering the human condition, care must be taken not to interpret every characteristic that exists in an organism to reflect the action of selection to produce adaptations. A useful distinction is that between 'selection of objects' and 'selection for properties'. 'Selection of' pertains to the effects of a selection process, whereas 'selection for' describes its causes. Linkages can be at the level of the phenotype (pleitropic) or at the level of the genotype (gene linkage), and the level has to be determined empirically if understanding is to be complete. The point is that systematic change can occur as a result of selection, but not be due to any direct adaptive advantage of the trait that was selected.

## Factors influencing selection

There are several important factors that influence the effects of selection. One is the structure of the gene pool on which selection can work to carve individual genotypes. The size of the inter-breeding population, called a deme, is of great importance when the factors determining the structure of the gene pool are considered. If a breeding population is small, then random effects can have major influence, because the balance of gene frequencies can vary a great deal from deme to deme. This variability is the result of sampling error because the specific individuals in the population will represent only a selected proportion of the total gene pool. Thus, chance historical factors can be of paramount importance with small demes, and the effects of selection will be of relatively less importance as determiners of the characteristics of the deme. On the other hand, if demes are large they will show less variability across the demes, and chance historical factors assume a lesser role than does selection.

Seldom does selection act alone in a frequency independent manner. Because selection usually occurs within a context in which fitness values depend on relative frequencies of genes, or organismic traits, that characterize the different individuals in a group (are frequency dependent), no general statement can be made regarding improvement in adaptation. Thus, organisms might achieve a higher relative fitness level and fail to improve further, or to move toward optimality; an adaptation might not go through the expense of genetic fine-tuning to reach optimality if the existing adaptations are useful enough to produce a higher relative fitness than its competitors possess. As Sober (1984) suggested, Herbert Spencer's slogan of 'the survival of the fittest' would have been less misleading, although less striking, if it had been phrased as 'the survival of the fitter'.

## Adaptation

Adaptation is defined in terms of traits that have emerged through a process of natural selection. A trait can secondarily enhance adaptedness without being a directly selected adaptation if the forces of pleitropy or gene-linkage are involved. A trait can be an adaptation, in the sense that it is selected, but not contribute to adaptedness because it works to the overall detriment of the possessors. A trait that enhances adaptedness, no matter how it arose, can undergo secondary natural selection and become an adaptation. Thus, adaptation is an historical concept, and in order to invoke it one should know the origin of the trait under question. In order to deny that adaptation has occurred, it is also necessary to know the origin of the trait, and because behavior does not leave fossils an evolutionary account of behavior can often be a bit dicey.

One further basic distinction is the norm of reaction, which is defined as the different phenotypes a genotype will produce as a function of the sort of environment in which it develops. There is no such thing as a gene or protein for any specific property or trait. Fitness is not an intrinsic property of organisms, but is a property that exists only in the relationship of the organism to the specific environments in which fitness has been tested. To establish fitness values the ecological factors that test the genes must be considered, and any generalizations regarding fitness must be expressed within that range. If the norm of reaction has been established in a wide range of ecological circumstances, then it will be possible to make educated estimates of the probability distribution of future states.

## All power to sexual recombination

The fact that sexual reproduction exists so widely is a problem that has concerned evolutionists for some time. If the game of life is played to maximize one's contribution to the genes of succeeding generations why doesn't the female just clone herself, so that all of her offsprings' genes are the same as her own? Why have sexual reproduction, thereby sharing half of the genetic makeup of offspring with a sexual partner?

It is agreed that heritable adaptation is the fuel that powers adaptive evolution. There must be a wide range of genotypes present in order for the gene pool to respond to changes in selection pressures, and sexual recombination is one way to assure that continual variation is present in each generation. As Michod and Levin (1988) pointed out, all agree that recombination, especially the generation of new combinations of existing alleles at multiple, homologous loci, is of primary importance in evolutionary processes.

Environments often change suddenly, especially when considered in the frame of geological time, because of radical alterations of the physical characteristics of the ecology, or due to the introduction of infectious diseases, such as through the action of parasites. W. D. Hamilton and his colleagues have championed the parasite model as reason for the existence of sexual recombination (Seger and Hamilton, 1988; Hamilton et al., 1990; Zuk, 1992). The parasite model notes that hosts usually have generation times that are longer than those of parasites, whose generation times are sometimes orders of magnitude shorter than those of their hosts. When this asymmetry exists, parasites can evolve improved methods of attack much faster than their hosts can evolve improved methods of defense. The host's best defense will be based on maintaining a broad range of genetic diversity. If there is sexual recombination in each generation, as Seger and Hamilton (1988, p. 176) vividly state, the host organisms "...can present to the parasites what amounts to a continually moving target". Continual recombination will result in organisms with a wide range of genetic diversity, and this diversity will make it difficult for parasites that have specialized on current host characteristics to exploit the diverse host offspring. This argues that there will be a benefit for hosts that have differing genotypes because they will be less exploitable by parasites.

In general, then, extinction is less likely for those genetic systems that practice sex than would otherwise be the case. I want to emphasize that this is not an argument that involves group selection; all effects are at the level of changes in gene frequencies of individuals, but their effects can be detected, and are effective, at the level of breeding populations.

# The human condition

There seems to be a general consensus that initial communities of Homo sapiens consisted of relatively small breeding populations of related individuals. If so, chance historical factors might be expected to have played an important role in determining the characteristics of the different demes because of sampling variability in regards to their available genotypes, and the attendant differential response to new ecological niches that pioneers would occupy. It might be expected, then, that the contemporary human gene pool has survived the tests of a wide range of environmental factors: the norm of reaction should have been established through history by exposure to a wide range of ecological circumstances.

Sexual reproduction tends to prevail in old, stable environments, especially if the organisms involved are large and complex, as is the case with Homo sapiens. Because humans have a relatively long generation time, diversity would be important to defeat short-lived parasites, and sexual recombination would permit the inter-generational repair of deleterious mutations. Thus, many factors seem to favor sex for humans, and I would hazard that sex is here to stay.

It is important to reconstruct the nature of the probable social environment of evolutionary adaptation for humans. The best estimate is that when human nature evolved, the reproductive system was one in which mateships were predominantly monogamous, paternal investment was important to enhance the survival of young, and the variance in reproductive success was slightly greater among men than among women. Such a system is found in almost all relict human societies occupying nonagricultural ecological niches, and a similar pattern of reproductive systems exists in the face of a wide diversity of cultural and technological characteristics. Wilson and Daly (1992, p. 254) suggest that this affords "...windows on the sociosexual milieu in which the human mind evolved and on the adaptive problems to which our species-typical social and sexual motives, emotions, and way of thought constitute the solutions".

Clearly, the complex agricultural and industrial societies humans now occupy are very different from the environments of evolutionary adaptation. Yet, no matter what the structure of current societies, there seem to be common threads concerning aspects of sociosexuality. A few of the universal structural characteristics concern such things as the existence of some sort of pair bond with mutual obligation, the bond persists over prolonged periods of time, the bond is sanctioned by the rest of society, and there are codes to legitimize the offspring of the pair, and regulate the inheritance of goods.

Not only are universal structural characteristics found within human societies, but there are universal behavioral tendencies as revealed by patterns of homicide, patterns of jealousy, sex differences in the characteristics preferred for mates, and in differential reproductive strategies employed by males and females. These behavioral studies will be discussed below. Halliday (1980) suggested that even anatomical characteristics such as the sturdier physique of men are likely to have developed to enable the man to fulfill his parental role in a mating alliance, as well as for the usually emphasized reason that these physical characteristics exist in the interests of competition between men for the possession of women.

## Altruism

To achieve an adequate evolutionary psychology that is applicable to human behavior one must deal with the existence of altruism. Altruism is defined most simply as a trait that increases the fitness of a recipient at the expense of an actor's fitness. If such traits exist (and everyone agrees that they are universal in human societies) then how could evolutionary theory account for the existence of such a costly trait? At first glance this poses a dilemma as profound as the question of "why sex".

Kin selection can be an important driving force in evolution because if one is predisposed to help others at one's own expense, one's own inclusive fitness can be increased due to the survival of kin with similar genetic structure. If the immediate community group consists of a number of kin, then helping members of that community will lead to an increase in inclusive fitness, even though there has been no 'calculation' of genetic similarity. The only important consideration is that kin are affected differentially because they are members of the community, not because people know about relative coefficients of relatedness. For kin selection to be effective, then, there only has to be tendencies for significant social interactions that are nonrandom with respect to kinship. The effects of frequency dependent individual selection would be powerful in demes of small starting size, and would generate differences between different demes through the effects of sampling error, and the differences would be perpetuated because there should be considerable inbreeding within demes.

There is agreement that human societies in the environment of evolutionary adaptation probably were small, that breeding predominantly was within the group, and that most of the group members were at least distantly related kin. Altruism might be expected to develop within such groups because it would enhance inclusive fitness through benefits to kin, and those groups within which altruism developed would be expected to have higher relative fitness when compared to groups that have a lower proportion of altruists. Thus, existence of altruism and a tendency toward reciprocal altruism between even unrelated group members would augment the absolute fitness of the population to which the individual actor belongs. As Masters (1982) has pointed out, rather than leading to a view that behavior is controlled by rigid instinct, inclusive-fitness models emphasize the importance of the influence of experience and learning, if only because accurate identification of close relatives and even friends should have a high pay-off in terms of increased reproductive success.

## Gender and sexuality

From an evolutionary perspective one would expect evolutionary mechanisms to have their greatest influence on traits related to reproduction, and, indeed, that is the case as indicated by a large number of empirical studies of human sexuality. One of the most common complaints regarding the use of evolutionary principles to explain human behavior is that there is a selective use of evidence, and inadequate consideration or exploration of alternative explanations. Buss (1989), in reply to commentaries of his article on sex differences in human mate preferences, pointed out that none of the several critical commentators provided any alternative hypotheses for three of the five specific hypotheses and predictions that were advanced in his article. Tooby and Cosmides (1989) developed the point that theorists emphasizing the importance of cultural influences confidently rest their case on the uncertain ground that evolutionary hypotheses about human nature must establish that there is universality across cultures. They point out that usually any degree of cross-cultural variability is assumed to establish that the behavior in question is the product of 'culture' rather than of 'biology'. They suggest, and I concur, that cultural theorists must specify the mechanisms and processes that determine how equipotential, domain-general mechanisms predict the statistical distribution of existing societies. As it stands, culture theory predicts the null hypothesis: differences between cultures are random and due to the vicissitudes of acculturation mechanisms. From this perspective, sex differences should occur as frequently in one direction as the other, and they do not. It is not acceptable to offer a plausible alternative (say psychoanalytic, alliance, or an economic powerlessness hypothesis) that is able to account for a specific outcome, but which is unable to accommodate the broad range of instances that evolutionary explanations can cover, and, on the basis of a single failure to obtain an evolutionarily predicted outcome, conclude that the evolutionary model must be rejected. Such a procedural gambit represents an inadequate scientific methodology, and sets an unreasonable standard for any complex network of hypotheses such as those that constitute the theory of evolution on which the emerging evolutionary psychology is based. Claims based on an acceptance of the null hypothesis are impossible to evaluate unless a reasonable estimate can be made of the statistical power of the test in question, and such estimates are rarely provided. Let me now consider some of the research of the recent generation of evolutionary psychologists.

## Patterns of homicide

In their book, Homicide, Daly and Wilson (1988) developed a selectionist argument to understand patterns of human homicide. They analyzed the extensive police files from Detroit and Canada, supplemented by available data from other cities and countries, as well as the existing ethnographic data. Without going into detail, their intensive analyses supported the hypothesis that, as evolutionary theory would predict, there are few instances where individuals kill close genetic kin, because such killing would lower inclusive fitness: conflicts tend to be increasingly severe and dangerous the more distantly related are the principals. When homicides do occur between cohabitants the victims are seldom genetic kin.

In general, their analyses support several conclusions. Selection shapes behavioral control mechanisms to increase fitness, to enhance nepotism, and to enable individuals to be effective reproductive competitors. Species-typical motives have evolved to promote genetic posterity such that murder is rare among genetic relatives. When infanticide occurs by males it is generally when paternity is uncertain, and by both males and females when the child is of poor phenotypic quality or is unlikely to survive. The risk of infanticide is greater at all ages when there is a step-parent than when there are two natural parents. When infanticide occurs by natural parents the rate is greater early in the infant's life (when parental investment is still low). There is also a sex difference in human competition and violence in terms of reproductive competition leading to homicide between individuals of the same sex; there is an extremely high incidence of male-male homicide as compared to female-female (over nine to one). The pattern of male-male homicide that was found supports the hypothesis that men compete for control over reproductive capacities of women, and that children are the currency regulating the competition.

Daly and Wilson examined alternative explanations that have been offered by social scientists and psychoanalysts to account for their data and found each alternative explanation inadequate to account for more than the specific instance it was designed to explain. If social scientists want to offer plausible alternatives to evolutionary explanations the alternatives they employ must be developed to accommodate a broad range of the relevant facts. Similarly, evolutionary psychology should be developed at a depth to encompass more than the few aspects of behavior (usually reproduction) with which it deals. Buss (1989) argues that the task for evolutionary psychologists is to identify basic psychological mechanisms and to specify the adaptive problems they solve in order to study overt behavior within the context of important features of the ecology.

## Age preferences for mates

Buss (1989) reported an extensive study of sex differences in human mate preferences using questionnaire data based on 37 samples from 33 countries, located on six continents and five islands, with a sample size of 10,047 people. Buss predicted that males should prefer as mates females who are in their mid-teens to early 20's, and they should value youth and physical attractiveness which would signal health, and, thus, higher reproductive value. Females should prefer males with greater resources and, because male fertility is less steeply age graded from puberty, physical appearance, which could be used to gauge fertility, should be valued less. These predicted differences should transcend cultural variations.

He found that females valued males who had "good financial prospects", were ambitious, and industrious. Males preferred younger mates and females older ones. Buss interprets the results to support two major points: (1) All 37 societies in the study placed tremendous value on kindness-understanding and intelligence in potential mates, and it is reasonable to characterize these traits, provisionally, as species-typical, sexually monomorphic, mate preferences; and (2) In all societies males showed significant differences in the value they attached to physical attractiveness and females valued good financial capacity. He interprets these latter findings to support the contention that these aspects of human psychology are sexually dimorphic.

Kenrick and Keefe (1992) examined sex differences in the preferred age of mates based on hypotheses derived from evolutionary theory. They hypothesized that two factors should be important in determining mate choice. The first was the partner's reproductive potential, given that the goal of mating is reproduction, and the second was the partner's similarity to the individual's own age, which would enhance the likelihood of common and cooperative parental effort. They hypothesized that males would overvalue youth and physical attractiveness in females (as did Buss), and that this would lead them to prefer younger females. Again, this hypothesis is based on the assumption that younger women have a greater reproductive value, and that physical attractiveness is a marker of health and vigor. In addition, they hypothesized that females would overvalue the ability of males to provide economic resources, which would lead them to prefer older males.

Males should prefer females with higher reproductive potential, but there should be some modulation due to a similarity factor. Because the reproductive potential of females declines more rapidly than does that of males, the age of the preferred partner should change as the male ages, with teenage males showing little or no discrimination against females somewhat older than they, middle-aged males showing a greater bias toward younger females, and older males preferring progressively older women, but still ones who are younger than themselves. Women should begin with a preference for older men and, compared to men, show less variation in that preference over the life span.

These hypotheses were tested in several studies using three basic types of data. The first was an analysis of classified personal advertisements in singles newspapers in Arizona, Germany, Holland, and India: indicators of preference. The second was an examination of marriage age statistics in Seattle (1986), Phoenix (for both 1923 and 1986), and an isolated island in the Philippines (1913 to 1939): indicators of behavioral choice. The third set of data was an analysis of those personal ads in theWashingtonian magazine that provided information regarding the wealth and social status of the advertiser.

All of their analyses supported all of the major hypotheses, and were the same for individuals of high and low socioeconomic status. Kenrick and Keefe (1992, p. 16) concluded, "...age preferences are more complex than earlier social psychological models led us to expect. Earlier studies suggested a simple relationship: males seek younger females, and females seek older males. Our results are consistent with half of that generalization: females tend to seek males who are slightly older than they are. For males, however, the preference for younger females is weak or nonexistent during early years, but becomes increasingly pronounced with age".

It is clear that these analyses of homicide and of mate preference support a framework that is consistent with that expected on the basis of evolutionary predictions, and it is difficult to account for all of them with any single competing hypothesis. It should also be pointed out that all of these studies considered the data at the level of the individuals, as must be done if evolutionary mechanisms are to be brought into play.

There are a host of studies, all consistent with the expectations based on evolutionary biology, but which are more difficult to interpret because they are based on analyses of data from the Human Relations Area Files or ethnographies for societies in the Standard Cross Cultural Sample. Although evolutionary conclusions based on such data are more difficult to evaluate, the expectations of these studies support evolutionary expectations quite well. Among the excellent studies that exist are those by Betzig (1986) on despotism and differential reproduction, and by N. W. Thornhill (1991) on rules regulating human inbreeding and marriage.

# Human nature

To understand environmental influences on the developing and functioning organism it is necessary to take into account the innately specified relationship between the environment and the expression of behavioral and psychological traits. This set of universal innate psychological mechanisms and developmental programs constitute what is meant by human nature. There is a great deal of flexibility, and many complex interactions, that must be considered when seeking to understand human nature. It is clear that there are both species-typical monomorphisms and gender-specific dimorphisms that can be understood within an evolutionary framework.

There are several promising directions for theory development and empirical research to take. Evolutionary theory developed quickly when the naturalistic based views of Darwin were synthesized with the newly developed science of genetics during the middle of this century. The next major influence was to invest the synthetic theory of evolution with an ecological perspective and to view the development of traits at the level of population genetics. The insights provided by this amalgamation led to a recognition of the necessity to consider individuals as members of groups, and to understand the significance of such things as frequency dependent selection.

A recent development has been to extend this thinking to the understanding of the relationship between evolutionary processes and a cultural evolution that is separate from individual learning processes, being based more on culturally transmitted cognitive principles. Boyd and Richerson (1985) developed ideas regarding cultural evolution based on qualitative analogies and formal mathematical models that organize existing data, and they suggest the kinds of data that should be gathered to understand human nature within a perspective that permits the expression of both evolutionary and cultural influences. The innovative aspect is that they have taken the formal principles of Mendelian and population genetic models and extended them to cultural transmission. This type of unification has promise to provide a set of highly specific functional principles that apply to molar human cultures and complex animal societies, and which were derived from molecular and population genetics.

## An empirical study of moral intuitions

With two of my students Patricia O'Neill and Matt Jorgensen, I have been conducting an extensive series of studies of the organization and coherence of people's moral intuitions, using both an evolutionary perspective and insights based on the arguments of moral philosophers to direct the inquiry. A questionnaire was constructed which contained two dilemmas used by moral philosophers to delineate moral attitudes. One of these dilemmas is called the "trolley problem". In this dilemma a participant is told to imagine that a trolley is hurtling down a track out of control. If it continues on the track it will kill the beings on the track ahead of it. However, there is a switch that can be thrown which will shunt the trolley to a spur, but the beings on the spur track will be killed. The composition of the beings on the main and spur tracks can be varied and the participant asked to make a life and death choice by deciding to allow the train to continue or to throw the switch.

A second fantasy dilemma is the "lifeboat problem". In this dilemma a ship has sunk, there is a lifeboat with survivors, but some have to be thrown over due to the limited capacity of the lifeboat. Again, the composition of the lifeboat occupants can be varied and a participant asked to choose who is to drown. We included dimensions that have been suggested by philosophers and biologists to regulate the choices people might use to arrive at moral decisions.

We also inquired into stated beliefs concerning some basic moral issues, and obtained some demographic information about the participants. In the first study the participants were all University of California undergraduate students. While this is a highly restricted population it was an appropriate one to use to evaluate the adequacy of the testing method through the psychometric operations necessary to determine if the dimensions in which we are interested are involved in the resolution of the dilemmas.

Two different classes were tested: a General Introductory Psychology class, N=387, and an Introductory Psychology class required of all sophomore pre-medical students, N=60. There were nine questions regarding both the circumstances when abortion should be legal, and when they personally would have (or encourage their significant other to have) an abortion. Eight questions were asked regarding the conditions under which they approve of capital punishment, and seven questions regarding approval of using animals for purposes such as for medical research, and of dissection to train surgeons, or to teach students at various levels. Finally, demographic data were obtained regarding gender, ethnicity, age, and religious affiliation.

The questions were coded using eight basic dimensions: Action/Inaction; Numbers; Social Contract (narrowly construed, such as an employee of the trolley company); Nazi (abhorrent political philosophy); Inclusive Fitness; Elitism; Species; Endangered Species. The questions were coded for each appropriate dimension. For example, there was a choice between throwing the switch to kill one person vs doing nothing and killing five endangered gorillas: this was coded for Action/Inaction, Numbers, Species, and Endangered Species.

The stated beliefs of the participants were strongly related to their expressed religious affiliation, but related only weakly or not at all to other demographic variables. The questions most influenced by religious affiliation were those pertaining to abortion and contraception, issues that are highly topical, and on which many organized religions have taken strong stands. In general, there were two religious clusters that differed significantly: one was Catholics, Protestants, and Christian Fundamentalists; the other was Jews and those indicating no religious preference. The latter two groups were consistently more permissive on all questions in their levels of approval of abortion and less inclined to approve of capital punishment than were the former. There were almost no gender differences regarding abortion, and none in attitudes toward contraception or capital punishment. There were no ethnic differences when differences in religious preference were controlled.

The analyses of the dilemmas indicated that, with our dimensions, we captured a high proportion of the variance for most individuals (multiple R-squared was significant for 90% of the individuals with a mean R-squared of 0.52 for that

90%). When all of the dimensions were included in the analysis, three of them were highly important: Species, Inclusive Fitness, and Nazis. Two dimensions were of moderate importance in this analysis: Social Contract, and Numbers. One other dimension, Action/Inaction, was of lesser importance, and Endangered Species and Elitism were of negligible importance. (Details of these analyses are presented in Petrinovich et al., In Press).

Analyses indicated that there was no relationship between religious preference, ethnicity, and dilemma choices, and only a slight tendency for females to favor a more egalitarian approach. In general, then, there were few differences in the resolution of the dilemmas as a function of religion, ethnicity, or gender. However, there were large differences in stated beliefs related to religion, and a few related to gender.

To extend the generality of our findings, we gathered data on 173 Taiwanese University students, and another sample of 120 University of California students. These two samples differed in one major characteristic: for the Taiwanese sample 52% were affiliated with an Eastern Religion (as compared to only 8% for the U.S. sample), and only 10% with a traditional Western Religion (compared to 71% for the U.S.). This high proportion of Eastern religious affiliation is what we had hoped for with the Taiwan sample.

For political reasons the questionnaire used for the Taiwan study did not include the Nazi or the Endangered Species dimensions. When the earlier U.S. data were analyzed without those two dimensions the Species and Inclusive Fitness dimensions still were large. One difference that appeared is that the Action/Inaction effect now was large. It was found that the rank order and magnitude of the other effects were almost identical for all groups of subjects tested, with one exception: The Numbers effect, which was moderate for the U.S. samples, was small for the Taiwanese. The Taiwanese seemed not to use Numbers as a dimension to resolve the dilemmas. It appears, then, that the relative importance of the dimensions with the Taiwanese sample is similar to that found for the U.S. samples. The order remains Species, Inclusive Fitness, Action/Inaction, Numbers, Social Contract, and Elitism. Thus, there are no obvious differences between those affiliated with Western or Eastern religions in the resolution of the dilemmas, attesting further to the generality of our findings across humans.

Finally, I consider it to be of prime importance to understand the biases in behavioral traits that have been built into human nature (to paraphrase the song, what is human nature all about, Alfie?). It is essential to know what it's all about to develop the kinds of moral principles and laws that represent what ought to be the structure of society. Social institutions and practices need not follow biology. If there is a tendency toward male violence toward females, a society could devote its energies toward achieving such things as sexual equality by encouraging male nurturance while moderating male violence and encouraging and developing mechanisms to enable females to stand against such violence. It is my belief that such social engineering best can be done with an understanding of the human nature with which we must contend, and then design our interventions to take advantage of any desirable biases and counteract those undesirable ones. I continue to be optimistic concerning the imminent progress we can expect toward the construction of a rational and biologically sound moral system.

# References

Betzig, L. L. (1986). *Despotism and Differential Reproduction: a Darwinian View of History*, Aldine Press, New York.

Boyd, R. and Richerson, P. J. (1985). *Culture and the Evolutionary Process*, University Chicago Press, Chicago and London.

Buss, D. M. (1989). Sex differences in human mate preferences: evolutionary hypotheses tested in 37 cultures. *Behav. Brain Sci.,* **12** : 1-49.

Daly, M. and Wilson, M. (1988). *Homicide*, Aldine Press, New York.

Halliday, T. (1980). *Sexual Strategy*, University Chicago Press, Chicago. IL.

Hamilton, W. D., Axelrod, R. and Tanese, R. (1990). Sexual reproduction as an adaptation to resist parasites (a review). *Proc. Natl. Acad. Sci. USA,* **87** : 3566-3573.

Kenrick, D. T. and Keefe, R. C. (1992). Age preferences in mates reflect sex differences in reproductive strategies. *Behav. Brain Sci.,* **14** : 75-133.

Masters, R. D. (1982). Is sociobiology reactionary? The political implications of inclusive-fitness theory. *Quart. Rev. Biol.,* **57** : 275-292.

Michod, R. E. and Levin, B. R. (1988). Introduction. In: Michod, R. E. and Levin, B. R. (Eds.), *The Evolution of Sex: An Examination of Current Ideas*, Sinauer Associates, Sunderland, MA, pp. 1-6.

Petrinovich, L., O'Neill, P. and Jorgensen, M. (1992). An empirical study of moral intuitions: toward an evolutionary ethics. *J. Pers. Soc. Psychol.,* in press.

Seger, J. and Hamilton, W. D. (1988). Parasites and sex. In: Michod, R. E. and Levin, B. R. (Eds.), *The Evolution of Sex: An Examination of Current Ideas*, Sinauer Associates, Sunderland, MA, pp. 176-193.

Sober, E. (1984). *The Nature of Selection*, MIT Press, Cambridge and London.

Thornhill, N. W. (1991). An evolutionary analysis of rules regulating human inbreeding and marriage. *Behav. Brain Sci.,* **14** : 247-293.

Tooby, J. and Cosmides, L (1989). The innate versus the manifest: how universal does universal have to be? *Behav. Brain Sci.,* **12** : 36-37.

Wilson, M. and Daly, M. (1992). The man who mistook his wife for a chattel. In: Barkow, J., Cosmides, L. and Tooby, J. (Eds.), *The Adapted Mind*, Oxford Univiversity Press, London, pp. 243-276.

Zuk, M. (1992). The role of parasites in sexual selection: current evidence and future directions. In: *Advances in the Study of Behavior*, New York: Academic Press, pp. 39-68.

# Sex and the Mutant Mouse: Strategies for Understanding the Sexual Differentiation of the Brain

K. L. OLSEN

*Neuroendocrinology Program, National Science Foundation, Washington, DC 20550, USA*

Sexual dimorphism in the central nervous system (CNS) of vertebrates is clearly established. Structural, biochemical and pharmacological differences exist between males and females (reviewed in Arnold and Gorksi, 1984; Arnold and Jordan, 1988; Baum, 1979; Döhler, 1991; Nottebohm, 1987; Schumaker et al., 1987; Tobet and Fox, 1992; Whalen, 1982). Moreover, evidence is accumulating that strongly links some of the sex differences in the CNS with function (e.g. Balthazart and Surlemont, 1990; DeVoogd, 1984; Nordeen and Nordeen, 1988; Whalen and Olsen, 1980; Yahr et al., 1982).

It is also clearly established that, in mammals, hormones secreted by the testes during a limited, sensitive stage of development differentiate the neural substrates underlying sexual dimorphisms. The hormonal effects are independent of the genetic sex since exposing females to testosterone can mimic the action of the testes on brain and behavior (Phoenix et al., 1959; Whalen, 1982). Conversely, males castrated at birth show similar behavioral responses as normal females in adulthood (Grady et al., 1965). While much of this work has concentrated on sexual differentiation of neural tissues regulating sexual behavior patterns and pituitary function, sex differences resulting from perinatal hormonal exposure are not limited to only reproductive capacities; a number of reviews have emphasized the importance of the early hormonal milieu in underlying nonreproductive behaviors and sensory functioning (Beatty, 1992; Velle, 1987; Williams and Meck, 1991).

While it is clearly established that testicular hormones are critical in determining sex differences in brain and behavior, which steroid hormone underlies or mediates this action is not always readily apparent. One problem is that testosterone (T), the primary testicular hormone, is rapidly metabolized in both peripheral and neural tissues (Hutchison and Steimer, 1984; Naftolin et al., 1975; Whalen et al., 1985) For example, T, dihydrotestosterone (DHT), androstenedione, androstandiols and estradiol (E) are recovered in neural tissues following an injection of T (Reddy et al., 1974; Weisz and Gibbs, 1974).

255

*M. Haug et al. (eds.), The Development of Sex Differences and Similarities in Behavior, 255–278.*

Therefore, since T is metabolized into E and other androgens within neural regions that either show sexual dimorphisms and/or are critical for sexually dimorphic behaviors, it can not be assumed that this androgen is the primary differentiating steroid.

The active steroid may also differ depending upon the particular sexual dimorphism being examined. For example, in rats, androgens are directly involved in the organization of the spinal nucleus of the bulbocavernosus, a sexually dimorphic group of motoneurons in the fifth and sixth lumbar segments, (Breedlove and Arnold, 1981; Breedlove, 1986) whereas E, formed from the intracellular aromatization of T, is thought to mediate the masculinization of sexually dimorphic nuclei in the medial preoptic area (Döhler, 1991). This is also true for organization of sexually dimorphic behaviors. While E is the steroid hormone underlying suppression of the development of female-typical mating behaviors, such as lordosis (behavioral defeminization) (Olsen, 1979a; Vreeburg et al., 1977), androgen is necessary for the enhancement of masculinization of play (Meaney et al., 1983).

Finally, the identity of the steroid hormone for a particular sexual dimorphism may differ depending upon the species and/or strain of animals being examined. Masculinization of sexual behavior, which is defined by an enhancement of male typical behaviors that includes mounts, intromissions and ejaculation towards a receptive female, is an excellent example. While E is a potent masculinizing agents in hamsters, (Etgen and Whalen, 1979), androgens *per se* are needed, possibly in combination with its estrogenic metabolite, in rats and mice (Clemens et al., 1978; Olsen, 1983; 1992; Vreeburg et al., 1977). Moreover, neonatal exposure to testosterone propionate (TP) increased male-typical mating responses in C57BL/6 and BALB/C mice but did not affect the behavior of other strains of mice, including DBA/2, BDF and the A strain (Batty, 1979; Campbell and McGill, 1970; Vale et al., 1973; 1974). Thus, the role of androgens and their estrogenic metabolites in CNS differentiation may differ depending upon the species, the strain, or the specific sexual dimorphism being examined.

Since the identity of the differentiating hormone is the first step towards elucidating the mechanisms underlying the sexual dimorphism, it is important to determine the unique role that androgens and estrogens play. Obviously, examining a sexual dimorphism following an injection of T or TP does not provide any conclusive information on the differentiating hormone given that this steroid is readily metabolism in the CNS. Moreover, conclusions drawn from the injections of E during perinatal development are confounded since some species have a blood-borne protein, alphafoetoprotein, that selectively binds estrogen relative to androgen (Raynaud et al., 1971; Whalen and Olsen, 1978). Consequently, different approaches were developed to separate androgen and estrogen activity (see reviews: Baum, 1979; McEwen et al., 1977; Olsen, 1983; Whalen, 1982) As shown in Table I, these approaches include using 1. nonaromatizable androgens, 2. hormone antagonists, 3. aromatase inhibitors and 4. mutant strains of rats and mice.

**Table I** Four research approaches used to identify the steroid hormone(s) mediating the defeminization and masculinization of sexual behavior.

| Treatment - DEVELOPMENT RATS | Behavioral Consequences [*] ADULTS | |
|---|---|---|
| | FEMALE | MALE |
| FEMALE | ++ | + |
| MALE | – | +++ |
| DHT <----Testosterone ----->Estrogen | | |
| | | |
| **1. NON-AROMATIZABLE ANDROGENS** | | |
| DHT ---\--->ESTROGEN ? | ++ | ++ |
| R1881---\--->ESTROGEN | + | ++ |
| | | |
| **2. AROMATIZATION INHIBITORS** | | |
| TESTOSTERONE---\---> ESTROGEN | +++ | ++ |
| ATD, ADT | | |
| | | |
| **3. STEROID ANTAGONISTS** | | |
| TESTOSTERONE -------> ESTR\OGEN | ++ | ++ |
| CI 628, MER 25, Nafoxidine | | |
| TESTOSTERONE ------>ESTROGEN | +++ | + |
| Cyproterone Acetate, Flutamide, Sch-16423 | | |
| | | |
| **4. ANDROGEN-INSENSITIVE (*Tfm*) MUTANTS** | – | --- ------> ++ |

[*] -- = No behavior
+++ = Full copulatory response

Each approach presents a number of caveats that must be recognized and considered in the interpretation of the findings. For example, DHT has been routinely used to distinguish the nature of the active hormone since it is not metabolized into estrogen (McDonald et al., 1970). DHT, however, is rapidly metabolized to other androgens which have proven to be weakly androgenic. Thus, the ineffectiveness of DHT in mediating an androgenic response may result from its rapid conversion to other androgen metabolites rather than from its inability to be aromatized to E (Gay, 1976). The synthetic androgen, R1881, overcomes the problems associated with administering DHT, since it is not apparently metabolized into either other androgens or estrogens (Doering and Leyra, 1984). Moreover, R1881 binds with high affinity to putative androgen receptors but not E receptors in the CNS. This compound, however, is also a very potent progestin and progestins can inhibit androgen action (Olsen, 1985; Olsen and Etgen, 1983). Hormone antagonists present some problems since they can act as agonists depending upon the dose (Etgen, 1987). Finally, aromatase inhibitors may not only block T's conversion to E but also interfere with androgen action. For example, ATD, a popular aromatase inhibitor, competes for hypothalamic androgen receptors (DeBold et al., 1981; Kaplan and McGinnis, 1989). Regardless of the problems associated with these approaches, the data have been extremely valuable in providing important new information about the direct role of androgens and estrogens.

# Testicular feminization mutation *(Tfm)*

A different approach is to use the androgen-insensitive testicular feminization (Tfm) mutation as a means to investigate the direct role of androgens. This mutation has been crucial in elucidating the molecular basis of sexual dimorphism (Bardin and Catterall, 1981; French et al., 1990), identifying and subsequently cloning androgen receptors (Charest et al., 1991; Fox, 1975; Fox et al., 1983; Gaspar et al., 1991; He et al., 1990; Lubahn et al., 1988; Wieland et al., 1978; Yarbrough et al., 1990), and in understanding the regulation of androgen receptor message and gene expression (Catterall et al., 1986; Kerrigan et al., 1991; Quarmby et al., 1990). Moreover, it plays an invaluable role in identifying the hormones mediating sexual differentiation of CNS and behavior (Arnold and Gorski, 1984; Beach and Buehler, 1977; Breedlove, 1986; Breedlove and Arnold, 1981; Fox et al., 1982; Krey et al., 1982; Meany et al., 1983; Olsen, 1979a, 1979b, 1983, 1992) as well as the induction of various hormone-regulated proteins and enzymes in adults (MacLusky et al., 1988; McQueen et al., 1990; Olsen et al., 1989; Roselli et al., 1987).

The testicular feminization mutation (Tfm) was initially described in humans (Morris, 1953), and later in rats (Stanley et al., 1973), mice (Lyon and Hawkes, 1970), cattle (Nes, 1966) and chimpanzees (Eil et al., 1980). It is caused by an X-linked recessive gene defect. Genetic males with this mutation are insensitive to androgens secreted by their testes and develop phenotypically as females. These individuals have a blind vagina pouch and small phallus instead of a scrotum and a penis. There is no internal genitalia since the insensitivity to androgens prevent the Wolffian duct system from developing and the presence of Müllerian duct inhibiting substance causes the Müllerian duct system to be reabsorbed.

The inherited non-responsiveness to androgens results from quantitative and qualitative defects in the androgen receptor. Androgen binding is reduced in the brain by 80%-90% in both Tfm rats and Tfm mice as compared to wild-type male siblings (Attardi et al., 1976; Fox, 1975; Fox et al., 1982; MacLusky et al., 1988). This is important since it is generally believed that the binding of steroid hormones to specific high-affinity receptors in hormone responsive cells, including neurons, is an initial step in the mechanism of action (see review: Clark et al., 1985). Moreover, there is strong evidence to suggest that the mouse Tfm receptor is qualitatively different from the wild-type receptor protein (Fox et al., 1982, 1983; Fox and Wieland, 1981; Wieland and Fox, 1979; Wieland et al., 1978; Young et al., 1989). This is in contrast to findings in the rat that suggests the Tfm receptor is qualitatively similar to the wild-type receptor (Wieland and Fox, 1981).

Indeed, with the availability of sophisticated molecular biological techniques, a heterogenous group of receptor abnormalities have been noted in humans (see review: French et al., 1990). In rats, the genetic defect is a point mutation resulting in a single amino acid change from arginine 734 to glutamine in the androgen receptor steroid binding domain. Arginine 734 is highly conserved among the family of steroid receptors and appears important for normal androgen binding and transcriptional activation (Yarbrough et al., 1990). In Tfm mice, the gene defect is a single base deletion in the N-terminal domain of the androgen receptor gene. This results in a frameshift mutation that destabilizes androgen receptor mRNA. There is a premature termination of the translation of protein for the receptor and this results in a truncated androgen receptor protein deficient in both DNA-and steroid binding domains (Charest et al., 1991; Gaspar et al., 1991; He et al., 1990; Lubahn et al., 1988).

The Tfm mutation is selective for androgen receptors since E binding activity appears to be normal (Fox, 1975; Fox et al., 1982; Krey et al., 1982; MacLusky et al., 1988; Olsen and Whalen, 1981; Wieland et al., 1978). Moreover, neural tissue from CNS of androgen-insensitive rats and mice are capable of aromatizing T into E (Naftolin et al., 1974; Roselli et al., 1987; Rosenfeld et al., 1977) Given that receptor binding activity is critical for hormone action and these Tfm mutants have a selective defect in androgen and not the estrogen receptor system, they provide an excellent model to separate the action of these two steroid hormones. We have used these mutants to define the active hormone during development (see reviews: Olsen, 1983, 1992), and, more recently, as a means to identify specific proteins in discrete brain regions (Olsen et al., 1989; Olsen et al., 1990).

# Testicular feminization mutation and sexual behavior

The goal of our studies is to capitalize upon the differences and similarities between Tfm mutants and their respective wild-types as well as between the rat (Tfm) and mouse (Tfm) mutation. These comparisons are depicted in Table II. Using this genetic model system, some interesting behavioral differences were reported between the two mutant which can be correlated with what we now know about the receptor defect.

## Development of female mating behavior

Androgen-insensitive rats and mice are defeminized by the presence of their testes during perinatal development (Olsen, 1979a; Olsen and Whalen, 1981; Krey et al., 1982). Similar to wild-type males, the androgen-insensitive rats and mice do not readily display lordosis when treated with ovarian hormones in adulthood (Beach and Buhler, 1977; Ohno et al., 1974; Shapiro et al., 1976). If castrated within 24 hrs of birth, the rat and mouse mutants are capable of showing lordosis when administered estradiol benzoate (EB) and progesterone as adults.

In rats, both the androgen-insensitive and wild-type males castrated on the day of birth show very high levels of female sexual behavior. The average lordosis quotient (number of lordotic responses/mounts with thrusts x 100) of 91% and individual ranges between 75-100% are similar for the two genotypes. Lordosis, however, is not readily induced in the mutant and wild-type males if castration is delayed until 10 days postpartum or if these males

**Table II** Summary of intraspecies and interspecies comparisons.

INTRASPECIES COMPARISONS:

| MUTANT | | LITTERMATE | SEX |
|---|---|---|---|
| *Tfm* Rats | vs | King-Holtzman | Male (Wild type) |
| *Tfm* Mice | vs | *Ta/y* | Male (Wild type) |
| | | *Ta/Ta* | Female(Wild type) |
| | | *Tfm/Ta* | Female (Carrier) |

INTERSPECIES COMPARISONS:

| MUTANT | | MUTANT | SEX |
|---|---|---|---|
| *Tfm* Rats | vs | *Tfm* Mice | Male |

are castrated and exposed to high levels of TP (500 μg) or EB (25 or 250 μg) at birth (Olsen and Whalen, 1981).

In mice, comparisons are made between the following genotypes: Tfm/Y (mutant males), Ta/Y (wild-type males), Tfm/Ta (carrier females), Ta/Ta (wild-type female littermates) and C57Bl/6J. The nonlittermate C57Bl/6J females are included in the study to provide a baseline since this strain of mice can reliably display lordosis when ovariectomized and treated with EB and progesterone as adults. The testing paradigm and scoring procedures for all of the mouse studies are similar to that developed and used by McGill (1962).

The Tfm or wild-type males castrated at 60 days of age and treated with ovarian hormones do not display lordosis. In contrast, the females exhibit lordosis, and both the quality and frequency of response increased during the 5 weekly mating tests. The average lordosis quotient and individual ranges on the last mating test is approximately 70% for C57BL/6J (30-100%) and Tfm/Ta - carrier (0-100%) females, and 50% for Ta/Ta - wild-type (10-90%) females. While androgen-insensitive and wild-type males castrated at birth display more lordosis than males castrated 10 days later, the scores are never as high as the females and there is enormous variability. Thus, there is a difference between male rats and mice in the effectiveness of neonatal castration on the ability to display lordosis following treatment with EB and progesterone in adulthood. One possibility is that there is a species difference in the critical period for defeminization. Regardless, the data support the hypothesis that E derived from circulating androgens mediate behavioral defeminization.

# Development of male sexual behavior

We also found that both androgen-insensitive rats and mice are not fully masculinized by their testes during perinatal development. Gonadally intact mutant rats mounted receptive females but only 20% displayed the ejaculatory pattern. Our findings are similar to that originally reported by Beach and Buhler (1977). In contrast, gonadally intact Tfm mice do NOT mount (see Figure 1). Although the data presented in the Figure 1 are for only 40 mice, we have tested over 75 gonadally intact androgen-insensitive mice and never observed mounting towards a receptive female.

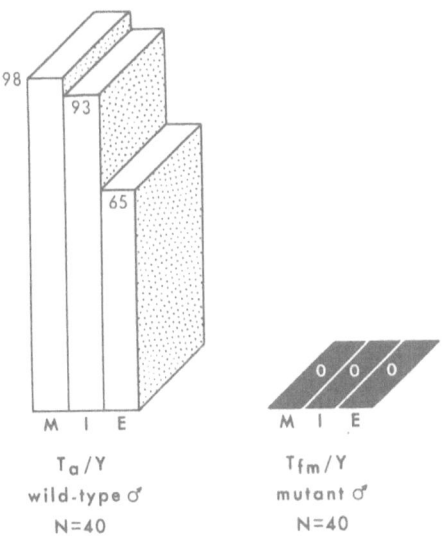

**Figure 1** The percent of wild-type (Ta/Y) and androgen-insensitive (Tfm/Y) male mice mounting (M), intromitting (I) or ejaculating (E) on the mating test.

Adult castrated Tfm rats treated with daily injections of TP, EB, EB + DHT but not DHT alone mounted and displayed the intromission pattern (Olsen, 1979b). In contrast, very few of the Tfm mice exposed to similar hormonal treatments mounted a receptive female (Olsen, 1992). Only DHT + EB injections are slightly effective in stimulating Tfm mice to show male behavior. It was found that 30% of these androgen-insensitive mice exhibited the ejaculatory pattern at least once during the six mating tests but the behavior is still inferior when compared with wild-type males (Ta/Y) as well as their female siblings (Tfm/Ta; Ta/Ta). For example, adult castrated Ta/Y males given daily injections of TP (200 µg), or EB (1 µg) + DHT (250 µg) ejaculated in over 70% of the mating tests (n = 48). Although wild-type male mice injected with only EB (1 µg), DHT (250 µg) or oil vehicle ejaculated on at least one of the six mating tests, total number of tests positive for this behavior is lower than the other two treatments (TP or EB+DHT). The females (Tfm/Ta, Ta/Ta) readily mounted and displayed intromission pattern following TP, EB, or EB + DHT treatment. In contrast, DHT and oil control are ineffective in stimulating male copulatory behavior in these females. A summary of these data are presented in a review by Olsen (1992). Since the androgen-insensitive rats and mice show reduced male mating responses in comparison to their respective wild-type controls, these data are interpreted to suggest a direct involvement of androgens in mediating behavioral masculinization.

It has been previously postulated that the behavioral differences in mounting behavior between the Tfm rats and Tfm mice is related to relative responsiveness to androgens resulting from "qualitative" differences in the androgen receptor defect (Fox et al., 1982; Fox and Wieland, 1981; Olsen, 1983, 1992; Wieland and Fox, 1979). Indeed, there are reports that Tfm rats show induced preputial gland growth (Bardin and Catterall, 1981) and partial reduction in LH levels when administered large doses of TP or DHT (Naess et al., 1976). In contrast, Tfm mice are considered to be relatively insensitive to androgen effects (Bardin and Catterall, 1981; Lyon et al., 1973). Since several laboratories have found a qualitative defect in addition to the quantitative defect in the putative Tfm mouse androgen receptor (Fox et al., 1982; Wieland et al., 1978; Young et al., 1989), the possibility exists that this may explain the differences in responsitivity. A similar explanation has been proposed for patients that exhibit different degrees of androgen insensitivity with either similar levels of binding activity or with no apparent reduction in the number of receptors (Pinksy, 1981; Wilson et al., 1983). Since the cloning of the human and rat androgen receptors (Chang et al., 1988; Lubahn et al., 1988), it has opened the door to elucidating the molecular basis of androgen-insensitivity. The bottom line is that there is not one common defect. A number of mutations, both point mutations and deletions, of the androgen receptor gene have been identified (see recent review, French et al., 1990). Better knowledge of the various molecular defects that result in differential responsiveness to androgens may open new doors into elucidating the important functional roles of androgens.

Another explanation for the behavioral difference in mounting behavior between Tfm rats and Tfm mice is that the testes do not secrete sufficient levels of androgens during the sensitive period of development. Indeed, differences in testosterone levels can explain why adult gonadally intact Tfm mice do not mount (see Figure 1). Unlike the rats and humans with this mutation that have normal to elevated levels of testosterone (Purvis et al., 1977), adult Tfm mice have very low levels of plasma testosterone (Amador et al., 1986; Olsen and Gladue, unpublished findings). Since the presence of the testes during development is correlated with the suppression of female typical behaviors, the testes must be functional at this time. However, given that T levels in these perinatal mice are unknown, we decided to measure male sexual behavior in Tfm mice exposed at birth to exogenous androgens and E. Our findings provide additional support for a direct role of androgens in masculinization. Tfm mice given TP or DHT at birth, mounted and displayed the ejaculatory pattern more frequently in response to DHT + EB treatment than similarly treated Tfm mice exposed perinatally to oil. Perinatal androgen treatment, however, is only

ffective in facilitating masculine behavior in about 50% of the mice. It is not
:lear why some of the Tfm mice responded while others did not but it may
eflect differences in their residual receptors or the underlying molecular defect.
\lthough these mice should possess the same mutation, Fox and his
:olleagues have reported at least three different types of residual receptors in
he various Tfm mutants that their laboratory has studied (Fox et al., 1983;
ʳolitch et al., 1988).

In summary, the androgen-insensitive rats and mice serve as a model system
o identify the steroid hormone(s) underlying the suppression of female sexual
ᵉehaviors and the enhancement of male sexual behaviors in rats and mice.
ſhe data indicate that aromatization of T into E plays a critical role in the
ᵈefeminization of sexual behavior while androgens *per se* are involved in the
ᵐasculinization of sexual behavior. In rats, androgens are most likely acting in
ᵉynergy with estrogens to differentiate the neural structures regulating
ᵉjaculatory behavior. Identifying the hormones that mediate these behavioral
:hanges are crucial for our eventual understanding of the neural mechanisms
ᵂhich underlie sexual differentiation.

# Testicular feminization mutation
# and the identification of specific neural proteins

The second part of this chapter is devoted to more recent work in which Tfm
mice are used as a tool to identify specific proteins in the CNS that may be
related to androgen-regulated functions (Olsen et al., 1989; Olsen et al., 1990).
It is clearly established that the primary mechanism by which steroid hormones
exert their widespread effect is by altering the rate of synthesis of proteins
within target cells (Clark et al.,1985). Initially, steroids enter cells by diffusion. In
hormone responsive cells, the steroids bind to intracellular protein receptors
which complex to acceptor sites in the nucleus and this results in an alternation
of gene expression (i.e. induction of RNA and proteins synthesis).

Since steroid-induced effects are thought to be mediated by increases and/or
decreases in proteins, it is reasonable to expect that the genetic sex and
hormone levels will influence the specific neural proteins to be found in the
brain areas important for steroid-induced functions. Indeed, this is the case.
Sex differences are found in the preoptic area (POA) and in the ventromedial
hypothalamus (VMH) (Angelbeck and Dubrul, 1983; Gold et al., 1983; Scouten
et al.,1985), two principal sites of steroid activity. The POA is considered to be
the most critical brain area for mediating the effects of androgens on male
sexual behavior and the VMH is a key site in which E + progesterone act to
facilitate female sexual behaviors. Not only are sex differences apparent but
gonadal hormones influence the density of specific proteins in these two brain
nuclei since changes in concentration are seen following gonadectomy
(Scouten et al., 1985). Moreover, estrogen treatment influences the
incorporation of amino acids into individual proteins (McEwen et al., 1987;
Rodriguez-Sierra et al., 1987) and the concentration of specific proteins in
specific hypothalamic nuclei (Jones et al., 1988; Lauber and Pfaff, 1990;

Rodriguez-Sierra et al., 1986). Except for the induction of the progestin receptor, the identity of specific proteins which change in response to E treatment are still unknown.

In contrast to E, androgens effect on neural proteins have not been widely studied, although elegant work in peripheral target tissues indicate that androgens act by modulating RNA and protein synthesis. Moreover, in the peripheral system, a number of androgen regulated proteins have been identified (e.g. ornithine decarboxylase, KAP, β-glucuronidase) and are being extensively studied (Bardin and Catterall, 1981; Catterall et al., 1986).

## Testicular feminization mutation and quantification of proteins

As a first step in the identification of possible androgen-regulated neural proteins, the Tfm mutation was used. These studies were done in the laboratory of Dr. Jacobowitz in collaboration with Dr. Heydorn, Dr. Rodriguez-Sierra, and Mr. Creet (Olsen et al., 1989). Using silver stained two-dimensional gel electrophoresis in combination with scanning densitometry, the densities of 195 protein spots from the POA, VMH and cortex (CX) were compared between Tfm and Swiss-Webster male mice. The Tfm mutation significantly (at least $P <$ .025) influenced the mean optical densities of 17 proteins measured on gels of POA tissue, 21 proteins on gels of VMH and 11 proteins on gels of CX. Figure 2 presents the mean optical density of the protein spots. Proteins labelled with numbers are believed to correspond to the original proteins number system developed from CNS of rats (Heydorn et al., 1983; Jacobowitz and Heydorn, 1984). Proteins labelled with letters A through G did not have molecular weights and isoelectric points which matched proteins from this atlas.

In Figure 3, the density of six protein spots generated from the POA for Tfm and Swiss-Webster mice are illustrated. From this photograph, it is clear that there are striking quantitative differences between the two genotypes. These proteins were selected to be illustrated because similar quantitative changes are also found for these protein spots in the VMH.

In summary, using two-dimensional gel electrophoresis and scanning densitometry, we have revealed a number of proteins which are influenced by the mutation. Further work is necessary to identify those proteins that could possibly be under regulatory control of androgens.

## Testicular feminization mutation and the glial fibrillary acidic protein (GFAP)

One protein that has been identified is the glial fibrillary acidic protein (GFAP), an intermediate filament protein found in astrocytes (Bignami et al., 1972; Eng, 1985; Eng et al., 1971). This protein spot corresponds to number 17 in Figure 3. The identity of GFAP was verified by transferring the proteins to nitrocellulose paper and staining immunologically for GFAP (Olsen et al., 1989).

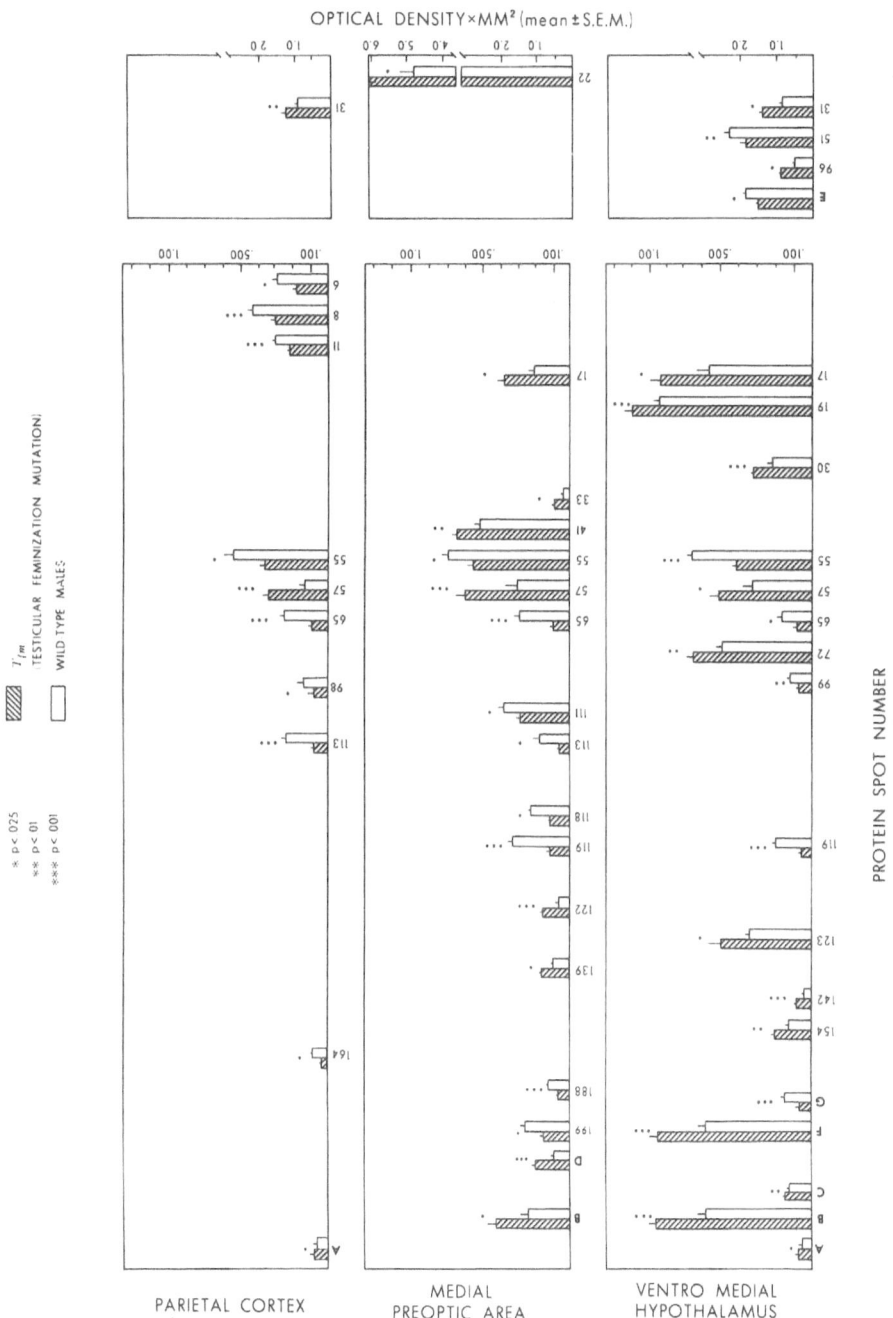

**Figure 2**    Mean (± S.E.M) optical density x mm² of protein spots in the ventromedial hypothalamus, medial preoptic area and parietal cortex that were found to be significantly different between *Tfm* and Swiss-Webster males. (From Olsen et al., 1989, with permission of S. Karger AG, Basel, Publishers.)

266

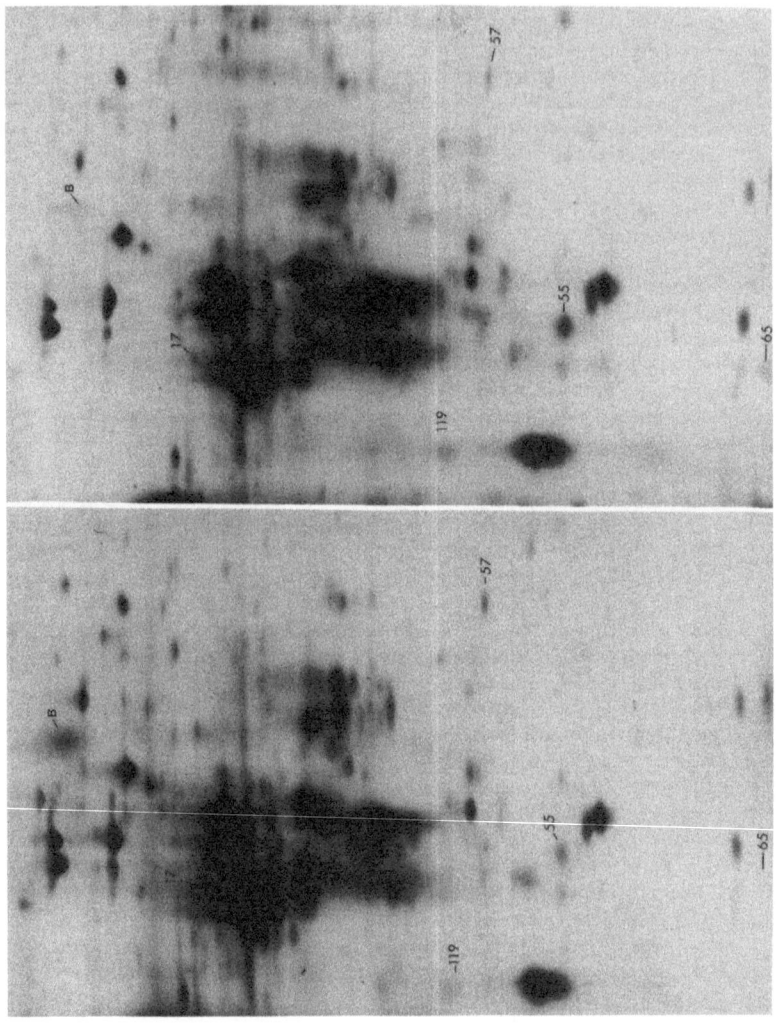

**Figure 3** Composite photograph showing the differences in densities of six protein spots isolated from medial preoptic area of *Tfm* (left) and Swiss-Webster (right) male mice. (From Olsen et al., 1989, with permission of S. Karger AG, Basel Publishers.)

The concentration of GFAP is significantly higher in POA and VMH but not CX of the androgen-insensitive Tfm mice. We (Olsen et al., 1990) and others (McQueen et al., 1990) have found that the increase in GFAP protein can be demonstrated by immunohistochemistry and appears to be highly localized to regions within the preoptic-hypothalamic area. Differences in the level of immunoreactive GFAP activity are not found between Tfm and normal male mice in the hippocampus or cortex. Interestingly, two other proteins that are also significantly enhanced in CNS of Tfm mice are believed to be associated with glial cells (Olsen et al., 1989). In Figure 2, Protein 122 is believed to be the acid charge isomer of GFAP and Protein 31 may correspond to non-neuronal enolase (NNE), an enzyme located in glial cells (Marangos et al., 1978).

Evidence from a variety of studies indicate that the astrocytic environment may have important roles in CNS function (Barres, 1991; Vernadakis, 1988). During development, glial cells are possibly involved in neuronal migration (Bignami and Dahl, 1974), in constructing the form and pattern within the brain (Steindler and Cooper, 1987), regulating morphology of the neurons and synaptic density (Meshul and Seil, 1988) and in providing neurotrophic support (Nieto-Sampedro et al., 1988). Astrocytes may also influence neuronal functioning by affecting ion and neurotransmitter concentrations and release (Martin, 1992). Finally, astrocytes play a major role in response to CNS injury (Brock and O'Callaghan, 1987; Hatten et al., 1991; Reier and Houle, 1988). A dramatic proliferation and hypertrophy of astrocytes occurs following insult and one important consequence is that the reactive astrocytes increase their synthesis of GFAP.

What is the significance of the increase in GFAP and other glial-associated proteins in discrete brain regions of androgen-insensitive Tfm mice? Since the glial hypertrophy is not found throughout the CNS but appears to be concentrated within the preoptic-hypothalamic region, then possibly the up-regulation of the filament protein in Tfm mice is not associated with degenerative neuronal changes but rather may reflect physiological events. While we can, at this stage, only speculate that the changes are related directly to the deficiency in androgen activity, there is precedence in the literature to suggest that steroid hormones influence glial proteins (García-Segura et al., 1988, 1989; Kumar and de Vellis, 1988; O'Callaghan et al., 1989; Schipper et al., 1990; Tranque et al., 1987). Furthermore, the recent finding by Langub and Watson (1992) that E receptors are located on hypothalamic glial cells supports a possible direct interaction between steroids and glial activity. Moreover, astrocytes play a dynamic role in control of hormone synthesis and release (see reviews: Hatton et al., 1984; Montagnese et al., 1988). Using immunocytochemistry, these investigators report that dehydration and lactation, two states that stimulate the production and release of vasopressin and oxytocin, profoundly affect the staining pattern of GFAP suggesting morphological changes within the hypothalamo-neurohypophysial system. Electron microscopic studies have shown that the neurohypophysial astrocytes surround the neurons at the level of the terminals and these astrocytic processes are retracted from the neurons upon demand for hormone. These data provide strong support that astrocytic glial cells play an important role in

268

neuronal functions of neuroendocrine systems.

This brings us back to the question of why would the Tfm mice have higher concentration of GFAP, a marker for astrocytes, in gonadal steroid-sensitive brain regions? I would like to propose that up-regulation of this protein is associated with normal "cellular elements in the hypothalamus". While emphasize that it may be premature at this point of our knowledge to theorize, one possibility is that dramatic differences represent consequences of normal occurring cell death in the absence of androgen. Indeed elegant work in the insect nervous system demonstrates a relationship between steroid hormones and cell death (Schwartz and Truman, 1982). This idea is also based on the exciting findings emerging from studies on song nuclei of the bird brain (Arnold and Gorski, 1984; DeVoogd, 1984; Nottebohm, 1987), and the spinal nucleus of the bulbocavernosus (Arnold and Gorski, 1984; Arnold and Jordan,1988; Breedlove, 1986; Nordeen et al., 1985); two model systems that have contributed greatly to our understanding of cellular mechanisms underlying hormone action. The major findings are 1. that androgens prevent the normally occurring cell death in these sexually dimorphic nuclei (Nordeen et al., 1985); and, 2. that circulating gonadal steroids in adulthood influence structural reorganization (somata size; dendritic length; synaptic input) of these structures (Arnold and Gorski, 1984; Arnold and Jordan, 1988; Breedlove, 1986; Kurz et al., 1986; Leedy et al., 1987; DeVoogd, 1984; Nottebohm, 1987; Olsen et al., 1988). Work with the Tfm rats and mice provide support for these findings since the sexually dimorphic nucleus in the spinal cord of Tfm rat and mouse mutants is markedly reduced (Breedlove and Arnold, 1981; Olsen et al., 1989; Sengelaub et al., 1989) and its size can be increased by specific hormone treatments in adulthood (Olsen et al., 1988). The increase in GFAP levels in hypothalamic nuclei of androgen-insensitiv Tfm mice may reflect normal events underlying androgen involvement in functional changes within the CNS. Three recent reports provide support for such a role. First, supplementing cultures from brain cells of day 14 mouse embryos with dehydroepiandrosterone and dehydroepiandrosterone sulfate, precursors for androgens, increased neuronal survival and reduced astroglial proliferation (Bologna et al., 1987). Second, castration of adult male rats increases GFAP in the dentate gyrus (Day et al., 1991). Finally, ultrastructural changes in neurohypophysis involving astrocytic glial elements are found following castration and testosterone replacement (Tweedle et al., 1988).

What is the significance of our findings that the concentration of GFAP and other glial-related proteins are enhanced in hypothalamic nuclei of Tfm mice? Is the androgen deficiency directly related to this increase in glial activity? Can GFAP activity be manipulated by early hormonal environment? Does the increase in glial proteins reflect an increase in the number of astrocytes or reflects a hypertrophy of these cells? At what age does the difference appear? Is there a relationship between male sexual behavior and glial proteins? Providing answers to some of these questions will provide a better understanding of the interactions between androgens, astrocytic glial cells and neuronal functions.

# Acknowledgements

This research was supported by NIH Grant HD-18893 to KLO and NSF DIR-9022207 to David Kingsbury. I am especially grateful to Kathleen Hock and Christine Stark for providing expert technical assistance on the behavioral studies and to Joe Creek for generating the beautiful silver-stained two dimensional gels. In addition, I thank my collaborators Joseph DeBold, Anne Etgen, Thomas Fox, David Jacobowitz, William Heydorn, David Kingsbury, Robert Moore, Jorge Rodriguez-Sierra, Joan Speh, Karen Geary and Richard Whalen who participating in the studies presented in this chapter.

# References

Amador, A. G., Parkening, T. A., Beamer, W. G., Bartke, A. and Collins, T. J. (1986). Testicular LH receptors and circulating hormone levels in three mouse models for inherited diseases (Tfm/y, lit/lit and hyt/hyt). *Endocrin. Exper.,* **20** : 349-358.

Angelbeck, J. H. and DuBrul, E. F. (1983). The effect of neonatal testosterone on specific male and female patterns of phosphorylated cytosolic proteins in the rat preoptic-hypothalamus, cortex and amygdala. *Brain Res.,* **264** : 277-283.

Arnold, A. P. and Gorski, R. A. (1984). Gonadal steroid induction of structural sex differences in the central nervous system. *Ann. Rev. Neurosci.,* 7 : 413-442.

Arnold, A. P. and Jordan, C. L. (1988) Hormonal organization of neural circuits. In: Martini, I. and Ganong, W. F. (Eds.), *Frontiers in Neuroendocrinology,* **10** : 185-214.

Attardi, B., Geller, L. N. and Ohno, S. (1976). Androgen and estrogen receptors in brain cytosol from male, female, and testicular feminized (tfm/ y). *Endocrinology,* **98** : 864-874.

Balthazart, J. and Surlemont, C. (1990). Copulatory behavior is controlled by the sexually dimorphic nucleus of the quail POA. *Brain Res.,* **25** : 7-14.

Bardin, C. W. and Catterall, J. F. (1981). Testosterone: a major determinant of extragenital sexual dimorphism. *Science,* **211** : 1285-1294.

Barres, B. (1991). New roles for glia. *J. Neurosci.,* **11** : 3685-3694.

Batty, J. (1979). Influence of neonatal injections of testosterone propionate on sexual behavior and plasma testosterone levels in male house mouse. *Dev. Psychobio.,* **12** : 231-238.

Baum, M. J. (1979). Differentiation of coital behavior in mammals: a comparative analysis. *Neurosci. Biobehav. Rev.,* **3** : 265-284.

Beach, F. A. and Buehler, M. G. (1977). Male rats with inherited insensitivity to androgen show reduced sexual behavior. *Endocrinology,* **100** : 197-200.

Beatty, W. W. (1992). Gonadal hormones and sex differences in nonreproductive behaviors. In: Gerall, A., Moltz, H. and Ward, I. L. (Eds.), *Sexual Differentiation, Handbook of Behavioral Neurobiology,* Plenum Press, New York, pp. 85-112.

Bignami, A. and Dahl, D. (1974). Astrocyte-specific protein and radial glia in the cerebral cortex of newborn rat. *Nature,* **252** : 55-56.

Bignami, A., Eng, L. F., Dahl, D. and Uyeda, C. T. (1972). Localization of the glial fibrillary acidic protein in astrocytes by immunofluorescence. *Brain Res.,* **43** : 429-435.

Bologa, L., Sharma, J. and Roberts, E. (1987). Dehydroepiandrosterone and its sulfated derivative reduce neuronal death and enhance astrocytic differentiation in brain cell cultures. *J. Neurosci. Res.,* **17** : 225-234.

Breedlove, S. M. (1986). Cellular analyses of hormone influence on motoneuronal development and function. *J. Neurobio.,* **17** : 157-176.

Breedlove, S. M. and Arnold, A. P. (1981). Sexually dimorphic motor nucleus in the rat lumbar spinal cord: response to adult hormone manipulations, absence in androgen-insensitive rats. *Brain Res.,* **225** : 297-307.

Brock, T. O. and O'Callaghan, J. P. (1987). Quantitative changes in the synaptic vesicle proteins synapsin 1 and P38 and the astrocyte-specific protein glial fibrillary acidic protein are associated with chemical-induced injury to the rat central nervous system. *J. Neurosci.,* **7** : 931-942.

Campbell, A. B. and McGill, J. (1970) Neonatal hormone treatment and sexual behavior in male mice. *Horm. Behav.,* **1** : 145-150.

Catterall, J. F., Watson, C. S., Kontula, K. K., Janne, O. A. and Bardin, C. W. (1986). Differential regulation of specific gene expression in mouse kidney by androgens and antiandrogens. In: Chrousos, G. P., Loriaux, D. L. and Lipsett, M. B. (Eds.), *Steroid Hormone Resistance,* Plenum Publishing Corporation, New York, pp. 213-226.

Chang, C., Kokontis, J. and Liao, S. (1988). Molecular cloning of human and rat complementary DNA encoding androgen receptors. *Science,* **240** : 324-326.

Charest, N. J., Zhou, Z., Lubahn, D. B., Olsen, K. L., Wilson, E M. and French, F. S. (1991). A framework mutation destabilizes androgen receptor messenger ribonucleic acid in the Tfm mouse. *Molec. Endocrin.,* **5** : 573-581.

Clark, J. H., Schrader, W. T. and O'Malley, B. W. (1985). Mechanisms of steroid hormone action. In: Wilson, J. D., Foster, D. W. (Eds.), *Williams Textbook of Endocrinology,* W.B. Saunders, Philadelphia, pp. 33-75.

Clemens, L. G., Gladue, B. A. and Coniglio, L. P. (1978). Prenatal endogenous androgenic influences on masculine sexual behavior and genital morphology in male and female rats. *Horm. Behav.,* **10** : 40-53.

Day, J. R., Laping, N. J., Lampert-Etchells, M., McNeill, T. H. and Finch, C. E. (1991). Castration of adult rats increases astrocyte reactivity (GFAP) in the molecular layer of the dentate gyrus. *Soc. Neurosci. Abstr.,* New Orleans p. 564.

DeBold, J. F., Fox, T. O. and Olsen, K. L. (1981). Inhibition of androgen binding by ATD and flutamide. *Soc. Neurosci. Abstr.,* Los Angeles, p. 7.

Doering, C. H. and Leyra, P. T. (1984). Methyltrienolone (R1881) is not aromatized by placental microsomes or rat hypothalamic homogenates. *J. Ster. Biochem.,* **20** : 1157-1162.

Döhler, K. D. (1991). The pre- and postnatal influence of hormones and neurotransmitters on sexual differentiation of the mammalian hypothalamus. *Internat. Rev. Cytol.,* **131** : 1-57.

DeVoogd, T. J. (1984). The avian song system: relating sex differences in behavior to dimorphism in the central nervous system. *Prog. Brain Res.,* **61**: 171-184.

Eil, C., Merriam, G. R., Bowen, J., Ebert, J., Tabor, E., White, B., Douglass, E. C. and Loriaux, D. L. (1980). Testicular feminization in the chimpanzee. *Clin. Res.,* **28** : 624A.

Eng, L. (1985). Glial fibrillary acidic protein (GFAP): the major protein of glial intermediate filaments in differentiated astrocytes. *J. Neuroimmunol.,* **8** : 203-214.

Eng, L. F., Vanderhaeghen,J. J., Bignami, A. and Gerstl, B. (1971). An acidic protein isolated from fibrous astrocytes. *Brain Res.,* **26** : 351-354.

Etgen, A. M. (1987). Steroid hormone antagonists, brain receptor systems and behavior. In: Agarwal, M. K. (Ed.), *Receptor Mediated Antiestrogen Action,* Walter de Gruyter, Berlin, pp. 405-434.

Etgen, A. M. and Whalen, R. E. (1979). Masculinization and defeminization induced in female hamsters by neonatal treatment with estradiol, RU-2858 and nafoxidine. *Horm. Behav.,* **15** : 282-288.

Fox, T. O. (1975). Androgen-and estrogen-binding macromolecules in developing brain: biochemical and genetic evidence. *Proc. Nat. Acad. Sci. USA,* **72** : 4303-4307.

Fox, T. O., Blank, D., and Politch, J. A. (1983). Residual androgen binding in testicular feminization (Tfm). *J. Ster. Biochem.,* **19** : 577-581.

Fox, T. O., Olsen, K. L., Vito, C. C. and Wieland, S. J. (1982). Putative steroid receptors: genetics and development. In: Schmitt, F. O., Bloom, F. E. and Bird, S., (Eds.), *Molecular Genetics and Neurosciences: A New Hybrid,* Raven Press, New York, pp. 289-306.

Fox, T. O. and Wieland, S. J. (1981). Isoelectric focusing of androgen receptors from wild-type and Tfm mouse kidneys. *Endocrinology,* **109** : 790-797.

French, F. S., Lubahn, D. B., Brown, T. R., Simental, J. A., Quigley, C. A., Yarbrough, W. G., Tan, J. A., Sar, M., Joseph, D. R., Evans, B. A. J., Hughes, I. A., Migeon, C. J. and Wilson, E. M. (1990). Molecular basis of androgen insensitivity. In: Clark, J. H. (Ed.), *Recent Progress in Hormone Research,* Academic Press, New York, pp. 1-42.

Garcia-Segura, L. M., Suarez, I., Segovia, S., Tranque, P. A., Cales, J. M., Aguilera, P., Olmos, G. and Guillamon, A. (1988). The distribution of glial fibrillary acidic protein in the adult rat brain is influenced by the neonatal levels of sex steroids. *Brain Res.,* **456** : 357-363.

Garcia-Segura, L. M., Torres-Aleman, I. and Naftolin, F. (1989). Astrocytic shape and glial fibrillary acidic protein immunoreactivity are modified by estradiol in primary rat hypothalamic cultures. *Dev. Brain Res.,* **47** : 298-302.

Gaspar, M. L., Meo, T., Bourgarel, P., Guenet, J. L. and Tosi, M. (1991). A single base deletion in the Tfm androgen receptor gene creates a short-lived messenger RNA that directs internal translation initiation. *Proc.Natl. Acad.Sci.,* **88** : 8606-8610.

Gay, V. L. (1976). Species variation in the metabolism of dihydrotestosterone : correlation with reported variations in behavioral response. *Soc. Study Reprod. Abstr.,* Philadelphia, p. 9.

Gold, M. A., Heydorn, W. E., Creed, G. J. and Jacobowitz, D. M (1983). Sex differences in specific proteins in the preoptic medial nucleus of the rat hypothalamus. *Neuroendocrinology, 37* : 470-472.

Grady, K. L., Phoenix, C. H. and Young, W. C. (1965). Role of the developing rat testis in differentiation of the neural tissues mediating mating behavior. *J. Comp. Physiol. Psych., 59* : 176-182.

Hatten, M. E., Liem, R. K. H., Shelanski, M. L. and Mason,C. A. (1991). Astroglia in CNS injury. *Glia, 4* : 233-243.

Hatton, G. I., Perlmutter, L. S., Salm, A. K. and Tweedle, C. D. (1984). Dynamic neuronal-glial interactions in hypothalamus and pituitary: implications for control of hormone synthesis and release. *Peptides, 5* : 121-138.

He, W. W., Young, C. Y. F. and Tindall, D. J. (1990) The molecular basis of the mouse testicular feminization (Tfm) mutation: a frameshift mutation. *Endocr. Soc. Abstr.*, Atlanta, p. 72.

Heydorn, W. E., Creed, G. J., Goldman, D., Kanter, D., Merril, C. R. and Jacobowitz, D. M. (1983). Mapping and quantification of proteins from discrete nuclei and other areas of the rat brain by two-dimensional gel electrophoresis. *J. Neurosci., 3* : 2597-2602.

Hutchinson, J. B. and Steimer, Th. (1984). Androgen metabolism in the brain : behavioral correlates. In: De Vries, G. J., de Bruin, J. P. C., Uylings, H. B. M. and Corner, M. A. (Eds.), *Progress in Brain Research, Volume 61,* Elsevier Science Publishers B.V., Amsterdam, pp. 23-51 .

Jacobowitz, D. M. and Heydorn, W. E. (1984). Two-dimensional gel electrophoresis used in neurobiological studies of proteins in discrete areas of the rat brain. *Clin. Chem., 30* : 1996-2002.

Jones, K. J., McEwen, B. S. and Pfaff, D. W. (1988). Quantitative assessment of early and discontinuous estradiol-induced effects on ventromedial hypothalamic and preoptic area proteins in female rat brain. *Neuroendocrinology, 48* : 561-568.

Kaplan, M. E. and McGinnis, M. Y. (1989). Effects of ATD on male sexual behavior and androgen binding: a re-examination of the aromatization hypothesis. *Horm. Behav., 23* : 10-27.

Kerrigan, J. R., Martha, Jr., P. M., Krieg, Jr., R. J. Queen, T. A., Monahan, P. E. and Rogol, A. D. (1991). Augmented hypothalamic proopiomelanocortin gene expression with pubertal development in the male rat : evidence for an androgen receptor-independent action. *Endocrinology, 128* : 1029-1035.

Krey, L. C., Lieberburg, I., MacLusky, N. J., Davis, P. G. and Robbins, R. (1982). Testosterone increases cell nuclear estrogen levels in the brain of Stanley-Gumbreck pseudohermaphrodite male rat: implications for testosterone modulation of neuroendocrine activity. *Endocrinology, 110* : 2168-2176.

Kumar, S. and de Vellis, J. (1988). Glucocorticoid-mediated functions in glial cells. In: Kimelberg, H. K. (Ed.), *Glial Cell Receptors,* Raven Press, New York, pp. 243-264.

Kurz, E. M., Sengelaub, D. R. and Arnold, A. P. (1986). Androgens regulate the dendritic length of mammalian motoneurons in adulthood. *Science, 232* : 395-398.

Langub, Jr. M. C. and Watson, Jr. R. E. (1992). Estrogen receptor-immunoreactive glia, endothelia, and ependyma in guinea pig preoptic area and median eminence: electron microscopy. *Endocrinology*, **130** : 364-372.

Lauber, A. H. and Pfaff, D. (1990). Estrogen regulation of mRNAs in the brain and relationship to lordosis behavior. *Cur.Top. Neuroendocr.*, **10** : 115-147.

Leedy, M. G., Beattie, M. S. and Bresnahan, J. C. (1987). Testosterone-induced plasticity of synaptic inputs to adult mammalian motoneurons. *Brain Res.*, **424** : 386-390.

Lubahn, D. B., Joseph, D. R., Sullivan, P. M., Willard, H. F., French, F. S. and Wilson, E. M. (1988). Cloning of human androgen receptor complementary DNA and localization to the X chromosome. *Science*, **240** : 327-330.

Lyon, M. F. and Hawkes, S. G. (1970). X-linked gene for testicular feminization in the mouse. *Nature*, **227** :1217-1219.

Lyon, M. F., Hendry, I. and Short, R. V. (1973). The submaxillary salivary glands as test organs for response to androgen in mice with testicular feminization. *J. Endocrinol.*, **58** : 357-362.

MacLusky, N. J., Luine, V. N., Gerlach, J. L., Fischette, C., Naftolin, F. and McEwen, B. S. (1988). The role of androgen receptors in sexual differentiation of the brain : effects of the testicular feminization (Tfm) gene on androgen metabolism, binding, and action in the mouse. *Psychobiology*, **16** : 381-397.

Marangos, P. J., Parma, A. M. and Goodwin, F. K. (1978). Functional properties of neuronal and glial isoenzymes of brain enolase. *J. Neurochem.*, **31**: 727-732.

Martin, D. L. (1992). Synthesis and release of neuroactive substances by glial cells. *Glia*, **5** : 81-94.

McDonald, P., Beyer, C., Newton, F. Brien, B., Baker, R., Tan, H. S., Sampson, C., Kitching, P., Greenhill, R. and Pritchard, D. (1970). Failure of 5α-dihydrotestosterone to initiate sexual behavior in the castrated rat. *Nature*, **227** : 964-965.

McEwen, B. S., Jones, K. J. and Pfaff, D. W. (1987). Hormonal control of sexual behavior in the female rat : molecular, cellular and neurochemical studies. *Biol. Reprod.*, **36** : 37-45.

McEwen, B. S., Lieberburg, I., MacLusky, N. and Plapinger, L. (1977). Do estrogen receptors play a role in the sexual differentiation of the rat brain? *J. Ster. Biochem.*, **8** : 593-598.

McGill, T. G. (1962). Sexual behavior in three inbred strains of mice. *Behaviour*, **19** : 341-350.

McQueen, J. K., Wright, A. K., Arbuthnott, G. W. and Fink, G. (1990). Glial fibrillary acidic protein (GFAP)-immunoreactive astrocytes are increased in the hypothalamus of androgen-insensitive testicular feminized (Tfm) mice. *Neurosci. Lett.*, **118** : 77-81.

Meaney, M. J., Stewart, J., Poulin, P. and McEwen, B. S. (1983). Sexual Differentiation of social play in rat pups is mediated by the neonatal androgen-receptor system. *Neuroendocrinology*, **37** : 85-90.

Meshul, C. K. and Seil, F. J. (1988). Transplanted astrocytes reduce synaptic density in the neuropil of cerebellar cultures. *Brain Res.*, **441** : 23-32.

Montagnese, C., Poulain, D. A., Vincent, J. D. and Theodosis, D. T. (1988).

Synaptic and neuronal-glial plasticity in the adult oxytocinergic system in response to physiological stimuli. *Brain Res. Bull.,* **20** : 681-692.

Morris, J. M. (1953). The syndrome of testicular feminization in male pseudohermaphrodites. *Amer. J. Obst. Gyn.,* **65** : 1192-1211.

Naess, O., Haug, E., Attramadal, A., Aakvaag, A., Hansson, V. and French, F. (1976). Androgen receptors in the anterior pituitary and central nervous system of the androgen "insensitive" (Tfm) rat : correlation between receptor binding and effects of androgens on gonadotropin secretion. *Endocrinology,* **99** : 1295-1303.

Naftolin, F., Ryan, K. J., Davies, I. J., Reddy, V. V., Flores, F., Petro, Z., Kuhn, M., White, R. J., Takaoka, Y. and Wolin, L. (1975). The formation of estrogens by central neuroendocrine tissues. In: Creep, R. O. (Ed.), *Recent Progress in Hormone Research,* Academic Press, New York, pp. 295-318.

Nes, N. (1966). Testikulaer feminisering hos storfe. *Norwegian Veter. Med.,* **18** : 19-29.

Nieto-Sampedro, M., Saneto, R. P., deVellis, J. and Cotman, C. W. (1985). The control of glial populations in brain changes in astrocyte mitogenic and morphogenic factors in response to injury. *Brain Res.,* **343** : 320-328.

Nordeen, E. J. and Nordeen, K. W. (1988). Sex and regional differences in the incorporation of neurons born during song learning in Zebra Finches. *J. Neurosci.,* **8** : 2869-2874.

Nordeen, E. J., Nordeen, K. W., Sengelaub, D. R. and Arnold, A. P. (1985). Androgens prevent normally occurring cell death in a sexually dimorphic spinal nucleus. *Science,* **229** :671-673.

Nottebohm, F. (1987). Plasticity in adult avian central nervous system : possibly relation between hormones, learning, and brain repair. In: Mountcastle, V., Plum, F. and Geiger, S. (Eds.), *Handbook of Physiology, Amer. Physiol. Soc.,* Bethesda, MD, pp. 85-108.

O'Callaghan, J. P., Brinton, R. E. and McEwen, B. S. (1989). Glucocorticoids regulate the concentration of glial fibrillary acidic protein throughout the brain. *Brain Res.,* **494** : 159-161.

Ohno, S., Geller, L. N. and Younglai, E. V. (1974). Tfm mutation and masculinization versus feminization of the mouse central nervous system. *Cell,* **3** : 235-242.

Olsen, K. L. (1979a). Androgen-insensitive (tfm) rats are defeminized by their testes. *Nature,* **279** : 238-239.

Olsen, K. L. (1979b). Induction of male mating behavior in androgen-insensitive (tfm) and normal (King-Holtzman) male rats : effects of testosterone propionate, estradiol benzoate and dihydrotestosterone. *Horm. Behav.,* **13** : 66-84.

Olsen, K. L. (1983). Genetic determinants of sexual differentiation. In: Balthazart, J., Prove, E. and Gilles, R. (Eds.), *Hormones and Behavior in Higher Vertebrates,* Springer-Verlag, Heidelberg, pp. 138-158.

Olsen, K. L. (1985). Aromatization : is it critical for differentiation of sexually dimorphic behaviors? In: Gilles, R. and Balthazart, J. (Eds.), *Neurobiology,* Springer-Verlag, Berlin Heidelberg, pp. 149-164.

Olsen, K. L. (1992). Genetic influences on sexual behavior differentiation. In:

Gerall, A., Moltz, H. and Ward, I. L. (Eds.), *Sexual Differentiation : A Life-Span Approach*, Handbook of Behavioral Neurobiology, pp. 1-40.

Olsen, K. L. and Etgen, A. M. (1983). Specificity of methyltrienolone (R-1881) binding in brain and pituitary. *Soc. Neurosci. Abstr.*, Boston, p. 9.

Olsen, K .L., Heydorn, W. E., Rodriguez-Sierra, J. F. and Jacobowitz, D. M. (1989). Quantification of proteins in discrete brain regions of androgen-insensitive testicular feminized Tfm mice. *Neuroendocrinology*, **671**: 392-399.

Olsen, K. L., Speh, J. C. and Moore, R. Y. (1990). Glial fibrillary acidic protein (GFAP) immunoreactivity is increased in the hypothalamus of androgen-insensitive (Tfm) mice. *Soc. Neurosci. Abstr.*, New Orleans, p. 16.

Olsen, K. L., Wagner, C. K. and Clemens, L. C. (1988) Relationship between male sexual behaviors and dorsomedial spinal nucleus in androgen-insensitive Tfm mice. *Soc. Neurosci. Abstr.*, Toronto, p. 14.

Olsen, K. L. and Whalen, R. E. (1981). Hormonal control of the development of sexual behavior in androgen-insensitive (tfm) rats. *Physiol. Behav.*, **27** : 883-886.

Olsen, K. L. and Whalen, R. E. (1982). Estrogen binds to hypothalamic nuclei of androgen-insensitive (tfm) rats. *Experientia*, **38** : 139-140.

Olsen, K. L. and Whalen, R. E. (1980). Sexual differentiation of the brain : effects of mating behavior and [3]H-estradiol binding by hypothalamic chromatin in rats. *Biol. Reprod.*, **22** : 1068-1072.

Phoenix, C. H., Goy, R. W. Gerall, A. A. and Young, W. C. (1959). Organizing action of prenatally administered testosterone propionate on the tissues mediating mating behavior in the female guinea pig. *Endocrinology*, **65** : 369-382.

Pinsky, L. (1981). Sexual differentiation. In: Collu, R., Ducharme, J. R. and Guyda, H. (Eds.), *Pediatric Endocrinology*, Raven Press, New York, pp. 231-239.

Politch, J. A., Fox, T. O., Houben, P., Bullock, L. and Lovell, D. (1988). TfmLac : a second isolation of testicular feminization in mice. *Biochem. Genet.*, **26** : 213-221.

Purvis, K., Haug, E., Clausen, O. P. F., Naess, O. and Hansson, V. (1977). Endocrine status of the testicular feminized male (TFM) rat. *Mol. Cell. Endocrin.*, **8** : 317-334.

Quarmby, V. E., Yarbrough, W. G., Lubahn, D. B., French, F.S. and Wilson, E. M. (1990). Autologous down-regulation of androgen receptor messenger ribonucleic acid. *Mol. Endocrin.*, **4** : 22-28.

Raynaud, J. P., Mercier-Bodard, C. and Baulieu, E. E. (1977). Rat estradiol binding plasma protein (EBP). *Steroids*, **18** : 767-788.

Reddy, V. V. R., Naftolin, F. and Ryan, K. J. (1974). Conversion of androstenedione to estrone by neural tissues from fetal and neonatal rats. *Endocrinology*, **94** : 117-121.

Reier, P. J. and Houle, J. D. (1988). The glial scar: its bearing on axonal elongation and transplantation approaches to CNS repair. In: Waxman, S. G. (Ed.), *Advances in Neurology, Vol 47, Neurological Disease*, Raven Press, New York, pp. 87-138.

Rodriguez-Sierra, J. F., Heydorn, W. E., Creed, G. J. and Jacobowitz, D. M. (1986). Isolation of specific proteins affected by estradiol in the arcuate-median eminence of prepuberal female rats. *Brain Res.*, **399** : 379-382.

Rodriguez-Sierra, J. F., Heydorn, W. E., Creed, G. J. and Jacobowitz, D. M. (1987). Incorporation of amino acids into proteins of the hypothalamus of prepuberal female rats after estradiol treatment. *Neuroendocrinology*, **45** : 459-464.

Roselli, C. E., Salisbury, R. L. and Resko, J. A. (1987). Genetic evidence for androgen-dependent and independent control of aromatase activity in the rat brain. *Endocrinology*, **121**: 2205-2210.

Rosenfeld, J. M., Daley, J. D., Ohno, S. and Younglai, E. V. (1977). Central aromatization of testosterone in testicular feminized mice. *Experientia*, **33** : 1392-1393.

Schipper, H. M., Lechan, R. M. and Reichlin, S. (1990). Glial peroxidase activity in the hypothalamic arcuate nucleus : effects of estradiol valerate-induced persistent estrus. *Brain Res.*, **507** : 200-207.

Schumacher, M., Legros, J. J. and Balthazart, J. (1987). Steroid hormones, behavior and sexual dimorphism in animals and men : the nature-nurture controversy. *Exper. Clin. Endocrin.*, **90** : 129-156.

Schwartz, L. M. and Truman, J. W. (1982). Peptide and steroid regulation of muscle degeneration in an insect. *Science*, **215** : 1420-1421.

Scouten, C. W., Heydorn, W. E., Creed, G. J., Malsbury, C. W. and Jacobowitz, D. M. (1985). Proteins regulated by gonadal steroids in the medial preoptic and ventromedial hypothalamic nuclei of male and female rats. *Neuroendocrinology*, **41**: 237-245.

Sengelaub, D. R., Jordan, C. L., Kurz, E. M. and Arnold, A. P. (1989). Hormonal control of neuron number in sexually dimorphic spinal nuclei of the rat: II. Development of the spinal nucleus of the bulbocavernosus in androgen-insensitive (Tfm) rats. *J. Comp. Neurol.*, **280** : 630-636.

Shapiro, B. H., Goldman, A. S., Steinbeck, H. F. and Neumann, F. (1976). Is feminine differentiation of the brain hormonally determined? *Experientia*, **32** : 650-651.

Stanley, A. J., Gumbreck, L. G., Allison, J. E. and Easley, R. B. (1973). Part I. Male pseudohermaphroditism in the laboratory Norway rat. *Rec. Prog. Horm. Res.*, **29** : 43-64.

Steindler, D. A. and Cooper, N. G. F. (1987). Glial and glycoconjugate boundaries during postnatal development of the central nervous system. *Dev. Brain Res.*, **36** : 27-38.

Tobet, S. A. and Fox, T. O. (1992). Sex differences in neuronal morphology influenced hormonally throughout life. In: Gerall, A., Moltz, H. and Ward, I. L. (Eds.), *Sexual Differentiation, Handbook of Behavioral Neurobiology*, Plenum Press, New York, 11: pp. 41-83.

Tranque, P. A., Suarez, I., Olmos, G., Fernandez, B. and Garcia-Segura, L. M. (1987). Estradiol-induced redistribution of glial fibrillary acidic protein immunoreactivity in the rat brain. *Brain Res.*, **406** : 348-351.

Tweedle, C. D., Modney, B. K. and Hatton, G. I. (1988). Ultrastructural changes in the rat neurohypophysis following castration and testosterone replacement. *Brain Res. Bull.,* **20** : 33-38.

Vale, J. R., Ray, D. and Vale, C. A. (1973). The interaction of genotype and exogenous neonatal androgen and estrogen : sex behavior in female mice. *Dev. Psychobiol.,* **6** : 319-327.

Vale, J. R., Ray, D. and Vale, C. A. (1974). Neonatal androgen treatment and sexual behavior in males of three inbred strains of mice. *Dev. Psychobiol.,* **7** : 483-488.

Velle, W. (1987). Sex differences in sensory functions. *Pers. Biol. Med.,* **30** : 490-522.

Vernadakis, A. (1988). Neuron-glia interactions. *Intern. Rev. Neurobiol.,* **30** : 149-224.

Vreeburg, J. T. M., van der Vaart, P. D. M. and Van der Schoot, P. (1977). Prevention of central defeminization but not masculinization in male rats by inhibition neonatally of oestrogen biosynthesis. *J. Endocrinol.,* **74** : 375-382.

Weisz, J. and Gibbs, C. (1974). Metabolites of testosterone in the brain of newborn female rat after injection of tritiated testosterone. *Neuroendocrinology,* **14** : 72-86.

Whalen, R. E. (1982). Current issues in the neurobiology of sexual differentiation. In: Vernadakis, A. and Timiras, P. S. (Eds.), *Hormones in Development and Aging,* Spectrum Publications, New York, pp. 273-304.

Whalen, R. E. and Olsen, K. L. (1978). Prednisolone modifies estrogen-induced sexual differentiation. *Behav. Biol.,* **24** : 549-553.

Whalen, R. E. and Olsen, K. L. (1981). Role of aromatization in sexual differentiation : effects of prenatal ATD treatment and neonatal castration. *Horm. Behav.,* **15** : 107-122.

Whalen, R. E., Yahr, P. and Luttge, W. G. (1985). The role of metabolism in hormonal control of sexual behavior. In: Adler, N., Pfaff, D. and Goy, R. W. (Eds.), *Handbook of Behavioral Endocrinology,* Plenum Press, New York, pp. 609-663.

Wieland, S. J. and Fox, T. O. (1979). Putative androgen receptors distinguished in wild-type and testicular-feminized (Tfm) mice. *Cell,* **17** : 781-787.

Wieland, S. J. and Fox, T. O. (1981). Androgen receptors from rat kidney and brain: DNA-binding properties of wild-type and Tfm mutant. *J. Ster. Biochem.,* **14** : 409-414.

Wieland, S. J., Fox, T. O. and Savakis, C. (1978). DNA-binding of androgen and estrogen receptors from mouse brain : behavior of residual androgen receptor from Tfm mutant. *Brain Res.,* **140** : 159-164.

Williams, C. L. and Meck, W. H. (1991). Organizational effects of gonadal steroids produce sexually dimorphic spatial ability. *Psychoneuroendocrinology,* **16** : 157-177.

Wilson, J. D., Griffin, J. E., Leshin, M. and McDonald, P. C. (1983). The androgen resistance syndromes : 5α-reductase deficiency, testicular feminization, and related disorders. In: Stanbury, J. B. (Ed.), *The Metabolic Basis of Inherited Disease,* McGraw-Hill, New York, pp. 1001-1026.

Yahr, P., Commins, D., Jackson, J. C. and Newman, A. (1982). Independent control of sexual scent marking behaviors of male gerbils by cells in or near the medial preoptic area. *Horm. Behav.,* **16** : 304-322.

Yarbrough, W. G., Quarmby, V. E., Simental, J. A., Joseph, D. R., Sar, M., Lubahn, D. B., Olsen, K. L., French, F. S. and Wilson, E. M. (1990). A single base mutation in the androgen receptor gene causes androgen insensitivity in the Testicular Feminized rat. *J. Biol. Chem.,* **265** : 8893-8900.

Young, C. Y. F., Johnson, M. P., Prescott, J. L. and Tindall, D. J. (1989). The androgen receptor of the testicular feminized (Tfm) mutant mouse is smaller than wild-type receptor. *Endocrinology,* **124** : 771-775.

# Sexualisation of Behavior During Development in the Pig

J. P. SIGNORET

*INRA/CNRS URA 1291, Comportement Animal, 37380 Nouzilly, France*

In most mammalian species, the female appears as able to display the male patterns of sexual behavior spontaneously especially during estrus. Moreover, the complete repertoire of male sexual behavior as well as non sexual although sex-specific behaviors are presented as a consequence of a treatment by steroid hormones mimicking the male endocrine balance. Conversely, the study of homosexual activity in mammalian males is limited to the observation of the display of sexual behavior directed towards another male, without considering the possibility for displaying female specific responses. The hormonal treatment that induces estrous behavior in the ovariectomized female has been first described as uneffective in the male gonadectomized as adult. More recent studies show the possibility for steroid hormone treatments to induce female-specific respopnses in the adult gonadectomized male. However, such responses require specific conditions of doses, sensory stimulation, and differ between strains, and are markedly different from those of ovariectomized females. The activational effect of steroid hormones appears as depending on established sex differences. A defeminization of the male - loss of the capacity to display female-specific patterns of sexual behavior - appears as the most obvious sex difference. Numerous experiments involving more than 10 mammalian species establish that the critical determinant of such permanent sex differences result from the effects of sex steroids to which the fetuses or neonates have been exposed (Goy and McEwen, 1980).

It has generally been found that the organizational effects of sex steroids take place during early development, during middle or late pregnancy and up to the first 5 days of life in rats (Whalen and Edwards, 1967). However, various neural processes (synaptogenesis, growth, regulation of receptors etc..) have been shown to be influenced by steroids throughout the whole life (Arnold and Breedlove, 1985). Consequently, the dichotomy between the permanent organizational action of steroid during development and reversible activation in adulthood is questionable. According to these authors, species diversity in steroid effect on behavior could be of great interest, in providing experimental models to analyze the general mechanisms of steroid action on sex differences. A series of experiments dealing with the responses to sex steroids in the domestic pig suggest that this species could be one of these interesting models.

*M. Haug et al. (eds.), The Development of Sex Differences and Similarities in Behavior, 279–289.*
© 1993 *Kluwer Academic Publishers.*

# The sexualization of the sexual behavior capacities in the pig

## The female sexual responses of the pig: hormonal induction and measure

Both aspects of pig female sexual reactions - proceptivity and receptivity - have been described and can be reliably assessed. The proceptivity or active searching for the male is measured by the preference for a male opposed to a female or a castrate in a T maze situation. The posture of receptivity - active immobilization when mounted by the male - is especially obvious as lasting for several minutes. In both cases, the sensory stimulations eliciting the response have been determined (Signoret, 1970).

The sexual reactions can be induced in the ovariectomized female by a single injection of estradiol. An effective treatment has been designed involving dose of .5 to 1 mg of estradiol benzoate given intramuscularly at an interval similar to that of the estrous cycle, i.e. 3 weeks (Signoret, 1970). No progesterone is required, and reliable responses are obtained during successive artificial cycles. A dose-response is observed on the duration of estrous behavior whereas neither the proceptive reaction nor the conditions for eliciting the immobilization are modified.

## The female sexual responses of castrated male pigs

In pilot experiments, male pigs, castrated between 2 and 4 weeks of age, have been compared with ovariectomized females after an injection of estrogen designed to induce estrous behavior. During the week after the treatment the animals were presented daily to a sexually active adult male to test the female posture of immobilization when mounted. On the same days, they were tested in a choice situation (T maze) for their preference for approaching an adult male opposed to an anestrous female. The castrates reacted exactly as did ovariectomized females, with typical estrous 'behavior responses of immobilization and of proceptivity (Figure 1).

At the age at castration - 2 to 4 weeks - piglets are well developped, what suggested the possibility for a process of sexualization extended later than in rodents.

## Evolution of the sexualization of the male pig during development

A series of experiments were then designed to determine the evolution of the sexual capacities during the development. Castration of male pigs were performed at various ages, from 1 hour after birth to 8 months, that is long after puberty that takes place between the ages of 5 and 6 months (Van Straaten and Wensing, 1977; Meusy-Dessolle, 1985).

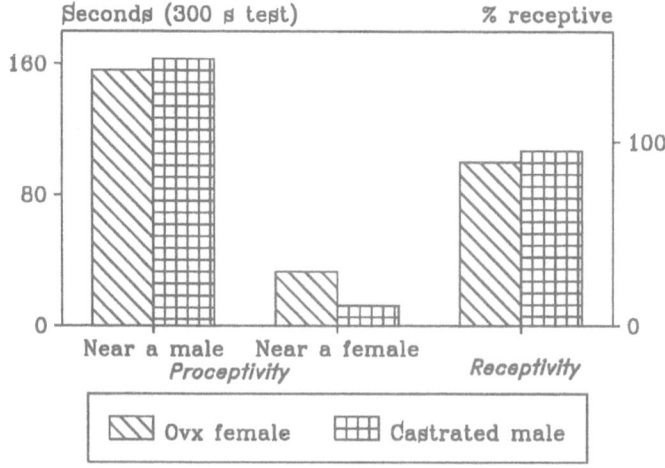

**Figure 1** Receptivity and proceptivity in the pig: comparison of the reactions of the female and the castrated male. (adapted from Ford, 1982; and Berry and Signoret, 1984).

The results (Figure 2) show that the first reduction in the immobilization rate in the male, when compared to ovariectomized females, appears as late as around the time of puberty (Ford, 1982; 1983a; Berry and Signoret, 1984). However, the sexual preference - proceptivity - símilar in females and males castrated during the first month of life, disappears completely when castration is performed at 3 months of age (Ford, 1983a; Signoret, 1990).

## Hormonal control of sexualization in the male pig

Genetic sex is established at conception, but the sexual development of males depends on the endocrine signals from the developping testis, whereas females' development takes place without major influence of the ovarian secretions. In the male, testosterone and its metabolites are critical for the development of the genital anatomy. At the level of the brain, the endocrine secretions of the developing testis account for the reduction of the hypothalamic feed back response of LH to estrogens. In most mammalian species studied, these hormonal secretions during foetal and perinatal life account for the reduction of the capacity for female sexual behavior, and for an eventual enhancement of the masculine response to hormonal stimulation as adults. In the pig, the castration experiments suggest that the action of sexual steroids could take place later than in most of the species investigated so far, at a period when most of the physiological development is considered as completed.

In male pigs, the circulating testosterone is higher than in females throughout gestation. This is already observed during and especially at the end of the second month of gestation (Colenbrander et al.,1978; Ford et al., 1980; Meusy-

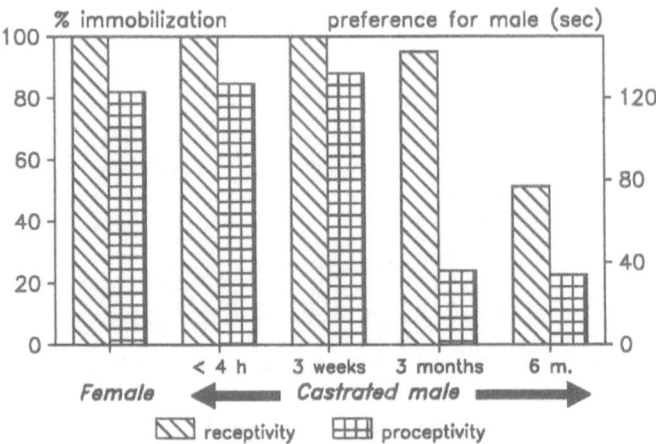

**Figure 2** Effect of sex and age at castration on female receptivity response in male and female pigs. (adapted from Ford, 1982; and Berry and Signoret, 1984).

Dessolle, 1985). At parturition, testosterone is high in males and decreases after the first weeks. It increases and rises again from the 4th month to reach the adult level at puberty (Figure 3).

Adult male pigs are known to produce high levels of estradiol (160 pg/ml: Ford, 1983b), higher than in estrous females (40 pg/ml: Henricks et al., 1972). The production of estradiol is elevated during the first postnatal weeks, decreases for some weeks and rises again around 4 months of age (Ford, 1983b; Meusy-Dessolle, 1985). In postnatal females estrogens rapidly decrease and remains low until the approach of puberty (Elsaesser, 1972).

The absence of sexualization due to androgens during gestation has been experimentally verified in females: when treated *in utero* at dosages that induce masculinization of external genitalia, the sexual responses of females as adult remain normal. Conversely, testosterone treatment of neonatally castrated males between 3 to 6 months of age reduces the immobilization response after estradiol treatment (Ford and Christenson, 1987).

The presence of high levels of circulating estradiol in the male pig throughout the period from birth to puberty could also contribute to defeminization. Estrogen derived from testosterone by aromatization has been shown to be active in brain sexualization in other species such as rats (McEwen, 1981), as well as birds (Balthazart and Schumacher, 1983). Implants of estradiol benzoate (Figure 4) given from 3 to 5.5 months of age resulted in a defeminization of both ovariectomized females and early castrated males (Adkins-Regan et al., 1989).

In conclusion, the experimental analysis of the process of sexualization of the male pig shows a late and progressive loss of the capacity of female receptivity as a response to an estrus-inducing hormonal treatment. Most of the males

MALE

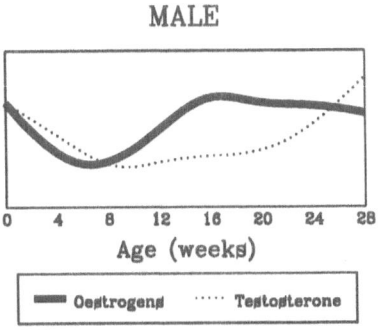

FEMALE

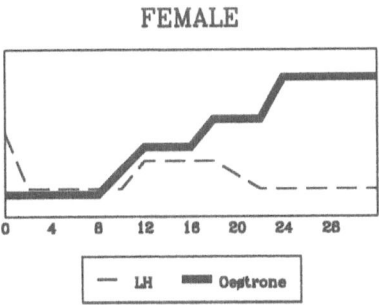

**Figure 3** Evolution of endocrine secretions during development in pigs. (adapted for males from Meusy-Dessolle, 1985; and Berry and Signoret, 1984; and for females from Camous et al., 1985).

castrated when physiological puberty has been reached - production of an ejaculate with motile spermatozoa - and treated with estrogens, are still able to display the typical female immobilization when mounted by a male. Conversely, the proceptivity, or capacity of the estrous sow to actively search for contact with the boar, disappears in the male before the 3rd month of age. Both characteristics of the sexualization - independent evolution for receptivity and proceptivity, and a slow and delayed process - makes the pig an very original model.

# Evolution of endocrine secretions and occurence of prepubertal sexual behavior

During development, the young pig appears as not sexualized. However, in the male, the production of sex steroids is variable, but generally high. The possibility for these endocrine secretion to induce prepubertal sexual activity

284

RECEPTIVITY

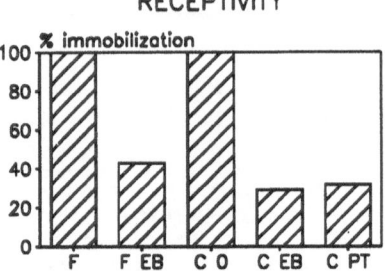

PROCEPTIVITY

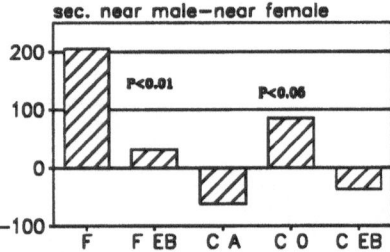

**Figure 4** Effects of steroid treatments on female-like responses in pigs. (adapted from Ford and Christenson, 1987; and Adkins-Regan et al., 1989).

has been investigated at different stages of the development in males and in females.

## Prepubertal sexual activity

As puberty is approaching, male patterns of sexual activity could be observed with an increasing frequency, without any possibility of actual consumatory act. This has been considered as a part of the normal evolution of the process of puberty, but has never been studied *per se*. The prepubertal male pig has high levels of circulating estradiol as well as testosterone at a period where the sexualization is not completed. The occurrence of female posture of receptivity could thus be theoretically possible.

To test this hypothesis, it would be necessary to have prepubertal pigs interacting with adult sexually active partners. The existence of differences in size between breeds makes it possible to test the male or female sexual responses in prepubertal animals: chinese Mei-shan adult males and females are of similar weight as Yorkshire pigs of 3-5 months of age.

Intact and early castrated males and intact females yorkshire pigs were presented twice a week successively to an active male and to an estrous female of the Mei-shan breed, between the ages of 3 and 5.5 months (Figure 5). Only a few mounting attempts were made by the castrates and the females, but all the intact prepubertal males mounted the estrous females that reacted by immobilization. The percentage of subjects mounting and the frequency of mounts did not change significatively with increasing age. Thus, the intact prepubertal males display complete and organized sexual postures towards a receptive female as early as at 3 months of age. The capacity to react adequately to the specific stimuli from the estrous female is thus present long before the capacity for fertilization (Signoret et al., 1989).

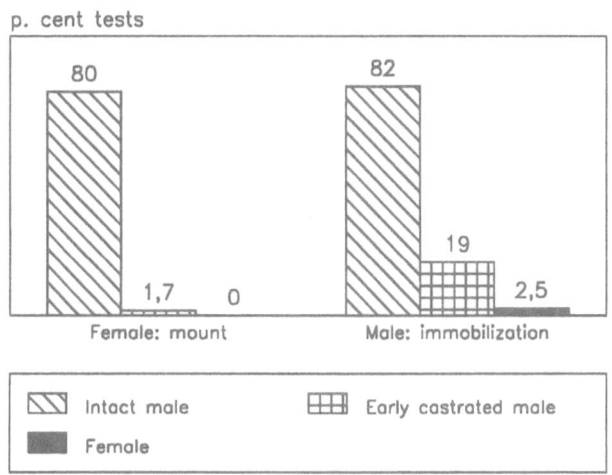

**Figure 5** Sexual responses to an adult active partner in the prepubertal pig. (adapted from Signoret, Adkins-Regan, and Orgeur, 1989).

Mounting by the adult mei-shan male did not occur in all tests. It elicited escape and vocalizations in castrates and females. In contrast, a high proportion of the intact prepubertal males reacted to mount by the typical female immobilization display (Signoret et al., 1989). The frequency of this reaction did not change with age.

Such observations are in agreement with the results of castration experiments that demonstrate the persistence of a bisexual capacity throughout the prepubertal period of the male pig. The presence of high levels of circulating steroids thus allows both male and female sexual reactions in the prepubertal male. The response depends on the stimuli provided by the partner. However, in most tests with the adult stimulus boar, the intact prepubertal males began by agonistic interactions, suggesting that they first reacted as males. However it was only when the adult male succeeded in mounting that suddenly, they stood and displayed the typical female "receptive" posture until the end of the test. The presence of such homosexual interactions has been observed in several species as a part of social interactions among males (monkeys , cats, etc...). Mounting of a subadult has be considered as a manifestations of dominance from an adult male. However, in free ranging conditions, the adult male pigs tend to isolate, and, when in contact, to interact agressively rather than with sexual-like displays. However, when boars are kept in groups from an early age true homosexual relations appear but they have not been described as related with social dominance. The origin of such a spontaneous homosexuality could be found in the complete bisexual capacity of peripubertal male pigs.

## Early presence of sexual patterns or "sexual play"

During the first post-natal months, male-like patterns of sexual behavior are observed, mostly mounts sometimes with with pelvic movements. These activities generally occurred in series involving several individuals, and are often associated with sudden running and gambolling. No obvious stimulation could account for trigerring of such a sequence, and for its end. These criteria are considered as characteristic of play activity. Males and females are both involved as mounters and mountees.

The average frequencies of mounting were observed as significantly different with age (Berry and Signoret, 1984) reaching a maximum during the second month of life (Figure 6). The evolution was similar in both sexes, but the frequency of mount was 3-4 time higher in males. The occurrence of sexual play, the sex differences and its evolution are similar to what has been observed in sheep by Orgeur (1982).

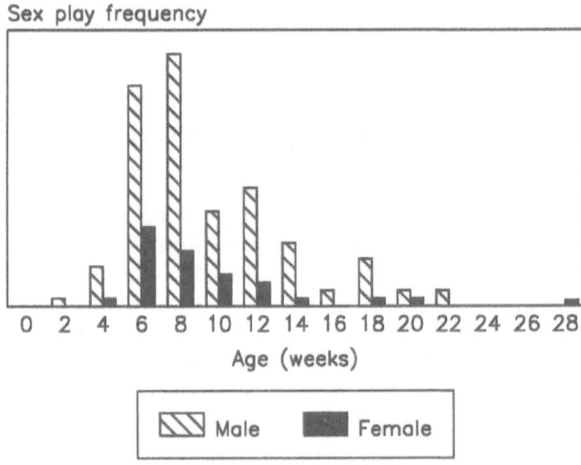

**Figure 6** Sex play during development in pigs. (adapted from Berry and Signoret, 1984).

The testicular hormonal secretions influence the sexual play: castration performed within the first hour of birth considerably reduces the occurrence of sex play. The relatively high levels of testosterone as well as estradiol around birth in males could account for the sex difference and the evolution of sexual play (Figure 7).

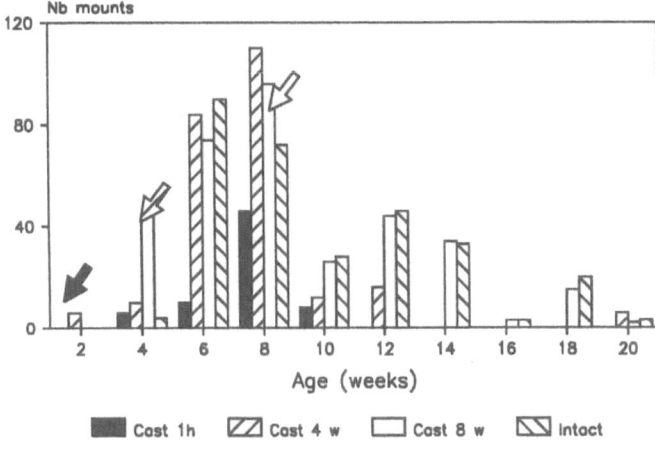

**Figure 7** Effect of age at castration on the evolution of sexual play in the male pig. The arrow indicates the time of castration. (adapted from Berry and Signoret, 1984).

This sexual play could have a functional role in organizing the postural realisation of the adult sexual patterns. In fact, social deprivation - rearing male pigs without any contact with other pigs from 20 days of age until puberty - that eliminates the possibility of this sexual play, considerably reduces the sexual performance in adulthood (Hemsworth et al., 1977).

In summary, during early periods of life, the steroid secretions of the male pig testis account for the presence of an intense sexual play that could contribute to the organization of adult patterns of sexual behavior. During the prepubertal period - from 3 to 5 months of age - a complete bisexuality is observed in the male, whereas the aggressive behavior towards same-sex opponents develops slowly. None of such phenomena could be observed in females.

# Discussion and conclusion

The major characteristics of the sex differences and their origin in the pig are i) the slow and progressive process of defeminization that terminates as late as after puberty itself, ii) the differential evolution of the capacities of proceptivity and receptivity, and iii) the existence of an activation of male behavior by sex steroids during prepubertal life.

The organizational effects of steroids are classically considered as permanent, occurring during a limited critical or "sensitive" period of development, and inducing structural irreversible changes in the brain. However, it has been shown recently that sexual differentiation of pig hypothalamus continues during and after puberty. No morphological difference has been observed before puberty in vasopressin and oxytocin containing nucleus, and supraoptic nucleus of hypothalamus. However both develop sexual dimorphism under steroid influence during and after puberty (van Eerdenburg, 1991). The evolution of the sexualization of brain structures in this species could account for the exceptionally late process of defeminization.

However, the differentiation of brain structures *per se* could not be the only factor involved in the sexual differentiation of adult behavior: the male pig reaches adulthood after an important experience of prepubertal sexual interactions. In pigs as in many other species (rats, dogs, primates), the acquisition of adequate postures of the adult sexual behavior depends on the experience acquired through early interindividual contacts. The socio-sexual interactions during development could similarly contribute to shift the reactions from a bisexual capacity to more or less strictly sex-specific sexual behavior. The development of the male social role in the pig social organization, involving aggressive reactions and progressive isolation from other males could also account, at least partially for the reduction or disappearance of female response in homosexual interactions. When boars are kept in permanent groups after puberty, homosexual interactions, involving acceptance to be mounted is observed. Such a situation of early and permanent association between males is known to reduce intermale aggressiveness, thus preventing or delaying the occurrence of the male social role, what could account for the increased possibility for homosexual activity.

In the model of the pig, it possible to hypothetize that the development of the sex-specific sexual behavior takes place through different and convergent processes: a late evolution of brain structures, associated with a progressive experience of the social roles of males and females. This interaction of the development of structural differentiation with experiential factors would make this species an interesting model for investigating the mechanisms of the organization of sexual behavior, especially for the studies on homosexuality in general.

# References

Adkins-Regan, E., Orgeur, P. and Signoret, J. P. (1989). Sexual differentiation of reproductive behavior in pigs: defeminizing effects of pubertal estradiol. *Horm. Behav.*, **23** : 290-303.

Arnold, A. P. and Breedlove, S. M. (1985). Organizational and activational effects of sex steroids on brain and behavior : a reanalysis. *Horm. Behav.*, **19** : 469-498.

Balthazart, J. and Schumacher, M. (1983). Testosterone metabolism and sexual differentiation in quail. In: J. Balthazart, E. Pröve, R. Gilles (Eds.),*Hormones and Behavior in Higher Vertebrates*, Springer Verlag, Berlin, pp. 237-260.

Berry, M. and Signoret, J. P. (1984). Sex play and behavioral sexualization in the pig. *Reprod. Nutr. Dev.*, **24** : 507-513

Colenbrander, B., De Jong, F. H. and Wensing, C. J. G. (1978). Changes in serum testosterone concentrations in the male pig during development. *J. Reprod. Fertil.*, **53** : 377-380.

Elsaesser, F. (1982). Endocrine control of sexual maturation in the female pig and sexual differentiation of the stimulatory estrogen feedback mechanism. In

Cole, D. J. A. and Foxcroft, G. R. (Eds.), *Control of Pig Reproduction*. Butterworth Scientific Publishers, London, pp. 93-116.

Ford, J. J. (1982). Testicular control of defeminization in male pigs. *Biol. Reprod.*, **27** : 425-430.

Ford, J. J. (1983a). Postnatal differenciation of sexual preferences in male pigs. *Horm. Behav.*, **17** : 152-162.

Ford, J. J., (1983b) Serum estrogen concentrations during post-natal development in male pigs. *Proc. Soc. Exp. Biol. Med.*, **174** : 160-174.

Ford, J. J. and Christenson, R. K. (1987). Influences of pre- and postnatal testosterone treatment on defeminization of sexual receptivity in pigs. *Biol. Reprod.*, **36** : 581-587.

Ford, J. J., Christenson, R. K. and Maurer, R. R. (1980). Serum testosterone concentrations in embryonic and fetal pigs during sexual differentiation. *Biol. Reprod.*, **23** : 583-587.

Goy, R. W. and McEwen, B. S. (1980).*Sexual Differentiation of the Brain*, MIT Press, Cambridge, M. A.

Henricks, D. M., Guthrie, H. D. and Handlin, D. L. (1972). Plasma estrogen, progesterone and luteinizing hormone lmevels during the estrous cycle in pigs. *Biol. Reprod.*, **6** : 210-218.

Hemsworth, P. H. and Beilharz, R. G. (1977). Influence of social conditions during rearing on the sexual behavior of the domestic boar. *Anim. Prod.* , **24** : 245-251.

McEwen, B. S. (1981). Neural gonadal steroid actions. *Science*, **211** : 1303-1311.

Meusy-Dessolle, N. (1985). *Contribution à l'étude du fonctionnement endocrine du testicule et de ses régulations au cours du développement chez le porc domestique (Sus scrofa) et le macaque crabier (Macaca fascicularis) depuis la différenciation sexuelle jusqu'à l'âge adulte*. Thèse de Doctorat es Sciences, Université de Paris VI.

Orgeur, P. (1982). *Ontogénèse du comportement sexuel mâle chez les ovins domestiques. Effet de l'environnement social*. Thèse de Doctorat es Sciences, Université de Tours.

Signoret, J. P., Adkins-Regan, E. and Orgeur, P. (1989). Bisexuality in the prepubertal male pig. *Behav. Proc.*, **18** : 133-140.

Signoret, J. P. (1970). Swine behavior in reproduction. In :*Effects of Disease and Stress on Reproductive Efficiency in Swine*, Symposium proceedings 70-0, Extension Service, University of Nebraska College of Agriculture, pp. 28-45.

Signoret, J. P. (1990). Différenciation des capacités de conduites sexuelles de type femelle - proceptivité et réceptivité - au cours du développement chez le porc mâle. *C. R. Acad. Sci., Paris*, **311**: 281-285.

Van Eerdenburg, F. (1991). *Postnatal development of some nuclei in the pig hypothalamus. A morphometric and immunocytochemical study*. Thesis University of Utrecht.

Van Straaten, H. W. M. and Wensing, C. J. G. (1977) Histomorphic aspects of testicular morphogenesis in the pig. *Biol. Reprod.*, **17** : 467-472.

Whalen, R. E. and Edwards, D. A. (1967). Hormonal determinants of the development of masculine and feminine sexual behavior in male and female rats. *Anat. Rec.*, **157** : 173-180.

# Some Genetic Considerations in the Development of Sexual Orientation

**M. DIAMOND**

*University of Hawai'i, John A. Burns School of Medicine, Department of Anatomy and Reproductive Biology, 1951 East-West Road, Honolulu, Hawai'i 96822 USA*

This last several years has seen several studies which have caught popular attention. Bouchard and colleagues (e.g., Bouchard et al., 1990) demonstrated uncanny similarities in behavior of twins reared apart. LeVay (1991), demonstrated the existence of a particular portion of the hypothalamus in homosexual men to be smaller than it is in heterosexual men but the same size as found in heterosexual women. And Bailey and Pillard (1991) and Whitam, Diamond and Martin (1993) showed a significant concordance for homosexuality among twins, more so for monozygotic twins than dizygotic. These studies renewed focus on nature-nurture issues in the etiology of behavior.

This paper will attempt to provide one window for viewing the contributions of genetics and the environment to aspects of sexual behavior. Primarily under consideration will be the development of sexual orientation.

## Chicken and egg: nature and nurture

### Mammals

It is well accepted that many aspects of mammalian sexual behavior are genetically controlled and transmitted from generation to generation. McGill and colleagues (e.g., 1963, 1969), for example, have shown that for male mice stable behavioral traits include almost every aspect of sexual behavior from mount latency, intromission latency, thrusts per intromission, to post castration retention of ejaculatory ability. Jakway (1959) has shown comparable strain differences in male guinea pigs and Goy and Jakway (1959) have shown strain differences in the sexual behavior of female guinea pigs. Such might be measured by latency to estrus, duration of estrus, likelihood of coming into estrus and so on. Other investigators have shown similarly in male and female rats, cattle (see Price 1987 for review) and other mammalian species.

*M. Haug et al. (eds.), The Development of Sex Differences and Similarities in Behavior, 291–309.*
© 1993 *Kluwer Academic Publishers.*

Commercial male sheep have been studied by Perkins and her colleagues (Perkins and Fitzgerald, 1992; Miller, 1990). Not only were high and low "drive" found inheritable in the males of this species but so too was homosexual activity implicated as heritable[1.]

Those who study non-human mammalian development accept that sexual differentiation and attendant subsequent behaviors come about by a well known string of events. Genetic forces initiated by fertilization lead to gonadal processes, the maturation of testes or ovaries and release of their subsequent hormones (or their absence) that bias the developing nervous system organizing it to behavioral effects to be seen after puberty. Each step of this process is subject to genetic mediation (see George and Wilson, 1988; Olsen, 1992 and other chapters in this volume for reviews). All subsequent environmental and maturational events in the individual's development are superimposed on this bias.

## Amphibia and teleosts

Looking at amphibia and teleosts offers a very different perspective. In these species the environmental influences are often the most important superimposition on the animals genetics to determine sexual differentiation. Among species of turtles, for instance, high incubation temperatures result in the hatching primarily of females while males are produced with low temperatures (Pieau, 1975; Bull, 1983). The reverse is typically true in alligators (Ferguson and Joanen, 1982) and lizards (Charnier, 1966). And in some turtles females develop at extreme hot and cold temperatures and males at intermediate temperatures (Yntema, 1976; Bull, 1983; Gutzke and Paukstis, 1984). These developments occur at temperature ranges normally found in the home territories of these species.

Among fish the environmental influences are even more "sophisticated". For examples I will use the work of two of my students. Robert Ross (Ross et al., 1983) found that in the saddleback wrass *Thalasoma duperrey* individuals born as females and producing eggs will switch to being male, producing sperm and mating as males, if two conditions are met. There must not be any larger male in her visual vicinity and there must be at least one smaller conspecific, visually present. The work of Marvin Lutnesky (1992) found that among the angelfish *Centropyge potteri* , also a protogyneous species (individuals start life as females and later can become males) the number of social interactions and population density in which the female finds herself will determine if she changes sex. The female with the most encounters with other males and females, usually the largest female in the harem, will become a male. Individuals of these species become male after they have already matured and produced young as females. Then, if induced to change, they "father" subsequent generations. Among other species - such as fish of the genus *Amphiprion* - the animals are protoandrous and the individuals start out as males with the postmaturational environmental stimuli inducing switch to the female sex. These sorts of phenomena are termed "sequential hermaphroditism".

"Prematurational sex change" also occur in certain species such as the minnows (family *Cyprinidae*). Here all individuals start out life as females. From the total population, a portion, for reasons yet undetermined, begin to develop testicular tissue and mature as males. The rest of the young mature as females (Takahashi, 1977; Takahashi and Shimizu, 1983).

To add interest to this non mammalian story, among other teleost species, the deep sea bass *Serranidae Tigrinus*, for instance, simultaneous hermaphroditism exists. These animals form stable pair bonds, defend territory together and mate each day, once as a male and once as a female (Pressley, 1981). Other aspects of the normal physical environment can influence sex determination in teleosts. For example pH can effect differentiation in *cichlids* and *poeciliids* (Rubin, 1985) and day length may effect differentiation in the Siamese fighting fish, *Betta splendens* (Forselius, 1957). A review of these fascinating developmental styles is given in Francis (1992).

The string of events in this second set of examples from amphibia and fish is thus quite different from that first seen with mammals. Among amphibia and fish we have species without sex chromosomes but with autosomes which contain genes of sex distinguishing behavioral characteristics that mesh with environmental events to differentiate the nervous system. This in turn organizes development of the gonads. Certainly, for these animals as well as mammals, genetics are part of every step; just in a different way to the observer. Genetics "primes" the animal to which environmental stimuli it must respond. In mammals, differentiation of the gonads induced by internal genetic events, leads to brain differentiation and subsequent appropriate sexual behavior. In contrast, in fish and amphibia, brain differentiation, induced by external environmental events, leads to gonadal development and then appropriate sexual behavior.

## Manipulating development

At first glance, in mammals constitutional factors seem to be most important for sexual development and in amphibia and fish it seems environmental events are most significant. A moments reflection shows that both genetic and environmental factors are crucial for both. If the environment in which a mammal finds itself changes, for instance, it may show different strain typical behavior. The copulatory patterns observed under standard testing conditions would be markedly altered should there be a hungry fox in the vicinity. And obviously it is the genetic differences between the species that had the environment's visual cues crucial for *Thalasoma* and social cues crucial for *Centropyge*. As biologists have known since the 1920s, for each species the heredity-environment interaction has to be studied separately for each trait [2,3].

Regrettably the links are not always simply revealed. Without testing there is no way to know how any trait will be transmitted. Commercial breeders often see this when they attempt to breed out male "duds" in favor of "studs" or do similarly for the female counterparts, without sacrificing the commercial nature of the product they are trying to obtain. The goal of these breeders is a better "crop" or yield. They are not always successful; the enhancement or manifestation of one trait often diminishes another.

Endocrine manipulation (changing the internal environment) has also been used commercially to modify behavioral development. The best known example here is the use of castration to pacify or stop the sexual activity of adult or preadult animals. The mirror to this is the administration of steroids to songbirds to stimulate singing or to fighting animals (e.g. game cocks, fighting dogs) to enhance pugnaciousness.

Laboratory experiments are also well known for manipulating the prenatal, neonatal or post-pubertal environment, particularly with hormones, drugs or other environmental challenges to alter sexual development and subsequent behavior. Thus the issue can no longer logically be whether the environment or genes can influence sexual development. The goals are to unravel which genetic and environmental factors mold development and how do they do so.

# Sexual orientation

Proponents of a strong environmental component to human sexual orientation propose that one is taught or reinforced to be heterosexually or homosexually oriented. Let us examine these sorts of evidence and compare them with more pointed genetic studies.

## Environmental contributions

### The fixedness of effeminacy in males: non reinforced western cultures: family influence

Green (1987) reported on boys prepubertally seen as obviously effeminate. He studied them for 15 years and compared their development with "control" boys. Of the families involved with the "sissy" boys, most tried on their own to discourage the effeminate behavior and a minority of the parents even entered their sons into formal treatment programs to change their behavior. When interviewed as adults, *"two-thirds of the original group of 'feminine' boys reveal that three-fourths of them developed as homosexual or bisexual. By contrast, only one of the two-thirds [still in the study] of the previously 'masculine' (control) boys was homosexually or bisexually oriented".*

Bell et al. (1981) in the United States and Siegelman (1981) in Great Britain looked for features that might distinguish the family constellations and backgrounds of adult heterosexuals, homosexuals and bisexuals. No common parameter of family or upbringing could be linked causally to sexual orientation nor could any link be found between any aspect of an individual's childhood or adolescent experiences and their homosexual or bisexual activities.

Bell et al. (1981) cautiously conclude: *"Exclusive homosexuality seemed to be something that was firmly established by the end of adolescence and relatively impervious to change or modification by outside influences"* (p. 211), and *"..., our findings are not inconsistent with what one would expect to find if, indeed, there were a biological basis for sexual preference"* (p. 216 ; emphasis in original).

## Transsexuals

In many ways, transsexuals are the archetype to demonstrate that behavior can be independent of rearing and environmental influences. Despite being brought up in accordance with their bodily appearance, and against the wishes of their family and all social institutions, these individuals refuse to continue in the life to which they were assigned. If an XY individual brought up as boy, the transsexual feels to be a girl and wishes to develop into a women. If an XX individual brought up as a girl, the person feels to be a boy and develop into a man.

The individual's feeling about himself or herself, how he or she identifies as male or female (not masculine or feminine which is different), is independent of his or her sexual orientation. An individual's sexual orientation/partner preference can assort independently from his or her sexual identity[4]. One can be a transsexual who is heterosexual, homosexual or ambisexual. Also, children brought up by transsexual parents do not develop as transsexuals (Green, 1978). A more complete discussion of this is available (Diamond, 1976, 1979, 1980, 1992).

## Cross-cultural studies

Whitam and Mathy (1986) studied homosexuality in Brazil, Guatemala, The Philippines and the United States. Across these diverse societies they found many similarities in how homosexual life styles were manifest. Similar behaviors included preferences in occupational interests, involvement in entertainment and the arts and cross-dressing. These researchers concluded that the similarities were not culturally instituted but more likely the result of inherent biological tendencies manifest despite acceptance or rejection by the community. They conclude: *"... sexual orientation is not highly subject to redefinition by any particular social structural arrangement"* ( p. 31).

### The fixedness of heterosexuality western cultures: family influences

Mandel et al. (1979, 1980) followed the development of "role modeling" in boys raised in households where the parental influence was openly lesbian. They concluded: *"Analysis of the children's data has not revealed any sexual identity conflict or homosexual interest. Relationships with fathers and other males do not differ significantly [from that of boys reared in heterosexually parented families.]"*. They find: *"no evidence of gender conflict or poor peer relations"* for children reared by lesbian mothers (Hotvedt and Mandel, 1982). Boys growing up in households parented by openly gay males were heterosexually oriented without conflict or homosexual interest (Green, 1978).

### Cross-sex rearing

There are now at least three personally known instances, two sets of male twins and one singleton, in which an individual was reared as a female, with surgery and endocrine treatment to alter the biology to facilitate the transformation. The first case involved a set of twins extensively reported upon (Diamond, 1982; Money and Ehrhardt, 1972 ). As a result of a surgical accident during circumcision by cautery, one of the boys had his penis burned off. Believing that sexual identity would be based upon the sex of rearing the decision was made to rear this individual as a female (Money and Ehrhardt, 1972)[5]. Now, more than 20 years later, it is known that despite pediatric orchidectomy, treatment with female hormones, and psychotherapy to facilitate a female psyche, this individual has never accepted the female status or role as claimed by the early investigators (Diamond, 1982; Diamond, 1993b). Prior to puberty the twin, without ever being told of his previous history, rebelled against the imposition of a female status. At 18 years of age, this individual who was raised as a girl, sought and had phalloplastic and scrotal reconstruction surgery. Now, as a mature adult, he lives as a male and seeks females as sexual partners. His adjustment is not without difficulties but, to him, seems preferable to imposed life as a female.

The second set of identical twins involves two Samoan children who were brought to my attention when they were 6-years-old. One was causing a great deal of disorder at school. The "female" of this twin set was disruptive and picking fights, not only with female classmates but also males. Case records revealed that ambiguous genitalia at birth had prompted the surgeons then in attendance to reassign him as a female. With appropriate castration and hormonal follow-up, they convinced the parents to rear the child as a girl.

Despite the rearing as a female, even at this young age, the child rebelled against the parents' and teachers' admonitions to "act like a girl". The twin's typical play patterns and demeanor were those of a six year old rambunctious boy and such that the brother, often slipped into using the male pronoun when referring to his twin; e.g. "*He*, ugh, I mean *she*, swims better than me". Asked to draw a child, the misassigned twin drew an ambiguous figure he identified as male. The child spontaneously expressed the desire to grow up as a boy.

The third case is similar. In 1990 I was called to review the behavior and condition of a four-year-old child. Here again, the history revealed that due to the traumatic loss of a penis soon after birth, the decision was made to reassign the boy as a girl. Castration and therapy followed with with the advice to rear the child as a girl. In consultation with Dr. Richard Green of U.C.L.A. it became apparent that by the age of four this individual was exhibiting marked boyish behavior sufficient to disturb the parents and attending professionals. The child was not accepting the female role. The fixedness of behavior patterns along male lines, and aversion to the female role, was strong despite the contrary upbringing.

In these last two instances, the individuals were too young to express erotic interest in a sexual partner. I predict in these cases, as I did in regard to the first twin mentioned above (Diamond, 1976, 1978, 1979) that despite being reared as girls, they will be gynephilic. The postnatal removal of penis and testis, in a human, and imposition of a female rearing has never proven sufficient to overcome the inherent bias of a normal male nervous system.

### Cross-cultural studies

The work by Herdt (1981) and Stoller and Herdt (1985) report examples of environmental forces having little success in inducing long term homosexual activity. These researchers document a New Guinea culture where homosexual behavior is taught, encouraged and institutionalized to transfer masculinity from adults to adolescents. The young boys are institutionalized to fellate the adult men to obtain their semen. Moreover, female bodies are presented as unattractive, to be avoided and poisonous. Nevertheless, these boys, upon reaching adulthood choose females as regular sexual partners, and are almost always heterosexual. Neither youths nor men report impulses to suck penises nor engage in anal intercourse.

Schiefanhovel (1990) reports on a similar New Guinea culture. Here anal intercourse is used to transmit the masculinity-inducing semen between older men and younger boys. He too stresses that heterosexual, not homosexual or bisexual behavior is the preferred and exclusive outlet for these males when they mature. And this obtains despite a severe shortage of adult women due to female infanticide.

A third type of cross-cultural evidence supports an inherent sexual orientation independent of upbringing. Reports by Imperato-McGinley and colleagues (Imperato-McGinley and Peterson, 1976; Imperato-McGinley et al., 1979) describe a population in which, due to a now understood genetic enzyme defect, males were born without penises. They were assumed to be girls and raised accordingly. At puberty, when the enzyme began to appear, the individuals started to develop penises and respond to their own endogenous male hormones. Then, despite their rearing, the boys assumed male identities and patterns. Since these original reports many subsequent similar situations have been reported. Occasionally these studies have been criticized (e.g. Gooren et al., 1990) by saying this phenomenon had been understood by the natives in the population and the children reared appropriately from birth. Indeed that is now true. However, prior to the 1950's this was not so. In those earlier days the boys were reared as girls and then, with varying degrees of ease, switched to live as males. The prepubertal environmental forces failed to imprint feminine development.

In summary then, despite the supposed power of upbringing, role modeling and learning, there is no known case anywhere in which an otherwise normal individual has accepted rearing or life status in an imposed role of the sex opposite to that of his or her natural genetic and endocrine history nor accepted an imposed sexual orientation.

## Population data

There are societies in which homosexuality is not only illegal but subject to the death penalty (e.g. Iran). There are also societies in which the practice is tolerated or considered of no concern. And as we saw above, there are groups among which same-sex activities are encouraged as part of growing up. With these differences in mind it might be instructive to consider if the prevalence of

298

homosexual activity is correlated with some environmental factor we might call "social tolerance". These data below are more fully reported in Diamond, (1993a).

## United States of America

Data from eight studies in the United States between the years 1970 and 1991 indicate that approximately 4.8 percent of the adult male population engage in same-sex behavior (Table I). In comparison with these surveys, a 1984 survey found 9.9 % of San Franciscans identified themselves as homosexual or bisexual (Schreiner, 1986). It might be hypothesized that the population of this city, reputed to have the largest and most powerful gay, lesbian and bisexual communities in the United States, would have a dramatically different proportion of individuals engaging in same sex activities. This, however, is probably a function of the city attracting homosexually oriented individuals rather than "producing" them.

## Asia

Four national studies of japanese students, conducted from 1974 to 1987, found that same-sex contact which may include bisexual contact, was reported by

**Table I** Reports of United States Population Surveys.

| STUDY | MALE HM. BEHAVIOR |
|---|---|
| Davis and Smith (1988) | 2.4 |
| Diamond, Ohye and Wells (1993) | 3.0 |
| Dixon et al. (1991) | 7.3 |
| Fay et al. (1989) | 6.7 |
| Michael et al. (1988) | 3.2 |
| Rogers and Turner (1991) | 6.1 |
| Schreiner (1986) | 4.0/9.9* |
| Smith (1991) | 5.6 |
| Mean | 4.8 |

* This 9.9 % figure is for the San Francisco area. (see Diamond, 1993a....., for details)

an average of 5.8 % of the male sample and 4.0 % of the female respondents. In contemporary Japan there is a strong stigma against homosexuality.

Information from a total Philippine population is available. Anthropologist Donn Hart (1968) lived for years in the village of Caticugan on the island of Negros. In his village of 729 persons, Hart found six male homosexuals and no lesbians (< 2%). In the province of Siaton, which Hart also studied, with a population of 2,862, there were 12 male homosexuals and "several" lesbians (< 2%).

Hart (1968) writes *"it is believed that the number of covert homosexuals is very small ... the majority of residents of Siaton province and Caticugan are both lenient and indulgent of the local bayot [male homosexuals] and lakin-on [lesbians]"*. Others too have reported on the tolerance of the Filipino people toward homosexual behaviors (Guthrie and Jacobs, 1966; Whitam and Mathy, 1986).

Research from Thailand by Sittitrai et al. (1992) reports same-sex contact by 3.6 % of the males interviewed but only 0.4% consider themselves homosexuals (K = 4-6). Only 1.3 % of females had same-sex contact and 1.0% consider themselves as homosexual (K = 4-6).

A 10 percent random sample of the total population from the Republic of Pilau asked of sexual behavior for the preceding 12 months. After the age of 20, exclusive homosexual activity was reported by 1.9% of the males and 2.8% of

**Table II**  National population surveys of same-sex activity.

| STUDY | MALE |
|---|---|
| Great Britain | 5.0-9.0 |
| Japan | 5.8 |
| Netherlands | 7.8 |
| Philippines* | 2.0 |
| Pilau* | 4.7 |
| Thailand* | 3.6 |
| United States | 4.8 |
| Mean | 4.8-5.4 |

* = the 3 most relatively tolerant of homosexuality. (see Diamond, 1993a....., for details)

the females interviewed. Bisexual activity was reported by 2.8 % of the males and 0.7 % of the females. (Morens and Polloi, personal communication). Pilau too is relatively tolerant of same-sex expression.

## Europe and Great Britain

Research cited by Schover and Jensen (1988) for a randomly selected population of danish women found only 2 of 625 women from 22 to 70 years of age reporting having had a homosexual experience.

A british national study (Wellings et al., 1990) found 9% of men and 4% of women having had homosexual experience. Only 5% of men and 1% of women reported ever having a homosexual partner (Table II).

A 1991 study from the Netherlands (van Zessen and Sandfort, 1992) found only about 13 in 100 males admitted to ever having a homosexual experience and only about 3.3% would consider themselves homosexual (K=5-6). Among females, only 10 in 100 reported ever having had homosexual activity. Only some 0.4% of the women considered themselves homosexual.

While we have no data on the incidence of homosexuality in strongly repressive societies the findings we do have seem in the opposite direction from that which might be hypothesized on the basis of social tolerance. In the non homophobic societies we find reported among the lowest rates of same sex activity. Also, while lesbianism can be said to carry less stigma than male homosexuality, considering world wide research, almost all studies have found the incidence of male homosexual activity exceeds that of females, approximately by a factor of 2[6].

## Bisexuality

Directing attention now specifically to studies of self identified male homosexual populations we gain relevant information about bisexuality which will be germane to later discussion.

Study of homosexual males in the United States, the Netherlands and Denmark by Weinberg and Williams (1974) showed about one in five American homosexuals were bisexually active as K=2, 3 or 4 and about one in ten Dutch or Danish gay men were similarly active. More recent studies by Bell and Weinberg (1978), McWhirter and Mattison (1984) and Higa (1988) find about three or more out of four, claim to be exclusively homosexual and fewer than one in ten claim they ever had more than incidental sex with a female. Thus, considering Kinsey's 7 point scale, distribution for same-sex or opposite-sex activity is definitely bimodal (see Diamond, 1993b, for details).

# Genetic contributions

The literature on pedigrees and twin studies is large and a significant portion of it pertains to aspects of sexuality. This discussion will emphasize work related to sexual orientation. Details are available in Whitam et al. (1993).

## Non twins

Pillard and colleagues studied families having a known heterosexual or homosexual adult (Pillard et al.,1982; Pillard and Weinrich, 1986; Weinrich, 1987). They found that among brothers, if a family contained one index son who was homosexual, between 20 and 25 per cent of the brothers would also be. If

he index brother were heterosexual, the chance of other brothers being
iomosexual was only about 4 to 6 per cent.

## Twins

<allmann, in well known studies (1952a,b), reported nearly 100% concordance
or homosexual orientation in monozygotic (MZ) and about 10% concordance in
dizygotic (DZ) twins. Following these reports, however, MZ twins discordant for
iomosexual orientation were soon reported by many investigators (see
Puterbaugh, 1990 for review).

Significantly, in 1991 Bailey and Pillard found a 52% concordance rate for
iomosexual orientation in MZ male pairs and a 22% concordance rate for DZ
male pairs. King and McDonald in 1992 reported a 25 % concordance rate
among monozygotic twins and a 12 % concordance rate among dizygotic twins
and Whitam, Diamond and Martin (1993) reported finding a 65% concordance
among MZ male twins and 30% concordance among DZ male twins.

These observations of the last decade do not find the rates of concordance
'ound by Kallmann (1952a,b) but taken together are significantly high that a
strong genetic contribution for homosexuality can no longer seriously be
contested (Table III).

**Table III** Concordance for male homosexuality among twins (* Percentages).

| STUDY | N.PAIRS | MONOZYGT* | DIZYGOT* |
|---|---|---|---|
| Kallmann | 40/45 | 100 | 10 |
| Schlegal | 113 | 95 | 5 |
| Heston and Shields | 7/7 | 71 | 14 |
| Bailey and Pillard | 56/54 | 52 | 22 |
| King and McDonald | 20/25 | 25 | 13 |
| Whitam, Diamond and Martin | 34/27 | 65 | 30 |
| TOTALS | | 68 | 16 |

Among our MZ male twins, 29.4% were discordant for sexual orientation; the
most common pattern was the index twin K-6 and his brother K-0 (Whitam et al.,

1993). These bimodal findings are consistent with those of Bailey and Pillard (1991).

The concordance rate for Female MZ twins for homosexual orientation we found was 75% (Whitam et al., 1993). Our sample size for female twins is quite small and a larger number might well produce a different rate of concordance. However, these findings questions the notion that male homosexuality may be biologically derived while female homosexuality is learned (Eckert et al., 1986).

There are two types of Male DZ twins: those whose co-twin is male and those whose co-twin is female. The concordance rate for homosexuality in the former is 28.6% and in the latter 33.3%. The combined concordance rate for male DZ twins with either a homosexual brother or sister is 30.4% (Whitam et al., 1993).

## Triplets

Three sets of triplets appeared in our sample (Whitam et al., 1993). One set consisted of three females; a pair of MZ twins who are both lesbian and a third heterosexual sister. A second pair of triplets consisted of a MZ male pair, both homosexual, with a heterosexual sister. A third MZ male triplet set all reported same-sex orientation.

## Other genetic considerations

Two more items to consider will be mentioned. Using data from different types of studies they infer a biological component to homosexuality. Blanchard and Sheridan (1992) reported that,

*"homosexual men had significantly more siblings than ... homosexual women, who in turn, had significantly more siblings than ... nonhomosexual men. The sibling sex ratio of the homosexual men, 131 brothers per 100 sisters, was significantly higher than the sex ratio of live births for the population as a whole ...[also] the homosexual men had a significantly later birth order than the nonhomosexual men".*

The second item for consideration stems from the recent report of Turner (1992). He finds, after studying family genealogies, that,

*"in the absence of alcoholism ...[homosexuality] may depend upon a gene in the pseudoautosomal region of the X and Y chromosomes".*

If alcoholism is present he believes homosexuality to have a different genetic origin. He considers these findings the result of differential fetal wastage. This can also account for the Blanchard and Sheridan findings.

Lastly, many critiques of the biological nature of homosexuality question why the phenomenon persists since there is no obvious evolutionary benefit to it. This has been answered in many ways (see e.g. Hutchinson, 1959; Kirsch, 1982; Trivers, 1974; Wilson, 1975). While interesting to consider, anything said here is speculative.

Obviously any genetic patterning is complex because most parents of homosexuals are heterosexual and rear their children accordingly. The concept of pleiotropy must obviously be considered with recognition that traits selected for by a mating couple are typically independent of the sexual orientation of future children. And if genetics are involved why are not all MZ twins concordant?

In ways we do not yet understand, not all sibs of homosexual index individuals show homosexuality even among monozygotic twins. There is obviously more than one set of genes involved. And they apparently interact with genes of other traits and social forces to organize how the final behaviors will be manifest. And why, among MZ twin brothers that are not concordant for homosexuality, do only a minority show bisexual behavior and are exclusively heterosexual instead? Intuitively one might expect a higher ratio of bisexuals to heterosexuals. Sexual orientation is obviously manifest bimodally. Indeed, it may be that bisexuality is related to homosexuality and heterosexuality but quite different in its developmental pattern.

## Discussion and conclusions

The material presented in this chapter demonstrates that both the environment and genetic programming interact in the development of sexual orientation, and for different species, the interaction occurs in different ways. Only some fish among all those with a certain genetic pool, for instance, change sex when the environment clues dictate. In humans, while certain twins have the genetic predisposition to manifest homosexual orientation, only certain individuals seem subject to unique, yet unknown, stimuli to show this phenotype.

Sexual orientation may follow patterns of other behaviors assumed to have a strong genetic component and yet not display 100% concordance in MZ pairs. Kaij (1960) found, for example, the rate of concordance for alcoholism to be 54% in MZ pairs and 24% for DZ pairs. Nagylaki and Levy (1973), found MZ twins have more reversed asymmetries than DZ pairs; there is a larger proportion of discordance of handedness in MZ pairs. Bouchard et al. (1990) found many traits fixed by heredity but not all twins showed these traits equally.

We have not seen sexual orientation noticeably influenced by events typically thought of as environmentally significant in development (e.g. role modeling, reinforcement, etc.). Other types of events might, nevertheless, be of consequence. For instance *in utero* chorion conditions may effect the nervous system. Melnick et al. (1978) have suggested that monochorionic twins are more alike than dichorionic twins. However, the shared blood circulation of the common chorion may be more unfavorable for one twin than the other. And certainly sexual orientation may be biologically determined *in utero* by biochemical mechanisms - under genetic mediation - which remain to be identified. And certainly the social-sexual environment in which discordant twins develop, rather than being alike may actually be quite different. Even still-attached Siamese twins can have different personalities.

As proposed more than 25 years ago (Diamond, 1965) and many times since, sexual orientation is most probably the result of interacting inherent biological forces meshing with environmental pressures. The biology sets a predisposition, a bias, with which the individual interacts with his or her surround (Diamond, 1965, 1968, 1976, 1978, 1979, 1980, 1982, 1992, 1993b; Diamond and Karlen, 1980; Whitam and Mathy, 1986). And particular stages or "critical periods" in development seem more significant than others in organizing these behaviors.

A last word. Legal restrictions and social taboos or other motives can move an individual to exhibit behaviors and form sexual and emotional attachments to partners he or she would not otherwise desire, or refrain from relationships that would be preferred. But given free opportunity, an individual's true choice will be manifest (Diamond, 1978; Diamond, 1979). Our biological heritage has given most humans the flexibility to adjust. The more environmental freedom, the more genetics will be allowed to express itself.

For some persons the idea that sexual orientation is biologically biased is threatening. Some have expressed consternation that if the developmental biological forces for sexual orientation are known (or even suspected), governmental, religious, medical or social agencies might use the knowledge to force conformity to a dictated ideal or otherwise modify a potential homosexual outcome. Unfortunately, groups who have the end of homosexuality or ambisexuality as their goal, I fear need no scientific justification for their malignant ends. They are sufficient in their own ignorance and prejudice to further their aims. Indeed, the truth is more likely than not to benefit us all.

# Acknowledgements

Thanks to Ronald Johnson, University of Hawaii, for his assistance and access to his behavior genetics notes.

# Notes

1. Heritable is not the same as " inheritable" as understood in lay terminology. Heritability is the proportion of variance in a specified population, for a specific phenotype, which can be attributed to additive genetic factor. Thus heritability is the probability that two individuals in a population would mate and produce offspring that show this character. Note this speaks of a population. There is rarely any predictive value for any particular individual(s) or behavior. And heritability does not have a fixed value that more studies will better define. It is a characteristic of only the particular population studied.

If everyone in a population, like inbred strains of mice, were homozygous at every gene loci, heritability would approach zero. It would mean that there were no traits subject to additive change by one individual mating with a another. This assumes that environmental conditions change, the opportunity for new genetic expression would expand and decrease the heritability component since more influence will now be manifest by the environment.

High heritability does not preclude high environmental influence. In fact, those traits showing the highest heritability usually are the most accessible to environmental influence since the population variance is greater because genetic flexibility has not been "used up". Most importantly, traits contributing to "fitness", should show little additive variation since excessive variation would reduce the stability of the particular trait in the population and subject the species to risk.

2 . A simple formula used to represent this relationship is $P = Gv + Ev + f\ Cov\ G \times E$.

P = the phenotype of the trait

G = the genetic contribution

E = the environmental contribution

V = the variation in the population studied

f Cov = some function of the covariance of G and E. This takes care of the possibility that G and E are not independent.

3. It is obvious from this formula that increasing the variance in the environment decreases the "weight" of the genetic contribution to any trait. Thus reducing the restrictiveness of a population's environment might increase the "weight" of the environment in determining phenotypic expression within that population. If the geneic contribution to a behavior were zero and the behavior only due to the environment, it should be "simple" to change the environment and thus modify the behavior.

4. I have previously proposed that an individual's sexual profile has five basic levels. Sexual identity, the core sense of being male and female and sexual orientation/partner preference are two of the five. The other three are Reproduction, Patterns and Mechanisms (Diamond, 1976, 1979, 1980, 1984, 1992). These are usually in concert but can assort independently.

5. Sexual identity is internal and private. Gender indentity is public and reflects the individuals way of interacting with society. For most individuals they are the same but not so for transsexuals (Diamond, 1976, 1979, 1992).

6. It might be argued, as done by Rogers and Turner (1991) that the figures reported in surveys of homosexuality are minimums and that most individuals who engage in same-sex activities remain closeted. But evidence for this being widespread in the confidential surveys reported is not supported by the evidence (Diamond, 1993b). Also, it is difficult to hypothesize that the most "closeting" would occur in the more tolerant cultures.

# References

Bailey, J. M. and Pillard, R. C. (1991). A genetic study of male sexual orientation. *Arch. Gen. Psychiat.*, **48** : 1089-1096.

Bell, A. P. and Weinberg, M. (1978). *Homosexualities - A Study of Diversity Among Men amd Women* , New York : Simon and Schuster.

Bell, A. P., Weinberg, M. S. and Hammersmith, S. K. (1981). *Sexual Preference - Its Development in Men and Women*, Bloomington: Alfred C. Kinsey Institute of Sex Research.

Blanchard, R. and Sheridan, P. M. (1992). Sibling size, sibling sex ratio, birth order, and parental age in homosexual and nonhomosexual gender dysphorics. *J. Nerv. Ment. Diseases*, **180** : 40-47.

Bouchard, T. J., Lykken, D. T., McGue, M., Segal, N. L. and Tellegen, A. (1990). Sources of human psychological differences: a Minnesota study of twins reared apart. *Science*, **250** : 223-228.

Bull, J. J. (1983). *Evolution of Sex Determining Mechanisms*, Menlo Park : Benjamin/Cummings Publishing.

Charnier, M. (1966). Action de la temperature sur la sex-ratio chez l'embryon d'Agama agama (Agamidae, Lacertilien). *Soc. Biol. Quest. Af.*, **160** : 620-622.

Diamond, M. (1965). A critical evaluation of the ontogeny of human sexual behavior. *Quart. Rev. Biol.*, **40** : 147-175.

Diamond, M. (1968). Genetic-endocrine interaction and human psychosexuality. In: Diamond M. (Ed.), *Perspectives in Reproduction and Sexual Behavior*, Indiana University Press, Bloomington, pp. 417-443.

Diamond, M. (1976). Human sexual development: biological foundation for social development. In: Beach, F. A. (Ed.), *Human Sexuality in Four Perspectives* , The John Hopkins Press, pp. 22-61.

Diamond, M. (1978). Sexual identity and sex roles. *Humanist*, 4 : 16-19.

Diamond, M. (1979). Sexual identity and sex roles. In: Bullough, V. (Ed.), *The Frontiers of Sex Research* , Buffalo, New York Prometheus, pp. 33-56.

Diamond, M. (1982). Sexual identity, monozygotic twins reared in discordant sex roles and a BBC follow-up. *Arch. Sex. Behav.*, **11** : 181-185.

Diamond, M. (1992). *Sexwatching: Looking at the World of Sexual Behaviour, 2nd Ed,* Prion Books, London.

Diamond, M. (1993a). Homosexuality and bisexuality in different populations. *Arch. Sex. Behav.,* In Press.

Diamond, M. (1993b) Bisexualities: a biological perspective. In : Haeberle, E. (Ed.), *Bisexualities,* In Press.

Diamond, M. and Karlen, A. (1980). *Sexual Decisions* , Boston : Little Brown.

Eckert, E., Bouchard, T., Bohlen, J. and Heston, L. (1986). Homosexuality in monozygotic twins reared apart. *Brit. J. Psychiat.,* **148** : 421-425.

Ferguson, M. J. W. and Joanen, T. (1982). Temperature of egg incubation determines sex in Alligator mississippiensis. *Nature,* **296** : 850-853.

Forselius, S. (1957). Studies of Anabantid fishes I-III. *Zool. Bidr. Upps.,* **32** : 93-97.

Francis, R. C. (1992 ). Sexual liability in teleosts: developmental factors. *Quart. Rev. Biol.,* In Press.

George, F. W. and Wilson, J. D. (1988). Sex determination and differentiation. In: Knobil, E., Neill, J. et al. (Eds.), *The Physiology of Reproduction* , New York : Raven Press, pp. 3-26.

Gooren, L., Fliers, E. and Courtney, K. (1990). Biological determinants of sexual orientation. In: Bancroft, J. (Ed.), *Annual Review of Sex Research*, Lake Mills, Iowa: The Society for the Scientific Study of Sex, pp. 175-196.

Goy, R. W. and Jakway, J. S. (1959). The inheritance of patterns of sexual behaviour in female guinea pigs. *Anim. Behav.,* 7 : 142-149.

Green, R. (1978). Sexual identity of 37 children raised by homosexuals or transsexual parents. *Psychiatry,* **135** : 692-697.

Green, R. (1978). Thirty-five children raised by homosexual or transsexual parents. *Amer. J. Psychiat.,* **135** : 692-697.

Green, R. (1987). *The "Sissy Boy Syndrome" and the Development of Homosexuality* , New Haven and London: Yale University Press.

Guthrie, G. M. and Jacobs, P. J. (1966). *Child Rearing and Personality Development in the Philippines,* University Park : Pennsylvania State University Press

Gutzke, W. H. N. and Paukstis, G. L. (1984). A low temperature threshold for sexual differentiation in the painted turtle, Chrysemys picta. *Copeia*, pp. 546-547.

Hart, D. V. (1968). Homosexuality and transvestism in the Philippines. *Behav. Sci. Notes*, **3** : 211-248.

Herdt, G. H. (1981). *Guardians of the Flute: Idioms of Masculinity*, New York : McGraw-Hill.

Higa, D. (1988). *The Psychosocial Functioning of Individuals at Risk for AIDS.* Unpublished Doctoral Dissertation, University of Hawai'i.

Hotvedt, M. E. and Mandel, J. B. (1982). Children of lesbian mothers. In: Paul, W., Weinrich, J., Gonsiorek, C. and Hotvedt, M. E. (Eds.), *Homosexuality: Social, Psychological and Biological Issues*, Beverly Hills: Sage Publications, pp. 275-285.

Hutchinson, G. E. (1959). A speculative consideration of certain possible forms of sexual selection in man. *Amer. Natur.*, **93** : 81-91.

Imperato-McGinley, J. and Peterson, R. E. (1976). Male pseudohermaphroditism: the complexities of male phenotypic development. *Amer. J. Med.*, **61** : 251-272.

Imperato-McGinley, J., Peterson, R. E., Gautier, T. and Sturia, E. (1979). Androgen and evolution of male-gender identity among male pseudohermaphrodites with 5α-reductase deficiency. *New Engl. J. Med.*, **300** : 1233-1237.

Jakway, J. S. (1959). Inheritance of patterns of mating behaviour in the male guinea pig. *Anim. Behav.*, **7** : 150-162.

Kaij, L. (1960). *Alcoholism in Twins* , Stockholm : Alqvist and Wiksell.

Kallmann, F. J. (1952a). Twin and sibship study of overt male homosexuality. *Amer. J. Hum. Gen.*, **4** : 136-146.

Kallmann, F. J. (1952b). Comparative twin study on the genetic aspects of male homosexuality. *J. Nerv. Ment. Disease*, **115** : 283-298.

King, M. and McDonald, E. (1992). Homosexuals who are twins: a study of 46 probands. *Brit. J. Psychiat.*, **160** : 407-409.

Kirsch, J. A. W. and Rodman, J. E. (1982). Selection and sexuality: the darwinian view of homosexuality. In: William, J. D. W., Gonsio, P. J. C. and Hotvedt, M. E. (Eds.), *Homosexuality: Social, Psychological and Biological Issues* , Beverly Hills: Sage Publications, pp. 183-196.

LeVay, S. (1991). A difference in hypothalamic structure between heterosexual and homosexual Men. *Science*, **253** : 1034-1037.

Lutnesky, M. M. F. (1992). *Behavioral Ecology of Reproduction in the Pomacanthid Angelfish, Centropyge potteri,* Experimental Dissertation, University of Hawai'i.

Mandel, J. B. and Hotvedt, M. E. (1980). Lesbians as parents. *Huisarts and Praktijk*, **4** : 31-34.

Mandel, J. B., Hotvedt, M. E. and Green, R. (1979). The lesbian parents comparison of heterosexual and homosexual mothers and their children. *Annual Meeting of the American Psychology Association*, Sept. 4.

McGill, T. E. (1969). An enlarged study of genotype and recovery of sex drive in male mice. *Psychon. Sci.*, **15** : 250-251.

McGill, T. E. and Blight, W. C. (1963). The sexual behaviour of hybrid male mice compared with the sexual behaviour of males of the inbred parent strains. *Anim. Behav.*, **11** : 480-483.

McWhirter, D. P. and Mattison, A. M. (1984). *The Male Couple: How Relationships Develop* , Englewood Cliffs: Prentice-Hall.

Melnick, M., Myrianthopolos, N. C. and Christian, J. C. (1978). The effects of chorion on variation in I. Q. in the NCPP twin population. *Amer. J. Human Genet.*, **30** : 425-433.

Miller, K. (1990). Is your ram a stud or a dud. *Nat.Wool Grower*, **3** : 28-30.

Money, J. and Ehrhardt, A. (1972). *Man and Woman, Boy and Girl*. Baltimore: John Hopkins University Press.

Morens, D. M. and Polloi, H. O. (1992). *Comprehensive Health Survey in The Republic of Pilau*, Personal Communication, University of Hawaii, School of Public Health.

Nagylaki, T. and Levy, J. (1973). "Sound of one paw clapping" isn't sound. *Behav. Genet.*, **3** : 279-292.

Olsen, K. L. (1992). Genetic influences on sexual behavior differentiation. In: Gerall, A., Moltz, H. and Ward, I. L. (Eds.), *Sexual Differentiation*, New York : Plenum Press, pp. 1-40.

Perkins, A. and Fitzgerald, J. A. (1992). Luteinizing hormone, testosterone and behavioral response of male-oriented rams to estrous ewes and rams. *J. Anim. Sci.*, **70**, In Press.

Pieau, C. (1975). Temperature and sex differentiation in embryos of two chelonians, *Emys orbicularis L.* and *Testudo graeca L.* In: Reinboth, R. (Ed.), *Intersexuality in the Animal Kingdom*, Berlin: Springer Verlag, pp. 332-339.

Pillard, R. and Weinrich, J. (1986). Evidence of familial nature of male homosexuality. *Arch. Psychiat.*, **43** : 808-812.

Pillard, R., Poumadere, J. and Carretta, R. (1982). A family study of sexual orientation. *Arch. Sex. Behav.*, **11** : 511-520.

Pressley, P. H. (1981). Pair formation and joint territoriality in a simultaneous hermaphrodite: the coral reef fish, Serranus tigrinus. *Zeits. Tierpsychol.*, **56** : 33-46.

Price, E. O. (1987). Male sexual behavior. In : Price, E. O. (Ed.), *The Veterinary Clinics of North America*, Philadelphia : W.B. Saunders Co., pp. 405-461.

Puterbaugh, G. (1990). *Twins and Homosexuality: A Casebook*, New York and London : Garland Publishing, Inc.

Ross, R., Losey, G. and Diamond, M. (1983). Sex change in a coral-reef fish : dependence of stimulation and inhibition on relative size. *Science*, **221** : 574-575.

Rubin, D. A. (1985). Effect of pH on sex ratio in cichlids and a poeciliid (Teleostei). *Copeia*, pp. 233-235.

Schiefenhovel, W. (1990). Ritualized adult-male/adolescent-male sexual behavior in Melanesia : an anthropological and ethological perspective. In : Feierman, J. R. (Ed.), *Pedophilia - Biosocial Dimensions*, New York: Springer - Verlag, pp. 394-421.

Schlegel, W. S. (1962). Die konstitutionbiologischen grundlagen der homosexualitat. *Z. Menschl. Vererb. Konstit.*, **36** : 341-364.

Schover, L. R. and Jensen, S. B. (1988). *Sexuality and Chronic Illness: A Comprehensive Approach*, New York: The Guilford Press.

Schreiner, J. (1986). *Measuring the Gay and Lesbian Population* . Pamphlet of the National Organization of Gay and Lesbian Scientists and Technical Professionals, Chicago, Illinois.

Siegelman, M. (1981). Parental backgrounds of homosexual and heterosexual men : a cross national replication. *Arch. Sex. Behav.*, **10** : 505-513.

Sittitrai, W., Brown, T. and Virulrak, S. (1992). Patterns of bisexuality in Thailand. In : Tielman, R. (Ed.), *HIV and Bisexuality*, Buffalo: Promethious Books.

Stoller, R. and Herdt, G. (1985). Theories of origins of male homosexuality. *Arch. Gen. Psychiat.*, **42** : 399-404.

Takahashi, H. (1977). Juvenile hermaphroditism in the zebrafish, Brachydanio rerio. *Bull. Fac. Fish., Hokkaido University*, **28** : 57-65.

Takahashi, H. and Shimizu, M. (1983). Juvenile intersexuality in a cyprinid fish, the Sumatra barb, Barbus tetrazona. *Bull. Fac. Fish., Hokkaido University*, **34** : 69-78.

Trivers, R. L. (1974). Parent-offspring conflict. *Amer. Zool.*, **14** : 249-264.

Turner, W. J. (1992). Is homosexuality of genetic origin. *Nature*, In Press.

Van Zessen, G. and Sandfort, T. (1992). *Sex and AIDS in the Netherlands (Seksualiteit in Nederland)*, Amsterdam: Swets and Zeitlinger.

Weinberg, M. and Williams, C. (1974). *Male Homosexuals - Their Problems and Adaptations*, New York: Oxford University Press.

Weinrich, J. D. (1987). *Sexual Landscapes: Why we are what we are, Why we Love whom we Love*, New York: Charles Schribner's Sons.

Wellings, K., Field, J., Wadsworth, A. M., Johnson, A. M., Anderson, R. M. and Bradshaw, S. A. (1990). Sexual lifestyles under scrutiny. *Nature*, **348** : 276-278.

Whitam, F. L. and Mathy, R. M. (1986). *Male Homosexuality in Four Societies: Brazil, Guatemala, the Philippines, and the United States,* New York: Praeger.

Whitam, F., Diamond, M. and Martin, J. (1993). Homosexual orientation in twins. 61 twin pairs and three sets of triplets. *Arch. Sex. Behav.*, In Press.

Wilson, E. O. (1975). *Sociobiology: The New Synthesis,* Cambridge: Harvard University Press.

Yntema, C. L. (1976). Effects of incubation temperatures on sexual differentiation in the turtle, Chelhydra serpentina J. *J. Morph.*, **150** : 453-462.

# Morphological Correlates of Neuronal Plasticity to Gonadal Steroids: Sexual Differentiation of the Preoptic Area

Y. ARAI[1], M. NISHIZUKA[1], S. MURAKAMI[1], M. MIYAKAWA[1], M. MACHIDA[2] , H. TAKEUCHI[2] and H. SUMIDA[3]

[1]Departments of Anatomy and [2]Obstetrics and Gynecology, Juntendo University School of Medicine, Hongo, Tokyo 113, Japan, and [3]Research Laboratories, Nippon Kayaku Co. Ltd., Takasaki-City, Gumma 270-12, Japan

Gonadal steroids exert very complex influences on the brain. The neural circuitries participating in neuroendocrine control of the reproductive functions are under the direct control of the gonadal steroids throughout life. Further, in the developmental processes, the sex steroids affect brain sexual differentiation to produce major sex differences in neuroendocrine and behavioral functions. In this regard, recent studies indicate that the sex steroids modulate the number of neurons in certain brain areas and promote circuit formation. Synaptogenesis is also facilitated by estrogen. These organizational effects of the gonadal steroids appear to be regionally specific and correlate with the presence and topographic localization of the sex steroid-receptor containing neurons (Arai et al., 1986; Gorski, 1990).

For the expression of sexually dimorphic neuroendocrine and behavioral functions, it would be logical to expect that some quantitative and/or qualitative differences exist between males and females, and not only in the metabolism of the neurotransmitters but also in the neural circuitry, and considerable evidence now exists to suggest male-female differences in brain morphology. This article discusses the morphological correlates that have been found in the sexually dimorphic neuroendocrine brain, especially in the preoptic area (POA).

## Gonadal steroids and the structural sex differences in the POA and other areas of the neuroendocrine brain

The medial POA of the rat is one of the sexually dimorphic regions, and in this area, Gorski and his co-workers (l978) have described an intensely stained neuron group with a striking sex difference that they have termed the sexually

311

*M. Haug et al. (eds.), The Development of Sex Differences and Similarities in Behavior, 311–323.*
© 1993 *Kluwer Academic Publishers.*

dimorphic nucleus of the POA (SDN-POA). The SDN-POA occupies more neurons in males than in females. The characteristics of these neurons are dependent on the perinatal steroid conditions, suggesting the existence of a critical period during which the SDN-POA is most sensitive to androgen, since continuous prenatal exposure to androgen is not essential for stimulation of the developmemnt of the SDN-POA (Ito et al., 1986a).

Analogues of the SDN-POA also have been identified in gerbils (Commins and Yahr, 1984), ferrets (Tobet et al., 1986) and guinea pigs (Hines et al., 1985) and other species. In addition to these animals, two reports of a sex difference in the human POA-hypothalamus have appeared. Swaab and Fliers (1985) have reported on the existence of an SDN-POA of the human hypothalamus. In the other report, four hypothalamic nuclei in the human brain have been quantified by Gorski and his associates (Allen et al., 1989). Out of four interstitial nuclei of the anterior hypothalamus (INAH), INAH-2 and -3 were found to be statistically larger in the male brain. More recently, LeVay (1991) has analyzed human brains of male homosexuals who died from AIDS, and found that the volume of the INAH-3 was significantly smaller than that of heterosexual men, and comparable to the volume of females. The functional significance of these sexually dimorphic structures in the POA-hypothalamus still remains unclear, but it is presumably concerned with the control of masculine behavior.

Another sexually dimorphic cell group, which is referred to as the anteroventral periventricular nucleus of the POA (AVPVN-POA), has been identified in the periventricular gray of the POA just caudal to the organum vasculosum lamina terminalis (Bleier et al., 1982). This cell group is larger and more densely cellular in females than in males (Figure 1). This structure is thought to play a critical role in regulating the cyclic release of gonadotropins in female rats, because small lesions confined to this part have been found to block spontaneous ovulation, inducing anovulatory persistent estrous syndrome (Terasawa et al., 1980).

Recently, the nuclear volume of the AVPVN-POA has also been found dependent upon perinatal androgen (Ito et al., 1986b). As shown in Figure 2, the AVPVN-POA is significantly smaller in the female rats exposed to testosterone propionate (TP) for the first 7 days of life than in normal female rats, but the AVPVN-POA volume reduction in females given a single injection of TP at embryonic day 17 or 21 (E 17 or 21) is not as marked as in females injected with TP neonatally. In males prenatally treated with TP, the AVPVN-POA also seems to be affected by TP. Further, in males injected with TP at E 21, the AVPVN-POA volume decreased significantly, when compared to its size in normal males. However, the size of the male AVPVN-POA could not be altered by neonatal castration, and this failure of neonatal castration of males to reverse to a female size may be due to the organizational action exerted by the endogenous androgen before birth. A sex difference in the nuclear volume also has been found in the ventromedial nucleus (Matsumoto and Arai, 1983), the bed nucleus of the stria terminalis (Hines et al., 1985), the medial amygdaloid nucleus (Mizukami et al., 1983).

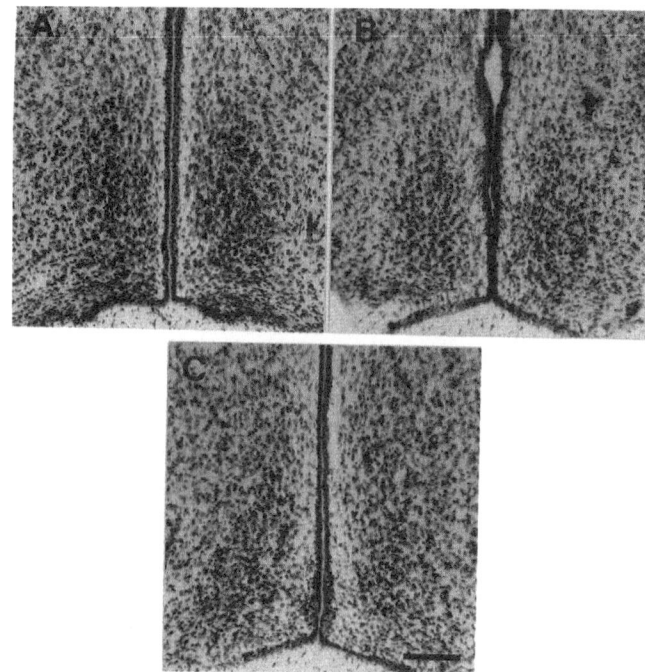

**Figure 1**  Histology of the AVPVN-POA. (A) AVPVN-POA of a normal adult female. (B) AVPVN-POA of a normal adult male. Note decrease in size. (C) AVPVN-POA of a female treated with TP for the first 7 days of life. The size is almost comparable to that of the male. Scale bar=125 μm.

## AVPVN-POA and the gonadal steroids

In the rat, estrogenic metabolites produced by the aromatization of testicular androgen are considered to be the masculinizing hormone. As shown in Figure 3, on treating female rats with 500 μg testosterone or 50 μg estradiol for the first 5 days of life, a significant reduction of the AVPVN-POA volume to that of the male level was achieved. However, nonaromatizable androgen, 5α-dihydro-testosterone injections, as well as simultaneous injections of the anti-estrogen tamoxifen with testosterone, could not reduce the volume of the AVPVN-POA. These results suggest the importance of aromatization from testicular androgen to estrogen in inducing sexually dimorphic changes in the developing rat AVPVN-POA.

In the SDN-POA, a perinatal treatment of females with androgen has been found to markedly increase the nuclear volume and neuronal number. Androgen also has been reported to prevent normally occurring cell death in the

314

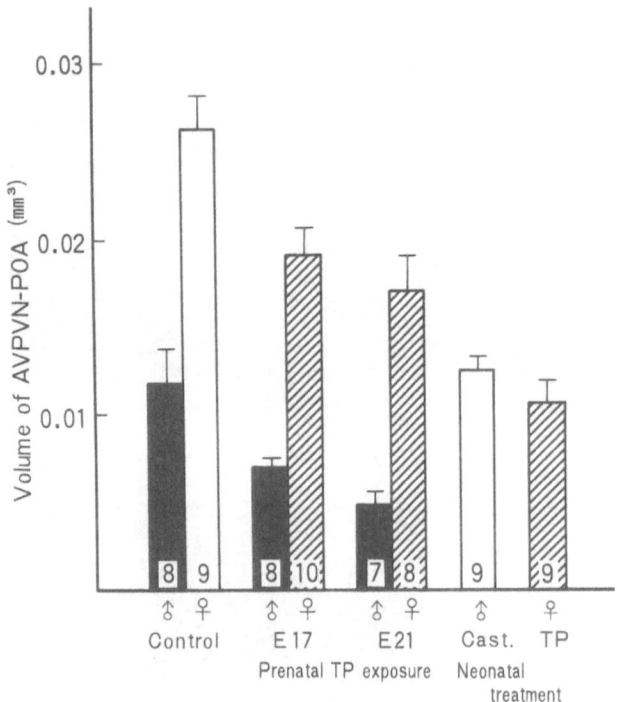

**Figure 2** Effect of prenatal androgen exposure on the volume of the AVPVN-POA. In the groups treated with TP prenatally, the animals were exposed to TP through the mothers at E 17 or 21. In the group receiving neonatal treatment, males were castrated on the day of birth (Cast) and females were injected with TP for the first 7 days (TP). Experimental and control animals were sacrificed at 90 days of age. Vertical bars indicate S.E.M. Numbers at the bottom of the columns refer to the number of rats examined.

spinal nucleus of the bulbocavernosus in the female rat (Nordeen et al., 1985), and a similar mechanism can be assumed to exist in the SDN-POA. In the AVPVN-POA of the female rat, however, a significant reduction in the volume to that of the male level was induced by a neonatal treatment of female rats with TP. This suggests that androgen may have caused a decrease in the number of AVPVN-POA neurons during the neonatal period. Thus, the same hormone appears to act on the AVPN in a reverse way than it does on the SDN-POA.

In a study to examine the effect of androgen on the neural substrates of the developing AVPVN-POA, the AVPVN-POA cell death pattern between normal and androgenized female rats was compared (Murakami and Arai, 1989). From the day of birth, female Wistar rats were treated with 50 μg of TP for 5 days, after which both the degenerating cells (pycnotic cells) and the normal cells in every third section were counted from days 1 to 13 of life. As shown in Figure 4, in the normal females pycnotic cells are found in the developing AVPVN-POA during the first 10 days of life. The incidence of pycnotic cells per 1000 cells is low at

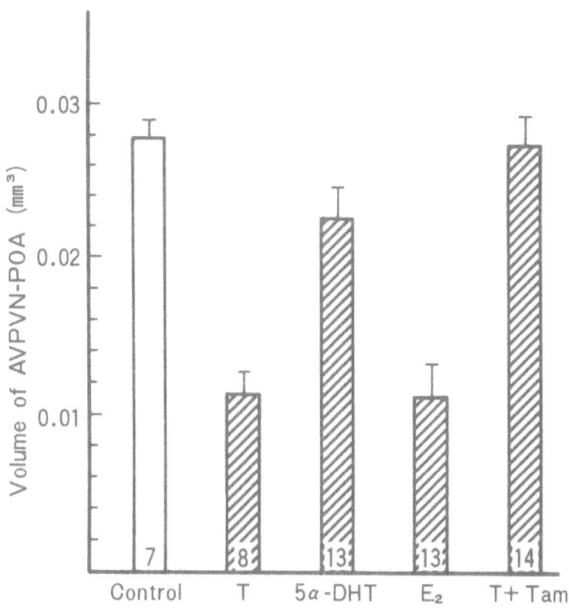

**Figure 3**   Effect of sex steroids given neonatally for the first 5 days of life on the volume of the AVPVN-POA. T: 500 μg of testosterone for the first 5 days of life. 5α-DHT: 500 μg of 5α-dihydrotestosterone for 5 days from the day of birth. E2: 50 μg of estradiol for 5 days from the day of birth. T+Tam: 100 μg of tamoxifen was injected concurrently with 500 μg testosterone for the first 5 days of life. Control and injected females were sacrificed at 90 days of age. Numbers at the bottom of the columns refer to the number of rats examined.

day 1, and reaches the maximal level at day 3, after which there is a gradual decrease to a rate of 0.83 per 1000 cells by day 10. In the TP-treated females, however, a high pycnotic rate level is maintained from days 3-7, followed by a gradual decrease to day 13. Although there is no significant difference in the pycnotic rate between normal and TP-treated females at days 3 and 5, the rate in the TP-treated females at day 7 is almost twice as high as that of the controls ($P < 0.001$). In both groups, however, the pycnotic rate at day 10 decreases to less than half of the value seen at day 7, respectively, but it remains significantly higher in the TP-treated females than in the normal females ($P < 0.001$). At day 13, pycnotic cells are still present in the TP-treated females, whereas they are almost absent in the normal females.

These results suggest that androgen effectively prolongs the active period for cell death in the developing AVPVN-POA, and it may be that this androgen sensitive degeneration of the AVPVN-POA neurons during early postnatal life contributes to a decrease in the nuclear volume. The possible factors responsible for neuronal death may be competition amongst the neurons for correct afferent and efferent synaptic contacts and a chemical environment that includes neurotrophic substances and hormones. However, the precise mode of action of the androgen on these AVPVN-POA neurons still remains unknown.

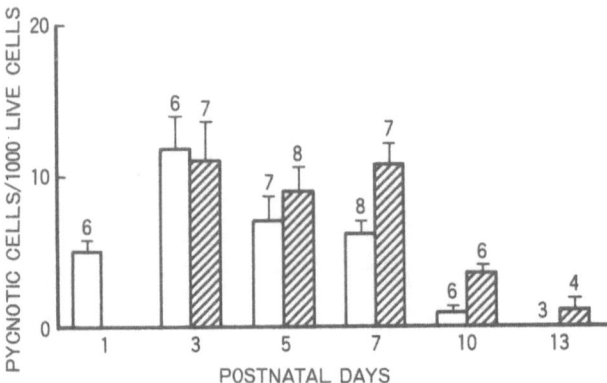

**Figure 4** Ratio of degenerating cells to 1000 normal cells in the AVPVN-POA of normal (open colum) and TP-treated (obliquelly lined column) female rats over the first 13 postnatal days. Numbers on the vertical lines refer to the number of rats examined.

# Prenatal development of AVPVN-POA and androgen

As shown in Figure 2, prenatal TP treatment of male and female rats significantly decreases the AVPVN volume. This indicates that the period during which the neural substrates of the AVPVN-POA are sensitive to androgen ranges from the prenatal to neonatal period.

Since neurogenesis of the AVPVN-POA neurons has been found to occur from E 13 to 18 (Nishizuka and Arai, 1987), the effect of androgen on the prenatal AVPVN-POA development was investigated. Pregnant female rats were injected with 2 mg of TP for 3 days (days 14-16 of pregnancy = E 14-16) and sacrificed at E 17. Other pregnant females were injected with 2 mg of TP for 5 days from E 14-18 or for 2 days from E 17-18 and sacrificed at E 21. In all rat groups, 50 mg of bromodeoxyuridine (BrdU), a thymidine analogue, was injected intraperitoneally at E 15.

The AVPVN-POA is identified in a small cluster of periventricular cells from the surrounding area in the fetal brain. As shown in Table I, male-female difference in the number of neurons in the AVPVN-POA is already detectable at E 21. TP given from E 14-18 (but not E 17-18) effectively reduced the number of neurons in the female AVPVN-POA. As to the distribution of BrdU-labeled neurons in the AVPVN-POA, no difference can be seen among males, androgenized females and normal females when examined at E 17 (Figure 5).

At E 21, however, a significant reduction in the number of BrdU-labeled neurons in the AVPVN-POA is observable in males and females treated with TP from E 1 4-18 (Figure 5). That the number of the BrdU-labeled neurons does not significantly differ between the normal and the androgenized females sacrificed at E 17 may indicate that the significant reduction of BrdU-labeled neurons

**Table I** Effect of prenatal androgen on incidence of pycnotic cells (per 100 cells) in the AVPVN-POA.

| Treatment | Pycnotic cells (%) E 17 | E 21 | Number of cells in AVPVN-POA E 21 |
|---|---|---|---|
| Oil-female | 0.2±0.1 | 0.4±0.1 | 302.2 ± 7.1 |
| Oil male | 0.2±0.1 | 0.9±0.2* | 221.3±13.9* |
| TP(E14-18)-female | 0.3±0.1 | 1.0±0.1* | 234.2± 8.6* |

* vs oil-female P < 0.05

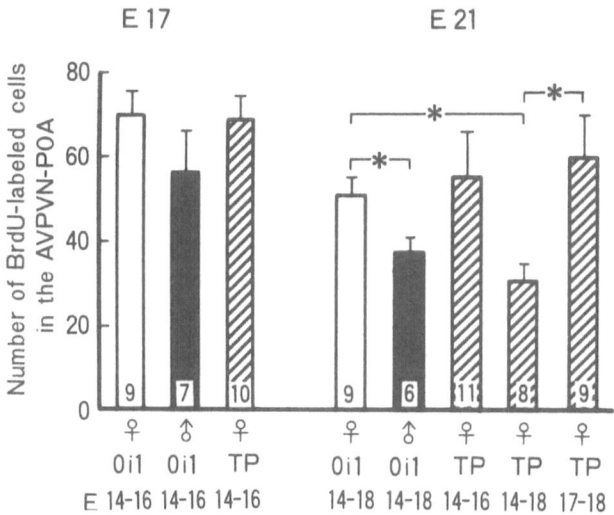

**Figure 5** Effect of androgen on the number of BrdU-labeled cells in AVPVN-POA during prenatal development. TP was given from E 14-18, E 14-16 or E 17-18. BrdU was given at E 15. Animals were sacrificed at E 17 or 2l. * P < 0.05.

observed at E 21 in the females injected with TP from E 14-18 is not the result of suppression of neurogenesis in the AVPVN-POA neurons by androgen, but rather due to the cell death of newly generated AVPVN-POA neurons.

At E 17, the incidence of pycnotic cells per 100 cells in the AVPVN-POA is not significantly different among males, females and females injected with TP from E 14-16 (Table I). When examined at E 21, however, the incidence of pycnotic cells in male and androgenized females significantly increases, when compared to that of the normal females. This suggests that testicular or exogenous androgen may stimulate cell death, which occurs more frequently after E 17.

Within the AVPVN-POA, sex-specific differences have been found to exist in the relative amounts of enkephalin- and peptide E-immunoreactive neurons (Simerly et al., 1988). A specific reduction of tyrosine hydroxylase immunoreactive neurons, which show a sexually dimorphic distribution in the AVPVN-POA, also has been found to be caused by neonatal androgen treatment (Simerly et al., 1985). Although it could not be determined whether the cell population of the androgen-sensitive degenerating cells in the TP-treated females is the same type of cell population in which cell death occurred neonatally in the control female rats, it could be speculated that androgen-sensitive degeneration in the AVPVN-POA might correlate with the reduction in these sexually dimorphic AVPVN-POA neurons.

# Synaptic sexual dimorphism in AVPVN-POA

At an electron microscopic level, sex difference in the synaptic organization are detectable in the AVPVN-POA. According to the site of the synaptic contact, three types of synapses have been roughly classified: a shaft synapse occurring on the dendritic shaft, a spine synapse on dendritic spine, and a somatic synapse on the cell body. In the AVPVN-POA, the number of both shaft and spine synapses is significantly greater in the male than in the female (Table II).

Table II Sexual dimorphism in synaptic number in the AVPVN-POA.

| Type of synapse | Male (6) per 9000 | Female (7) sq µm |
|---|---|---|
| Shaft synapse | 562 ± 33 * | 459 ± 30 |
| Spine synapse | 150 ± 13 * | 114 ± 11 |
| Somatic synapse | 39 ± 6 | 41 ± 5 |

* vs female P < 0.05

However, the number of somatic synapses is less and there is no significant difference between males and females. As the low neuronal density in the male AVPVN-POA (Table I) provides a larger neuropil area than in the female, this may account for the greater synaptic density in the male AVPVN-POA.

The neuropil matrix in the POA-hypothalamus and limbic brain is still in an immature state during the neonatal period, and the major neural circuit networks for operating postpubertal neuroendocrine and behavioral regulation have yet to be established at this period. Thus, the sexually undifferentiated neuropil of the neural substrates, which contain abundant steroid receptors, may be subjected to organizational action of gonadal steroids (Arai et al., 1986). As a matter of fact, estrogen is known to markedly stimulate axonal and dendritic differentiation and synapse formation during postnatal development. In the medial amygdaloid nucleus (Nishizuka and Arai, 1981a), for example, estrogen was found to specifically promote the formation of shaft synapses. This provides clear evidence of an underlying mechanism for the synaptic sexual differentiation of this nucleus, since the sex difference can be attributed to a significant increase in the number of shaft synapses in response to the organizational influence of the sex steroids in males (Nishizuka and Arai, 1981b).

# Neuronal plasticity of the AVPVN-POA to estrogen in the post-pubertal brain

In addition to the organizational effect of the sex steroids in the perinatal brain, estrogen has a facilitatory effect on synapse formation in peripubertal and adult rats. When a single dose of pregnant mare's serum gonadotropin (PMSG, 20 IU) is given to 28-day-old female rats, a precocious ovulation occurs 3 days later. Concurrently, the synaptic number in the rat arcuate nucleus increases and reaches an adult level within 3 days (Matsumoto and Arai, 1977). Since PMSG fails to increase the number of synapses in the arcuate nucleus of ovariectomized rats, the ovarian estrogen appears to play a facilitatory role in the maturation of synaptic organization in the arcuate nucleus of these animals. A similar precocious synaptogenesis in the arcuate nucleus has been reported in immature rats in which a precocious ovulation was induced by an administration of estrogen (Clough and Rodriguez-Sierra, 1983).

During the postnatal development of the AVPVN-POA, the volume of the AVPVN-POA is not yet marked enough to distinguish a sex difference between males and females. Subsequently, the volume of the female AVPVN-POA increases significantly around the onset of puberty, whereas no significant increase is seen in the male AVPVN-POA (Figure 6). Estrogen secretion at the onset of puberty may oscillate male-female difference in the AVPVN-POA, because castration prevents the female AVPVN-POA from increasing its volume following PMSG injection, whereas estrogen induces a significant increase in the AVPVN-POA volume in castrated females (Figure 7). Recently, however, a report has indicated that the AVPVN-POA volume was altered in castrated adult male rats by estrogen and progesterone treatment (Bloch and Gorski, 1988).

Estrogen can also affect synaptic remodelling in certain neuronal circuits which possess considerable plasticity and where vacated synaptic sites are made available by spontaneous degeneration or surgical deafferentation (Matsumoto and Arai, 1981; Arai et al., 1986). In some brain areas, the lateral septum for example, a sexually dimorphic synaptic plasticity to estrogen has been reported (Miyakawa and Arai, 1987). Furthermore, the dendritic spine density on adult hippocampal pyramidal neurons has been found to show cyclic fluctuations during the estrous cycle (Woolley et al., 1990).

These results suggest that even in the adult, gonadal steroids can have morphological effects. The effects of steroids in the adult animals, however, appear to be less dramatic than the impact they have during the development, and these effects may be plastic or to some extent reversible. However, the evidence that has been presented strengthens the possibility that the steroid hormones play a significant role in influencing the morphological development of the brain from the perinatal through the adult stage.

320

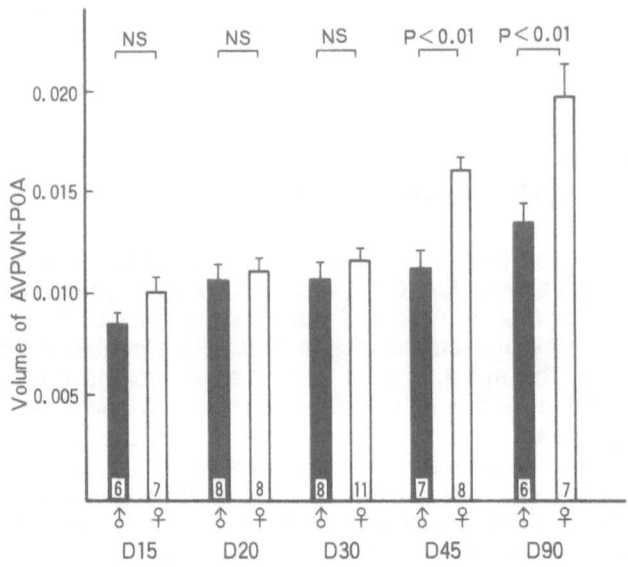

**Figure 6**    Age-related changes in the volume of the AVPVN-POA in male and female rats.

## Acknowledgements

The works reported from authors' laboratories were supported by research grants from the Japanese Ministry of Education, Culture and Science and the Ministry of Health and Welfare.

## References

Allen, L. S., Hines, M., Shryne, J. E. and Gorski, R. A. (1989).Two sexually dimorphic cell groups in the human brain. *J. Neurosci.*, **9** : 497-506.

Arai,Y., Matsumoto, A. and Nishizuka, M. (1986). Synaptogenesis and neuronal plasticity to gonadal steroid: implications for the development of sexual dimorphism in the neuroendocrine brain. In: Ganten, D. and Pfaff, D. (Eds.), *Current Topics in Neuroendocrinology 7*, Springer-Verlag, Berlin Heidelberg New York, pp. 291-307.

Bleier, R., Byne, W. and Siggelkow, I. (1982). Cytoarchitectonic sexual dimorphism of the medial preoptic area and anterior hypothalamuic areas in guinea pig, rat, hamster, and mouse. *J. Comp. Neurol.*, **212** : 118-183.

Bloch, G. J. and Gorski, R. A. (1988). Estrogen/progesterone treatment in adulthood affects the size of several components of the medial preoptic area in the male rat. *J. Comp. Neurol.*, **275** : 725-730.

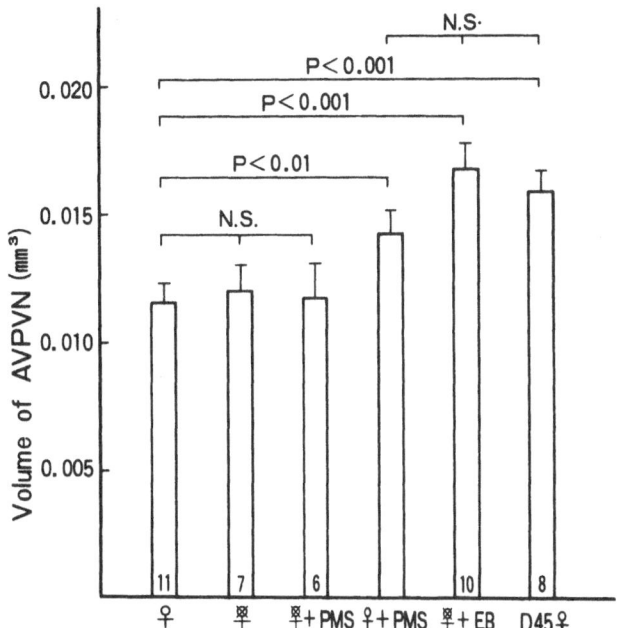

**Figure 7**   Effect of PMSG- and EB-induced precocious puberty on the volume of the AVPVN-POA in prepubertal female rats.

Clough, R. W. and Rodriguez-Sierra, J. F. (1983). Synaptic changes in the hypothalamus of the prepubertal female rat administered estrogen. *Am. J. Anat.*, **167** : 205-214.

Commins, D. and Yahr, P. (1984). Adult testosterone levels influence the morphology of a sexually dimorphic area in the mongolian gerbil brain. *J. Comp. Neurol.*, **224** : 132-140.

Gorski, R. A. (1990). Structural sexual dimorphism in the brain. In: Krasnegor, N. A. and Bidges, R. (Eds.), *Mammalian Parenting: Biological and Behavioral Determinants*, Oxford University Press, London / New York, pp.61-90.

Gorski, R. A., Gordon, J. H., Shryne, J. E. and Southam, A. M. (1978). Evidence for a morphological sex difference within the medial preoptic area of the rat brain. *Brain Res.*,**148** : 333-346.

Hines, M., Davies, F. C., Coquelin, A., Goy, R. W. and Gorski, R. A. (1985). Sexually dimorphic regions in the medial preoptic area and the bed nucleus of the stria terminalis of the guinea pig brain: a description and an investigation of their relationship to gonadal steroids in adulthood. *J. Comp. Neurol.*, **144** : 193-204.

322

Ito, S., Murakami, S., Yamanouchi, K. and Arai, Y. (1986a). Prenatal androgen exposure, preoptic area and reproductive functions in the female rat. *Brain Develop.*, **8** : 463-468.

Ito, S., Murakami, S., Yamanouchi, K. and Arai, Y. (l986b). Perinatal androgen exposure decreases the size of the sexually dimorphic medial preoptic nucleus in the rat. *Proc. Japan Acad.*, **62B** : 408-411.

LeVay, S. (1991). A difference in the hypothalamic structure between heterosexual and homosexual men. *Science*, **253** : 1034-1037.

Matsumoto, A. and Arai, Y. (1977). Precocious puberty and synaptogenesis in the hypothalamic arcuate nucleus in pregnant mare serum gonadotropin (PMSG) treated immature females. *Brain Res.*, **129** : 275-278.

Matsumoto, A. and Arai, Y. (1981). Neuronal plasticity in the deafferented hypothalamic arcuate nucleus of adult female rat and its enhancement by treatment with estrogen. *J. Comp. Neurol.*, **197** : 197-205.

Matsumoto, A. and Arai, Y. (1983). Sex difference in volume of the ventromedial nucleus of the hypothalamus in the rat. *Endocrinol. Japon.*, **30** : 277-280.

Miyakawa, M. and Arai, Y. (1987). Synaptic plasticity in the lateral septum of the adult male and female rats. *Brain Res.*, **436** : 184-188.

Mizukami, S., Nishizuka, M. and Arai, Y. (1983). Sexual difference in nuclear and its ontogeny in the rat amygdala. *Exp. Neurol.*, **79** : 569-575.

Murakami, S. and Arai, Y. (1989). Neuronal death in the developing sexually dimorphic periventricular nucleus of the preoptic area in the female rat: effect of neonatal androgen treatment. *Neurosci. Lett.*, **102** : 185-190.

Nishizuka, M. and Arai, Y. (l981a). Organizational action of estrogen on synaptic pattern in the amygdala: implications for sexual differentiation of the brain. *Brain Res.*, **213** : 422-426.

Nishizuka, M. and Arai, Y. (1981b). Sexual dimorphism in the synaptic organization in the amygdala and its dependence on neonatal hormone environment. *Brain Res.*, **212** : 31-38.

Nishizuka, M. and Arai, Y. (1987). Neurogenesis in the medial preoptic nucleus of the rat: bromodeoxyuridine (BrdU)- anti BrdU monoclonal antibody method. *Zool. Sci.*, **4** : 1082.

Nordeen, E. J., Nordeen, K. W,. Senglaub, D. R. and Arnold, A. P. (1985). Androgen prevents normally occurring cell death in a sexually dimorphic spinal nucleus. *Science*, **229** : 671-673.

Simerly, R. B., McCall, L. D. and Watson, S. D. (l988). Distribution of opioid peptides in preoptic region: immunochemical evidence for a steroid-sensitive enkephalin sexual dimorphism. *J. Comp. Neurol.*, 276 : 442-459.

Simerly, R. B., Swanson, L. W., Handa, R. J. and Gorski, R. A. (1985). Influence of perinatal androgen on the sexually dimorphic distribution of tyrosine hydroxylase-immunoreactive cells and fibers in the anteroventral periventricular nucleus of the rat. *Neuroendocrinol.*, **40** : 501-510.

Swaab, D. F. and Fliers, E. (1985). A sexually dimorphic nucleus in the human brain. *Science*, **228** : 1112-1115.

Terasawa, E., Wiegand, S. J. and Bridson, W. E. (1980). A role for the medial preoptic nucleus on afternoon of proestrus in female rats. *Am. J. Physiol.*, **238** : 533-539.

Woolley, C. S., Gould. E., Frankfurt, M. and McEwen, B. S. (1990). II.Naturally occurring fluctuation in dendritic spine density on adult hippocampal pyramidal neurons. *J. Neurosci.*, **10** : 4035-4039.

# Mating-Induced Expression of Immediate-Early Genes in the Male and Female Nervous System

**M. J. BAUM**

*Department of Biology, Boston University, 5 Cummington Street, Boston, MA 02215, USA*

The existence of sex dimorphisms in the structure of the vertebrate nervous system was first inferred from the results of studies (reviewed in Baum, 1979; Goy and McEwen, 1980; Whalen, 1974) showing that perinatal exposure to androgens permanently altered the ability of female mammals to express either hetero- or homotypical courtship behaviors in later life. Thus, for example, female guinea pigs exposed prenatally to testosterone propionate later showed reduced levels of lordotic responsiveness to ovarian steroids and enhanced levels of mounting behavior in response to testosterone given in adulthood (Phoenix et al., 1959). These authors inferred that neural tissues controlling the expression of these steroid-dependent reproductive behaviors were 'organized' as a result of prenatal steroid manipulations, in a manner analogous to the androgen-induced organization of the Wolffian duct structures into the internal male accessory sex organs. It was more than a decade after the publication of the pioneering study by Phoenix et al. (1959) that Raisman and Field (1971) demonstrated a clear-cut sex dimorphism in synaptic organization of neurons in the rat preoptic area (POA), and showed that the male phenotype could be created in females by neonatal administration of testosterone whereas the female phenotype was created in males by neonatal castration. In the subsequent years even more striking sex dimorphisms in the cytoarchitecture, dendritic arborization, and connectivity of various forebrain structures were documented in species representing essentially every vertebrate class (reviewed in Tobet and Fox, 1992). This work also showed that early exposure to gonadal steroids played a crucial role in the development of these neural dimorphisms. In some species the link between neural sex dimorphisms and behavioral capacity was clearly established. Thus, in zebra finches the ability of the male to sing during courtship has been linked to the greater size and connectivity of several telencephalic nuclei in this sex, as compared with females (reviewed in Nottebohm, 1987). In mammals, however, it has been more difficult to establish a functional link between sexually dimorphic features of neural organization and sex differences in behavioral capacity. Thus, for example, males' capacity to exhibit mounting and other masculine coital behaviors depends on the functional integrity of the medial preoptic nucleus

*M. Haug et al. (eds.), The Development of Sex Differences and Similarities in Behavior, 325–339.*
© 1993 *Kluwer Academic Publishers.*

(mPOA) (reviewed in Everitt and Stacey, 1987); however, lesions restricted to the sexually dimorphic portions of this structure generally have been found to cause little long-lasting disruption of males' coital capacity in rats and ferrets (reviewed in Cherry and Baum, 1990).

Neuroscientists have for years sought techniques, in addition to using destructive lesions or electrical/chemical stimulation of selected brain regions, to reveal the neural pathways which are activated in the context of particular behaviors. In some instances multiunit or single cell recordings from particular brain regions have been used to correlate altered cellular activity and behavioral expression. However, in all of these instances the investigator is limited by his hypotheses concerning which region should be studied in a particular behavioral context. Furthermore, it is technically difficult to record neuronal activity in multiple brain sites from awake, behaving animals. For these reasons it was with considerable anticipation that behavioral neuroscientists witnessed the advent of studies in which the increased expression of a particular class of gene (immediate-early genes; IEG's) in a limited number of brain regions occurred in response to specific, behaviorally relevant stimuli.

Immediate-early genes, including c-fos and c-jun, are cellular homologues of viral proto-oncogenes (reviewed in Curran et al., 1990). Expression of these cellular IEG's in neurons is activated by synaptic inputs, resulting in the rapid synthesis of proteins (FOS and JUN, respectively), which dimerize and bind to a nuclear acceptor protein (AP-1). These events initiate a cascade of further gene transcription and long-term changes in cellular activity. One of the most functionally revealing examples of stimulus-induced IEG expression occurs in the suprachiasmatic nucleus (SCN) of the hamster in response to light pulses. Light pulses, presented to hamsters which are showing free-running activity rhythms while housed under constant darkness, cause phase shifting of the activity cycle only when presented during subjective night. Likewise, it is only at these circadian times that light pulses induce c-fos mRNA, FOS protein, jun-B mRNA, and AP-1 activity (indexed by a gel mobility-shift assay which measures light-induced increases in AP-1 binding to DNA) in SCN neurons which receive direct retinal inputs (Rusak et al., 1990; Kornhauser et al., 1992). Thus, light-induced IEG expression serves as a marker for neurons in the SCN which mediate the synchronizing action of this stimulus on the circadian clock. More work is needed to determine whether increased gene transcription, caused by IEG's, is a prerequisite for the phase shifting of the circadian clock caused by appropriately timed light pulses. My co-workers and I have sought to use the expression of the IEG, c-fos, as a marker of increased neuronal activity in order to compare the effects of genital and other modalities of stimulation derived from coital and sociosexual contact on the rat and ferret nervous system. In both species we have compared the profile of induced c-fos responses in the two sexes in the hope of gaining insight into similarities and differences in the neural processing of sexually relevant stimuli in males and females. A condensed description of some of our findings follows.

# Rat studies

## Males

In an initial study (Baum and Everitt, 1992) we screened the brain and spinal cord for FOS immunoreactivity (IR) 1h after male rats achieved 1-2 ejaculations (preceeded by numerous mounts and intromissions) with an estrous female. All subjects were sexually experienced adult males which were housed alone. Control males were placed by themselves for 1 h in the same type of circular test chamber used to test mating behavior in mated males, and killed 1 h later. After ejaculation, intense FOS-IR was seen in the medial preoptic area (mPOA), the bed nucleus of the stria terminalis (BNST), the caudal-dorsal portion of the medial amygdaloid nucleus (mAMYG), and in the dorsal-lateral aspects of the tegmentum (central tegmental field; CTF). (See examples of FOS-IR in Figure 1).

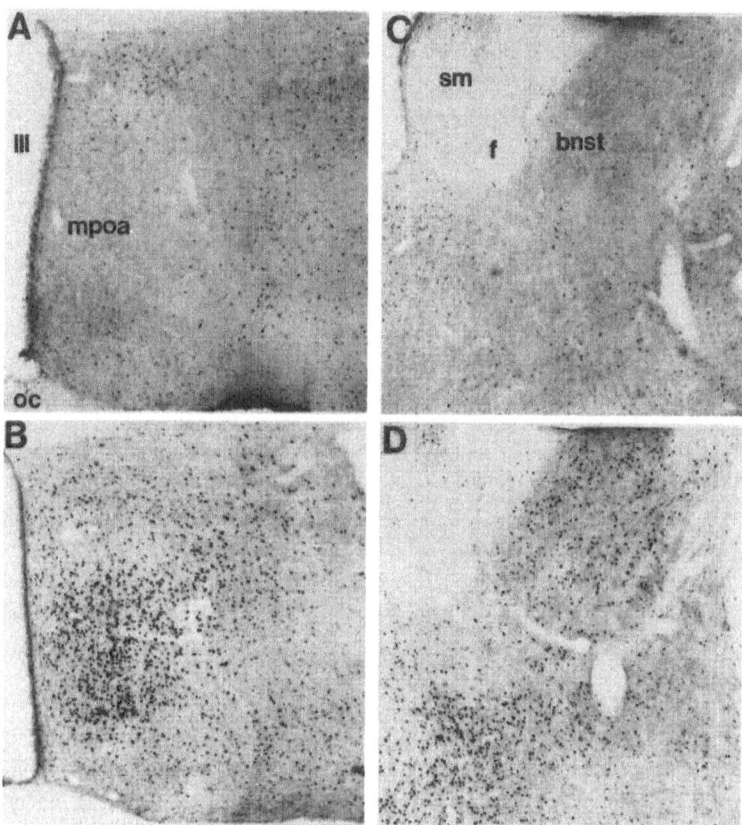

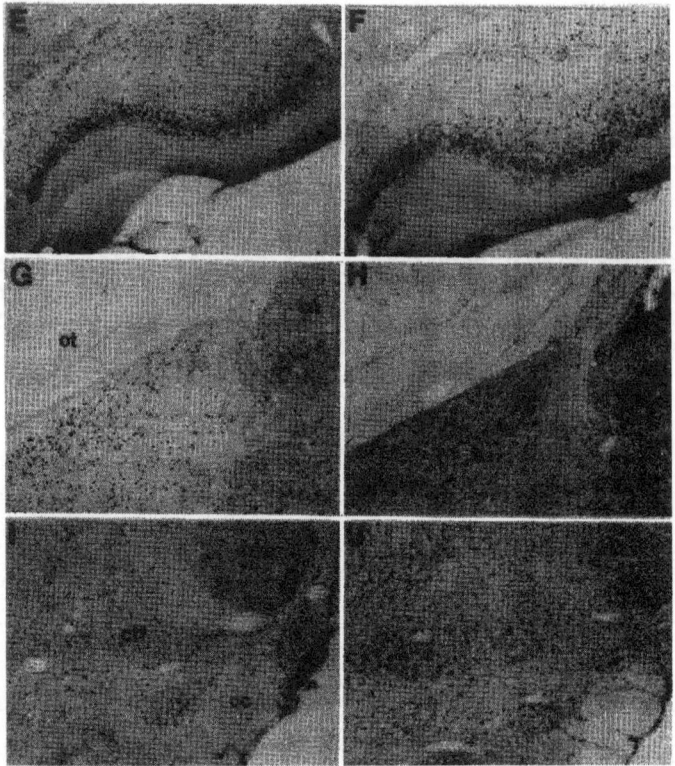

**Figure 1** Effect of mating on FOS-IR in rat brain. Photomicrographs of the medial POA (A,B), bed nucleus of the stria terminalis (C,D), piriform cortex (E,F), medial amygdala (G,H) and midbrain central tegmental field (I,J) from each of two rats, one naive male sacrificed 1h after spending 1h in an empty mating arena (A,C,E,G,I) and the other sacrificed 1h after ejaculation with an estrous female (B,D,F,H,J). In each site, except the piriform cortex, there is a marked increase in the number of FOS-IR nuclei following ejaculation. Abbreviations: III-third ventricle; cc-cerebral peduncle; cn-central amygdaloid nucleus; ctf-central tegmental field; f-fornix; mpoa-medial preoptic area; oc-optic chiasm; sm-stria medullaris; mgn-medial geniculate nucleus. Reproduced with permission from Baum and Everitt (1992).

A similar increase in FOS-IR was reported by Robertson et al. (1991) in the mPOA of male rats following numerous ejaculations. These workers also reported that FOS-IR was increased in the primary olfactory (piriform) cortex after ejaculation. In our experience, FOS-IR was always evident in piriform cortex even in males which were killed after exposure to an empty test arena. Robertson et al. (1991) compared FOS-IR in mated males and males which were simply taken from their home cages and killed. It seems likely that they mistook increased FOS-IR in piriform cortex, associated with a novel environment, for a response induced specifically by stimuli associated with mating with an estrous female.

In our studies (Baum and Everitt, 1992) graded increments in the number of FOS-IR neurons were obtained in the mPOA, BNST, and mAMYG as males were given increasing opportunity for direct physical contact with an estrous female. Thus, males which showed ano-genital sniffing and climbing over females (but no actual mounts or intromissions) had significantly more FOS-IR neurons in these brain regions. No such increments were seen in other males which were placed in a test arena containing a Plexiglas box (with holes around the base) into which an estrous female was placed. These data suggest that vomeronasal, as opposed to distal olfactory cues, may be required for the activation of c-fos in these brain regions. Indeed, in male hamsters application of vaginal secretions from estrous females directly to the nose was shown to increase FOS-IR in the above-mentioned sites (Fiber and Swann, 1991). Finally, we observed significant increments in FOS-IR in the midbrain CTF only in males which achieved several (5 or more) penile intromissions with the estrous female in the course of a test, suggesting that genital somatosensory stimuli are primarily responsible for the observed FOS response in this region.

Baum and Everitt (1992) have additional evidence that olfactory stimuli, derived from an estrous female, contribute to the observed increments in FOS-IR in the mAMYG. Numerous studies (reviewed in Winans et al., 1982) have established that both the primary and accessory olfactory bulbs project to the mAMGY, which in turn, projects to the BNST and on to the MPOA. We made large thermal lesions unilaterally in the olfactory peduncle, so as to interrupt both the primary and accessory olfactory inputs to the rest of the CNS. Several days later lesioned males were either allowed to ejaculate with an estrous female, or alternatively, were allowed only to mount (and occasionally intromit) with the female. This latter behavior was achieved by applying a local anesthetic paste (5% lidocaine) to the male's penis repeatedly prior to and during the behavioral test with an estrous female. Unilateral lesions of the olfactory peduncle significantly reduced FOS-IR in the ipsilateral piriform cortex (see Figure 2), confirming that these lesions effectively reduced olfactory inputs to the CNS in both groups of males. These olfactory lesions also significantly reduced FOS-IR ipsilaterally in the mAMYG, provided males only achieved mounts, and the occasional intromission, with their female partners (Figure 2). No further ipsilateral reductions in FOS-IR were seen in the BNST or mPOA of these males, suggesting that other types of sensory input, or contralateral olfactory inputs compensated for the lesion-induced loss of ipsilateral olfactory stimuli. Also, no lesion-induced assymetry in FOS-IR occurred in any brain region, including the mAMGY, of males which were allowed to ejaculate with the female. This suggests that genital, somatosensory stimuli readily compensate for any deficiency in olfactory inputs to the amgydala. Finally, FOS-IR in the midbrain CTF was significantly lower in males whose penes were smeared with lidocaine anesthetic, so as to prevent intromission and ejaculation, than in ejaculating males. This finding is consistent with, though not proof of, our earlier suggestion (see above) that the CTF FOS response to mating reflects primarily the action of genital, somasenory stimuli on these neurons.

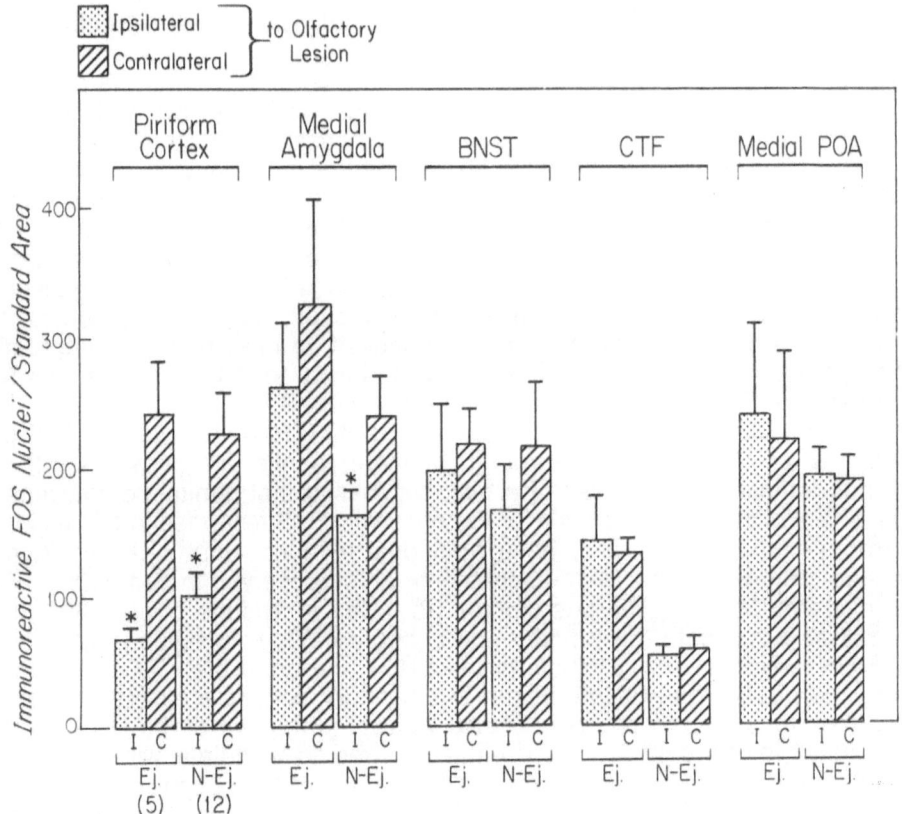

**Figure 2** Effect of unilateral, electrothermal lesions of the olfactory peduncle on mating-induced FOS-IR in brain regions ipsilateral and contralateral to the side of the olfactory lesion. Ej.-male rats which ejaculated with an estrous female 1h prior to sacrifice; no lidocaine anesthetic was applied to the penes of these males. N-Ej.-non-ejaculating males in which lidocaine was applied to the penes prior to and during mating tests, so that males displayed primarily mounts with thrusting, an occasional intromission, and no ejaculation. Males were killed 1h after completion of the behavioral test. Abbreviations: BNST-bed nucleus of the stria terminalis; CTF-central tegmental field. Data are expressed as mean ± SEM; the number of males in each group is given in parentheses. * P<0.05; Duncan's multiple range test comparisons with the contralateral side. Reproduced with permission from Baum and Everitt (1992).

The results described thus far all suggest that sensory stimuli, engendered in males as a result of physical (e.g., olfactory/vomeronasal and genital/somatosensory ) contacts with an estrous female augment c-fos expression in a polysynaptic circuit projecting to the mPOA. Baum and Everitt (1992) obtained further confirmation of this hypothesis by comparing the effects of excitotoxic lesions of these different FOS-responsive brain regions. In one study we found that placement of lesions (made with the NMDA receptor agonist, quinolinic ιcid) unilaterally in the mPOA failed to attenuate the ipsilateral FOS response to mating in either the mAMYG or midbrain CTF, although there was a reduction in FOS-IR in the ipsilateral BNST. By contrast, combined unilateral lesions of the nAMYG and midbrain CTF caused significant reductions in mating-induced FOS-IR in both the BNST and the mPOA. No such reduction in mating-induced FOS responses occurred in groups of males which received unilateral quinolinic acid lesions of either the mAMYG or the midbrain CTF. This suggests that parallel projections exist from the mAMYG and the midbrain CTF, respectively, and that heightened activity in either system can compensate for experimentally induced reductions in the other. Considered together, these data strongly suggest that the mating-induced FOS response in the mPOA depends on inputs from the mAMGY and midbrain CTF, and not the reverse.

The capacity of male rats to mate declines gradually over the weeks following castration and the resultant deprivation of steroid hormones (Davidson, 1966). Numerous studies (reviewed in Baum et al., 1987) suggest that estrogenic metabolites of circulating testosterone, formed directly in brain regions including the mPOA, contribute to this activational effect of sex steroid on males' sexual behavior. Several studies (Gibbs et al., 1990; Loose-Mitchell et al., 1988) suggest that estrogen stimulates c-fos mRNA and protein synthesis in rat uterus, and another study (Insel, 1990) points to a similar action of estradiol in the female rat mPOA and mAMYG. There is also evidence (Hyder et al., 1991) of an estradiol response region embedded in the mouse uterine c-fos oncogene. Finally, studies with male hamsters (Wood et al., 1992; Kollack and Newman, 1991) suggest that there is considerable overlap in the mAMYG cells which contain estradiol and androgen receptors and in which FOS-IR is elevated after mating. Both categories of neuron are located in the most caudal-dorsal portion of the mAMYG. Baum et al. (1992) asked whether testosterone, or its neural metabolites, estradiol and dihydrotestosterone, play a permissive role in the mating-induced activation of neural c-fos expression in the male rat? Sexually experienced male rats were castrated and treated daily with either testosterone propionate, estradiol benzoate, dihydrotestosterone propionate, or oil vehicle. Seven days later males were allowed to achieve 8 intromissions with an estrous female, whereupon they were killed 1h later and their brains processed for FOS-IR. We found that the number of FOS-IR neurons present in mPOA, mAMYG, and midbrain CTF was equivalent in all groups, suggesting that gonadal steroids contribute little, if anything, to the ability of sensory stimuli (i.e., olfactory/vomeronasal and genital/somatosensory) to augment neural c-fos expression.

## Females

Wersinger et al. (1992) recently compared the distribution of neural FOS-IR in the brains of male and female rats following mating, in order to determine whether the two sexes differentially process the resultant sensory stimuli. Male and female rats were gonadectomized and subsequently treated for 4 consecutive days with estradiol benzoate (5 µg/kg). On the morning of the fifth post-operative day, rats of both sexes received progesterone. Four hours later male-female pairs were placed together until the male ejaculated, whereupon both animals were killed 1 h later, and the brains processed for FOS-IR. Control male and female rats received the same sequence of endocrine treatments, but were killed after being placed alone in a test arena. We observed a striking similarity between the sexes in the localization and number of FOS-IR cells after mating, with intense responses being noted in the mPOA, mAMYG, BNST, and midbrain CTF. It seems likely that genital/somatosensory inputs, as opposed to olfactory/vomeronasal stimulation, were primarily responsible for the increased c-fos expression observed in this study. First, as already described (above) for males, when ejaculation was allowed to occur we were unable to reduce FOS-IR in forebrain sites by interupting olfactory afferents to these sites. Second, in females which received an ejaculation from a male, bilateral transection of the pelvic nerves completely blocked the activation of c-fos expression observed in the above-mentioned forebrain regions (Erskine and Rowe, 1992). Thus the neural circuits which respond to these genital/somatosensory inputs, at least as revealed by the observed patterns of c-fos response, are very similar in the two sexes. More work is needed to see whether the same is true of the pathways which process olfactory inputs to the CNS. We hypothesize that olfactory/vomeronasal stimuli more readily activate c-fos expression in the mAMYG, BNST, and mPOA of male than female rats.

# Ferret studies

In the rat and many other rodent species pre-ovulatory LH surges are normally induced in the female as a consequence of the action of estradiol and progesterone on forebrain LHRH neurons. Hoffman and co-workers have recently shown that these steroidal signals augment c-fos expression in LHRH neurons of the female rat. In one such study (Lee et al., 1990) this effect was noted in ovary-intact females on the night of proestrus, when the pre-ovulatory LH surge normally occurs. In another study (Lee et al., 1990a) exogenous estradiol and progesterone exerted similar effects on c-fos expression in forebrain LHRH neurons in juvenile female, but not male, rats. This sexual dimorphism corresponds nicely with the dimorphic response of gonadectomized, estrogen-primed male and female rats to the LH positive feedback actions of estradiol: only females respond (Neill, 1972).

Carroll et al. (1987) have pursued the question of sexually dimorphic control of LH secretion in a carnivore, the ferret, in which the female shows a preovulatory surge in LH secretion in response to somatosensory stimuli derived from receipt of a male's penile intromission as opposed to a steroidal signal. Receipt of an intromission provokes a massive surge in plasma LH in estrous female ferrets, which lasts for more than 12h. By contrast, in male ferrets achieving an intromission either inhibits or causes no change in the pituitary secretion of LH and the testicular secretion of testosterone (Carroll et al., 1987; Lambert and Baum, 1991). The results (Carroll et al., 1987) also show that pituitary responsiveness to exogenous LHRH is similar in male and female ferrets, suggesting that the observed sex dimorphism in LH-responsivess to intromissive stimulation results from a dimorphism in the ability of genital/somatosensory stimulation to activate forebrain LHRH neurons.

Results of two recent studies (Lambert et al., 1992, 1992a) support this view. In an initial study the mediobasal hypothalamus (including pituitary and pituitary stalk; MBH) was removed from female and male ferrets at different intervals after receipt of or achievement of an intromission, respectively, and perfused *in vitro* with oxogenated Kreb's-Ringer phosphate buffer. For each sex, the *in vitro* release of LHRH from MBH was thus compared in mated versus unpaired ferrets in breeding condition. In females the basal release of LHRH was significantly reduced in MBH tissues collected within .25h of intromission onset. No such reduction was seen in MBH taken from females 1 h after onset of intromission, and LHRH release actually tended to be higher in mated versus unpaired females killed 2.6h after onset of intromission. This profile of *in vitro* LHRH data suggests that receipt of an intromission by the female ferret causes an immediate outpouring of LHRH into the pituitary portal vessels, which depletes presynaptic MBH terminals of peptide such that the capacity for *in vitro* release .25h after onset of intromission is significantly reduced, compared with unpaired females. The lack of any difference between mated and unpaired females killed 1 or 2.6 h after mating suggests that by this time synthesis and / or post-translational processing of LHRH precursor peptide had compensated for the initial deficiency in releasable stores of the neuropeptide. In contrast to females, males killed .25h after onset of intromission showed a basal *in vitro* release of LHRH from the MBH which was equivalent to that seen in unpaired breeding males. This result suggests that no mating-induced release of LHRH from presynaptic MBH terminals occurs in the male.

The results of a second study, in which mating-induced increments in FOS-IR were studied in LHRH-IR neurons, provide further support for the hypothesis that intromissive stimulation selectively augments activity (and peptide secretion) of LHRH neurons in the female ferret forebrain. Photos of LHRH-IR neurons with and without co-labelled FOS-IR nuclei are shown in Figure 3. We found that the percentage of LHRH-IR neurons co-labelled with nuclear FOS-IR was significantly greater in mated versus unpaired females whereas no such effect was seen in mated males (Figure 4). Note that the significant stimulatory effects of mating on LHRH neuronal c-fos expression were evident at all levels of the female's preoptic-hypothalamic continuum. This suggests that a diffuse group of LHRH neurons contributes to the LHRH signal which reaches the anterior pituitary gland and stimulates LH secretion following mating. This distribution of co-labelled FOS and LHRH neurons differs from that seen in female rats, in which the co-labelled cells are primarily restricted to the organum vasculosum of the laminae terminalis and mPOA.

Perhaps not surprisingly, the ability of mating to induce FOS-IR in non-LHRH neurons differed in male and female ferrets (Lambert et al., 1992a). In females receipt of an intromission caused significant increments in FOS-IR in the mAMYG, mPOA, and BNST whereas in males intromission significantly augmented FOS-IR only in the mAMYG. Thus in the ferret, in contrast to the rat, there was a striking sex dimorphism in the ability of genital/somatosensory stimulation to augment c-fos expression in limbic and hypothalamic sites. More information about the effects of mating on the expression of c-fos in midbrain

334

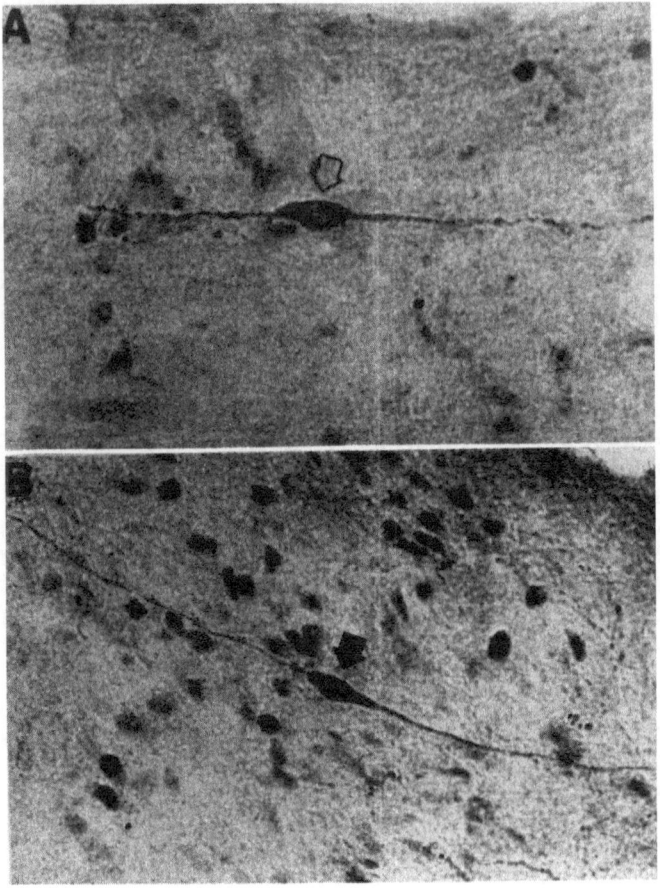

**Figure 3** Effect of mating on FOS-IR in LHRH and non-LHRH neurons of the female ferret forebrain. (A). An LHRH-IR neuron with reaction product in the cytoplasm but no immunoreactivity over the nucleus (i.e., no FOS-IR; open arrow). (B). An LHRH-IR neuron that also contains FOS-IR over the nucleus (closed arrow). These examples are from a mated, female ferret. Reproduced with permission from Lambert et al., 1992a.

sites (especially the CTF) is needed for ferrets of both sexes. Likewise, we need to determine whether olfactory, visual, or auditory stimuli (excluding genital/somatosensory stimuli) by themselves can augment neural c-fos expression in ferrets of either sex. The available data suggest that genital stimulation is conveyed in both male and female ferrets to the mAMYG. In

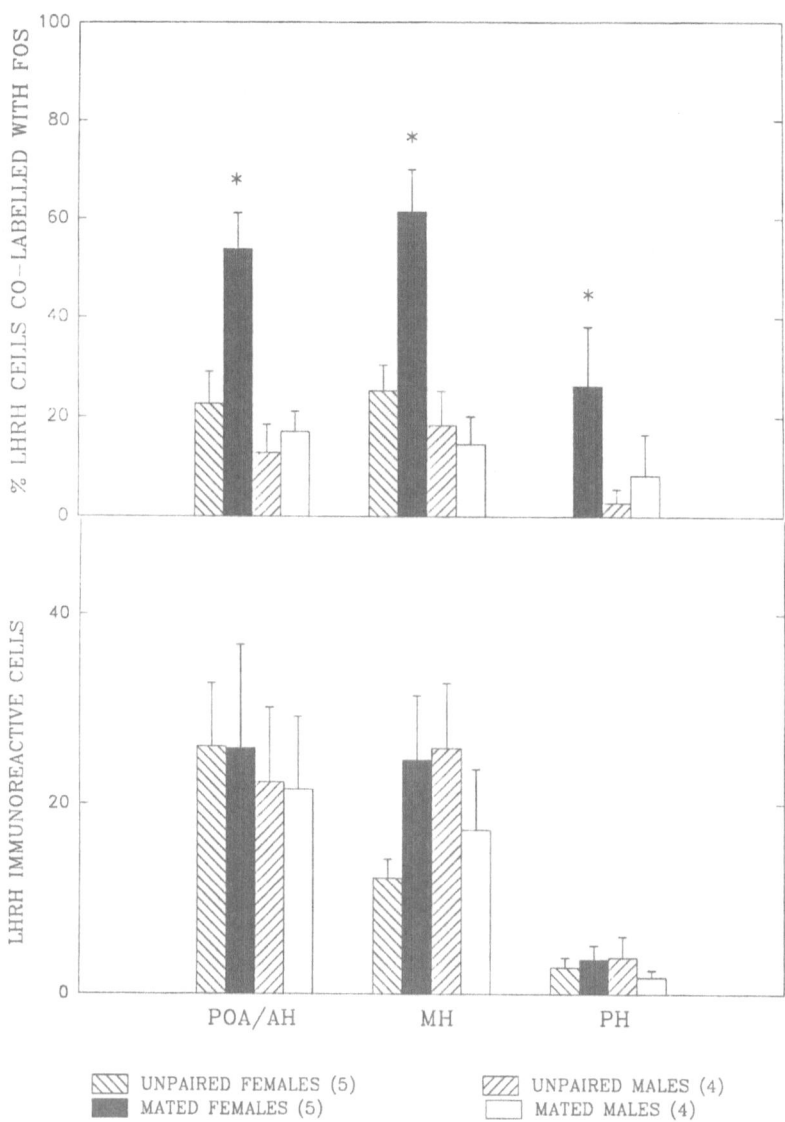

**Figure 4** Effect of mating on FOS-IR in LHRH neurons of male and female ferrets. The total number of LHRH-IR neurons (lower panel) and the percentage of LHRH-IR neurons which were co-labelled with nuclear FOS-IR (upper panel) in coronal sections from the preoptic/anterior hypothalamic area (POA/AH), the medial (MH), and posterior (PH) hypothalamus of mated and unpaired male and female ferrets. Data are presented as mean ± SEM. The number of ferrets in each group is given in parentheses. * P<0.05, Duncan's multiple range test comparisons with unpaired females. Reproduced with permission from Lambert et al., 1992a.

absence of an input mechanism to MBH LHRH neurons. Previous studies females such input is further projected to the BNST and mPOA, and then on to a diffuse network of LHRH neurons in the MBH. In males genital input appears to reach the mAMYG, but fails to go further either due to active inhibition or the (Tobet et al., 1986, 1986a) have established the existence in male ferrets of a nucleus of the dorsal POA/AH, which is not found in females. Descrete lesions of this male nucleus of the POA/AH in male ferrets augmented their proceptive responsiveness to increasing dosages of estradiol benzoate, suggesting that this structure may tonically inhibit this aspect of feminine responsiveness in males (Cherry and Baum, 1990). Future studies will explore the possible contribution of this male nucleus of the POA/AH to the inability of coital stimulation to activate LHRH neurons in this sex. For example, might unilateral neurotoxic lesions of the Mn-POA/AH facilitate the ability of intromission to stimulate c-fos expression in ipsilateral MBH LHRH neurons?

# Conclusion

Monitoring the neural expression of c-fos after exposure to stimuli associated with mating has provided a useful index of activation in neural pathways which convey sexually relevant sensory information into the male and female brain. The biological significance, if any, of the augmented expression of c-fos after mating has yet to be established. What is clear, however, is that useful information about differences and similarities between the sexes in the processing of sensory inputs derived from mating (either in specific cell types - e.g. LHRH - or in otherwise unspecified types of neurons) can be obtained using this method.

# Acknowledgments

I am grateful to numerous collaborators, including Barry Everitt, Rona Carroll, Mary Erskine, Stuart Tobet, Geralyn Lambert, James Cherry, Scott Wersinger, and Beverly Rubin for their important contributions to the work described herein. This research was supported by U.S. public health service grants HD21094 and MH00394.

# References

Baum, M. J. (1979). Differentiation of coital behavior in mammals : a comparative analysis. *Neurosci. Biobehav. Rev.*, **3** : 265-284.

Baum, M. J. and Everitt, B. J. (1992). Increased expression of c-fos in the medial preoptic area after mating in the male rat : role of afferent input from the medial amygdala and midbrain central tegmental field. *Neurosci.*, **50** : 627-646.

Baum, M. J., Kingsbury, P. A. and Erskine, M. S. (1987). Failure of the synthetic androgen, R1881, to duplicate the activational effect of testosterone on mating in castrated male rats. *J. Endocr.*, **113** : 15-20.

Baum, M. J., Wersinger, S. R. and Alvarez, J. C. (1992). Equivalent levels of mating-induced neural c-fos immunoreactivity in castrated male rats given androgen, estrogen, or no steroid replacement. *Soc. Neurosci. Abstr.*, **18** : 892.

Carroll, R. S., Erskine, M. S. and Baum, M. J. (1987). Sex difference in the effect of mating on the pulsatile secretion of luteinizing hormone in a reflex ovulator, the ferret. *Endocrinology*, **121** : 1349-1359.

Cherry J. A. and Baum, M. J. (1990). Effects of lesions of a sexually dimorphic nucleus in the preoptic/anterior hypothalamic area on the expression of androgen- and estrogen-dependent sexual behaviors in male ferrets. *Brain Res.*, **522** : 191-203.

Curran, T., Abate, C., Cohen, D. R., MacGregor, P. F., Rauscher I. F. J., Sonnenberg, J. L., Connor, J. A. and Morgan, J. I. (1990). Inducible proto-oncogene transcription factors : third messengers in the brain? Cold Spring Harbor Symposium, *Quant. Biol.*, **55** : 225-234.

Davidson, J. M. (1966). Characteristics of sex behaviour in male rats following castration. *Anim. Behav.*, **14** : 266-272.

Erskine, M. S. and Rowe, D. W. (1992). Induction of c-fos in the female rat brain in response to mating : role of afferent input via the pelvic nerve. *Soc. Neurosci. Abstr.*, **18** : 891.

Everitt, B. J. and Stacey, P. (1987). Studies of instrumental behavior with sexual reinforcement in male rats : II. Effects of preoptic area lesions, castration, and testosterone. *J. Comp. Psych.*, **101** : 407-419.

Fiber, J. M. and Swann, J. M. (1991). Female hamster vaginal secretion stimulates c-fos expression in the vomeronasal organ and olfactory mating behavior pathways in the male golden hamster. *Soc. Neurosci. Abstr.*, **17** : 1060.

Gibbs, R. B., Mobbs, C. V. and Pfaff, D. W. (1990). Sex steroids and fos expression in rat brain and uterus. *Mol. Cell. Neurosci.*, **1** : 29-40.

Goy, R. W. and McEwen, B. S. (1980). *Sexual Differentiation of the Brain*, MIT Press, Cambridge, MA.

Hyder, S. M., Stancel, G. M. and Loose-Mitchell, D. S. (1991). Presence of an estradiol response region in the mouse c-fos oncogene. *Steroids*, **56** : 498-504.

Insel, T. R. (1990). Regional induction of c-fos-like protein in rat brain after estradiol administration. *Endocrinology*, **126** : 1849-1853.

Lambert, G. M. and Baum, M. J. (1991). Reciprocal relationships between pulsatile androgen secretion and the expression of mating behavior in adult male ferrets. *Horm. Behav.*, **25** : 382-393.

Lambert, G. M., Rubin, B. S. and Baum, M. J. (1992). Sexual dimorphism in the effects of mating on the in vitro release of LHRH from the ferret medio-basal hypothalamus. *Physiol. Behav.*, **52** : 809-813.

Lambert, G. M., Rubin, B. S. and Baum, M. J. (1992a). Sex difference in the effect of mating on c-fos expression in LHRH neurons of the ferret forebrain. *Endocrinology*, **131** : 1473-1480.

Kollack, S. S. and Newman, S. W. (1991). Induction of c-fos immunoreactivity within the neural circuitry underlying copulatory behavior in the male Syrian hamster. *Soc. Neurosci. Abstr.*, **17** : 1059.

Kornhauser, J. M., Nelson, D. E., Mayo, K. E. and Takahashi, J. S. (1992). Regulation of jun-B messenger RNA and AP-1 activity by light and a circadian clock. *Science*, **255** : 1581-1584.

Lee, W. S., Smith, M. S. and Hoffman, G. E. (1990). LHRH neurons express Fos protein during the proestrous surge of LH. *Proc. Natl. Acad. Sci.*, **87** : 5163-5167.

Lee, W. S., Smith, M. S. and Hoffman, G. E. (1990). Progesterone enhances the surge of LH by increasing the activation of LHRH neurons. *Endocrinology*, **127** : 2604-2606.

Loose-Mitchell, D. S., Chiappetta, C. and Stancel, G. M. (1988). Estrogen regulation of c-fos messenger ribonucleic acid. *Mol. Endocr.*, **2** : 946-951.

Neill, J. (1972). Sexual differences in the hypothalamic regulation of prolactin secretion. *Endocrinology*, **90** : 1154-1159.

Nottebohm, F. (1987). Plasticity in adult avian central nervous sytem : possible relation between hormones, learning, and brain repair. In : Mountcastle, V., Plum, F. and Geiger, S. (Eds.), *Handbook of Physiology, Amer. Physiol. Soc.*, Bethesda, pp. 85-108.

Raisman, G. and Field, P. M. (1971). Sexual dimorphism in the preoptic area of the rat. *Science*, **173** : 731-733.

Robertson, G. S., Pfaus, J. G., Atkinson, L. J., Matsumura, H., Phillips, A. G. and Fibiger, H. D. (1991). Sexual behavior increases c-fos expression in the forebrain of the male rat. *Brain Res.*, **564** : 352-357.

Rusak, B., Robertson, H. A., Wisden, W. and Hunt, S. P. (1990). Light pulses that shift rhythms induce gene expression in the suprachiasmatic nucleus. *Science*, **248** : 1237-1240.

Phoenix, C. H., Goy, R. W., Gerall, A. A. and Young, W. C. (1959). Organizing action of prenatally administered testosterone propionate on the tissues mediating mating behavior in the female guinea pig. *Endocrinology*, **65** : 369-382.

Tobet, S. A. and Fox, T. O. (1992). Sex differences in neuronal morphology influenced hormonally throughout life. In : Gerall, A. A., Moltz, H. and Ward, I. L. (Eds.), *Handbook of Behavioral Neurobiology, vol. 11*, Plenum, New York, pp. 41-84.

Tobet, S. A., Zahniser, D. J. and Baum, M. J. (1986). Sexual dimorphism in the preoptic/anterior hypothalamic area of ferrets : effects of adult exposure to sex steroids. *Brain Res.*, **364** : 249-257.

Tobet, S. A., Zahniser, D. J. and Baum, M. J. (1986a). Differentiation in male ferrets of a sexually dimorphic nucleus of the preoptic/anterior hypothalamic area requires prenatal estrogen. *Neuroendocr.*, **44** : 299-308.

Wersinger, S. R., Baum, M. J. and Erskine, M. S. (1992). Similar increments in limbic and preoptic c-fos immunoreactivity after mating in male and female rats. *Soc. Neurosci. Abstr.*, **18** : 891.

Whalen, R. E. (1974). Sexual differentiation : models, methods, and mechanisms. In : Friedman, R. C., Richart, R. M. and Van de Wiele, R. L. (Eds.), *Sex Differences in Behavior*, Wiley, New York, pp. 467-481.

Winans, S. S., Lehman, M. N. and Powers, J. B. (1982). Vomeronasal and olfactory CNS pathways which control male hamster mating behavior. In : Breiphol, W. (Ed.), *Olfaction and Endocrine Regulation*, IRL Press, London, pp. 187-214.

Wood, R. I., Brabec, R. K., Swann, J. M. and Newman, S. W. (1992). Androgen and estrogen concentrating neurons in chemosensory pathways of the male Syrian hamster brain. *Brain Res.*, In press.

# The Development of Sex Differences and Similarities in Brain Anatomy, Physiology and Behavior is Under Complex Hormonal Control

K. D. DÖHLER[1], C. GANZEMÜLLER[2] and C. VEIT[2]

[1]Pharma Bissendorf Peptide, Karl-Wiechert-Allee 3, 3000 Hannover 61, Germany
[2]Department of Clinical Endocrinology, University School of Medicine, 3000 Hannover 61, Germany

A number of functions, which are controlled by the brain, are expressed differently in male and female mammalian organisms. The most obvious functional differences between male and female animals are those involved in reproductive physiology and reproductive behavior.

In female mammals, rising plasma titers of estrogens trigger a cyclic neural stimulus which activates the release of gonadotropin-releasing hormone (GnRH) from the hypothalamus (positive feedback). GnRH, in turn, stimulates the release of luteinizing hormone (LH) and follicle stimulating hormone (FSH) from the pituitary gland. The gonadotropins FSH and LH stimulate follicular maturation in the ovaries and trigger ovulation. In male mammals, rising plasma titers of estrogens or androgens are unable to stimulate the release of GnRH. The neural substrate which controls GnRH release has apparently developed differently in males and females.

The neural substrate which controls sexual behavior has also developed along different lines in males and females. Under the influence of estrogens and progesterone adult female rats will respond to the mounting attempts of a sexually active male by an arching of the back, the so-called lordosis reflex. Adult male rats will hardly show any lordosis behavior, even if given the same hormone treatment. Under the influence of testosterone, adult male rats will show vigorous mounting, intromission and ejaculatory behavior towards a receptive female, whereas female rats will show few or no such responses when so treated with testosterone.

In regard to brain structure a great number of sexual differences in neuronal connectivity, neurotransmitter distribution and receptor concentrations have been reported (for review see Döhler, 1991). The first discovery of a gross sexual dimorphism of the brain was made by Nottebohm and Arnold (1976) on

341

*M. Haug et al. (eds.), The Development of Sex Differences and Similarities in Behavior, 341–361.*
© 1993 *Kluwer Academic Publishers.*

two species of song birds. During a reinvestigation of the male and female rat brain Gorski et al. (1978) observed a striking sexual dimorphism in gross morphology of the medial preoptic region (Figure 1). The volume of an intensely staining area, now called the sexually dimorphic nucleus of the preoptic area (SDN-POA), is several times larger in adult male rats than in females. Analogous gross sexually dimorphic structures have subsequently been identified in a variety of other species such as the gerbil, guinea pig, ferret, quail, and also in the human (for review see Döhler, 1991). The development of this nucleus starts during late fetal life (Jacobson et al., 1980) and depends on the hormonal environment during the critical period of sexual differentiation (for review see Döhler, 1991).

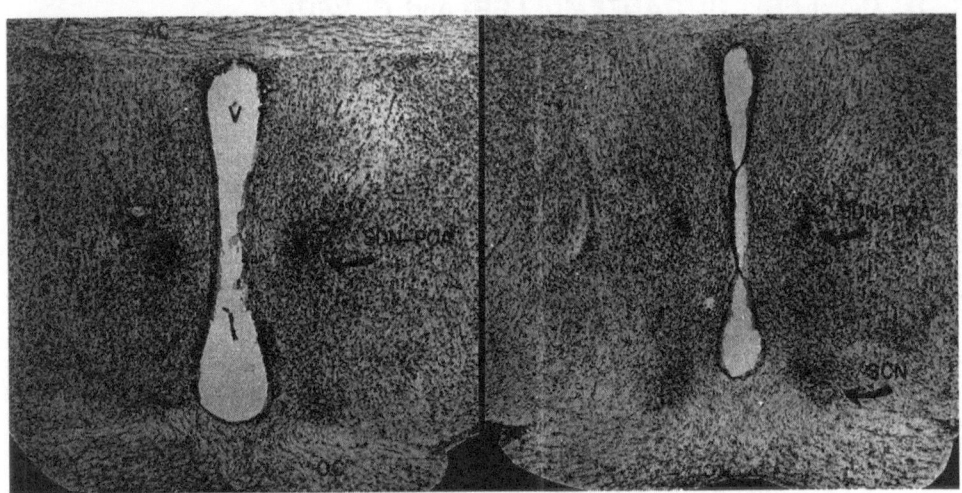

**Figure 1** Representative coronal sections through the sexually dimorphic nucleus of the preoptic area (SDN-POA) in a normal adult male rat (left) and in a normal adult female rat (right). AC, anterior commissure; OC, optic chiasma; SCN, suprachiasmatic nucleus; V, third ventricle.

# Sexual differentiation of brain structure and functions

In 1936, Pfeiffer presented evidence that there is a critical period during early postnatal development of the rat, during which differentiation of the pattern of anterior pituitary hormone secretion can be influenced permanently by testicular hormone action. He removed the testes of newborn male rats and replaced them with ovaries when the animals were adult. These male animals showed the female capacity to form corpora lutea in the grafted ovarian tissue. Newborn female rats, implanted with testes from littermate males, were unable to show estrous cycles or to form corpora lutea in their ovaries when adult.

Present knowledge of hormonal influences on the development of sexually dimorphic brain functions is based on a great number of studies, most of which have been carried out during the last 30 years. In summary, there is a sensitive developmental period during which sexual differentiation of neural substrates proceeds irreversibly under the influence of gonadal hormones. In the rat this period starts a few days before birth and ends approximately 10 days after birth. Female rats, treated during this sensitive period with high doses of androgens or estrogens, will permanently lose the capacity to release GnRH in response to estrogenic stimulation and will lose the capacity to show female lordosis behavior. The loss of female characteristics is termed "defeminization". Instead, female rats which are treated postnatally with androgens will develop the capacity to show the complete masculine sexual behavior pattern following administration of testosterone in adulthood. The acquisition of male characteristics is termed "masculinization".

If male rats are castrated shortly after birth, they become unable to display male sexual behavior patterns after treatment with testosterone in adulthood. The loss of male characteristics is termed "demasculinization". Instead, these rats will develop the capacity to show lordosis behavior and to respond in adulthood with a positive GnRH feedback to estrogen treatment. The acquisition of female characteristics is termed "feminization".

These studies indicate that androgens and/or estrogens, whether released by the testis or applied exogenously to rats during the perinatal period, will permanently defeminize and masculinize neural substrates controlling sexually dimorphic brain functions. The prevailing hypothesis indicates that androgens *per se* are not the primary stimulators of masculinization and defeminization of brain structure and functions. Instead, androgens seem to be a substrate, which has to be converted into estrogens before being able to influence sexual differentiation of the brain.

## Sexual differentiation of brain functions

Differentiation of male or female type of sexual behavior patterns is under similar influence of gonadal hormones very early in life as differentiation of the gonadotropin release pattern. Early postnatal gonadectomy of male or female rats will result in differentiation of the capacity for female lordosis behavior and cyclic pattern of gonadotropin release regardless of the genetic sex of the animals. Early postnatal implantation of testes into female rats or early postnatal treatment of female rats with aromatizable androgens or estrogens has been shown to interfere with differentiation of lordosis behavior and cyclic gonadotropin release and to result, instead, in differentiation of a tonic pattern of gonadotropin release and the capacity for male mounting, intromission and ejaculatory behavior (for review see Plapinger and McEwen, 1978; Goy and McEwen, 1980; Döhler, 1991). Pre- and postnatal inhibition of androgenic activity by treatment of male rats with the androgen antagonist cyproterone acetate was shown to result in differentiation of female behavior patterns and, after implantation of ovaries, in ovarian cyclicity (Neumann and Elger, 1966).

It is of particular interest that ring A-reduced androgens which cannot be aromatized to estrogens seem to be unable to disrupt cyclic differentiation of gonadotropin release or to interfere with differentiation of female behavior patterns when injected perinatally into female rats. Since only estrogens and such androgens, which can be aromatized into estrogens, seem to be active in sexual differentiation of the developing rat brain, it is generally assumed that disintegration of female sexual behavior patterns and differentiation of male sexual behavior patterns, as well as disintegration of the cyclic pattern and differentiation of the tonic pattern of gonadotropin release, are primarily under estrogenic, rather than androgenic control (for reviews see Plapinger and McEwen, 1978; Goy and McEwen, 1980).

Interactions between steroids and neurotransmitters are widely investigated in adult animals and have been described to operate also during the perinatal phase of sexual brain differentiation (for review see Döhler, 1991). The available data indicate that the adrenergic, the cholinergic, the serotoninergic, and the dopaminergic systems are involved in differentiation of male and female sexual behavior and in differentiation of the gonadotropin release pattern (for detailed review see Döhler, 1991).

## Development and differentiation of the sexually dimorphic nucleus of the preoptic area (SDN-POA)

Development of the SDN-POA was shown to start during late fetal life and to extend throughout the first ten days of postnatal life (Jacobson et al., 1980). This developmental period is identical with the period when sexual differentiation of brain function proceeds under the influence of gonadal hormones.

A series of studies was performed during recent years in order to test the influence of hormones perinatally on development and differentiation of the SDN-POA. The summarized results of these studies are listed in Figure 2. Neonatal castration of male rats reduced the volume of the SDN-POA permanently (Gorski et al., 1978). Reimplantation of a testis or treatment with a single injection of testosterone propionate (TP) up to 4 days after neonatal castration restored SDN-POA volume in male rats to normal (Rhees et al., 1990). Treatment of female rats with a single injection of TP postnatally (Gorski et al., 1978) increased SDN-POA volume significantly, however, the volume of the SDN-POA in these animals was still significantly smaller than that of normal male rats. Only the extended pre- and postnatal treatment of female rats with TP resulted in SDN-POA differentiation equivalent to that of normal males (Döhler et al., 1984 a). The treatment of male rats pre- and postnatally with TP did not increase the size of their SDN-POA above normal (Döhler et al., 1984 a).

Although pre- and postnatal treatment of rats with TP was shown to substitute fully for testicular activities in stimulating SDN-POA development, the prime candidates for the control of SDN-POA differentiation do not seem to be androgens as such, but rather estrogens. This conclusion is supported by several observations :-

1. Female rats, which had been treated pre- and postnatally with the synthetic estrogen diethylstilbestrol, developed a significantly enlarged SDN-POA which was similar in volume to that of control males (Döhler et al., 1984 a). This observation indicates that estrogens can stimulate SDN-POA development directly.

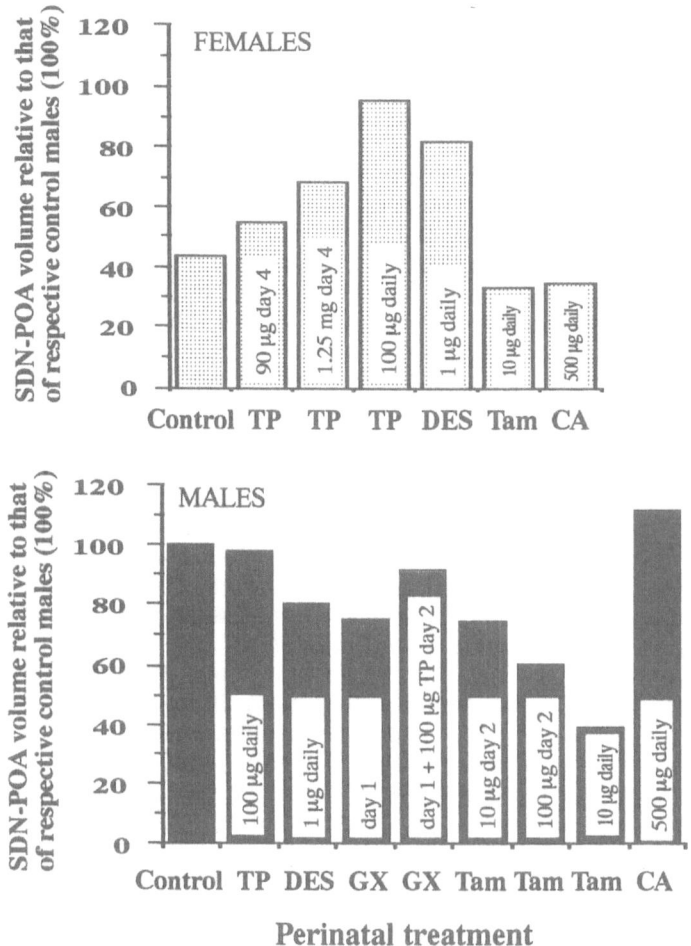

**Figure 2** Schematic representation of the hormonal environment perinatally on development and differentiation of the sexually dimorphic nucleus of the preoptic area (SDN-POA) in female (top) and male (bottom) rats. Female rats received treatment with either a single injection of 90 µg or 1.25 mg testosterone propionate (TP) on day 4 after birth, or daily treatment with TP, diethylstilbestrol (DES), the estrogen antagonist tamoxifen (Tam), or the androgen antagonist cyproterone acetate (CA) from day 16 of fetal life until day 10 after birth. Two groups of male rats were gonadectomized (GX) on the day of birth, one group received a single injection of 100 µg TP one day after GX. Two groups of male rats received a single injection of either 10 µg or 100 µg Tam on day 2 after birth. Four groups of male rats received daily treatment with TP, DES, Tam, or CA respectively from day 16 of fetal life until day 10 after birth. SDN-POA volume is indicated in percent as compared to SDN-POA volume of normal adult male rats (100 percent) from several different experiments (Gorski et al., 1978; Döhler et al., 1984 a; 1984 c; 1986).

2. Male rats, treated pre- and postnatally with the androgen antagonist cyproterone acetate, developed female genitalia, but the volume of their SDN-POA was not reduced (Döhler et al., 1986).

3. Male rats, treated pre- and postnatally with the estrogen antagonist tamoxifen, developed male genitalia, but the volume of their SDN-POA was significantly reduced and was similar to that of control female rats (Döhler et al., 1986). The normal development of male genitalia in these animals and the observation that pre- and postnatal treatment of male rats with tamoxifen did not influence serum levels of testosterone (Döhler et al., 1986), indicate that tamoxifen did not act via inhibition of testosterone release from the testes. Instead, the growth inhibiting influence of the estrogen antagonist on the SDN-POA, a brain area with known sensitivity to estrogens, seems most likely to be due to local interference with the activity of estrogens, which may have derived via enzymatic conversion from circulating androgens.

In the adult organism tamoxifen is known to bind to intracellular estrogen receptors and to prevent estrogen uptake as it inhibits cytosol receptor replenishment (Nicholson et al., 1976). Tamoxifen may act similarly in the developing organism. After aromatization of testicular androgens into estrogens tamoxifen may have interfered with estrogen uptake into cell nuclei of the SDN-POA by occupying intracellular estrogen receptors. The inhibitory effect of pre- and postnatal tamoxifen on growth and differentiation of the SDN-POA in male rats indicates that structural differentiation of the male rat brain may be dependent on aromatization of testicular androgens into estrogens and on the subsequent interaction of these estrogens with the nuclear material. The observation that the androgen antagonist cyproterone acetate did not interfere with growth and differentiation of the SDN-POA indicates, that androgens are not the primary stimulators of SDN-POA differentiation. Androgens seem to be the substrate, which has to be converted into estrogens before being able to activate SDN-POA differentiation.

The SDN-POA is sexually dimorphic not only in terms of its volume but also in terms of neurochemicals present in the cell-bodies of neurons comprising this nucleus and in the fibers innervating the nucleus and its vicinity (Commins and Yahr, 1984 a; Simerly et al., 1986). These differences are established during the critical pre- and postnatal period (Simerly et al., 1985) when sexual differentiation of the SDN-POA takes place. Thus, it seems that during the perinatal period gonadal steroids act not only as differentiation signals for morphological and functional parameters of the brain, but also influence neurotransmitter activity in the developing brain.

Concerning the SDN-POA, it was shown by Simerly et al. (1986) that in adult rats this nucleus is innervated by adrenergic fibers. In a series of studies our own group demonstrated that alteration of serotoninergic or adrenergic neurotransmission postnatally has profound effects on development and differentiation of the SDN-POA (Jarzab et al., 1990 a, b). Both, stimulation and inhibition of serotonin synthesis postnatally, was shown to provide a stimulus for SDN-POA morphogenesis in female rats. Adrenergic effects on differentiation of the SDN-POA are mediated mainly by alpha2- and beta2-adrenergic receptors (Jarzab et al., 1990 a, b). The alpha2-receptor agonist clonidine was shown to augment the stimulatory effect of TP on SDN-POA differentiation in female rats and the beta2-receptor agonist salbutamol causes the volume of the SDN-POA to increase in both sexes. The observed effects are independent from postnatal levels of circulating testosterone, as judged in male rats on day 3 of life (Jarzab et al., 1990 a).

Because of the sex difference in volume, its afferent and efferent connections, and its presence within the medial preoptic area, the SDN-POA has been hypothesized to be particularly involved in the regulation of reproductive functions. Conclusive data on functional aspects of the SDN-POA are rather scarce, however. Arendash and Gorski (1983) reported that small discrete lesions of the SDN-POA were unsuccessful in disrupting copulatory behavior in sexually experienced male rats. Lesions of the lateral sexually dimorphic area of adult male gerbils decreased mating behavior and interfered with open field scent marking (Commins and Yahr, 1984 b). Preslock and McCann (1987) made discrete lesions in the area of the SDN-POA of male rats and observed attenuation of the post-castration rise in LH and FSH levels and a significant decrease in the serum levels of prolactin. Hennessey et al. (1986) observed an increase in the capacity to show lordosis behavior after adult male rats had received lesions of the SDN-POA. Hennessey et al. (1986) concluded that cells of the preoptic area, which project to the ventromedial hypothalamus and from there to the midbrain central gray, exert a tonic inhibition over the display of lordosis which is terminated after destruction of the medial preoptic area.

Our own studies with the androgen antagonist cyproterone acetate (Döhler et al., 1986) indicate that the SDN-POA may not be involved in the control of female lordosis behavior or in the cyclic mechanism of gonadotropin release. Pre- and postnatal treatment of male rats with cyproterone acetate had previously been shown to stimulate differentiation of lordosis behavior and cyclic release of gonadotropins (Neumann and Elger, 1966). Our results demonstrate, however, that this same pre- and postnatal treatment did not "feminize" the SDN-POA (Döhler et al., 1986). Another finding which would speak against the SDN-POA being possibly involved in the control of lordosis behavior is the observation that beta-adrenergic stimulation postnatally increases both the volume of the SDN-POA and the capacity for lordosis behavior (Jarzab et al., 1990 a, b).

In conclusion, although many data concerning the perinatal influence of hormones and neurotransmitters on development and differentiation of the SDN-POA have been generated (for review see Döhler, 1991), very little is still known about the function of this nucleus and about its connection with other brain areas.

# A closer look at female differentiation of the brain

Sexual organization of the brain is thought to be inherently female unless male differentiation is superimposed by androgens or estrogens during a critical period of development. The organizational effects of androgens are thought to be mediated by intracellular conversion of these hormones in certain brain areas into estrogens. In other words, female differentiation is thought to proceed in the absence of specific hormonal influences, whereas male differentiation requires estrogenic stimulation.

The assumption that female sexual differentiation proceeds normally in the absence of gonadal hormones is based upon the early observations that gonadectomy of female rabbit fetuses (Jost, 1950), or gonadectomy of newborn female rats (Pfeiffer, 1936) does not interfere with female differentiation. Estrogen concentrations in mammalian fetuses and in newborn rats are known to be very high, often higher than during later reproductive life (for review see Döhler, 1991). It has been shown, however, that fetal and neonatal ovaries are in fact not the major source of estrogens found in the fetal and neonatal circulation. In the best studied species, the human, the primary source of estrogens during pregnancy are the fetal and the maternal adrenals. The adrenals secrete aromatizable androgens (mainly dehydroepiandrosterone sulfate) which are aromatized to estrogens in the placenta (Kime et al., 1980). There is, therefore, no reason to believe that fetal gonadectomy renders the fetus free from estrogens.

## The role of alpha-fetoproteins

It has also been shown that postnatal ovariectomy of rats does not clear the blood circulation of estrogenic hormones (Weisz and Gunsalus, 1973). This is due to the presence of high levels of estrogen-binding alpha-fetoproteins (AFP) (Nunez et al., 1971) which protect circulating estrogens from metabolism. The biological role of AFP during the fetal and neonatal period is rather speculative. It was originally assumed that AFP may prevent the high levels of perinatally circulating estrogens to interact with the developing brain, thus protecting the brain from defeminization.

This assumption becomes highly dubious in view of the intra-neuronal localization of AFP (Benno and Williams, 1978) and the observation that AFP does not appear to be synthesized within the brain (Schachter and Toran-Allerand, 1982). The available data favour the proposition that the biological purpose of AFP may actually be to protect estrogens from enzymatic degradation and to inhibit estrogen uptake by the liver, thus precluding metabolism and excretion (see Döhler et al., 1984b; Döhler, 1991 for reviews). Steroid-binding proteins, such as AFP, are known to protect steroids from being attacked by enzymes or chemical reagents such as oxygen.

The high levels of estrogens, observed in newborn male and female rats, were suggested to be remainders of maternal/placental origin from prenatal life (for discussion see Döhler et al., 1984b; Döhler, 1991). Due to the presence of estrogen-binding AFP, estrogens seem to be preferentially retained in the fetuses and are carried over into the postnatal period. By these means animals with a short gestation - such as the rat, mouse, and hamster - possess the unique ability to extend the prenatal intrauterine hormonal milieu into the postnatal period, where it is retained for at least several days, until the postnatal ovaries are able to produce their own estrogens. AFP may even act as carrier for the transport of estrogens into brain cells, as suggested by Döhler (1978) and by Toran-Allerand (1984). The overall result would be the conservation of vital estrogens which are crucial for brain development.

## The influence of estrogen antagonists

Studies about the hormonal influence on female differentiation of the brain have been hampered by the fact that gonadal and placental hormones cannot entirely be removed from the blood circulation of fetal mammals and of postnatal rats and mice. In a series of studies our group, therefore, adopted the approach of inactivating endogenous estrogens by treating newborn female rats with the estrogen antagonists tamoxifen or LY 117018 respectively. Both estrogen antagonists inhibit the biological effects of estrogens by competing with estrogens for intracellular estrogen receptor binding sites.

On days 1, 3, 5, and 7 after birth male and female rats were treated with either 0.1 µg, 1 µg, 10 µg or 100 µg of tamoxifen or LY 117018. Control rats were treated with the vehicle (oil) only. At 80 days of age all animals were gonadectomized and the gonads were inspected. At 90 days of age blood was taken at 2.30 p.m. from the retrobulbar venous plexus and the animals were treated with 20 µg estradiol benzoate (EB). 48 hours later another blood sample was taken and all animals received 2.5 mg of progesterone (P). Another 5 hours later, at 7.30 p.m., a third blood sample and on the following day at 2.30 p.m. a fourth blood sample were taken. Levels of LH were measured in the blood serum.

At 120 days of age all animals were treated with the same EB + P regimen, as described before. Five hours after treatment with P the rats were tested for lordosis behavior in the presence of sexually active male rats. At 140 days of age all animals were implanted subcutaneously with 30 mg of TP, embeded in 30 mm of silicone tubing. This type of implant had previously been tested in our laboratory and was shown to provide serum levels of testosterone in the physiological range of normal male rats. Five weeks later, when serum levels of testosterone were still in the physiological range, all animals were tested for male mounting, intromission and ejaculation behavior in the presence of receptive female rats.

In female rats postnatal treatment with tamoxifen (Figure 3) or LY 117018 (Figure 4) inhibited, in a dose-dependent way, differentiation of the capacity to show lordosis behavior. Neither treatment stimulated differentiation of the capacity to show male type of intromission behavior (Figures 3 and 4).

In male rats postnatal treatment with 0.1 µg and 1 µg LY 117018 stimulated significantly, in a dose-dependent way, differentiation of the capacity to show lordosis behavior (Figure 4). Higher doses of LY 117018 (10 µg and 100 µg) also stimulated the capacity to show lordosis behavior, but these doses were not more effective than the 1 µg dose. In male rats postnatal treatment with tamoxifen had a slight, but statistically insignificant, stimulatory effect on differentiation of lordosis behavior at the 1 µg dose (Figure 3). The 10 µg and 100 µg dose of tamoxifen inhibited lordosis differentiation (Figure 3). Postnatal treatment with tamoxifen inhibited differentiation of intromission behavior in

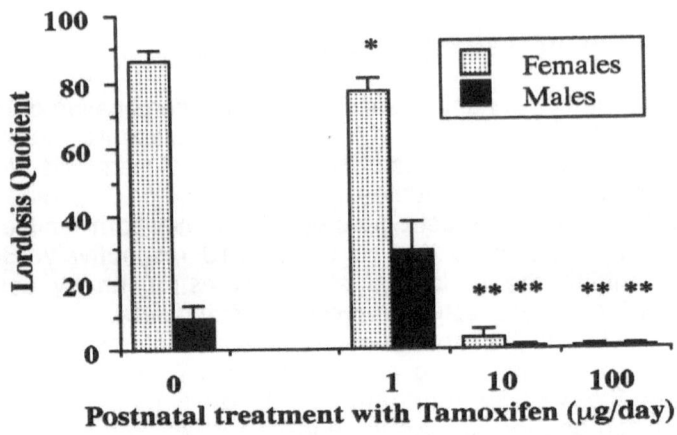

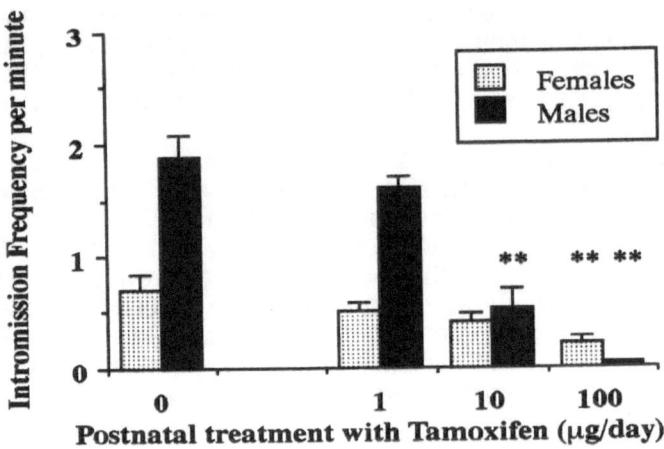

**Figure 3** Lordosis quotient (top) and intromission frequency (bottom) of adult gonadectomized and hormone-primed male and female rats which had been treated postnatally with the estrogen antagonist tamoxifen. Means ± SEM are indicated. Levels of statistical significance: *P<0.05, **P<0.01.

nale rats significantly and in a dose-dependent way (Figure 3). Postnatal reatment with LY 117018 inhibited differentiation of intromission behavior in nale rats only at the 10 µg dose (Figure 4).

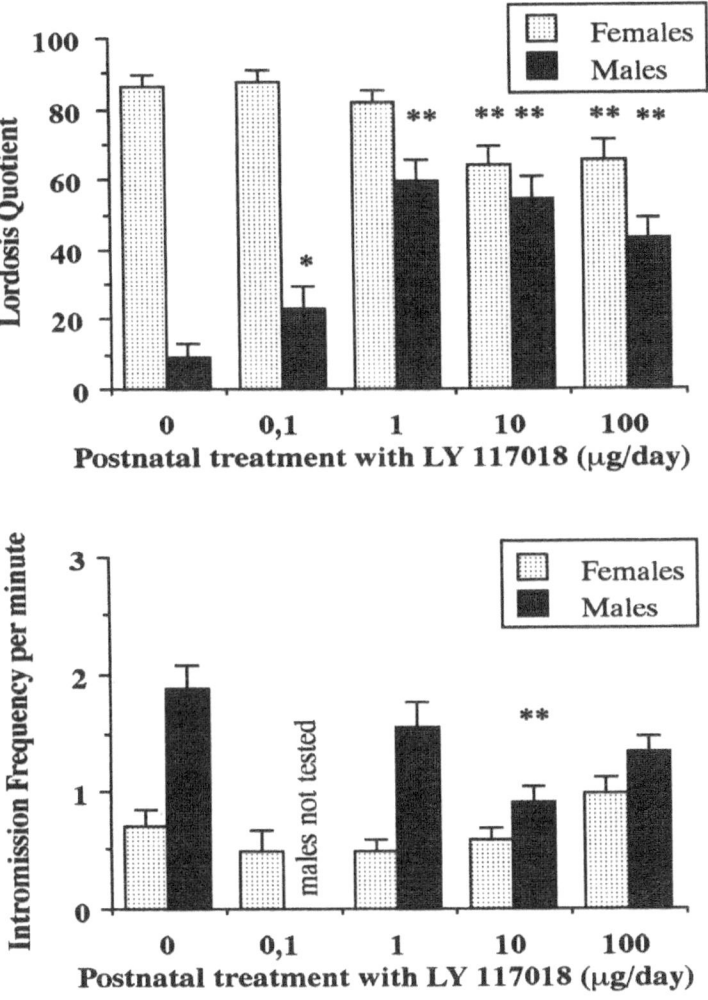

**Figure 4** Lordosis quotient (top) and intromission frequency (bottom) of adult gonadectomized and hormone-primed male and female rats which had been treated postnatally with the estrogen antagonist LY 117018. Means ± SEM are indicated. Levels of statistical significance: **P<0.01.

Postnatal treatment of female rats with tamoxifen inhibited significantly, in a dose-dependent way, the differentiation of a positive feedback mechanism for estrogen/progesterone-stimulated release of LH (Figure 5). Postnatal treatment

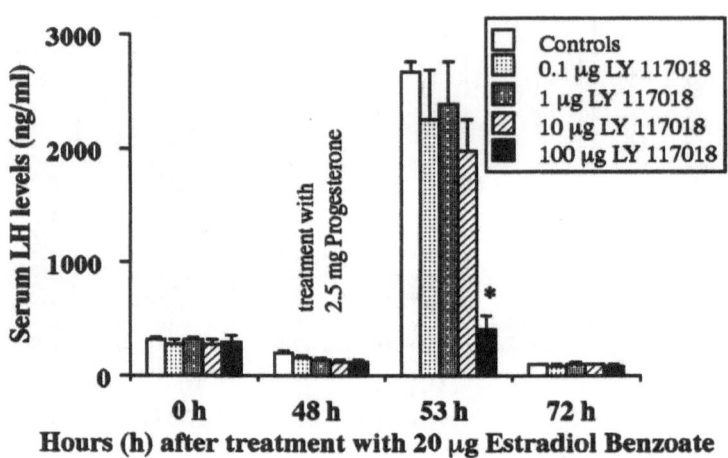

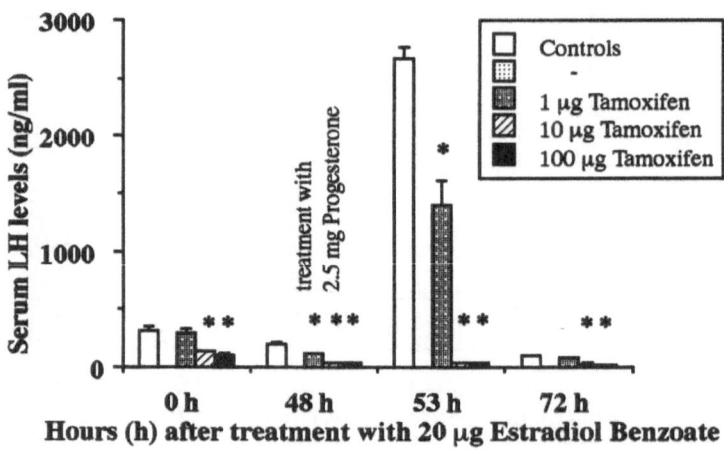

**Figure 5** Serum levels of luteinizing hormone (LH) in adult gonadectomized and estrogen/progesterone-primed female rats which had been treated postnatally with theestrogenantagonists LY 117018 (top) or tamoxifen (bottom). Means ± SEM are indicated. Levels of statistical significance: *P<0.05, **P<0.01.

of female rats with LY 117018 inhibited the differentiation of this positive feedback mechanism only at the 100 µg dose (Figure 5). Neither tamoxifen nor LY 117018 stimulated differentiation of a positive feedback for estrogen/progesterone-stimulated release of LH, when given to male rats postnatally (Figure 6).

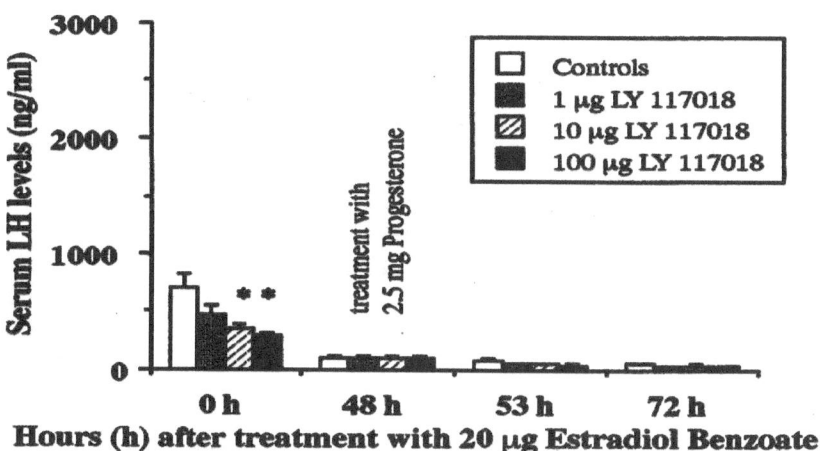

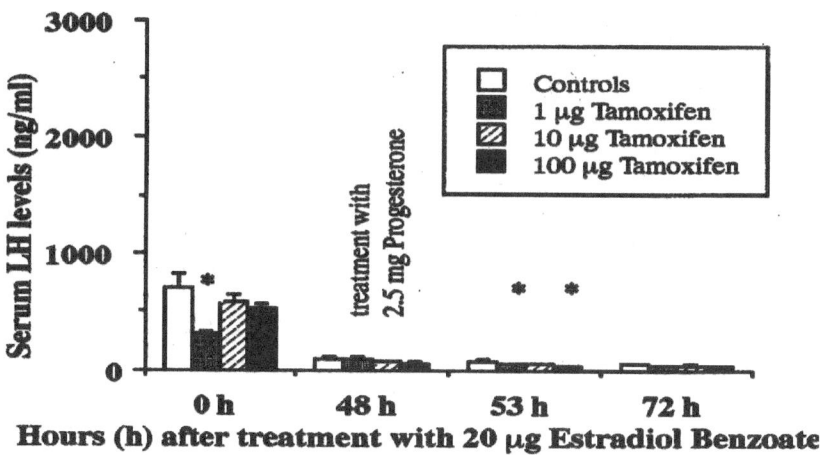

**Figure 6** Serum levels of luteinizing hormone (LH) in adult gonadectomized and estrogen/progesterone-primed male rats which had been treated postnatally with the estrogen antagonists LY 117018 (top) or tamoxifen (bottom). Means ± SEM are indicated. Levels of statistical significance: *P<0.05.

In summary, postnatal treatment of female rats with the estrogen antagonists tamoxifen and LY 117018 interfered with differentiation of the ovulation inducing positive LH-feedback and with the capacity to show lordosis behavior, but did not stimulate differentiation of the capacity for male-type intromission behavior. These results indicate, that differentiation of the mechanism for estrogen/progesterone-induced positive LH-feedback and differentiation of lordosis behavior only proceed under estrogenic influence. Interference by estrogen antagonists with the endogenous perinatal estrogenic environment interferes with differentiation of the ovulation-inducing positive LH-feedback and with differentiation of lordosis behavior.

Since postnatal treatment of female rats with either estrogen antagonist did not stimulate differentiation of the capacity for male mounting (data not shown), intromission, or ejaculation (data not shown) behavior, there is no reason to suggest that the two estrogen antagonists may have expressed their defeminizing capacity via a possibly intrinsic estrogenic activity. The conclusion that the two estrogen antagonists did not act like estrogens, but instead prevented the activity of estrogens postnatally, is supported by the findings that development and differentiation of the SDN-POA is stimulated by perinatal treatment with an estrogen, but inhibited by similar treatment with tamoxifen (Figure 2). Furthermore, the defeminizing effect of tamoxifen on organization of female sexual brain functions had previously been shown to be attenuated by concomitant treatment of postnatal female rats with estradiol (Döhler et al., 1984 b).

The observation that tamoxifen and LY 117018 interfered with lordosis differentiation in female rats but, particularly LY 117018, stimulated differentiation of the capacity for lordosis behavior in male rats, indicates that estrogens have a dual effect on differentiation of lordosis behavior. At low concentrations, which are normal physiologically in females, estrogens stimulate differentiation of lordosis behavior. At high concentrations, which are normal locally in male brains after conversion of testicular androgens, estrogens disintegrate differentiation of lordosis behavior. This conclusion explains why estrogen antagonists stimulate lordosis differentiation in males but inhibit lordosis differentiation in females (see also Figure 7).

The observation that tamoxifen and LY 117018 interfered with differentiation of the estrogen/progesterone-induced positive LH-feedback in female rats but did not stimulate differentiation of this positive feedback mechanism in male rats indicates that at low concentrations, which are normal physiologically in females, estrogens are necessary for differentiation of the positive LH-feedback mechanism, but at high concentrations, which are normal locally in male brains, estrogens do not seem to be the only parameter responsible for disintegration of this mechanism.

The conclusion that female sexual differentiation of the brain may not proceed without hormones, but may need estrogenic stimulation, is supported by the results from several other studies. Toran-Allerand (1976) demonstrated that hypothalamic neurons of newborn mice do not develop neurite processes in vitro when the culture medium is devoid of estrogens. Vom Saal et al. (1983) observed that female mice, which were located in utero between two other females, had higher levels of estradiol in their amnionic fluid and showed better

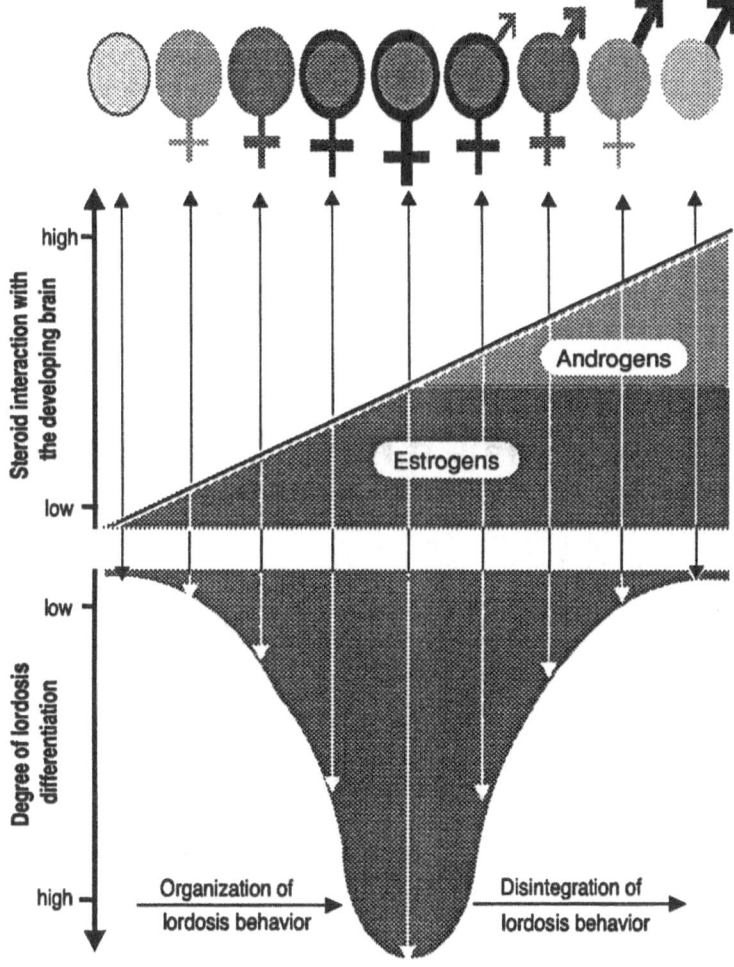

**Figure 7** Symbolic representation on how the capacity for female lordosis behavior might differentiate or disintegrate depending on the quantitative influence of estrogens and androgens perinatally. The embryonic brain, represented by the faint circular symbol at the top left, is as yet sexually undifferentiated. Under the influence of moderate levels of estrogens (of placental origin) the embryonic and postnatal brain elaborates neural substrates and circuitries which will be able, in adulthood, to respond to estrogens with lordosis behavior. Under the pre- and postnatal influence of high levels of estrogens and androgens the capacity for lordosis behavior disintegrates. Individual differences in the quantitative interaction of estrogens and androgens with the developing brain will lead to corresponding individual differences in differentiation of the capacity for lordosis behavior (redrawn from Döhler, 1991).

adult sexual performance than did their female litter mates which had been located in utero between two male fetuses.

In summary, the available data suggest (for review see Döhler, 1991), that female sexual differentiation of the brain, or even brain development per se, may require perinatal estrogenic stimulation for its full expression. Therefore, the capacity for the normal display of female sexual behavior and for the cyclic release of gonadotropins is not, as has been assumed, inherent to central nervous tissue, but depends on active hormonal induction during a sensitive period of development. Perinatal antagonism of estrogenic activity, thus, produces animals which are neither male nor female, behaviorally and physiologically speaking (Figure 7). In adulthood these animals respond neither to estradiol nor to testosterone. Requirements for estrogenic influences on male and female brain differentiation, functional and structural, may be quantitative (Figure 7) rather than qualitative.

# A closer look at male differentiation of the brain

The observation that only aromatizable androgens stimulate differentiation of male sexual behavior patterns in female rats, whereas non-aromatizable androgens seem to be without this capacity (for reviews see Plapinger and McEwen, 1978; Goy and McEwen, 1980), and the observation that masculinization of sexual behavior patterns can be inhibited by postnatal treatment of rats with estrogen antagonists (Figure 3 and Figure 4), seem to indicate that estrogens are the major effective hormones, which stimulate the differentiation of male sexual behavior patterns. However, this conclusion does not fit with the observation that perinatal treatment of male rats with an aromatization inhibitor did not inhibit differentiation of the capacity for male sexual behavior (Vreeburg et al., 1977), whereas perinatal treatment with an androgen antagonist inhibits differentiation of the capacity for male sexual behavior (Neumann and Elger, 1966), despite its inability to prevent aromatization of testicular androgens into estrogens (Döhler et al., 1986). The latter observations suggest that estrogens per se may be less important and androgens per se may be more important for organization of male sexual brain functions, than has been assumed.

Testosterone is known to enter androgen target cells in the brain. Within the target cells testosterone is subjected to aromatization or to $5\alpha$-reduction, the principal metabolites being estradiol and $5\alpha$-dihydrotestosterone (DHT). Both hormones are bound with high affinity to specific cytoplasmic receptor proteins and are then translocated into the cell nucleus where they stimulate a characteristic biological response. Cyproterone acetate does not prevent androgen entry into hypothalamic cells, nor does it influence androgen metabolism (Mainwaring, 1977). Its main antagonistic activity seems to be based on interference with intracellular androgen binding to specific androgen receptors in the cytosol and prevention of the translocation of the receptor-androgen complex into the cell nucleus (Mainwaring, 1977). Thus, the activity of cyproterone acetate is directed against androgen-mediated events, but not directed against estrogen-mediated events.

In reference to sexual differentiation of the brain, this discussion points to one necessary conclusion: masculinization and defeminization of sexual brain functions in the rat seem to be mediated not only by estrogens alone, but they also seem to require the participation of androgens per se. Both, androgenic and estrogenic components, seem to be required for complete masculinization and defeminization of sexual brain functions (Figure 7). Interference of hormone antagonists with one or the other component results in incomplete organization of the male brain (Figure 8).

Metabolism of non-aromatizable androgens is very rapid in the rat, but slow in the rhesus monkey (Goy and McEwen, 1980). The fact that non-aromatizable androgens are quite effective to stimulate differentiation of male sexual behavior patterns in monkeys (Plapinger and McEwen, 1978; Goy and McEwen, 1980), but not in rats, may be a result of the different speed of metabolism, rather than an indication for a different, species specific, mechanism of brain differentiation. The inefficacy of DHT, in contrast to TP, to stimulate male type of genital differentiation in female rats, when given at high daily doses during the last week of fetal life (Döhler et al., 1986), is a strong indication that the non-aromatizable androgen never reached the target organ. In conclusion, during differentiation of male sexual brain function estrogens may be supportive, rather than directive, to the primary action of androgens (Figure 8).

# Summary and conclusion

The brain of male and female mammals seems to be yet undifferentiated before the period of increased susceptibility to gonadal steroids and neurotransmitters starts. Feminization of brain structure and functions, e.g. establishment of the cyclic LH-surge mechanism and the expression of lordosis behavior, seems to depend on the moderate interaction of estrogens with the developing nervous system. Defeminization and masculinization of brain functions seem to be established during interaction of the developing nervous system with androgens, which have to be converted, at least in part, into estrogens. Structural differentiation of the male brain, e.g. the sexually dimorphic nucleus of the preoptic area (SDN-POA), seems to be exclusively estrogen dependent. During differentiation of male brain functions, however, estrogens may be supportive, rather than directive, to the primary action of androgens.

The molecular mechanisms of sexual differentiation of the brain are not yet fully understood. It seems, however, that the priming action of gonadal steroids during the period of increased susceptibility is either mediated by neurotransmitters, or neurotransmitters modulate the priming action of gonadal steroids. In particular the adrenergic, the serotoninergic, the cholinergic, and possibly the dopaminergic system were shown to have strong influences on sexual differentiation of brain structure and functions.

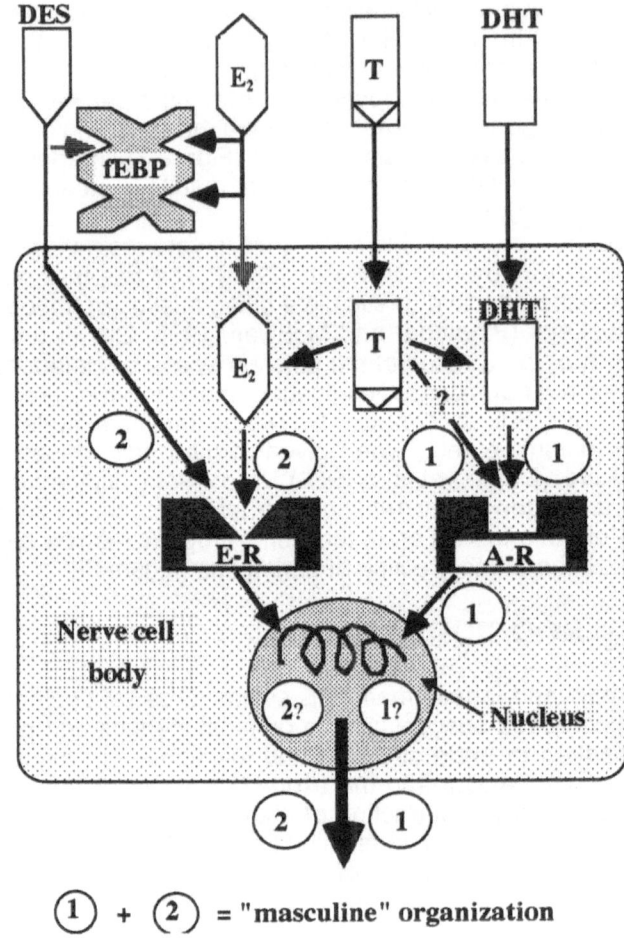

$\textcircled{1}$ + $\textcircled{2}$ = "masculine" organization

**Figure 8** Schematic representation of the androgenic and estrogenic hormone environments outside and inside neuronal compartments in the perinatal rat brain and their influence on masculine organization. The diagram indicates that interference with androgen action by the androgen antagonist cyproterone acetate (1), or interference with estrogen action by estrogen antagonists (2) will interfere with masculine organization of the brain. The possible steps of interference are indicated by (1) and (2). A-R, cytoplasmic androgen receptor; DES, diethylstilbestrol; DHT, $5\alpha$-dihydrotestosterone; E2, estradiol; E-R, cytoplasmic estrogen receptor; fEBP, fetal estrogen-binding protein; T, testosterone. Redrawn from Döhler et al. (1983).

# References

Arendash, G. S. and Gorski, R. A. (1983). Effects of discrete lesions of the sexually dimorphic nucleus of the preoptic area or other medial preoptic regions on the sexual behavior of male rats. *Brain Res. Bull.*, **10** : 147-154.

Benno, R. and Williams, T. (1978). Evidence for intracellular localization of alpha-fetoprotein in the developing rat brain. *Brain Res.*, **142** : 182-186.

Commins, D. and Yahr, P. (1984 a). Acetylcholinesterase activity in the sexually dimorphic area of the gerbil brain : sex differences and influences of adult gonadal steroids. *J. Comp. Neurol.*, **224** : 123-131.

Commins, D. and Yahr, P. (1984 b). Lesions of the sexually dimorphic area disrupt mating and marking in male gerbils. *Brain Res. Bull.*, **13** : 185-193.

Döhler, K.-D. (1978). Is female sexual differentiation hormone mediated? *Trends Neurosci.*, **1** : 138-140.

Döhler, K. D. (1991). The pre-and postnatal influence of hormones and neurotransmitters on sexual differentiation of the mammalian hypothalamus. *Int. Rev. Cytol.*, **131** : 1-57.

Döhler, K. D., Coquelin, A., Davis, F., Hines, M., Shryne, J. E. and Gorski, R. A. (1984 a). Pre- and postnatal influence of testosterone propionate and diethylstilbestrol on differentiation of the sexually dimorphic nucleus of the preoptic area in male and female rats. *Brain Res.*, **302** : 291-295.

Döhler, K. D., Coquelin, A., Hines, M., Davis, F., Shryne, J. E. and Gorski, R. A., (1983). Hormonal influence on sexual differentiation of rat brain anatomy. In : Balthazart, J. Pröve, R. and Gilles, R. (Eds.), *Hormones and Behaviour in Higher Vertebrates*, Springer, Berlin, pp. 194-203.

Döhler, K. D., Hancke, J. L., Srivastava, S. S., Hofmann, C., Shryne, J. E. and Gorski, R. A. (1984 b). Participation of estrogens in female sexual differentiation of the brain; neuroanatomical, neuroendocrine and behavioral evidence. In : De Vries, G. J., de Bruin, J. P. C., Uylings, H. B. M. and Corner, M. A. (Eds.), *Progress in Brain Research*, Elsevier Science Publication, Amsterdam, pp. 99-117.

Döhler, K. D., Srivastava, S. S., Shryne, J. E., Jarzab, B., Sipos, A. and Gorski, R. A. (1984 c). Differentiation of the sexually dimorphic nucleus in the preoptic area of the rat brain is inhibited by postnatal treatment with an estrogen antagonist. *Neuroendocrinology*, **38** : 297-301.

Döhler, K. D., Coquelin, A., Davis, F., Hines, M., Shryne, J. E., Sickmöller, P. M., Jarzab, B. and Gorski, R. A. (1986). Pre- and postnatal influence of an estrogen antagonist and an androgen antagonist on differentiation of the sexually dimorphic nucleus of the preoptic area in male and female rats. *Neuroendocrinology*, **42** : 443-448.

Gorski, R. A., Gordon, J. H., Shryne, J. E. and Southam, A. M. (1978). Evidence for a morphological sex difference within the medial preoptic area of the rat brain. *Brain Res.*, **148** : 333-346.

Goy, R. W. and McEwen, B. S. (1980). *Sexual Differentiation of the Brain*, The MIT Press, Cambridge, Massachusetts.

Hennessey, A. C., Wallen, K. and Edwards, D. A. (1986). Preoptic lesions increase the display of lordosis by male rats. *Brain Res.*, **370** : 21-28.

Jacobson, C. D., Shryne, J. E., Shapiro, F. and Gorski, R. A. (1980). Ontogeny of the sexually dimorphic nucleus of the preoptic area. *J. Comp. Neurol.*, **193** : 541-548.

Jarzab, B., Kaminski, M., Gubala, E., Achtelik, W., Wagiel, J. and Döhler, K. D. (1990 a). Postnatal treatment of rats with the beta2-adrenergic agonist salbutamol influences the volume of the sexually dimorphic nucleus in the preoptic area. *Brain Res.*, **516** : 257-262.

Jarzab, B., Kokocińska, D., Kaminski, M., Gubala, E., Achtelik, W., Wagiel, J. and Döhler, K. D. (1990 b). Influence of neurotransmitters on sexual differentiation of the brain : relationship between the volume of the SDN-POA and functional characteristics. In : Balthazart, J. (Ed.), *Hormones, Brain and Behaviour in Vertebrates. I. Sexual Differentiation, Neuroanatomical Aspects, Neurotransmitters and Neuropeptides*, Karger, Basel, pp. 41-50.

Jost, A. (1950). Sur le contrôle hormonal de la differenciation sexuelle du lapin. *Arch. Anat. Microscop. Morphol. Exp.*, **39** : 577-598.

Kime, D., Vinson, G., Major, P., and Kilpatrick, R. (1980). Adrenal-gonadal relationships. In : Jones, I. and Henderson, I. (Eds.), *General, Comparative and Clinical Endocrinology of the Adrenal Cortex*, Academic Press, New York 1980, pp. 183-264.

Mainwaring, W. I. P. (1977). Modes of action of antiandrogens : a survey. In : Martini, L. and Motta, M. (Eds.), *Androgens and Antiandrogens*, Raven Press, New York, pp. 151-161.

Nunez, E. A., Engelmann, F., Benassayag, C., Savu, L., Crepy, O. and Jayle, M. F. (1971). Mise en évidence d'une fraction protéique liant les oestrogènes dans le sérum de rats impubères. *C.R. Acad. Sci. Paris* , **272** : 2396-2399.

Neumann, F. and Elger, W. (1966). Permanent changes in gonadal function and sexual behavior as a result of early feminization of male rats by treatment with an antiandrogenic steroid. *Endokrinologie*, **50** : 209-224.

Nicholson, R. I., Golder, M. P., Davies, P. and Griffiths, K. (1976). Effects of oestradiol-17β and tamoxifen on total and accessible cytoplasmic oestradiol-17β receptors in DMBA-induced rat mammary tumours. *Eur. J. Cancer*, **12** : 711-717.

Nottebohm, F. and Arnold, A. P. (1976). Sexual dimorphism in vocal control areas of the songbird brain. *Science*, **194** : 211-213.

Pfeiffer, C. A. (1936). Sexual differences of the hypophysis and their determination by the gonads. *Am. J. Anat.*, **58** : 195-226.

Plapinger, L. and McEwen, B. S. (1978). Gonadal steroid - brain interactions in sexual differentiation. In : Hutchison, J. B. (Ed.), *Biological Determinants of Sexual Behaviour*, John Wiley and Sons, New York, pp. 153-218.

Preslock, J. P. and McCann, S. M. (1987). Lesions of the sexually dimorphic nucleus of the preoptic area : effects upon LH, FSH and prolactin in rats. *Brain Res. Bull.*, **18** : 127-134.

Rhees, R. W., Shryne, J. E. and Gorski, R. A. (1990). Termination of the hormone-sensitive period for differentiation of the sexually dimorphic nucleus of the preoptic area in male and female rats. *Dev. Brain Res.*, **52** : 17-23.

Schachter, B. and Toran-Allerand, C. D. (1982). Intraneural alpha-fetoprotein and albumin are not synthesized locally in developing brain. Develop. *Brain Res.*, **5** : 93-98.

Simerly, R. B., Swanson, L. W. and Gorski, R. A. (1985). Reversal of the sexually dimorphic distribution of serotonin immunoreactive fibers in the medial preoptic nucleus by treatment with perinatal androgen. *Brain Res.*, **340** : 91-98.

Simerly, R. B., Gorski, R. A. and Swanson, L. W. (1986). Neurotransmitter specifity of cells and fibers in the medial preoptic nucleus : an immunohistochemical study in the rat. *J. comp. Neurol.*, **246** : 343-363.

Toran-Allerand, C. D. (1976). Sex steroids and the development of the newborn mouse hypothalamus and preoptic area in vitro : implications for sexual differentiation. *Brain Res.*, **106** : 407-412.

Toran-Allerand, C. D. (1984). On the genesis of sexual differentiation of the central nervous system : morphogenetic consequences of steroidal exposure and possible role of alpha-fetoprotein. In : De Vries, G. J., de Bruin, J. P. C., Uylings, H. B. M. and Corner, M. A. (Eds.), *Progress in Brain Research*, Elsevier Science Publications., Amsterdam, pp. 63-98.

Vom Saal, F. S., Grant, W. M., McMullen, C. W. and Laves, K. S. (1983). High fetal estrogen concentrations : correlation with increased adult sexual performance and decreased agression in male mice. *Science*, **220** : 1306-1309.

Vreeburg, J. T. M., van der Vaart, P. D. M. and van der Schoot, P. (1977) Prevention of central defeminization, but not masculinization in male rats by inhibition neonatally of oestrogen biosynthesis. *J. Endocr.*, **74** : 375-382.

Weisz, J. and Gunsalus, P. (1973). Estrogen levels in immature female rats : true or spurious - ovarian or adrenal? *Endocrinology*, **93** : 1057-1065.

# Sexual Dimorphism in the Accessory Olfactory System

## A. GUILLAMON AND S. SEGOVIA

*Departamento de Psicobiologia, Universidad Nacional de Educacion a Distancia, Ciudad Universitaria, P.O.Box 50.487. 28040 Madrid, Spain*

The concept of a dual olfactory system (DOS) (Raisman, 1971; Scalia and Winans, 1975) refers to the existence of two morphologically and functionally different olfactory systems in vertebrate species. They are the main olfactory system (MOS) and the vomeronasal, or accessory olfactory system (AOS). Since Powers and Winans (1975) showed that the vomeronasal organ (VNO) has a functional role in the copulatory behavior of hamsters, a remarkable amount of research showing the functional participation of the AOS in mammalian reproduction has appeared (see e.g. Wysocki, 1979; Wysocki and Meredith, 1987; Halpern, 1987).

Several years ago we found that the rat VNO is a sexually dimorphic structure whose development is governed by gonadal hormones present shortly after birth (Segovia and Guillamon, 1982). This fact and two other considerations led us to hypothesize (Segovia and Guillamon, 1982,1986) that the AOS might be a sexually dimorphic complex network and that stimuli conveyed by a sexually dimorphic VNO most likely have relevance in reproductive behavior. First, examples of sexual dimorphism had already been found in some AOS structures such as the medial preoptic area (MPA) (Dörner and Staudt, 1968; Raisman and Field, 1971,1973; Gorski et al., 1978,1980), the ventromedial hypothalamic nucleus (VMH) (Dörner and Staudt, 1969; Matsumoto and Arai, 1983,1986), the ventral region of the premammillary nucleus (PMV) (Dörner, 1976) and the medial amygdaloid nucleus (Me) (Staudt and Dörner, 1976; Mizukami et al., 1983). The second consideration was the existence of steroid receptors in AOS structures (Stumpf and Sar, 1982). To verify the hypothesis three AOS structures needed to be studied, i.e. the accessory olfactory bulb (AOB), the bed nucleus of the accessory olfactory tract (BAOT) and the bed nucleus of the stria terminalis (BST).

In the following sections of this chapter evidence will be provided to show that the AOB, BAOT and BST are sexually dimorphic. In addition, the hormonal mechanisms that most likely control sex differences in the AOS will be addressed.

*M. Haug et al. (eds.), The Development of Sex Differences and Similarities in Behavior, 363–376.*
© 1993 *Kluwer Academic Publishers.*

# Sexual dimorphism in the vomeronasal organ

The rat VNO is a sexually dimorphic sensory organ controlled by sex steroids present soon after birth (Segovia and Guillamon, 1982). Males naturally have greater values than females with respect to VNO volume, neuroepithelium volume and number of olfactory receptors (Tables I and II). Orchidectomy of males and androgenization of females conducted on the day of birth (D1) abolished or inverted, respectively, this sexual dimorphism, as seen when the subjects were studied in adulthood (90 days old). D1 orchidectomized males did not differ from control females, but did differ from control males (Table I). Moreover, androgenized females were significantly different from control females, but not from control males. The area of the nuclei in the receptor cells was larger in the females than in the males. However, this sexual difference was abolished through the above mentioned treatments on D1. These results were confirmed in a later study (Segovia et al., 1984b) when we tried to determine whether sex differences in the VNO depended on the presence of gonadal steroids in adult animals (6 months). Gonadectomy of the adult rat produced a decrease in the neuroepithelial height in both males and females.
Thus the VNO undergoes a sexual differentiation process that depends on the appropriate sex hormones. This is at least the case on the first day of extrauterine life. Moreover, the structure of the VNO depends on the level of sexual steroids during adulthood.

# Sexual dimorphism in the accessory olfactory bulb

The AOB shows sexual dimorphism in several structural aspects (Tables I and II, c.f. Segovia et al., 1984a, 1986; Valencia et al., 1986; Roos et al., 1988; Caminero et al., 1991). Male rats show larger values for AOB volume and number of mitral cells than females (Segovia et al., 1984a; Valencia et al., 1986, Roos et al., 1988). Furthermore, they have larger mitral somata and a greater number of dendritic branches growing out from the main dendritic stalks (Caminero et al., 1991). However, the number of dendritic branches extending from the basal stalks was not greater in males than in females. Sexual dimorphism in all of these morphological measures was suppressed and/or reversed through experimental treatment (D1) of gonadectomy of males and androgenization of females (Segovia et al., 1984a; Valencia et al., 1986; Caminero et al., 1991).
The number of AOB granule cells is also sexually dimorphic (Segovia et al., 1986). Male rats have a larger number of light and dark granule cells than females. Gonadectomy of males and androgenization of females performed on D1 reverse the number of light granule cells, thereby causing the D1 gonadectomized males to have fewer light granule cells than the control males, but not than the control females. Moreover, androgenized females have a

| | MALES | | FEMALES | |
| --- | --- | --- | --- | --- |
| | Control | Orchidectomized | Control | Androgenized |
| VNO | 1.7263±0.071* | 1.0779±0.036† | 1.0811±0.068 | 1.6631±0.125† |
| VNO neuroepithelium | 0.1838±0.013* | 0.1141±0.011† | 0.1134±0.012 | 0.2023±0.011† |
| AOB | 0.211±0.050* | 0.113±0.030† | 0.137±0.040 | 0.231±0.090† |
| AOB layers VN-glomerular | 0.036±0.010* | 0.017±0.008† | 0.034±0.020 | 0.052±0.020† |
| mitral cells | 0.065±0.010* | 0.034±0.010† | 0.038±0.003 | 0.072±0.030† |
| plexiform | 0.032±0.006* | 0.020±0.006† | 0.020±0.006 | 0.036±0.013† |
| granular | 0.073±0.020* | 0.039±0.010† | 0.041±0.007 | 0.063±0.020† |
| BAOT | 0.030±0.001* | 0.027±0.0016† | 0.022±0.001 | 0.030±0.0017† |
| BST total | 1.078±0.069* | 1.148±0.048† | 1.145±0.072 | 1.266±0.047† |
| BSTMP | 0.389±0.019* | 0.303±0.004† | 0.327±0.020 | 0.441±0.031† |
| BSTMA | 0.264±0.017* | 0.399±0.021† | 0.362±0.034 | 0.393±0.020† |
| PS ✻ | 1.041±0.103* | 1.334±0.150† | 1.412±0.141 | 1.060±0.105† |
| LC ✻ | 0.050±0.002* | 0.053±0.001 | 0.059±0.002 | 0.053±0.001† |

**Table I** Sexual dimorphism in the volume of some AOS and non-AOS (*) structures and the effects of early postnatal male orchidectomy and female androgenization. See text for references and abbreviations. Data show means (mm3) ± SEM. At least $P<0.05$: * comparisons between control groups; + comparisons with respect to the control group of the same genetic sex.

larger number of light granule cells than the control females, but not compared to the control males (Segovia et al., 1986). On the other hand, the population of dark granule cells behaves differently after the same treatment on D1. Orchidectomy on D1 significantly reduces the number of dark granule cells compared to control males and no difference is found with respect to control females. However, androgenization of females on D1 did not cause any increment in the number of dark granule cells (Segovia et al., 1986).

It has been reported in the literature that AOB granule cells have two neurogenetic periods (Struble and Walters, 1982; Bayer, 1983). The first takes place prenatally (17-19 days after conception), while the second occurs postnatally between days 1-20 and is most intense between days 6-8. Since the percentage of dark AOB granule cells reported by Struble and Walters (1982) and by us (Segovia et al., 1986) in the same structure and species were similar to that found by Bayer (1983) for the AOB granule cells proliferated postnatally, and we were unable to affect the dark granule cells in females by the administration of testosterone on D1, we suspected they might be the same granule cells that proliferate postnatally. Thus, it was hypothesized that these cells have a period of maximum susceptibility to the organizational effects of androgens that is both different from and occurs later than in the light granule cells. In fact, the administration 14 days after birth of a single injection of testosterone propionate (TP) affected the female AOB granule cell population in a selective manner, increasing the number of these cells to a quantity not statistically different from that found in control males, but statistically higher than those observed in control females (Segovia et al., 1986).

| | MALES | | FEMALES | |
| | Control | Orchidectomized | Control | Androgenized |
|---|---|---|---|---|
| VNO | 37961±1438* | 31560±720† | 30175±1154 | 38819±1576† |
| AOB | | | | |
| mitral | 5646±536.36* | 3910±258.86† | 3850±339.56 | 7410±966.16† |
| light granule | 53340±3543.71* | 35208±3604.61† | 35936±3917.16 | 47260±3861.12† |
| dark granule | 8448±1309.06* | 3634±479.19† | 3910±502.91 | 3642±360.08 |
| BAOT | 1690±158.7* | 872±44.50† | 1033±104.8 | 1571±158.4† |
| BSTMP | 39769±2037.4* | 33662±670.4† | 30117±1218.4 | 40548±3443.5† |
| BSTLA✸ | 3828±252.5* | 4746±515.2† | 5434±95.7 | 4577±210.2† |
| LC✸ | 2178±78.9* | 2305±74.3 | 2605±69.5 | 2311±70.1† |

**Table II** Sexual dimorphism in the number of neurons in some AOS and non-AOS (*) structures and the effects of early postnatal male orchidectomy and female androgenization. See text for references and abreviations. Data show means ± SEM. At least P<0.05: * comparisons between control groups; + comparisons with respect to the control group of the same genetic sex.

These results show that the critical period for androgens differs in AOB dark and light granule cells. We came to this conclusion because TP administration on days 1 and 14, as opposed to day 1 only, was effective in selectively increasing the number of dark granule cells in the females. This explanation can also be extended to dark AOB granule cells in male rats since no statistically significant differences were found between the control males and the genetic females treated with TP on days 1 and 14.

In addition to these data, Roos et al. (1988) reported that the castration of males on postnatal days 20 or 30 also impairs the development of the AOB until day 60. Moreover, TP administration is able to completely restore AOB development in male rats castrated at postanatal day 20 (Roos et al., 1989). These facts indicate that AOB sexual differentiation appears to be due not only to the organizational action of the testicular secretion inmediatly after birth, but also to a late second phase of prepubescent testicular activity.

# Sexual dimorphism in the bed nucleus of the stria terminalis

Although the overall volume of the BST does not present sexual dimorphism, volumetric sex differences do appear in several smaller divisions of this nucleus (Table 1) (Del Abril et. al.,1987b). The volume of the medial posterior division of the BST (BSTMP) is larger in the male rat compared to the female (Del Abril et al., 1987b). Analogous sex differences were found in the guinea pig (Hines et al., 1985) and in human beings (Allen and Gorski, 1990). Sex differences are due to the sexual dimorphism in volume present in the so-called "small celled" or "encapsulated" region of the BSTMP and gonadal hormones present shortly after birth which control this sexual dimorphism (Del Abril et al., 1987b). On the other hand, in the medial anterior region of the BST (BSTMA) females showed greater measures for volume than male rats (Del Abril et al., 1987b). Male orchidectomy on D1 increased BSTMA volume to a size similar to that found in control females, while androgenization of females on D1 produced no change (Del Abril et al., 1987b).

With respect to neuronal population, males have more neurons in the BSTMP than females (Table II) . These sex differences are also circumscribed in the "small celled" region (Guillamon et al., 1988b). Neonatal treatments of gonadectomy to males and androgenization to females induced significant changes in the number of neurons and they also suppressed sex differences (Guillamon et al., 1988b).

The female BSTMA shows a higher number of neurons than that of males. D1 gonadectomy of males increased this number to a quantity statistically different from that of the control males and females, and androgenization of females on D1 brought about an increase in the number of neurons to a quantity higher than that of both control males and females (Del Abril et al., 1987a).

In the anterior region of the lateral division of the BST (BSTLA), a part of the MOS (De Olmos and Ingram, 1972; Saper, 1984), females have more neurons than males (Table II); however, neonatal treatments affected this region and the BSTMA differently (Guillamon et al., 1988b). D1 orchidectomy of males caused a significant increase in the number of neurons compared to control males but not control females. Yet, female androgenization on D1 significantly reduced the number of neurons compared to both control males and females (Guillamon et al., 1988b).

These results indicate that the BST is not a homogeneous structure in terms of sex differences as two patterns of sexual dimorphism take place. In some regions, males show greater morphometric values than females, while in others females show greater morphometric values than males.

# Sexual dimorphism in the bed nucleus of the accessory olfactory tract

The BAOT is a nucleus belonging to the AOS (Broadwell, 1975; Scalia and Winans, 1975) that is implicated at least in the control of maternal behavior (Del Cerro et al., 1991; Izquierdo et al., 1992). It shows sexual dimorphism (Collado et al., 1990) in that males have a larger volume and more neurons in this nucleus compared to females (Tables I and II). Male orchidectomy and female androgenization performed on the day of birth reversed these measures. This pattern of sexual dimorphism is similar to that described for the VNO (Segovia and Guillamon, 1982; Segovia et al., 1984b).

Collado et al. (1990) did not find sexual dimorphism with respect to glial cells. However, the ratio of neurons to glia presented a difference related to sex. The control males showed a larger ratio than the control females. Similar findings have been reported for the cortex (McShane et al., 1988). It should be remembered that BAOT neurogenesis in the rat is biphasic, with the largest surge of neurons (74%) occurring around embryonic days 12 and 13 and a later surge (17%) taking place on about day 15 (Bayer, 1980). If BAOT neurons proliferate between days 12 and 15, the effects of TP could be related to the *survival* of neurons in D1 androgenized females. The absence of gonadal hormones in D1 orchidectomized males also induces a clear loss in BAOT neurons. This, together with the effects of TP in the genetic female, indicates that testicular secretion of testosterone during this early postnatal period is necessary for males to achieve a greater number of neurons than females. This might occur through a process in which testosterone prevents neuronal death (Nordeen et al., 1985; Konishi et al., 1985; Segovia et al., 1986).

# Hormonal mechanisms controlling sexual dimorphism: facts, hypotheses and suggestions

The hormonal mechanisms that control the development of sexual dimorphism in the AOS and in other regions of the nervous system may account for the existence of two patterns of sexual dimorphism; one in which males present larger volumes and numbers of neurons than females and the opposite in which females show larger volumes and greater numbers of neurons than males. We believe that the simplest approach to this problem is to focus our effort on determining the hormone(s) that promote(s) a greater or lesser volume and/or number of neurons regardless of genetic sex. Thus, we will first take a look at the mechanisms that produce greater volume and number of neurons in both sexes, and later, at those that produce the opposite pattern.

The mechanism(s) promoting a greater volume and/or number of neurons seem(s) initially to be androgen-dependent and ultimately to be accomplished by estradiol produced by way of testosterone aromatization. The androgen dependent mechanism is evidenced by the fact that early postnatal orchidectomy to males decreases the number of cells and/or the volumetric neasures in the VNO, AOB, BSTMP, BAOT, SDN-POA and VMH (Figure 1) Gorski et al., 1978,1980; Segovia and Guillamon, 1982; Matsumoto and Arai, 983; Segovia et al., 1984a, 1986; Valencia et al., 1986; Del Abril et al., 1987b; Guillamon et al., 1988b; Collado et al., 1990). Early postnatal androgenization f females also increases the volume and/or number of neurons in the VNO, AOB, BSTMP, BAOT, and SDN-POA and VMH (Figure 1) (Gorski et al.,1978; acobson et al., 1981; Segovia and Guillamon, 1982; Matsumoto and Arai, 983; Segovia et. al., 1984a, 1986; Valencia et al., 1986; Del Abril et al., 987b; Guillamon et al., 1988b; Collado et al., 1990).

| STRUCTURE | PATTERN | ORCHIDECTOMY | ANDROGENIZATION | TESTING $E_2$ | AUTHORS |
|---|---|---|---|---|---|
| VNO | ♂>♀ | ↓ | ↑ | | Segovia & Guillamón, 1982 |
| AOB | ♂>♀ | ↓ | ↑ | + | Segovia et al., 1984, 1986<br>Valencia et al., 1986<br>Pérez-Laso et al., 1992 |
| BAOT | ♂>♀ | ↓ | ↑ | + | Collado et al., 1990<br>Collado et al., 1992 |
| BSTMP | ♂>♀ | ↓ | ↑ | | Del Abril et al., 1987<br>Guillamón et al., 1988 |
| Me | ♂>♀ | — | — | + | Mizukami et al., 1983 |
| SDN-POA | ♂>♀ | ↓ | ↑ | + | Gorski et al., 1978, 1980<br>Jacobson et al., 1981 |
| VMH | ♂>♀ | ↓ | — | | Matsumoto & Arai, 1983 |
| LC | ♀>♂ | N | ↓ | | Guillamón et al., 1988 |
| PS | ♀>♂ | ↑ | ↓ | | Del Abril et al., 1990 |
| BSTMA | ♀>♂ | ↑ | N | | Del Abril et al., 1987 |
| BSTLA | ♀>♂ | ↑ | ↓ | | Guillamón et al., 1988 |

Figure 1 Effects of early postnatal treatments on the number of neurons and/or volume in some neural nuclei in male and female rats. N: no effect; -: no study reported in the literature; testing E2: testing the aromatization hypothesis; +: positive.

The question of whether testosterone or estradiol (which is aromatized from testosterone) promotes a greater volume and/or number of neurons has been addressed for the SDN-POA (Gorski et al., 1981; Jacobson et al., 1981; Döhler et al., 1982a,1982b,1986), the Me (Mizukami et al., 1983) the AOB (Perez-Laso et al., in preparation) and the BAOT (Collado et al.,1992b). Estradiol promotes a greater volume and/or number of neurons in all of these structures in which males present a greater morphological pattern (Figure 1).

In the BSTMA, there is a larger volume and number of cells in females than in males (Del Abril et al., 1987a,b). A similar pattern of sexual dimorphism has also been found in such structures as the anteroventral periventricular nucleus (Byne and Bleier, 1987), the anterior part of the lateral division of the BST (BSTLA) (Guillamon et al., 1988b), the locus coeruleus (LC) (Guillamon et al., 1988a) and the parastrial nucleus (PS) (Del Abril et al., 1990). Estrogens play an active role in inducing sexual differentiation in the female brain (Shapiro et al., 1976; Döhler et al., 1984; Toran Allerand, 1984). Our studies concerning structures such as the BSTLA, LC and PS suggest that production of a larger volume and number of cells in the females might also be dependent on the ovaries (Figure 1).

Normal adult female rats show a larger volume and number of neurons than males in the LC (Guillamon et al., 1988a). Testosterone treatment of females on D1 after birth eliminated these differences by decreasing both measures. However, D1 castration of males affected neither of them. These data on the LC suggest that hormones from the ovaries might also induce differentiation of the LC during early postnatal life.

In the PS, females show larger volumes than males.When males were orchidectomized and females androgenized on D1, sexual dimorphism was reversed compared to control animals (Del Abril et al., 1990). These authors suggested an ovary-dependent mechanism(s) to account for the greater volume characteristic of females. However, since orchidectomy of males on D1 significantly increased the PS volume in males and androgenization of females decreased PS volume, it was suggested that testicular androgen secretion might be "inhibitory"; that is, it is promoting neuronal ingrowth.

The volume of the BSTMA is greater in females than males. Neonatal (D1) treatment with TP did not decrease this measure in the females, but D1 gonadectomy did increase it in the males (Table I and Figure 1) (Del Abril et al., 1987b). The promoting action of ovarian hormones in the female and an "inhibitory" one for testicular hormones in the males were also suggested to explain this pattern in the BSTMA (Del Abril et al., 1987b; Segovia and Guillamon, 1992).

Females have a greater number of neurons than males in the BSTLA (Guillamón et al., 1988b). Orchidectomy of males on D1 significantly increased this number, while TP treatment of females on the same day produced the opposite effect (Table II and Figure 1). Again the authors suggested an ovarian mechanism for the females while proposing that androgens might act as "inhibitors" during the development of sexual dimorphism in the male BSTLA (Guillamon et al., 1988b). All these data point out that in the SDN-POA, Me and BAOT, estradiol plays an important role in promoting a greater volume and/or number of neurons in male rats. For structures such as the VNO, AOB, BSTMP and VMH, a similar mechanism might be suggested for the male. Regarding the LC, BSTMA, BSTLA and PS, an ovarian-dependent mechanism was necessary to explain the greater volume and/or number of neurons seen in the female compared to males. Thus, the greater morphological pattern in both sexes is probably due to estradiol. Toran-Allerand (1984) addressed the way in which estradiol promotes this pattern, proposing a "cascade-hypothesis" to explain neuronal survival and the consequent greater number of neurons.

A different mechanism, in which males or females have lesser volume and/or number of neurons than the opposite sex in a particular structure, must be solved for a complete explanation of the mechanism(s) that induce sexual dimorphism in the nervous system. When males presented a smaller volume and/or number of neurons than females, as in the BSTMA, BSTL and PS (see above) early postnatal orchidectomy "increased" the volume and/or the number of neurons (Figure 1). Thus, it was necessary to suggest that androgens normally have an "inhibitory effect" on volume and/or number of neurons. A parsimonious approach to this problem would be to discard the aromatization of testoterone to estradiol and any effect of the latter hormone in order to concentrate on the alpha-reduction of testosterone to dihydrotestosterone (DHT) in some brain nuclei to explain the fact that one sex presents smaller volume and/or number of neurons than the other.

Regarding AOB volume, males treated with DHT from postnatal days 6 to 20 showed a drastic reduction in overall AOB volume and its constituent layers compared to intact an vehicle control males. AOB volumetric measures in DHT treated males did not differ, however, from those shown by intact females (Valencia et al., 1992). With respect to the BAOT, postnatally DHT treated males presented a statistically significant decrease in BAOT volume compared with control males and a similar volume compared with control females. Moreover, BAOT volume *increased* in females treated with cyproterone acetate (CA) from D6 to D20 (Collado et al., 1992a).

Since it is known that a progressive increment in DHT develops in the female hypophysis between postnatal days 5 to 20 (Denef et al., 1974), the above mentioned data indicate that DHT has a functional role in the sexual differentiation of the female and suggest that this non-aromatic androgen could also be involved in causing the sexually dimorphic pattern found in the BSTMA, BSTL and PS, in which the female rat has a greater volume and/or number of neurons than the male. However, it remains to be established whether alpha-reductase activity develops in the male BSTMA, BSTL and PS during the periods of sexual differentiation. The mechanim(s) causing DHT to produce a smaller volume is also still unknown. The perinatal effects of DHT might help to account for the production of this pattern, since it hinders the development of a greater volume in the male AOB and BAOT. DHT is counteracted during a critical period in CA treated females causing them to present an increment in BAOT volume similar to that of the males. It might be the case that DHT facilitates neuronal death, at least in structures that experience prenatal neurogenesis and postnatal differentiation (such as the AOB) and/or it may also be that DHT contributes to a general process that induces neuronal ingrowth.

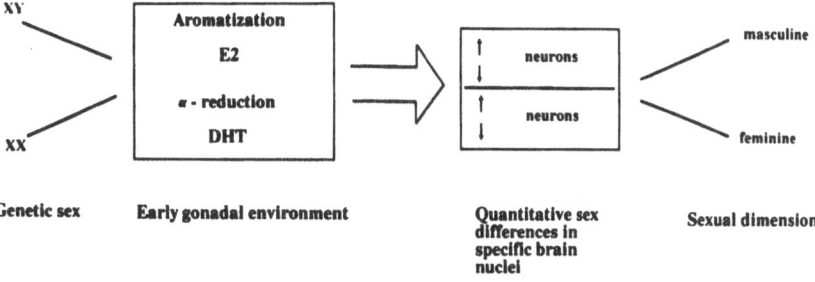

**Figure 2** A bidimensional model for the development of sexual dimorphism in the brain.

372

Much experimental data will be needed to test this hypothesis but we would like to present the suggestion that development of brain sex differences is not a linear process, dependent only on the level of E2 during different critical periods. It is rather a bidimensional process (Figure 2) in which the particular conditions of a group of cells (receptors, enzymes, neurotransmitters, critical periods etc.) and the hormone E2 promote neuronal survival while DHT, another hormone, facilitates neuronal death. This bidimensional process therefore determines different axes for males and females.

# References

Allen, L. S. and Gorski, R. A. (1990). Sex difference in the bed nucleus of the stria terminalis of the human brain. *J. Comp. Neurol.*, **302** : 697-706.

Bayer, S.A. (1980). Quantitative 3H-thymidine-radiographic analyses of neurogenesis in the rat amygdala. *J. Comp. Neurol.*, **194** : 845-875.

Bayer, S. A. (1983). 3H-thymidine-radiographic studies of neurogenesis in the rat olfactory bulb. *Exp. Brain Res.*, **50** : 329-340.

Broadwell, R. D. (1975). Olfactory relationships of the telencephalon and diencephalon in the rabbit. I. An autoradiographic study of the efferent connections of the main and accessory olfactory bulbs. *J. Comp. Neurol.*, **163** : 329-346.

Byne, W. and Bleier, R. (1987). Medial preoptic sexual dimorphisms in the guinea pig. I. An investigation on their hormonal dependence. *J. Neurosci.*, **7** : 2688-2696.

Caminero, A. A., Segovia, S. and Guillamon, A. (1991). Sexual dimorphism in accessory olfactory bulb mitral cells : a quantitative Golgi study. *Neuroscience.*, **45** : 663-670.

Collado, P., Guillamon, A., Valencia, A. and Segovia, S. (1990). Sexual dimorphism in the bed nucleus of the accessory olfactory tract in the rat. *Dev. Brain Res.*, **56** : 263-268.

Collado, P, Segovia, S., Cales, J. M., Perez-Laso, C., Rodriguez-Zafra, M., Guillamon, A. and Valencia, A. (1992a). Female's DHT controls sex differences in the rat bed nucleus of the accessory olfactory tract. *Neuro Reports.*, **3** :327-329.

De Olmos, J. S. and Ingram, W. R. (1972). The projection field of the stria terminalis in the rat brain : an experimental study. *J. Comp. Neurol.*, **146** : 303-334.

Del Abril, A., Guillamon, A. and Segovia, S. (1987a). El nucleo de la estria terminal de la rata : diferencias de sexo en la poblacion neuronal de la region medial anterior. *Trabajos Instituto. Cajal.*. LXXVI : 230.

Del Abril, A., Segovia, S. and Guillamon, A. (1987b). The bed nucleus of the stria terminalis in the rat : regional sex differences controlled by gonadal steroids early after birth. *Dev. Brain Res.*, **32** : 295-300.

Del Abril, A., Segovia, S. and Guillamon, A. (1990). Sexual dimorphism in the parastrial nucleus of the rat preoptic area. *Dev. Brain Res.*, **52** : 11-15.

Del Cerro, M. C. R., Izquierdo, M. A. P., Collado, P., Segovia, S. and Guillamon, A. (1991). Bilateral lesions of the bed nucleus of the accessory olfactory tract facilitate maternal behavior in virgin female rats. *Physiol. Behav.,* **50** : 67-71.

Denef, C., Magnus, C. and McEwen, B. S. (1974). Sex dependent changes in pituitary 5alpha-dihydrotestosterone and 3alpha-androstenediol formation during postnatal development and puberty in the rat. *Endocrinol.,* **94** : 1266-1275.

Döhler, K. D., Coquelin, A., Davis, F., Hines, M., Shryne, J. E. and Gorski, R. A. (1982a). Differentiation of the sexually dimorphic nucleus in the preoptic area of the rat brain is determined by the perinatal hormone environment. *Neurosci. Lett.,* **33** : 295-298.

Döhler, K. D., Coquelin, A., Davis, F., Hines, M., Shryne, J. E., Sickmoller, P. M., Jarzab, B. and Gorski, R. A. (1986). Pre-and postnatal influence of an estrogen antagonist and an androgen antagonist on differentiation of the sexually dimorphic nucleus of the preoptic area in male and female rats. *Neuroendocrinol.,* **42** : 443-448.

Döhler, K. D., Hancke,J. L., Srivastava, S. S., Hofman, C., Shryne, J. E. and Gorski, R. A. (1984). Participation of estrogens in female sexual differentiation of the brain : neuroanatomical, neuroendocrine and behavioral evidence In : De Vries, G. J., De Bruin, J. P. C., Uylings, H. B. M. and Corner, M. A. (Eds.), *Sex Differences in the Brain*, Progress in Brain Research, Elsevier, Amsterdam, pp.99-117.

Döhler, K. D., Hines, M., Coquelin, A., Davis, F., Shryne, J. E. and Gorski, R. A. (1982b). Pre- and postnatal influence of diethystilbestrol on differentiation of sexually dimorphic nucleus in the preoptic area of the female rat brain. *Neuroendocrinol.Lett.,* **4** : 361-365.

Dörner, G. (1976). *Hormones and Brain Differentiation*, Elsevier, Amsterdam.

Dörner, G. and Staudt, J. (1968). Structural changes in the preoptic anterior hypothalamic area of the male rat, following neonatal castration and androgen substitution. *Neuroendocrinol.,* **3** : 136-140.

Dörner, G. and Staudt, J.(1969). Structural changes in the hypothalamic ventromedial nucleus of the male rat, following neonatal castration and androgen treatment. *Neuroendocrinol.,* **4** : 278-281.

Gorski, R. A., Csermus, V. J. and Jacobson, C. D. (1981). Sexual dimorphism in the preoptic area. *Reprod. Dev. Adv. Physiol. Sci.,* **15** : 121-130.

Gorski, R. A., Gordon, J. H., Shryne, J. E. and Southam, A. M. (1978). Evidence for a morphological sex difference within the medial preoptic area of the rat brain. *Brain Res.,* **148** : 333-346.

Gorski, R. A., Harlan, R. E., Jacobson, C. D., Shryne, J. E. and Southam, A. M. (1980). Evidence for the existence of a sexually dimorphic nucleus in the preoptic area of the rat. *J. Comp. Neurol.,* **193** : 529-539.

Guillamon, A., De Blas, M. R. and Segovia, S. (1988a). Effects of sex steroids on the development of the locus coeruleus in the rat, *Dev. Brain Res.,* **40** : 306-310.

Guillamon, A., Segovia, S. and Del Abril, A. (1988b). Early effects of gonadal steroids on the neuron number in the medial posterior and the lateral divisions of the bed nucleus of the stria terminalis in the rat. *Dev. Brain Res.*, **44** : 281-290.

Halpern, M. (1987). The organization and function of the vomeronasal system. *Ann. Rev. Neurosci.*, **10** : 325-362.

Hines, M., Davis, F., Coquelin, A., Goy, R. W. and Gorski, R. A. (1985). Sexually dimorphic regions in the medial preoptic area and the bed nucleus of the stria terminalis of the guinea pig brain : a description and an investigation of their relationship to gonadal steroids in adulthood. *J. Neurosci.*, **5** : 40-47.

Izquierdo, M. A. P., Del Cerro, M. C. R., Collado, P., Segovia, S. and Guillamon, A. (1992). Maternal behavior induced in male rats by bilateral lesions of the bed nucleus of the accessory olfactory tract. *Physiol. Behav.*, In press.

Jacobson, C. D., Csernus, V. J., Shryne, J. E. and Gorski, R. A. (1981). The influence of gonadectomy, androgen exposure, or a gonadal graft in the neonatal rat on the volume of the sexually dimorphic nucleus of the preoptic area. *J. Neurosci.*, **1** : 1142-1147.

Konishi, M. and Akutagawa, E. (1985). Neuronal growth, atrophy and death in a sexually dimorphic song nucleus in the zebra finch. *Nature.*, **315** : 145-147.

Matsumoto, A. and Arai, Y. (1983). Sex difference in volume of the ventromedial nucleus of the hypothalamus in the rat, *Endocrin. Jpn.*, **30** : 277-280.

Matsumoto, A. and Arai, Y. (1986). Male-female difference in synaptic organization of the ventromedial nucleus of the hypothalamus in the rat, *Neuroendocrinol.*, **42** : 232-236.

McShane, S., Glaser, L., Greer, E. R., Houtz, J., Tong, M. F. and Diamond, M. C. (1988). Cortical asymmetry- a preliminary study : neurons-glia, female-male. *Exp. Neurol.*, **99** : 353-361.

Mizukami, S., Nishizuka, M. and Arai, Y. (1983). Sexual difference in nuclear volume and its ontogeny in the rat amygdala. *Experimental Neurol.*, **79** : 569-575.

Nordeen, E. J., Nordeen, K. W., Sengelaub, D. R. and Arnold, A. P. (1985). Androgens prevent normally occurring cell death in a sexually dimorphic spinal nucleus. *Science.*, **229** : 671-673.

Powers, J. B. and Winans, S. S. (1975). Vomeronasal organ : critical role in mediating sexual behavior of the male hamster. *Science,* **187** : 961-963.

Raisman, G. and Field, P. M. (1971). Sexual dimorphism in the preoptic area of the rat. *Science.*, **173** : 731-733.

Raisman, G. and Field, P. M. (1973). Sexual dimorphism in the neuropil of the preoptic area of the rat and its dependence on neonatal androgen. *Brain Res.*, **54** : 1-29.

Roos, J., Roos, M., Schaeffer, C. and Aron, C. (1988). Sexual differences in the development of accessory olfactory bulbs in the rat. *J. Comp. Neurol.*, **270** : 121-131.

Roos, J., Roos, M., Schaeffer, C. and Aron, C. (1989). Prepubescent hormonal control of the development of accessory olfactory bulbs in male rat. *Dev. Brain Res.*, **47** : 309-312.

Saper, C. B. (1984). Organization of cerebral cortical afferent system in the rat. II. Magnocellular basal nucleus. *J. Comp. Neurol.,* **222** : 313-342.

Scalia, F. and Winans, S. S. (1975). The differential projections of the olfactory bulb and accessory olfactory bulb in mammals. *J. Comp. Neurol.,* **161** : 31-56.

Segovia, S. and Guillamon, A. (1982). Effects of sex steroids on the development of the vomeronasal organ in the rat. *Dev. Brain Res.,* **5** : 209-212.

Segovia, S. and Guillamon, A. (1986). Effects of sex steroids on the development of the vomeronasal system in the rat. In : Breipohl, W. (Ed.), *Ontogeny of Olfaction in Vertebrates,* Springer-Verlag, Berlin Heidelberg, pp. 35-41.

Segovia, S. and Guillamon, A. (1992). Sexual dimorphism in the vomeronasal pathway and sex differences in reproductive behaviors. *Brain Res. Rev.,* Submited.

Segovia, S., Orensanz, L. M., Valencia, A. and Guillamon, A. (1984a). Effects of sex steroids on the development of the accessory olfactory bulb in the rat : a volumetric study. *Dev. Brain Res.,* **16** : 12-314.

Segovia, S., Paniagua, R., Nistal, M. and Guillamon, A. (1984b). Effects of postpuberal gonadectomy on the neurosensorial epithelium of the vomeronasal organ in the rat. *Dev. Brain Res.,* **14** : 289-291.

Segovia, S., Valencia, A., Cales, J. M. and Guillamon, A. (1986). Effects of sex steroids on the development of two granule cell subpopulations in the accessory olfactory bulb. *Dev. Brain Res.,* **30** : 283-286.

Shapiro, B. H., Goldman, A. S., Steinbeck, H. F. and Neuman, F. (1976). Is feminine differentiation of the brain hormonally determined? *Experientia,* **32** : 650-651.

Staudt, J. and Dörner, G. (1976). Structural changes in the medial and central amygdala of the male rat, following neonatal castration and androgen treatment. *Endocrinol.,* **67** : 296-300.

Struble, R. G. and Walters, C. P. (1982). Light microscopic differentiation of two populations of rat olfactory bulb granule cells. *Brain Res.,* **236** : 237-251.

Stumpf, W. E. and Sar, M. (1982). The olfactory system as a target organ for steroid hormones. In : Breipohl, W. (Ed.), *Olfaction and Endocrine Regulation,* IRL Press, London, pp. 11-21.

Toran-Allerand, C. D. (1984). On the genesis of sexual differentiation of the central nervous system : morphogenetic consequences of steroidal exposure and possible role of alfa-fetoprotein. In : De Vries, G. J., De Bruin, J. P. C., Uylings, H. B. M. and Corner, M. A. (Eds.), *Sex Differences in the Brain, Progress Brain Research.,* Elsevier, Amsterdam, pp. 63-98.

Valencia, S., Segovia, A. and Guillamon, A. (1986). Effects of sex steroids on the development of the accessory olfactory bulb mitral cells in the rat. *Dev. Brain Res.,* **24** : 287-290.

Valencia , A., Collado, P., Cales, J. M., Segovia, S., Perez-Laso, C., Rodriguez-Zafra, M. and Guillamon, A. (1992). Postnatal administration of dihydrotestosterone to the male rat abolishes sexual dimorphism in the accessory olfactory bulb : a volumetric study. *Dev. Brain Res.*, **68** : 132-135.

Wysocki, Ch. J. (1979). Neurobehavioral evidence for the involvement of the vomeronasal system in mammalian reproduction. *Neurosci. Biobehav. Rev.*, **3** : 301-341.

Wysocki, Ch. J. and Meredith, M. (1987). The vomeronasal system. In : Finger, T. E. and Silver, W. L. (Eds.), *Neurobiology of Taste and Smell*, John Wiley and Sons, New York, pp. 125-150.

# Sex Differences in the Rat Cerebral Cortex

**J. M. JURASKA**

*Department of Psychology, University of Illinois, 603 E. Daniel Street, Champaign, IL 61820, USA*

Sex differences are evident in the human cerebral cortex both in normal functioning and after damage (eg. Witelson, 1991), yet little is known about sex differences in the human cortex, especially at the cellular level. One approach to investigating sex differences in the cortex is to study sex differences in a simpler cortex - that of the rat. Even in the rat, the cortex is involved with diverse behaviors (Kolb and Tees, 1990). My students and I have been examining sex differences in the posterior (visual cortex) cortex of the hooded rat and the concomitant portion of the corpus callosum, the splenium (Figure 1a and b). An intricate series of differences are unfolding in these regions. There is also an added complication that the cerebral cortex is plastic in response to various environmental conditions. Thus the nature of sex differences can change depending on the environment to which rats have been exposed.

## Gross size

In order to get an overall picture of the generality of cortical sex differences, we measured the thickness of the cortex in every major cytoarchitectonic area of 90 day old rats, all of which had been housed socially. We found that male rats had thicker cortices in 16 of the 24 sites examined (Reid and Juraska, 1992a). Thus sex differences are widespread in the rat cortex. This does not mean, however, that sex differences are uniform throughout the cortex. By performing a slightly finer analysis, we found that not all layers are sexually dimorphic in thickness even in cortical areas that are dimorphic in overall thickness. Additionally, there is variability between cortical areas in which layers were sexually dimorphic in thickness (Figure 2a and b). Thus, while sex differences are widespread in the rat cortex, sweeping generalizations about their presence are not appropriate and cytoarchitectonic areas must be dealt with separately.

We have found that hemispheric asymmetries are erratic in rats of either sex (Reid and Juraska, 1992a; Juraska and Reid, unpublished manuscript; Seymoure and Juraska, 1992). We find no consistency in the appearance, direction or location of asymmetries. It is interesting to note that there are

*M. Haug et al. (eds.), The Development of Sex Differences and Similarities in Behavior, 377–388.*
© 1993 *Kluwer Academic Publishers.*

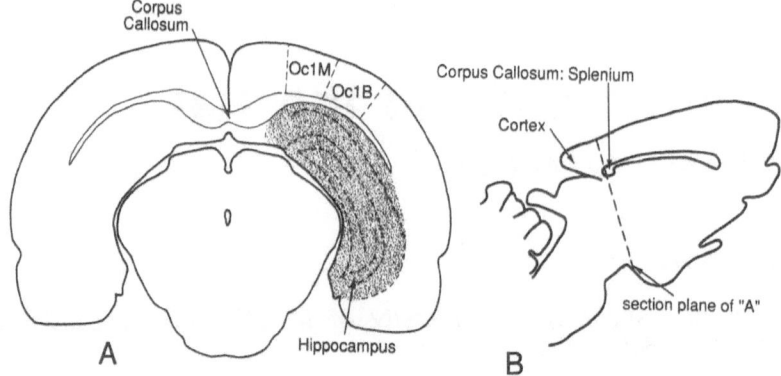

**Figure 1a**   A coronal section illustrating the location of the primary visual cortex (Oc1B and Oc1M), and the splenium of the corpus callosum.

**Figure 1b**   A sagittal section near the midline of the rat brain that illustrates the location and shape of the corpus callosum. The hatched line represents the approximate plane of section of the coronal Figure in 1a above.

inconsistencies among studies in the location of asymmetries even from a laboratory that claims general hemispheric asymmetries in male rats (Diamond et al., 1981; Dowling et al., 1982; Diamond, 1987).

Sex differences in the size of large areas of the brain such as the cerebral cortex and corpus callosum are often treated as proportional to the size of the brain as a whole or to the size of the body. While it is true that larger animals tend to have larger brains, there is no evidence that such proportions hold within a species (Jerison, 1979). Apart from regions of the nervous system that are obviously related to body size (eg, somatosensory cortex), these proportions do not enlighten us about the meaning of differences between brain areas of different sizes. Do larger areas have more cells or are the cells simply larger? What are the implications for the number and types of synaptic connections? Ultimately, what are the implications for the functioning of the area? These questions are more relevant than the question of the proportion between the size of a brain area and body size.

# Cell number

To begin to understand the implications of sex differences in the gross thickness of the cortex, we focused on one cytoarchitectonic area to count the number of neurons in 90 day old rats (Reid and Juraska, 1992b). The binocular area of the visual cortex (Oc1B) had been found to be sexually dimorphic in thickness

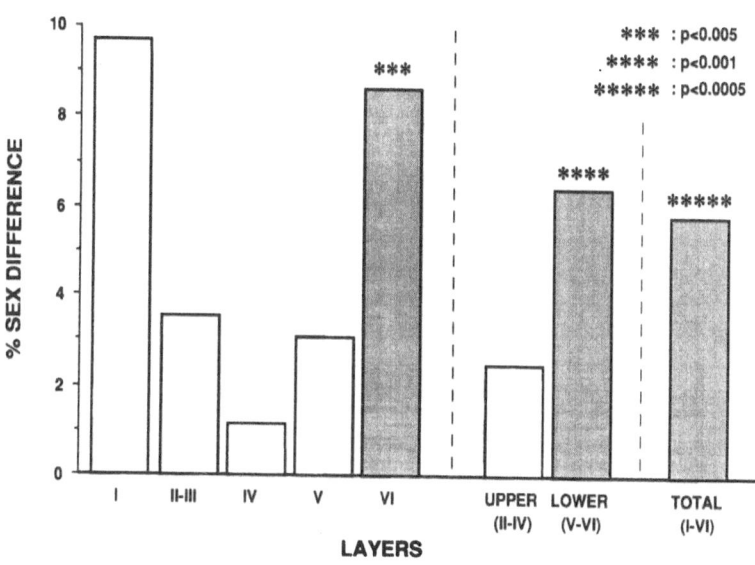

**Figure 2a** The percent difference between the sexes for layer thickness in the forelimb field of the sensori-motor cortex (FL). Percent sex difference: (male-female)/[male + female]/2. From Reid and Juraska (1992a).

(Figure 2b) and we were able to parcellate the borders of Oc1B from the surrounding regions of Oc1M and Oc2 (Reid and Juraska, 1991). Through this parcellation, we found that male hooded rats had a larger volume of Oc1B than female rats (Figure 3). (It is interesting to note that we found that Oc1B is more dimorphic than the cortex as a whole, which speaks to the importance of examining each area separately.) There were no sex differences in neuronal density (number of neurons per unit area) as calculated with the stereological technique, the disector. However, when neuronal density was multiplied by volume to determine the total number of neurons in the area, males had 18% more neurons in the Oc1B area than females. This sex difference was found in every layer except IV, the thalamic input layer. Thus, the number of neurons (and glia) are responsible to a great degree for the larger size of Oc1B in male rats.

It is interesting to speculate that this sex difference in neuron number may have arisen through differences in cell generation or cell death. Biochemical assays have demonstrated that estrogen receptors are present in the rat cortex from late in gestation through the second postnatal week (eg, MacLusky et al., 1979), and postnatal cell death has been described in the rat cortex between days 4 and 10 (Ferrer et al., 1990). Although the appearance of estrogen receptors is too late to influence neuronal proliferation (Miller, 1988), they could play a role in cell death and, therefore, create sex differences. This would be consistent with cell

**OC1B (PRIMARY VISUAL CORTEX - BINOCULAR FIELD)**

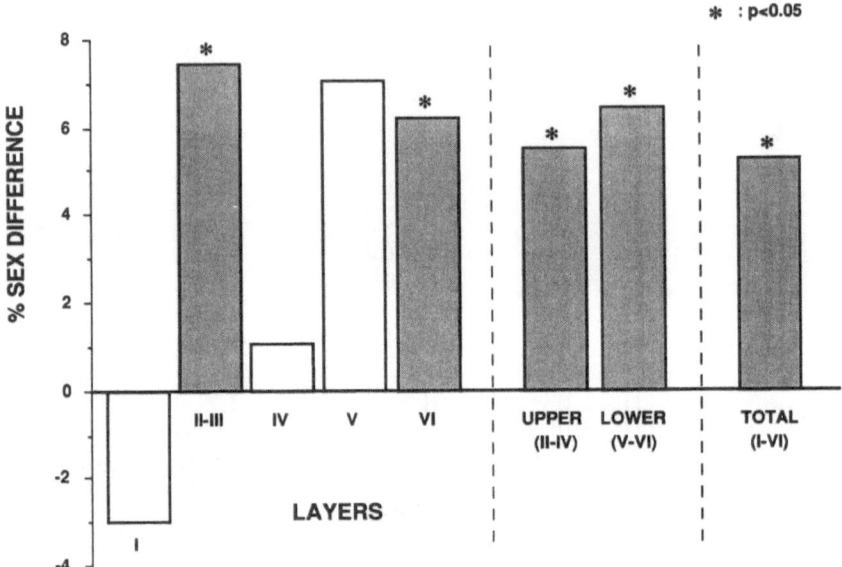

**Figure 2b** The percent difference between the sexes for layer thickness in the binocular field of the primary visual cortex (Oc1B). From Reid and Juraska (1992a).

death as the mechanism for sex differences in other areas such as the spinal cord and the superior cervical ganglion (Nordeen et al., 1985; Wright and Smolan, 1987).

The lack of sex differences in neuronal density in Oc1B suggests that there probably are few sex differences in the number of synapses associated with each neuron in Oc1B. We investigated this by counting synapses and measuring their length (Reid and Juraska, unpublished manuscript). Although we found no sex differences in synaptic density, synaptic length or the number of synapses per neuron varies with more subtle environmental manipulations such as rearing in a stimulating, complex environment as opposed to individual housing (Turner and Greenough, 1985). Therefore, the present pattern of a greater number of synapses in the Oc1B area in males might be different in other environments, as experiments below will illustrate.

# Dendritic branching

It has long been established that male rats reared post-weaning in a complex environment (social housing with a changing set of objects) have larger dendritic fields in the visual cortex (Oc1) than rats housed alone (Volkmar and

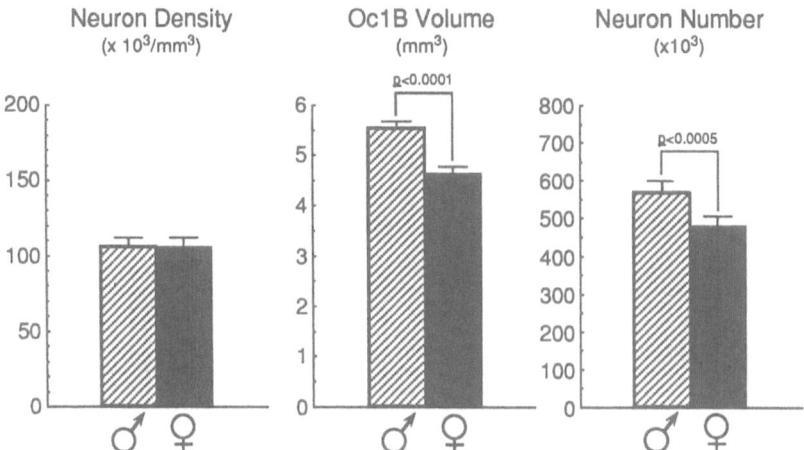

**Figure 3**    A summary of the measurements from Oc1B as a whole: neuron density, Oc1B volume and neuron number. Adapted from Reid and Juraska (1992b).

Greenough,1972). I have found that there are sex differences in the degree of plasticity exhibited in some neuronal populations with this paradigm (Juraska, 1984). In both layer III pyramidal neurons and layer IV stellate neurons, there was more plasticity (i.e. differences between environmental groups) in males than in females. (In contrast, I should note that female rats exhibit more plasticity in the dendritic fields of hippocampal dentate granule neurons than male rats (Juraska et al., 1985)). These sex differences in dendritic plasticity in the visual cortex also influence the sex differences within an environment (Figure 4). There are no significant sex differences in the dendritic fields in rats from the isolated environment, but males have larger dendritic trees than females in the complex environment in some neuronal populations.

We have subsequently examined the state of the basilar dendritic tree of layer III neurons at weaning age, when the rats are placed in the complex and isolated environments (Seymoure and Juraska, 1992). There are few sexual dimorphisms in the dendritic tree at this age and those that exist are opposite (female > male) to those found in young adults (Figure 5). Thus it is clear that both types of post-weaning environments shape the occurrence and form of dendritic sex differences. We found an added complication in that the appearance of sex differences varied between the monocular (Oc1M) and binocular (Oc1B) regions of the primary visual cortex. This is a distinction that was not made in the adult study (Juraska, 1984) in which all of Oc1 was sampled, but it certainly needs to be dealt with in future work. It is consistent with a study by Kolb and Stewart (1991) in which they found that the pattern of sex differences in dendritic branching varies with the individual cytoarchitectonic area within the prefrontal cortex.

We have begun to investigate the hormonal basis for the sex differences in plasticity in response to the post-weaning environment. We castrated or sham

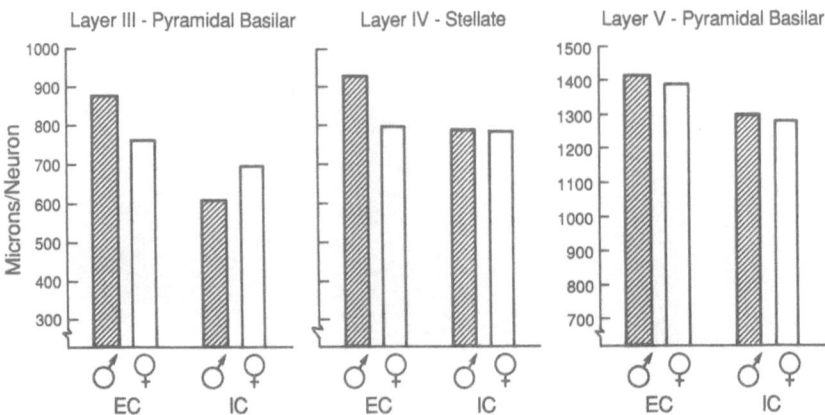

**Figure 4** The total dendritic length for three populations of neurons within the visual cortex (Oc1). There was a significant interaction (P<.01) between sex and environment for the basilar dendrites of layer III pyramidal neurons; there also was a significant environment effect (P<.00001). Layer IV stellate neurons had significant sex (P<.05) and environment (P<.05) effects. There was only an environment effect (P<.006) for the basilar dendrites of layer V pyramidal neurons. From Juraska (1991).

operated littermate sets of male rats at birth and after weaning raised them in either an isolated or complex environment. Our preliminary data indicate that neonatal castration was without effect on the dendritic plasticity of layer III pyramidal neurons (Seymoure et al., 1992). This is especially surprising because we had previously found that neonatal castration of male rats reversed their lack of dendritic plasticity to these environments in hippocampal granule neurons (Juraska et al., 1988). It is also without precedent for neonatal gonadal steroids not to play a role in sex differences (Toran-Allerand, 1986). It may be that testosterone affects the properties of layer III cortical neurons prenatally at a time that precedes their migration into the cortex.

# Corpus callosum

Sex differences in no other region of the brain has evoked such widespread interest as the corpus callosum. The corpus callosum does represent a unique opportunity to study an axon pathway in a quantitative manner because its component axons are clumped into a distinguishable mass. This mass can be traced and multiplied by axonal density to calculate the number of axons in the whole pathway or some part of it. Unfortunately, axonal density is arduous to determine, requires electron microscopy and is almost never available in humans where considerable work on the gross size of the structure has been done.

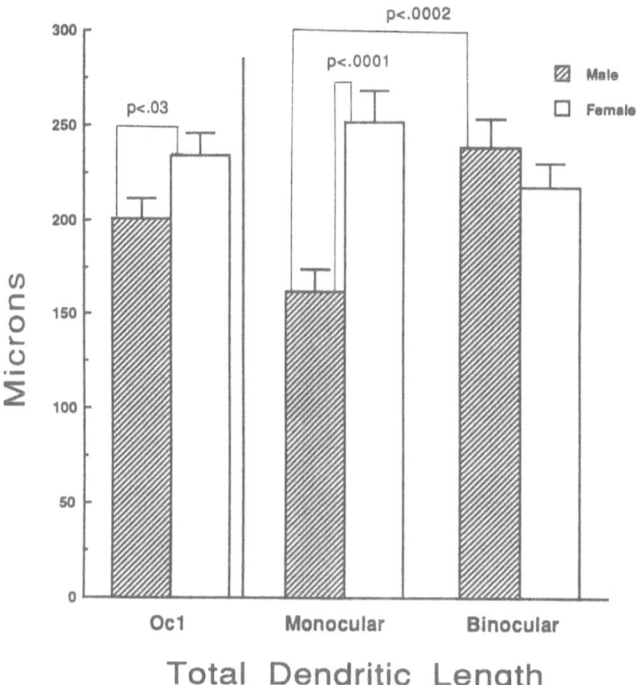

**Figure 5** Total dendritic length of oblique branches along the apical shaft of layer III pyramidal neurons in the primary visual cortex (Oc1) and its subfields: the monocular (Oc1M) and binocular (Oc1B) regions. From Seymoure and Juraska (1992).

The investigations into sex differences in the corpus callosum started with a report by DeLacoste-Utamsing and Holloway (1982) that human females had a more bulbous splenium (posterior corpus callosum) than human males in autopsy tissue. Many other laboratories have tried to replicate this phenomenon and failed in both autopsy tissue and MRI images (eg, Bell and Variend, 1985; Witelson, 1985; Bleier et al., 1986; Kertesz et al., 1987). Both Clarke et al. (1989) and Allen et al. (1991) found that the ratio of the splenium to the more anterior body of the corpus callosum was larger in females but there were no sex differences in size. This indicates a sex difference in the shape of the corpus callosum in humans. How this translates into possible cellular differences is unknown. It may be that in females the same number of axons are bent into a different shape because of the smaller female cranium in which case there may be no implications for axon number and function at all.

Furthermore, we have evidence that the lack of sex differences in the gross size of the rat splenium does not predict axonal numbers. We measured the gross size of the callosum as a whole and as percentages of its overall length, and found no sex differences (Juraska and Kopcik, 1988). We did find that the gross size of the corpus callosum varied with the post-weaning environment such that rats of both sexes that were reared in a more complex environment had a larger corpus callosum overall and in the splenial region than rats reared in individual cages.

In order to determine axonal density, we quantified the axonal composition of the splenium (posterior fifth) through electron microscopy and found that within each environment (complex or isolated) females had more axons than males (Figure 6). This was consistently true in both environments for the unmyelinated axons that make up approximately 90% of the axons in the splenium (females had more myelinated axons than males only in the complex environment). We have also confirmed this pattern of sex differences in the splenium (female > male) in rats socially housed post-weaning (Kim and Juraska, unpublished observations). Thus, sex differences in axonal composition of the splenium are not reflected in sex differences in gross size of the area. This casts a new light on the controversy surrounding the gross size of the human corpus callosum.

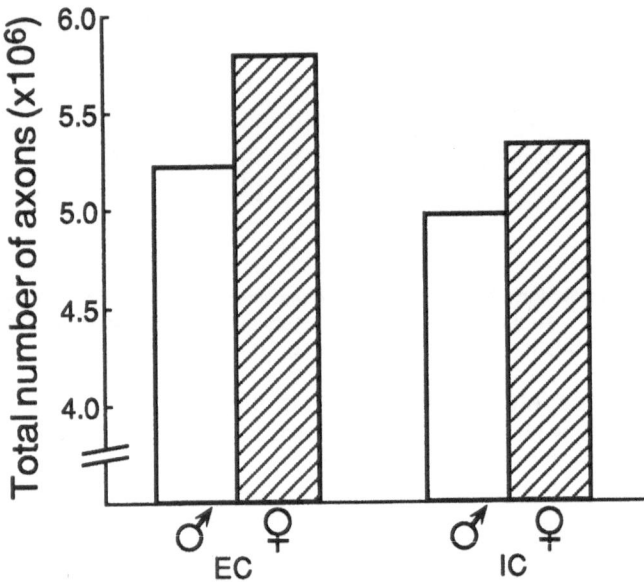

**Figure 6**  The total number of axons (myelinated and unmyelinated) in the rat splenium (posterior fifth) of the corpus callosum. Both sex (P<.002) and environment (P<.05) factors are significant.

From where do the larger number of axons in the female rat's splenium originate? Callosal projection neurons are not evenly spread across the posterior cortex. Many, perhaps most, are concentrated along the 17/18a border in the visual cortex in what is Oc1B for the most part (Olivarria and Van Sluyters, 1985). It should be recalled that we have found that males have more neurons in Oc1B. This makes the greater number of axons in females even more puzzling. We hypothesized that females might have an extra region of callosal projection neurons in comparison to males that would be the source of their greater number of splenial axons. To examine this idea, we filled the posterior cortex on one side (varied right or left) with horseradish peroxidase (HRP) and examined the pattern of retrogradely labelled neurons. We did not find any sex differences in the location of callosal projection neurons in the posterior cortex (Kopcik et al., 1992). This leaves the question of the source of the greater number of axons in females unanswered. It may be that females simply have a higher proportion (or density) of callosal projection neurons in their visual cortex. HRP and other retrograde tracers are ill suited to the type of quantification (i.e. cell counts) that could reveal this.

In trying to understand the location of neurons that contribute to the greater number of axons in the female rat splenium, one other relevant question is to what degree is the posterior fifth of the rat corpus callosum comprised of fibers from the visual cortex? Also, can we localize the axons from specific areas within the visual cortex, such as Oc1B, within the splenium? To answer these questions we are currently locating the course of axons from various small HRP injections within the corpus callosum (Kim et al., 1992). To date we have found that axons from the visual, and to a lessor extent, the temporal cortex are contained in the posterior fifth of the corpus callosum. While there is some anterior-posterior and lateral-medial organization, the axons from any given part of the visual cortex (e.g. Oc1B) cannot be localized to a smaller portion of the splenium.

We have also done some preliminary investigation of the development of the sex differences in axonal numbers in the splenium. According to prior studies that have examined patterns of neurons filled with retrograde HRP, callosal projection neurons are widespread in the developing visual cortex but there is pruning back to the adult locations of projection neurons by postnatal day 15 (Lund et al., 1984; Olavarria and Van Sluyters, 1985). This suggested that axon number was mature by this age. We counted axons in electron micrographs at postnatal days 15, 25 and 60 and found that sex differences were not apparent in the splenium at 15 days but did appear at 25 days. Furthermore, there was an increase in the number of axons in females between 15 and 25 days of age (Kim and Juraska, 1990). This is very late for the addition of axons to a major pathway! It is unclear whether this indicates that only females have such late growth or whether males have more axon withdrawal in addition to their growth of axons which results in no net change. We view these data as preliminary for two reasons. First, we have evidence that different regions within the rat splenium have somewhat different axonal densities and how extensively one samples the splenium will influence the results. We intend to reexamine all three ages (15, 25 and 60) and sample more widely. Second, the gross size of the structure is very important in the calculation of total axon number from axonal density. We have recently been devising ways of staining the developing corpus callosum en block that result in as clear a boundary for the structure as our methods in adults. These are technical innovations that should help to refine our data to better understand the development of sex differences in axon numbers in the splenium.

In summary, there is no one generalization that describes sex differences in the rat cerebral cortex. It is evident that these cellular sex differences can change during the course of development and are not to be inferred from measures of gross size. Further work is needed on the role of hormones in the formation of these differences. Also the behavioral implications require exploration and, given how ubiquitous sex differences are, will be multidimensional. These cellular sex differences in the cerebral cortex need to be understood to grasp the underpinnings of sex differences in cognitive behavior.

# Acknowledgements

Work not yet published in refereed journals was supported by NSF grant BNS 89-09164.

# References

Allen, L. S., Rickey, M. F., Chai, Y. M. and Gorski, R. A. (1991). Sex differences in the corpus callosum of the living human being. *J. Neurosci.*, **11** : 933-942.

Bell, A. D. and Variend, S. (1985). Failure to demonstrate sexual dimorphism of the corpus callosum in childhood. *J. Anat.*, **143** : 143-147.

Bleier, R., Houston, L. and Byne, W. (1986). Can the corpus callosum predict gender, age, handedness, or cognitive differences? *Trends in Neurosci.*, **9** : 391-394.

Clarke, S., Kraftsik, R., Van Der Loos, H. and Innocenti, G. M. (1989). Forms and measures of adult and human corpus callosum : is there sexual dimorphism? *J. Comp. Neurol.*, **280** : 213-230.

de Lacoste-Utamsing, M. C. and Holloway, R. L. (1982). Sexual dimorphism in the human corpus callosum. *Science*, **16** : 1431-1432.

Diamond, M. C. (1987). Sex differences in the rat forebrain. *Brain Res. Rev.*, **12** : 235-240.

Diamond, M. C., Dowling, G. A. and R. E. Johnson (1981). Age-related morphological cerebral cortical asymmetry in male and female rats. *Exp. Neurol.*, **71** : 261-268.

Dowling, G. A., Diamond, M. C., Murphy, G. M. Jr. and R. E. Johnson (1982). A morphological study of male rat cerebral cortical asymmetry. *Exper. Neurol.*, **75** : 51-67.

Ferrer, I., Bernet, E., Soriano, E., Del Rio, T. and Fonseca, M. (1990). Naturally occurring cell death in the cerebral cortex of the rat and removal of dead cells by transitory phagocytes. *Neuroscience*, **39** : 451-458.

Jerison, H. J. (1979). The evolution of diversity in brain size. In : Hahn, M. E., C. Jensen and Dudek, B. C. (Eds.), *Development and Evolution of Brain Size, Behavioral Implications*, Academic Press, New York, pp. 29-57.

Juraska, J. M. (1984). Sex differences in dendritic response to differential experience in the rat visual cortex. *Brain Res.*, **295** : 27-34.

Juraska, J. M. (1991). Sex differences in "cognitive" regions of the rat brain. *Psychoneuroendocrinology*, **16** : 105-119.

Juraska, J. M., Fitch, J., Henderson C. and Rivers, N. (1985). Sex differences in the dendritic branching of dentate granule cells following differential experience. *Brain Res.*, **333** : 73-80.

Juraska, J. M. and Kopcik, J. R. (1988). Sex and environmental influences on the size and ultrastructure of the rat corpus callosum. *Brain Res.*, **450** : 1-8.

Juraska, J. M., Kopcik, J. R., Washburne D. L. and Perry, D. L. (1988). Neonatal castration of male rats affects the dendritic response to differential environments in hippocampal dentate granule neurons. *Psychobiology*, **16** : 406-410.

Kertesz, A., Polk, M., Howell, J. and Black, S. E. (1987). Cerebral dominance, sex and callosal size in MRI. *Neurology*, **37** : 1385-1388.

Kim, J. H. Y. and J. M. Juraska (1990). Sex differences in the ultrastructural development of the rat corpus callosum. *Soc. Neurosci. Abstr.*, **15** : 321.

Kim, J. H. Y., Ellman A. B. and Juraska, J. M. (1992). Topographical organization of axons in the splenium of the rat corpus callosum. *Soc. Neuro. Abstr.*, **18** : 300.

Kolb, B. and Stewart, J. (1991). Sex-related differences in dendritic branching of cells in the prefrontal cortex of rats. *J. Neuroendocrinol.*, **3** : 95-100.

Kolb, B. and Tees, R. C. (1990). *The Cerebral Cortex of the Rat.*, MIT Press, Cambridge, MA.

Kopcik, J. R., Seymoure, P., Schneider, S. K., Kim-Hong J. and Juraska, J. M. (1992). Does the distribution of callosal projection neurons reflect the sex difference in the number of axons in the rat corpus callosum? *Brain Res. Bull.*, **29** : 493-497.

Lund, R. D., Chang, F. L. F. and Land, P. W. (1984). The development of callosal projections in normal and one-eyed rats. *Dev. Brain Res.*, **14** : 336-347.

MacLusky, N. J., Lieberburg, I. and McEwen B. S. (1979). The development of estrogen receptor systems in the rat brain : perinatal development. *Brain Res.*, **178** : 129-142.

Miller, M. W. (1988). Development of projection and local circuit neurons in neocortex. In : Peters, A. and Jones, E. G. (Eds.), *Cerebral Cortex, Vol. 7, Development and Maturation of Cerebral Cortex*, Plenum Press, New York, pp. 133-175.

Nordeen, E. J., Nordeen, K. W., Sengelaub, D. R. and Arnold, A. P. (1985). Androgens prevent normally occurring cell death in a sexually dimorphic spinal nucleus. *Science*, **229** : 671-673.

Olavarria, J. and Van Sluyters, R. C. (1985). Organization and postnatal development of callosal connections in the visual cortex of the rat. *J. Comp. Neurol.*, **239** : 1-26.

Reid, S. N. M. and Juraska, J. M. (1991). The cytoarchitectonic boundaries of the monocular and binocular areas of the rat primary visual cortex. *Brain Res.*, **563** : 293-296.

Reid, S. N. M. and Juraska, J. M. (1992a). Sex differences in the gross size of the rat neocortex. J. Comp. Neurol., 321 : 442-447.

Reid, S. N. M. and Juraska, J. M. (1992b). Sex differences in neuron number in the binocular area of the rat visual cortex. *J. Comp. Neurol.*, **321** : 448-455.

Seymoure, P., Jang, J., Pluskwa, J. and Juraska, J. M. (1992) What is the influence of testosterone on rat visual cortex dendritic plasticity? *Soc. Neuro. Abstr.*, **18** : 231.

Seymoure, P. and Juraska, J. M. (1992). Sex differences in cortical thickness and the dendritic tree in the monocular and binocular subfields of the rat visual cortex at weaning age. *Dev. Brain Res.*, **69** : 185-189.

Toran-Allerand, C. D. (1986). Sexual differentiation of the brain. In : Greenough, W. T. and Juraska, J. M. (Eds.), *Developmental Neuropsychobiology*, Academic Press, Orlando, pp. 175-211.

Turner, A. M. and Greenough, W. T. (1985). Differential rearing effects on rat visual cortex synapses. I. Synaptic and neuronal density and synapses per neuron. *Brain Res.*, **329** : 195-203.

Volkmar, F. R. and Greenough, W. T. (1972). Rearing complexity affects branching of dendrites in the visual cortex of the rat. *Science*, **176** : 1445-1447.

Witelson, S. F. (1985). The brain connection : the corpus callosum is larger in left-handers. *Science*, **229** : 665-668.

Witelson, S. F. (1991). Neural sexual mosaicism : sexual differentiation of the human temporo-parietal region for functional asymmetry. *Psychoneuroendocrinology*, **16** : 131-153.

Wright, L. L. and Smolen, A. J. (1987). The role of cell death in the development of the gender difference in the number of neurons in the rat superior cervical ganglion. *Int. J. Dev. Neurosci.*, **5** : 305-311.

# Sexual Dimorphisms in Regulatory Systems for Aggression[1,2]

**N. G. SIMON, S. F. LU, S. E. McKENNA[3], X. CHEN[4] and A. C. CLIFFORD**

*Department of Psychology and Center for Molecular Bioscience and Biotechnology, Lehigh University, Bethlehem, PA 18015, USA*

Characterization of the hormonal processes that mediate the development and expression of sexual dimorphisms in regulatory systems for conspecific, male-typical aggression has provided a model for elaborating the cellular processes that underlie these sex differences. The ability to pursue these relationships, however, is more than simply the product of methodological advances. While the development of receptor assays, highly specific antibodies, and gene probes have vastly expanded the capabilities of neuroscientists, the systematic description of steroidal effects on aggression represents an essential prerequisite if a functional role is to be ascribed to particular molecular events. Our studies on the regulation of aggression in mice have evolved along these lines over the past fifteen years. They have focused on defining active neuroendocrine pathways in adult males and females from various genotypes. Descriptions of similarities and differences between sexes and among strains provided the basis for developmental investigations that sought to define both the specific roles of the androgenic and estrogenic metabolites of testosterone in the differentiation of these regulatory systems and the precise time frame during the perinatal period when they were established. These data, in turn, generated models for evaluating specific aspects of steroid receptor function in the brain that were potentially linked to observed differences in behavioral sensitivity/insensitivity to the aggression-promoting property of gonadal steroids. The intent of the following discussion will be to review our current understanding of these relationships and, additionally, to identify the kinds of information that will be needed to develop a comprehensive model of the molecular processes that underlie sexual dimorphisms in steroid-sensitive pathways regulating aggressive behavior.

## Hormonal activation of aggression

The critical role of testosterone in facilitating the display of aggressive behavior has been well-established in non-primate mammals (for reviews see Archer, 1988; Brain, 1979; Gandelman, 1980). The robust nature of this relationship has engendered considerable interest in the possible relationship between

*M. Haug et al. (eds.), The Development of Sex Differences and Similarities in Behavior, 389–408.*
© 1993 *Kluwer Academic Publishers.*

testosterone and aggressiveness in human males, although results of these studies are less clear due to methodological constraints (Archer, 1991). An additional factor, which has received considerable attention in rodent models but virtually none in primates, is the relative contribution of the major metabolites of testosterone to behavioral activation. More specifically, T is converted by aromatase to estradiol ($E_2$) and by $5\alpha$-reductase to dihydrotestosterone (DHT) in neural target tissues (Naftolin et al., 1975; Celotti et al., 1987, 1991). As shown in Figure 1, it only has been by defining the effects of each of these metabolic products that a picture of sexual dimorphisms in neuroendocrine regulatory systems has emerged. Clearly, the issue is far more complicated than simply examining the effect of testosterone itself in each sex.

## Neuroendocrine Regulatory Systems for Aggression

|        | Androgen Sensitive | Estrogen Sensitive | Combined or Synergistic |
|--------|:------------------:|:------------------:|:-----------------------:|
| Male   | + +                | + +                | + +                     |
| Female | +                  | -                  | -                       |

+ +  highly sensitive
+    moderately sensitive
-    insensitive

**Figure 1**  A summary of the relative sensitivity of male and female mice to the aggression-promoting property of androgens or estrogens alone or in combination. ++ = highly sensitive; + = moderately sensitive; - = insensitive.

In males, there appear to be three potential activational pathways, with genotype serving as the factor determining the functional system. This model was developed through a series of studies that compared the aggression-promoting effects of specifically acting androgens (methyltrienolone (R1881), DHT) and estrogens (diethylstilbestrol (DES), $E_2$ in low doses) to those seen with T in castrated males from several strains (Simon and Gandelman, 1978; Simon and Whalen, 1986; Simon and Masters, 1987). In CF-1 males, for example, both estrogen-sensitive and androgen-sensitive systems are present. In contrast, aggression in CFW males is under estrogenic control, because both DES and $E_2$ are highly effective in restoring fighting behavior while R1881 and DHT were inactive. Rockland-Swiss males also have an estrogen-responsive system and other investigators also have reported similar findings with estrogen treatments (Edwards and Burge, 1971; Simon and Gandelman, 1978). The wealth of data demonstrating that $E_2$ can restore aggression has been viewed as strongly supporting the aromatization hypothesis, which holds that $E_2$ is the active agent mediating the behavioral effects of T in males. Yet findings with CD-1 males demonstrate that the concept is inadequate. These males were relatively insensitive to estrogen replacement but responded to DHT or R1881 at levels obtained with T. However, the most effective treatment was a combined DES + DHT regimen (Simon and Masters, 1987), in accord with an earlier report by Finney and Erpino (1976). These observations identify both androgen-regulated and combined hormonal pathways in males. It thus seems that while estrogen-sensitive pathways are present in males from several genotypes, both androgen-sensitive and combined estrogen-androgen systems also can be functional.

Studies with ovariectomized adult females have provided a very different picture. Until the early 1970's it was believed that females were incapable of responding to the aggression-promoting property of T, a position driven largely by the organization-activation model (Young et al., 1964). However, Svare et al. (1974) showed that administration of T for about 22 days resulted in the display of male-like fighting behavior by over 80% of ovariectomized, non-neonatally hormone treated R-S mice toward olfactory bulbectomized stimulus males. This result demonstrated that the sexual dimorphism in adulthood was in sensitivity to the aggression-promoting effect of T because gonadectomized adult males responded far more rapidly (about 2-3 days). While this was a singularly important finding, it did not address how aggression was induced in females; was it an androgenic, estrogenic, or combined action of the metabolites of T? Studies with several strains of female mice showed clearly that it was a direct androgenic effect that mediated behavioral activation (Schechter et al., 1981; Simon and Gandelman, 1978; Simon, et al., 1985; Simon and Masters, 1987). In ovariectomized CF-1, R-S, and C57BL/6J mice, even chronic estrogen administration at pharmacological levels failed to activate fighting behavior while T, DHT, and R1881 were highly effective in the R-S and CF-1 strains. In C57 females, only T itself was effective; no other androgen, estrogen, or combined treatment led to male-like fighting. These observations established that the female mouse CNS had an androgenic regulatory system for aggression.

In sum, males and females differ along several dimensions in neuroendocrine regulatory systems for aggression. First, there are multiple systems in males, while only an androgen-sensitive system has been identified in females. Second, the androgenic systems exhibit a relative sexual dimorphism. When present in males, it is highly responsive, requiring only 2-3 days of hormone administration to restore aggression after gonadectomy. In females, extended androgen treatment is required to activate fighting behavior, with mean durations ranging from about 14 days for CF-1 females to 22 days for R-S females after ovariectomy. Third, there is an absolute sexual dimorphism in the estrogen-sensitive pathway. It is found only in males; female mice are completely insensitive to the aggression-promoting effect of estrogens.

# Sexual differentiation of regulatory systems for aggression

The expression of a masculine or feminine pattern of steroid sensitivity in adulthood is the product of differences in the hormonal environment during the perinatal period. Conceptual models describing the effects of the presence or absence of testicular androgens have evolved from the organization-activation model, which was drawn from studies of somatic differentiation (see Griffin and Wilson, 1989), to the currently accepted sensitization model, which emphasized that the effect of perinatal testosterone exposure was the production of relative rather than absolute differences in neural sensitivity to the behavioral effects of steroids during adulthood (Gandelman, 1980). Our research in this area (Klein and Simon, 1991; Simon and Cologer-Clifford, 1991; Simon and Whalen, 1987; Suarez et al., 1992) has focused on two issues. One was to characterize the contribution of each of the metabolites of T in establishing the androgen-sensitive and estrogen-sensitive systems. The other was to more precisely define the time when these systems are masculinized. In mice, rats, and other short gestation mammals, this issue involves a consideration of whether hormonal stimulation prenatally, early in postnatal development, or throughout the entire perinatal period is needed to masculinize the neural substrates for these systems.

Masculinization of the androgen-sensitive and estrogen-sensitive pathways appears to be independently controlled by specific metabolites of T ( Figure 2; Simon and Whalen, 1987). This concept was based on the finding that Day 1

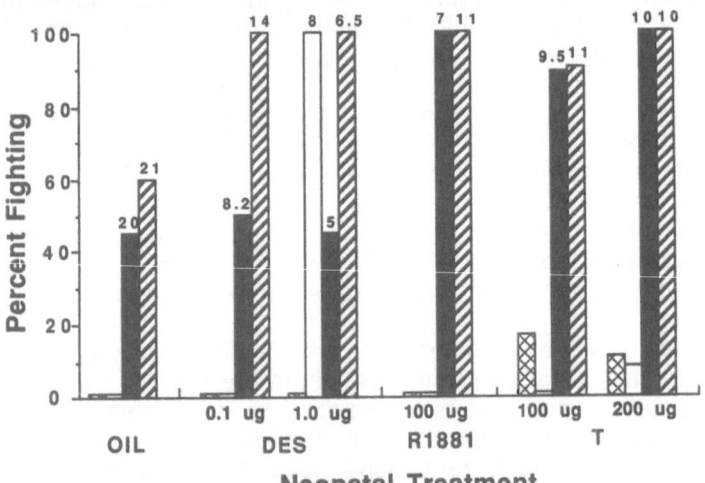

**Figure 2** The effects of Day 1 administration of T, R1881, DES, or oil vehicle on the subsequent response to DES or R1881 administered in adulthood. Numbers above each bar represent the mean treatment duration required to activate aggression among those animals within each group that actually fought. Data are adapted from Simon and Whalen, 1987.

administration of DES, but not R1881, to newborn CF-1 females established the capacity to respond to the aggression-promoting effect of estrogens in adulthood. In a complementary fashion, R1881 administration on Day I led to a more rapid, i.e., male-like response to specific androgenic treatment in adulthood. Estrogenic stimulation neonatally only had a slight masculinizing effect on responsiveness to androgens.

While the results described above defined sufficient conditions for masculinizing the two systems, several questions remained unanswered. Specifically, could the time frame for establishing the systems be narrowed and could the effects produced in females by exogenous hormone administration be validated by gonadectomizing males around the time of birth? The latter question was pivotal because males represent the natural model for masculinization and, in the previous study, T administration on Day 1 did not establish an estrogen-responsive pathway. In regard to the time frame issue, the estrogen-responsive system seems to be established early in postnatal development. Three lines of evidence support this concept. First, the system normally is absent in adult females, which argues against an effect of prenatal hormones. Second, female CF-1 mice given T on Day 1-3 postpartum exhibited aggression in response to DES as adults; administration on Days 4-6 or 7-9 were ineffective (Klein and Simon, 1991; Figure 3). Third, males delivered by

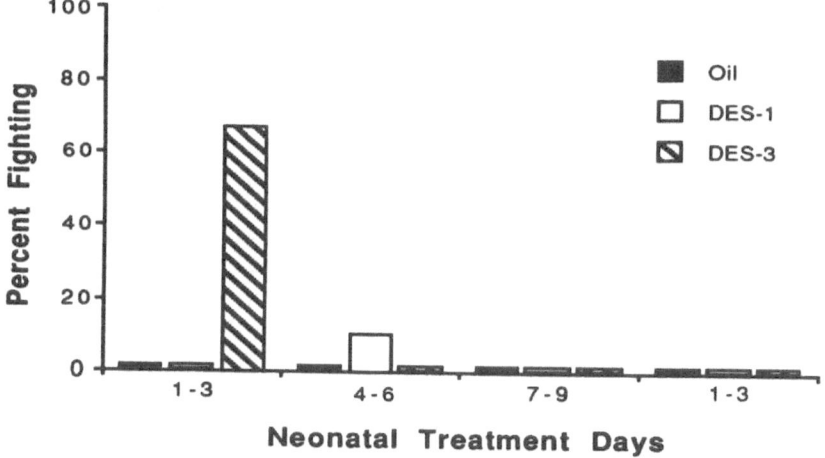

**Figure 3** The proportion of ovariectomized CF-1 females that fought in response to 1 or 3µg DES/day after neonatal exposure to 200µg T on Day 1-3, 4-6, or 7-9 postpartum. Control females received vehicle only. Mean latency for those females that fought in the T 1-3 + DES-3 condition is shown above the bar. Data are from Klein and Simon, 1991.

caesarean section and castrated immediately are insensitive to the aggression-promoting effect of estrogens as adults. Castration on Day 5 results in about 30% of males responding to estrogens while full masculinization of the system was seen if gonadectomy was conducted on Day 10 postpartum (Suarez et al.,

1992; Figure 4). An important aspect of the latter findings is that they demonstrated the utility of the proposed model under naturally occurring T exposure.

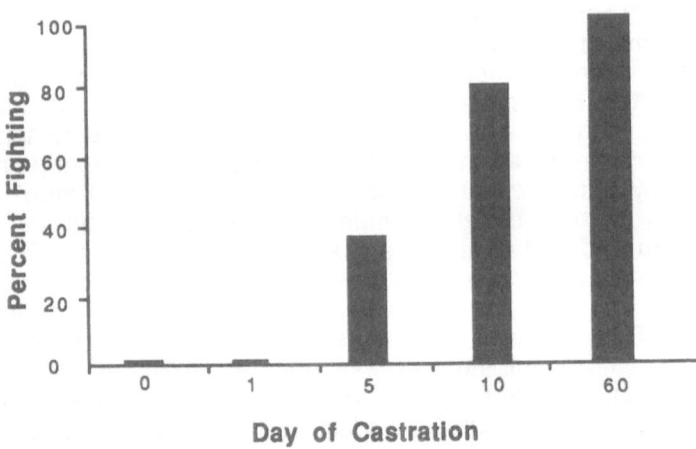

**Figure 4** Aggressive behavior exhibited by CF-1 males in response to 2μg $E_2$ /day after gonadectomy at the time of delivery by caesarean section or 1, 5, 10, or 60 day postpartum. Mean latencies for those males that fought are shown above each bar. Data are from Suarez et al, 1992.

Timing of the masculinization of the androgen-sensitive pathway appears to be somewhat more complicated, largely due to a controversy about the effects of uterine position. In mice, Gandelman and co-workers (1977) and vom Saal and Bronson (1980) reported that contiguity to two males *in utero* led to enhanced sensitivity to the aggression-promoting property of androgens in R-S and CF-1 females in comparison to females that were adjacent to two females. More recently, however, we found no effect of uterine position on T sensitivity in CF-1 females (Simon and Cologer-Clifford, 1991). It is thus unclear whether prenatal androgen exposure contributes to masculinization of the androgen-responsive pathway and it may be that these effects are genetically constrained. Early postnatal androgen exposure, on the other hand, does lead to a rapid, male-like response to the aggression-promoting property of androgen in adulthood (Bronson and Desjardins, 1968; Edwards, 1969; Simon and Whalen, 1987).

In sum, the androgenic and estrogenic metabolites of T exert specific effects in masculinizing the androgen-sensitive and estrogen-sensitive regulatory systems. The estrogen responsive pathway is masculinized early in postnatal development in mice and exposure to testicular hormones normally appears to be required for ten days if this system is to be fully differentiated. Early postnatal exposure to androgens will fully masculinize the androgen-responsive pathway, but whether or not prenatal androgenic stimulation has a contributory function remains unclear. An interesting feature of these observations is that while development of the androgen-sensitive system follows the sensitization concept, differentiation of an estrogen-sensitive pathway for aggression seems to be consistent with the notion of an organized response.

# Steroid receptor function in the regulation of aggression

The sequence of events involved in the production of steroid-dependent effects is shown in Figure 5. After entering a cell, a steroid i) binds to a specific

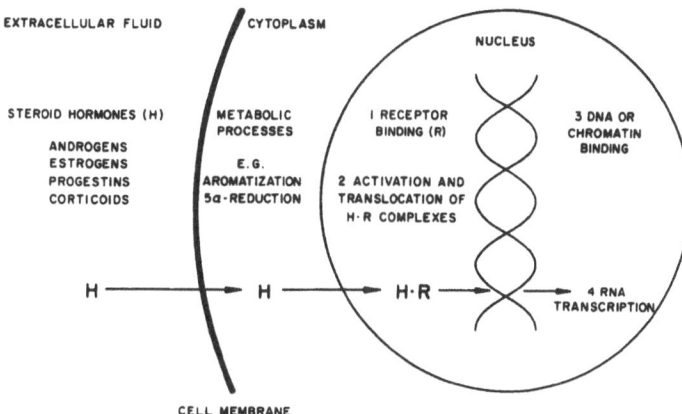

**Figure 5** A graphic representation of the steps involved in gene regulation by steroid hormones. After entering a target cell, steroids (androgens, estrogens, progestins, corticosteroids) i) bind to specific intracellular receptor proteins, ii) the complex undergoes a temperature-dependent conformational shift, termed activation, that increases affinity for genomic binding sites, iii) the activated complex translocates to DNA and/or chromatin acceptor sites, and iv) this receptor-acceptor interaction regulates RNA and subsequent protein synthesis through gene activation.

intracellular receptor protein, forming a hormone-receptor complex; ii) this unit undergoes a temperature-dependent conformational shift, termed activation, that results in increased affinity for DNA; iii) the ligand-activated receptor then binds to genomic acceptor sites; iv) this interaction enhances transcription of specific promoter genes, which then (v) influence gene translation and subsequent protein synthesis (see Yamamoto, 1985, and Beato, 1989, for reviews). Syndromes of steroid resistance have shown that alterations in receptor function at any of these steps can affect target cell responsiveness (Brinkmann et al., 1992; Griffin and Wilson, 1989; Chrousos et al., 1982, 1983; Linder and Thompson, 1989). Therefore, the potential role of each must be considered to fully characterize receptor mechanisms that may potentially regulate neural sensitivity to the aggression-promoting property of androgens and estrogens. Our own work in this area to date has focused primarily on biochemical aspects of receptor function (steps i and ii) and these studies provide some insights as to potential sources of sexual dimorphisms in regulatory systems for aggression. Newer methods now have made it possible to examine the cellular distribution of receptors and changes in gene translation in response to steroid stimulation, and examples of relevant studies will be incorporated although a comprehensive review is not our intent. In essence, the goal of this section will be to describe not only what is known about receptor mechanisms that may contribute to sexual dimorphisms in regulatory systems for aggression, but also to identify other aspects of receptor function that will need to be evaluated to understand the molecular basis(es) for these differences.

Perhaps the most basic question that should be addressed concerns the number of receptors and the affinity of ligand-receptor binding in the neural substrate for aggression (from available lesion and hormone implant studies in mice, this includes the septal region, preoptic area, and the anterior hypothalamus (Lisciotto et al., 1990; Owen et al., 1974; Slotnick and McMullen, 1972; see Table I). The importance of these receptor functions has been established through a form of androgen resistance related to a deficiency in receptor number and a syndrome of cortisol resistance attributable to low binding affinity (Griffin and Wilson, 1989; Chrousos et al., 1982, 1983). In this context, it is important to recognize that these parameters are more likely tied to the dimorphism in the androgen-responsive system because adult females have the capacity to respond to estrogens, although not its aggression-promoting effect.

**Table I**  A summary of the effects of TP implants in various brain regions in gonadectomized male R-S mice. Pellets were introduced via 27 or 30g cannulae and males were tested for aggression toward olfactory bulbectomized stimulus males.

| IMPLANT SITE | PROPORTION FIGHTING |
|---|---|
| Septum | 9/14 |
| Preoptic Area/Anterior Hypothalamus | 6/11 |
| Ventromedial nucleus, olfactory bulbs, hippocampus, caudate putamen | 1/14 |
| Cholesterol (in SPT or POA/AH) | 0/3 |

Studies of CF-1 mice have shown that males have about a 3-fold higher basal androgen receptor (AR) concentration (7.8 vs 2.5 fmol/mg protein) than females in combined hypothalamic-preoptic-septal cytosol. Interestingly, chronic T administration via silastic implant for 29 days induced a significant increase (2.5 fold) in AR in neural tissue from females (Simon and Masters, unpublished data). Additional time points will be needed to determine whether the increase is progressive or if it occurs within a narrow window, but the possibility remains that some minimal AR concentration is required before aggression can be activated. Concerning the affinity of androgen-AR binding, comparisons of three strains of male mice (CD-1, CF-1, CFW) indicated that lower or higher affinity binding was not linked to behavioral sensitivity (Simon and Whalen, 1986; Chen and Simon, 1990). While it thus appears that affinity is not critical, it would be of interest to learn whether this parameter changes in female neural tissue over the course of chronic androgen exposure. This concept of hormonal state, i.e., exposure to elevated T levels, influencing binding affinity was suggested by observed changes in uterine estrogen and progestin receptor affinity during pregnancy (Padayachi et al., 1987).

A related issue raised by the finding of receptor induction is the distribution of AR. This question can be addressed immunocytochemically and we are currently developing a monoclonal antibody that will permit these studies in mice. Basically, it is important to know whether chronic androgen exposure leads to enhanced receptor synthesis in the same cells, whether additional cells begin to express AR, or if a combination of these effects are produced. These possibilities, which are yet to be examined in neural tissue, were suggested by studies of AR distribution in the lateral, ventral, and dorsal prostatic lobes in rats (Prins, 1989) and in mouse kidney (Crozat et al., 1992). The former showed that the post-castration loss and androgen-induced up-regulation of AR were limited to the ventral and dorsal lobes, while the latter report found that androgen treatment served to enhance AR mRNA synthesis only in cells where receptors initially were present.

The sexual dimorphism in estrogen responsiveness may be linked to the relative stability of activated receptor complexes. This aspect of receptor function is determined by evaluating dissociation kinetics, and studies of peripheral tissues from rats, rabbits, mice, and humans have shown that a more rapid dissociation rate can attenuate target tissue responsiveness and, in severe cases, lead to complete insensitivity (see Griffin and Wilson, 1989, for a review). In neural tissue, we have obtained preliminary evidence indicating that activated $E_2$-ER complexes dissociate faster in females than males (Figure 6). Whether this dimorphism contributes to the functionality of the estrogen-sensitive regulatory system is unclear at this time, but one possibility is that rates of gene activation might differ as a consequence of receptor stability. This could affect neural target cell responsiveness, as has been shown in comparisons of estrogenic effects in uterine ER preparations from mice and rabbits of different ages (Belisle et al., 1986, Chilton et al., 1987).

Androgen resistance also has been linked to abnormal dissociation kinetics in several studies (Evans et al., 1984; Pinsky et al., 1984; Griffin and Wilson, 1989). Interestingly, the functional changes in AR in affected individuals have provided a model that has led to the identification of specific amino acid substitutions that underlie the defect (Brinkmann et al., 1992; Brown et al., 1990; Zoppi et al., 1992). Whether there is a sexual dimorphism in neural AR dissociation kinetics is currently unknown, in part because of technical limits associated with these studies in neural receptor preparations (see Chen and Simon, 1991).

Interactions with nuclear acceptor sites constitute the next level that could contribute to sexual dimorphisms. Until recently, these studies in neural tissue consisted primarily of examining potential relationships between the amount of

398

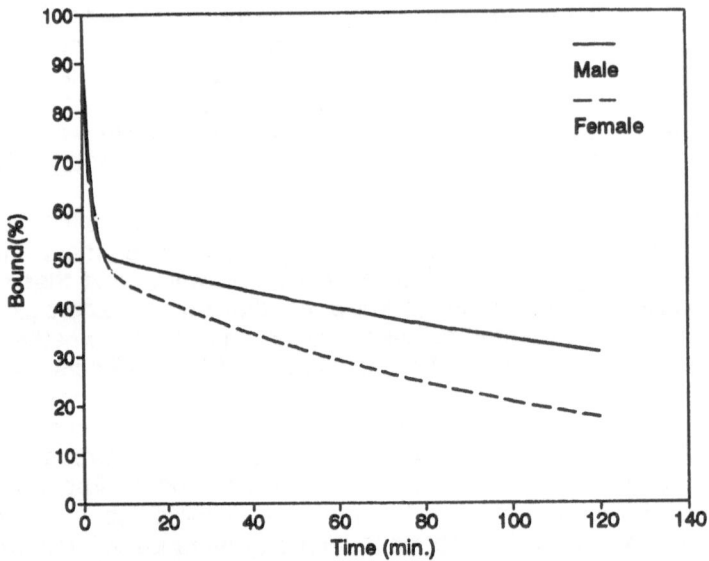

**Figure 6** Dissociation kinetics of activated neural ER from CF-1 male and female mice. Receptors were equilibrated with 15 nM [$^3$H]E$_2$ and activated by warming at 29°C for 15 min. The dissociation reaction was initiated by adding a 300-fold excess of unlabeled E$_2$. Data are expressed as a percentage of binding seen in control incubations where competitor was not introduced and are corrected for loss over the 150 minute sampling period. Results from females and males are from Chen and Simon, 1991, and from Simon and Chen, unpublished data, respectively.

nuclear bound receptor and a behavioral or physiological response. For example, Brown and coworkers (1990) found sex differences in nuclear ER in the preoptic area and ventromedial nucleus in rats across several age groupings. In some of these nuclei a dimorphism in progestin receptor induction was observed, suggesting a functional relationship between amount of binding and target cell responsiveness. In others, however, differences in nuclear ER binding did not result in differential PR induction. A comparable dissociation between amount of nuclear binding and behavioral outcomes also was described for the regulation of male sexual behavior in rats (McGinnis and Dreifuss, 1989). The pattern of nuclear ER and AR binding in several limbic nuclei was measured in intact males and compared to that seen in T-treated gonadectomized males that were behaviorally active and E$_2$ + DHT-treated males that did not show copulatory behaviors other than mounting. Testosterone treatment resulted in lower levels of nuclear ER than in intact males, while the E$_2$ + DHT regimen produced similar ER and AR levels in hypothalamus, preoptic area, and septum. These observations suggest a cautionary note, which is that a functional consequence of differences in amount of nuclear receptor needs to be identified before significant import can be ascribed to quantitative differences. Alternatively, it may be that a limitation of the exchange assay approach is that much of detectable nuclear binding is to non-specific DNA sites (Yamamoto, 1985). An emerging body of literature suggests that the nuclear matrix contains the majority of specific acceptor sites (Barrack, 1983; Metzger et al., 1991; Metzger and Korach, 1990; Mowszowicz et al., 1987) for both ER and AR in peripheral tissues. Although it represents a small fraction of total nuclear DNA and nuclear protein, several reports have demonstrated tissue-specific, high affinity, saturable receptor binding to these sites (see reviews by Nelson et al., 1986; and Rories and Spelsberg, 1989). These findings suggest that comparisons of sex differences in AR and ER binding in neural nuclear matrix may be needed to characterize functional differences linked to behavioral regulation. To date, there have not been any studies of this kind with neural preparations, and this more refined acceptor site preparation could overcome some of the limits of current exchange assay methodologies.

A more direct approach for assessing the functional consequences of receptor-acceptor site interactions is to measure gene translation products via *in situ* hybridization. This procedure is finding increasing use in neural preparations, particularly in relation to ER-regulated events. For example, a sexual dimorphism in basal ER-mRNA levels and in the response to estrogen treatment after castration has been described in both the ventromedial and arcuate nuclei (Lauber et al., 1991a; Simerly and Young, 1991). In gonadectomized females, rapid down-regulation of ER-mRNA was observed after $E_2$ administration while a response in castrated males required three days of T exposure (Simerly and Young, 1991) or was not detected (Lauber et al., 1991a). The potential behavioral significance of these differences in ER effects on gene translation was suggested by a sexual dimorphism in PR-mRNA production. In the same regions $E_2$ treatment produced about a 3.5-fold increase in PR message in females it had no effect in males (Lauber et al., 1991b). Comparable studies of ER effects on gene translation have not been conducted in mouse brain or in regions that appear to regulate the expression of aggressive behavior. Given that regional sexual dimorphisms in ER-mRNA distribution have been described in rat brain (Simerly et al., 1990) and that tissue-specific differences in ER-mRNA regulation have been demonstrated in rat pituitary, liver, and uterus (Shupnik et al., 1989), these studies may well be critical for understanding the sex difference in the capacity to utilize estrogens for the promotion of aggression.

The detection of gene translation products also appears to hold promise for understanding the androgen-sensitive regulatory pathway. There has been only one study of AR-mRNA distribution in neural tissue to date and this investigation used rats (Simerly et al., 1990)[5]. Interestingly, no overt sexual dimorphisms were dectected. However, studies of androgen-regulated gene expression in mouse and rat kidney (e.g. Caterall et al., 1986; Crozat et al., 1992) appear to provide some insights into a potential source of the sexual dimorphism in behavioral sensitivity to androgen. The utility of this model lies in the fact that the kidney, like the brain, is an androgen-responsive, non-dependent tissue where hyperplasia is not seen. Specifically, androgenic effects on the enzymes ornithine decarboxylase (ODC) and B-glucuronidase (BGD) were evaluated. Two aspects of the data were noteworthy. First, a species difference in ODC-mRNA expression in response to androgen was noted (Crozat et al., 1992). In rats, the response peaked within 8 hrs, while in mice the response was still increasing 72 hrs into the period of hormone exposure, which was the last time point assayed. Even more remarkably, BGD-mRNA levels continued to increase over 15 days of androgen exposure in mice. These sustained, incremental increases in androgen-regulated gene expression in mice, especially that described for BGD, parallel the time course for the activation of aggression by androgens in adult females (Svare et al., 1974; Simon et al., 1985; Simon and Cologer-Clifford, 1991). The demonstration of comparable changes in neural tissues from females, coupled with a more rapid peak in males, would suggest a basis for the sex difference in sensitivity.

The domain-specific transcriptional activating functions (TAF) of receptors also may be involved in sexually dimorphic responses to steroids. This aspect of receptor biology was investigated in relation to the mechanism of action of antiestrogens (Berry et al., 1990; Green, 1990) and it appears to have potentially significant implications for elaborating a basis for the estrogen-responsive regulatory pathway. Basically, ER consists of three domains - a variable length N-terminal, a DNA binding domain, and a steroid binding domain, termed regions A/B, C, and E, respectively (Green, 1990; Green and Chambon, 1988). Studies of various receptor mutants revealed two transcriptional activating functions, termed TAF1 and TAF2, that were located in different domains. TAF1 is in the N-terminal and is constitutive, that is, its ability to activate transcription is ligand-independent, while TAF2 lies in the steroid-binding domain and requires estrogen binding before transcriptional enhancement is seen (Green, 1990). Further, the relative activity of TAF1 and TAF2 were cell and gene specific based on comparative effects in HeLa and CEF cells (Berry et al. ,1990). Subsequent investigations comparing the effects of tamoxifen (TAM), an antiestrogen, and estradiol showed that the antagonist action of TAM was due to suppression of TAF2 and that its partial agonist effects were produced by TAF1 (Berry et al., 1990; Green, 1990). These observations were most interesting from our perspective because behavioral and biochemical studies of TAM in mouse brain showed antagonism in females and agonism in males (McKenna and Simon, 1992; Simon and Perry, 1987). More specifically, $E_2$-activated lordotic behavior and progestin receptor induction were blocked in CF-1 (Figures 7 and 8). These effects now can be reconciled based on our understanding of TAFs and their potential roles in behavior. First, the neuroanatomical substrates for aggression and female sexual behavior differ; the former includes the septum, preoptic area, and anterior hypothalamus, while the latter is regulated at the level of the ventromedial nucleus (Rubin and Barfield, 1983; Lisciotto et al., 1990; Owen et al., 1974; Slotnick and McMullen, 1972). This raises the possibility of cell-specific effects of TAF1 and TAF2 in the brain comparable to those described for HeLa and CEF cells. Perhaps more importantly, however, it is possible to suggest that each behavior is primarily regulated by different TAFs. For example, female-typical responses to estrogens, which are blocked by TAM in mice, could be regulated by TAF2, which is ligand-dependent. Aggressive behavior, in turn, which was potentiated by TAM, could primarily involve TAF1. The relative activities of these factors can vary with the target gene promoter as well as the cell type (Berry et al., 1990; Shull et al., 1992) which provides an additional basis for cellular variation in estrogenic effects. It therefore seems reasonable to suggest that an analysis of domain-specific transcriptional activating functions could help explain the basis for the estrogen-sensitive regulatory path.

## Summary and conclusions

The central nervous systems of adult female and male mice are differentially responsive to the aggression-promoting properties of testosterone and its major metabolites, estradiol and 5α-dihydrotestosterone. These sexual dimorphisms

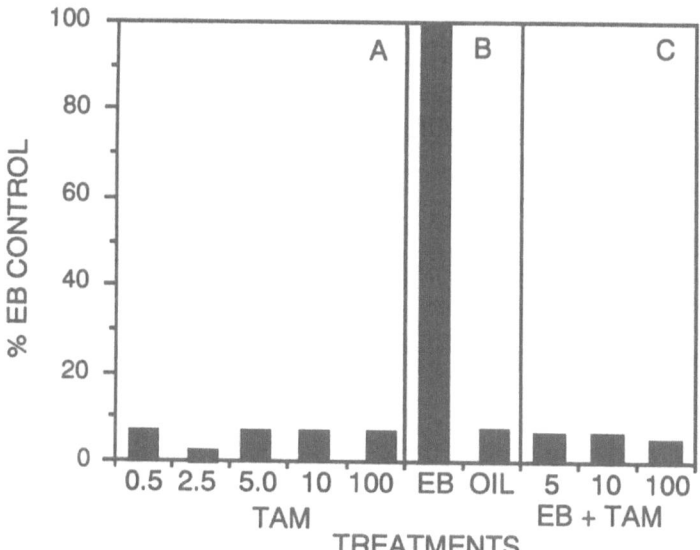

**Figure 7** Effects of tamoxifen (TAM) either alone or in combination with EB on progestin receptor induction in ovariectomized female CF-1 mice. Treatments consisted of EB (5µg), Oil vehicle, TAM (0.5-100 µg), or EB + TAM (5,10, or 100 µg), plus 500µg progesterone weekly for 4 weeks. On week 5, progesterone was not given and animals were sacrificed 42 hr after EB, Oil, TAM, or EB + TAM treatment. Data are expressed as a percentage of the PR level seen in EB + P females. For details, see McKenna and Simon 1992.

have led to the description of four neuroendocrine regulatory pathways for aggression: androgen-sensitive, estrogen-sensitive, a combined androgen-

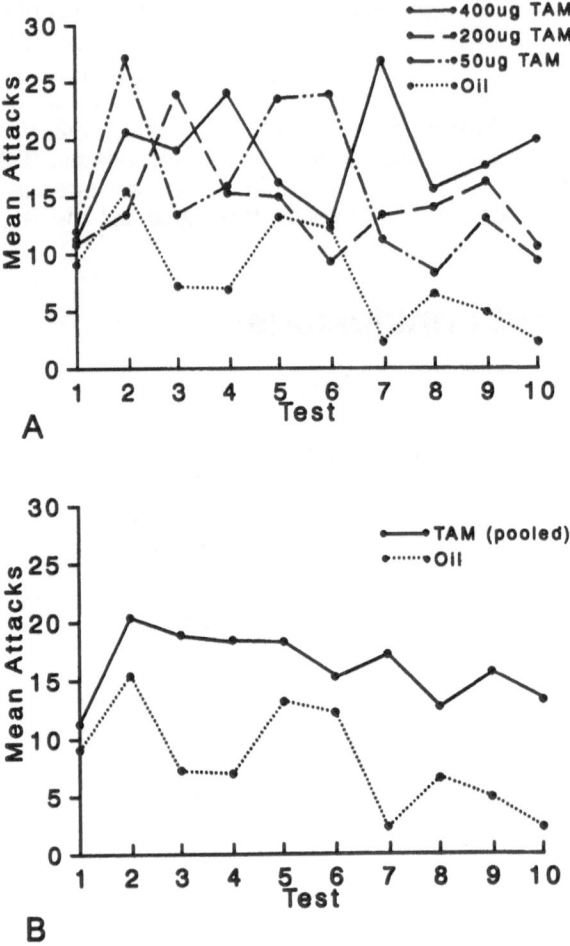

**Figure 8** The mean number of attacks by intact CF-1 males while receiving daily treatment with tamoxifen. (A) behavior of each group is shown separately; (B) data were pooled across the 3 tamoxifen doses. Results are from Simon and Perry (1988), Pharm. Biochem. Behav., 30, Medroxyprogesterone acetate and tamoxifen do not decrease aggressive behavior in CF-1 male mice, pp; 829-833, and are reprinted with permission from Pergamon Press Ltd, Headington Hill Hall, Oxford OX3 OBW, UK.

estrogen system, and a direct testosterone-activated path. In females, only the androgenic systems are present and these are less sensitive than in males; the estrogenic pathway is absent. In males, the functional system is determined genetically and can be any of the four. Under normal developmental conditions, specific actions of the androgenic and estrogenic metabolites of testosterone during sexual differentiation mediate the establishment of the androgen-sensitive and estrogen-sensitive pathways, respectively.

Few studies have attempted to characterize the biochemical and molecular biological processes that underlie the different regulatory pathways and the sexual dimorphisms in responsiveness. At the receptor level, it appears that the concentration of androgen receptors is a factor in the function of the androgen-sensitive pathway, although several other aspects of receptor biology (stability, nuclear binding, gene activation) also need to be examined. For the estrogen-sensitive system, it appears that efforts should be directed toward examining sexual dimorphisms in receptor distribution, the dynamics of nuclear binding, and the specific functions of each domain of of the estrogen receptor. The completion of these studies, which are now possible given advances in methodology, should facilitate development of a comprehensive model of the cellular processes mediating sensitivity to the aggression-promoting property of androgens and estrogens.

## Notes

[1] Supported in part by grants from the National Institutes of Health, the Ben Franklin Partnership, and the Lehigh University Research Fund to NGS.
[2] The position of the second through fifth authors was determined by lot.
[3] Suzanne E. McKenna is a NIH predoctoral fellow in biotechnology funded by grant #T32 GM08351..
[4] Xiang Chen is a Harry Frank Guggenheim Foundation Dissertation Fellow.
[5] The absence of such studies may be due to poor signal detection with cDNA probes. It may be that cRNA probes will be needed to assess AR gene translation (Simerly, personal communication, and see Quarmby et al., 1990)

## References

Archer, J. (1991). The influence of testosterone on human aggression. *Brit. J. Psychol.*, **82** : 1-28.
Archer, J. (1988). *The Behavioral Biology of Aggression*. Cambridge, Cambridge University Press.
Barrack, E. (1983). The nuclear matrix of the prostate contains sites for androgen receptors. *Endocrinology*, **113** : 430.
Beato, M. (1989). Gene regulation by steroid hormones. *Cell*, **56** : 335-344.
Belisle, S., Bellabarba, G., Lehoux, J-G. Robel, P., and Baulieu, E. (1986). Effect of aging on the dissociation kinetics and estradiol receptor nuclear interactions in mouse uteri: correlation with biological effects. *Endocrinology*, **118** : 750-758
Berry, M., Metzger, D., and Chambon, P. (1990). Role of the two activating domains of the oestrogen receptor in the cell type and promoter-context

dependent agonistic activity of the anti-oestrogen 4-hydroxytamoxifen. *EMBO Journal*, **9** : 2811-2818.

Brain, P.F. (1979). *Hormones and Aggression. Annual Research Reviews* **2**, Montreal, Eden Press.

Brinkmann, A., Kuiper, G., Ris-Stalpers, C., van Rooij, H. Romalo, G., Trifiro, M., Mulder, E., Pinsky, L., Schwikert, H., and Trapman, J. (1991). Androgen receptor abnormalities. *J. Steroid Biochem. Mol. Biol.*, **40** : 349-352.

Brinkmann, A., Jenster, G., Kuiper, G., Ris, C., van Laar, J.H., van der Korput, J., Degenhart, H., Trifiro, M., Pinsky, L., Romalo, G., Schweikert, H., Veldscholte, J., Mulder E., and Trapman, J. (1992). The human androgen receptor: Structure/ function relationship in normal and pathological situations. *J. Steroid Biochem. Mol. Biol.*, **41** : 361-368.

Bronson, F. and Desjardins, C. (1968) Aggression in adult mice: modification by neonatal injection of gonadal hormones. *Science*, **161** : 705-706.

Brown, T., Lubahn, D., Wilson, E., French, F., Migeon, C. and Corden, J. (1990). Functional characterization of naturally occurring mutant androgen receptors from subjects with complete androgen insensitivity. *Mol. Endocrinol.*, **4** : 1759-1772.

Brown, T., MacLusky, N., Shanabrough, M., and Naftolin, F. (1990). Comparison of age- and sex-related changes in cell nuclear estrogen-binding capacity and progestin receptor induction in the rat. *Brain Endocrinol.*, **126** : 2965-2972.

Catterall , J., Kontula, K., Watson, C., Seppanen, P., Funkenstein, B., Melanitou, E., Hickock, N., Bardin, C., and Janne, O. (1986). Regulation of gene expression by androgens in murine kidney. *Rec. Prog. Horm. Res.*, **42** : 71-109.

Celotti, F., Melcangi, R., Negri-Cesi, P., and Poletti, A. (1991). Testosterone metabolism in brain cells and membranes. *J. Steroid Biochem. Mol. Biol.*, **40** : 673-678.

Celotti, F., Melcangi, R., Negri-Cesi, P., Ballabio, M., and Martini, L. (1987). Differential distribution of the 5α-reductase in the central nervous system of the rat and the mouse: are the white matter structures of the brain target tissue for testosterone action? *J. Steroid Biochem.*, **26** : 125-129.

Charest, N., Zhou, Z.X., Lubahn, D., Olsen, K., Wilson, E., and French, F. (1991). A frameshift mutation destabilizes androgen receptor messenger RNA in the Tfm mouse. *Mol. Endocrinol.*, **5** : 573-581.

Chatterjee, B. Roy, A. (1990). Changes in hepatic androgen sensitivity and gene expression during aging. *J. Steroid Biochem. Mol. Biol.*, **37** : 437-445.

Chen, X. and Simon, N. (1990). Genetic variation in hypothalamic methyltrienolone (R1881) binding in male mice. *Physiol. Behav.*, **47** : 589-592.

Chen, X., and Simon, N. (1991). Dissociation kinetics of hypothalamic estrogen receptors. *Soc. Neurosci. Abstracts*, **17** : 571.

Chilton, B., Williams, N., Cobb, A., and Leavitt, W. (1987). Ligand-receptor dissociation: a potential mechanism for the attenuation of estrogen action in the juvenile rabbit uterus. *Endocrinology*, **120** : 750-757.

Chrousos, G., Renquist, D., Brandon, D. Eil, C., Pugeat, M., Vigersky, R., Cutler, G., Jr., Loriaux, D., and Lipsett, M. (1982) Glucocorticoid hormone resistance during primate evolution: receptor-mediated mechanisms. *Proc. Natl. Acad. Sci. USA*, **79** : 2036-2040.

Chrousos, G., Loriaux, D., Brandon, D., Tomita, M., Vingerhoeds, A., Merriam, G., Johnson, E., and Lipsett, M. (1983). Primary cortisol resistance: a familial syndrome and an animal model. *J. Steroid Biochem.*, **19** : 567-575.

Crozat, A., Palvimo, J., Julkunen, M., and Janne, O. (1992). Comparison of androgen regulation of ornithine decarboxylase and S-adenosylmethionine decarboxylase gene expression in rodent kidney and accessory sex organs. *Endocrinology*, **130** : 1131-1144.

Edwards, D. (1969). Early androgen stimulation and aggressive behavior in male and female mice. *Physiol. Behav.*, **4** : 333-338.

Edwards, D., and Burge, K., (1971). Estrogenic arousal of aggressive behavior and masculine sexual behavior in male and female mice. *Horm. Behav.*, **2** : 239-245.

Evans, B., Jones, T., Hughes, I. (1984). Studies of the androgen receptor in dispersed fibroblasts: investigation of patients with androgen insensitivity. *Clin. Endocrinol.*, **20** : 93-105.

Finney, H., and Erpino, M. (1976). Synergistic effect of estradiol benzoate and dihydrotestosterone on aggression in mice. *Horm. Behav.*, **7** : 391-400.

Gandelman, R. (1980). Gonadal hormones and the induction of intraspecific fighting in mice. *Neurosci. Biobehav. Rev.*, **4** : 133-140.

Gandelman, R., Vom Saal, F., Reinisch, J. (1977). Contiguity to male foetuses affects morphology and behaviour of female mice. *Nature*, **266** : 722-744.

Green, S. (1990). Modulation of oestrogen receptor activity by oestrogens and anti-oestrogens. *J. Steroid Biochem. Mol. Biol.*, **37** : 747-751.

Green, S. and Chambon, P. (1988). Nuclear receptor enhance our understanding of transcription regulation. *Trends Genet.*, **4** : 309-314.

Griffin, J. and Wilson, J. (1989). The androgen resistance syndromes. In: Scriver, C., Beaudet, A., Sly, W. and Valle, D. (Eds.). *The Metabolic Basis of Inherited Disease*. McGraw Hill, New York, pp 1919-1944.

Klein, W. and Simon, N. (1991). Timing of neonatal testosterone exposure in the differentiation of estrogenic regulatory systems for aggression. *Physiol. Behav.*, **50** : 91-93.

Lauber, A., Mobbs, C., Muramatsu, M., and Pfaff, D. (1991a). Estrogen receptor messenger RNA expression in rat hypothalamus as a function of genetic sex and estrogen dose. *Endocrinology*, **129** : 3180-3186.

Lauber, A., Romano, G., and Pfaff, D. (1991b). Sex difference in estradiol regulation of progestin receptor mRNA in rat mediobasal hypothalamus as demonstrated by *in situ* hybridization. *Neuroendocrinology*, **53** : 608-613.

Linder, M. and Thompson, E. (1989). Abnormal glucocorticoid receptor gene and mRNA in primary cortisol resistance. *J. Steroid Biochem.*, **32** : 243-249.

Lisciotto, C., Debold, J., Haney, M., and Miczek, K. (1990). Implants of testosterone into the septal forebrain activate aggressive behavior in male mice. *Aggress. Behav.*, **16** : 249-258.

Marcelli, M., Tilley, W., Wilson, C., Griffin, J., Wilson, J. and McPhaul, M. (1990). Definition of the human androgen receptor structure permits the identification of mutations that cause androgen resistance: premature termination of the receptor protein at amino acid residue 588 causes complete androgen resistance. *Mol. Endocrinol.*, **4** : 1105-1116.

McGinnis, M., and Dreifuss, R. (1989). Evidence for a role of testosterone-androgen receptor interactions in mediating masculine sexual behavior in male rats. *Endocrinology*, **124** : 618-626.

McKenna, S., and Simon, N. (1992). An assessment of the agonist/antagonist effects of tamoxifen in the female mouse brain. *Horm. Behav.*, in press.

Metzger, D., Curtis, S., and Korach, K. (1991). Diethylstilbestrol metabolites and analogs: differential ligand effects on estrogen receptor interactions with nuclear matrix sites. *Endocrinology*, **128** : 1785-1791.

Metzger, D. and Korach, K. (1990). Cell-free interaction of the estrogen receptor with mouse uterine nuclear matrix: evidence of saturability, specificity, and resistance to KCl extraction. *Endocrinology*, **126** : 2190-2195.

Mowszowicz, I., Doukani, A., Giacomini, M. (1988). Binding of the androgen receptor to the nuclear matrix of human foreskin. *J. Steroid Biochem.*, **6** : 715-719.

Naftolin, F., Ryan, K., Davies, I., Reddy, V., Flores, F. Petro, Z., Kuhn, M., White, R. and Takaoka, Y. (1975). The formation of estrogens by central neuroendocrine tissues. *Rec. Prog. Horm. Res.*, **31** : 295-319.

Nelson, W., Pienta, K., Barrack, E., and Coffey, D. (1986). The role of the nuclear matrix in the organization and function of DNA. *Ann. Rev. Biophys. Chem.*, **15** : 457.

Owen, K., Peters, P., and Bronson, F. (1974). Effects of intracranial implants of testosterone propionate on intermale aggression in castrated mice. *Horm. Behav.*, **5** : 83-92.

Padayachi, T., Pegoraro, R., Hofmeyr, J., Joubert, S., and Norman, R. (1987). Decreased concentrations and affinities of oestrogen and progesterone receptors of intrauterine tissue in human pregnancy. *J. Steroid Biochem.*, **26** : 473-479.

Pinsky, L., Kaufman, M., Killinger, D., Burko, B., Shatz, D. and Volpe, R. (1984). Human minimal androgen insensitivity with normal dihydrotestosterone-binding capacity in cultured genital skin fibroblasts: evidence for an androgen-selective qualitative abnormality of the receptor. *Am. J. Hum. Genet.*, **36** : 965-978.

Prins, G. (1989). Differential regulation of androgen receptors in the separate rat prostate lobes: androgen independent expression in the lateral lobe. *J. Steroid Biochem.*, **33** : 319-326.

Quarrmby, V., Yarbrough, W., Lubahn, D., French, F. and Wilson, E. (1990). Autologous down-regulation of androgen receptor messenger ribonucleic acid. *Mol. Endocrinology*, **4** : 22-28.

Rories, C. and Spelsberg, T. (1989). Ovarian steroid action on gene expression. *Ann. Rev. Physiol.*, **51** : 653-681.

Rubin, B., and Barfield, R. (1983). Progesterone in the ventromedial hypothalamus facilitates estrous behavior in ovariectomized, estrogen-primed rats. *Endocrinology*, **113** : 797-804.

Schechter, D., Howard, S., and Gandelman, R. (1981). Dihydrotestosterone promotes fighting behavior in female mice. *Horm. Behav.*, **5** : 233-237.

Shull, J., Beams, F., Baldwin, T., Gilchrist, C. and Hrbek, M., (1992). The estrogenic and antiestrogenic properties of tamoxifen in GJ4C1 pituitary tumor cells are gene specific. *Mol. Endocrinol.*, **6** : 529-535.

Shupnik, M., Gordon, M., and Chin, W. (1989). Tissue-specific regulation of rat estrogen receptor mRNAs. *Mol. Endocrinol.*, **3** : 660-665.

Simerly, R., Chang, C., Muramatsu, M., and Swanson, L.W. (1990). Distribution of androgen and estrogen receptor mRNA-containing cells in the rat brain: An in situ hybridization study. *J. Comp. Neurol.*, **294** : 76-95.

Simerly, R. and Young, B. (1991). Regulation of estrogen receptor messenger ribonucleic acid in rat hypothalamus by sex steroid hormones. *Mol. Endocrinol.*, **5** : 424-432.

Simon, N. and Whalen, R. (1987). Sexual differentiation of androgen-sensitive regulatory systems for aggressive behavior. *Horm. Behav.*, **21** : 493-500.

Simon, N. and Cologer-Clifford, A. (1991). In-utero contiguity to males does not influence morphology, behavioral sensitivity to testosterone, or hypothalamic androgen binding in CF-1 female mice. *Horm. Behav.*, **25** : 518-530.

Simon, N. and Gandelman, R. (1978). The estrogenic arousal of aggressive behavior in female mice. *Horm. Behav.*, **10** : 118-127.

Simon, N. and Masters, D. (1988). Activation of intermale aggression by combined estrogen-androgen treatment. *Aggress. Behav.*, **14** : 291-295.

Simon, N. and Gandelman, R. (1978). Aggression-promoting and aggression-eliciting properties of estrogen in male mice. *Physiol. Behav.*, **21** : 161-164.

Simon, N. and Masters, D. (1987). Activation of male-typical aggression by testosterone but not its metabolites in C57BL/6J female mice. *Physiol. Behav.*, **41** : 405-407.

Simon, N. and Perry, M. (1988). Medroxyprogesterone acetate and tamoxifen do not decrease aggressive behavior in CF-1 male mice. *Pharmacol. Biochem. Behav.*, **30** : 829-833.

Simon, N. and Whalen, R. (1986). Hormonal regulation of aggression: evidence for a relationship among genotype, receptor binding, and behavioral sensitivity to androgen and estrogen. *Aggress. Behav.*, **12** : 255-266.

Simon, N., Whalen, R., and Tate, M. (1985). Induction of male-typical aggression by androgens but not by estrogens in adult female mice. *Horm. Behav.*, **19** : 204-212.

Slotnick, B. and McMullen, M. (1972). Intraspecific fighting in albino mice with septal forebrain lesions. *Physiol. Behav.*, **8** : 333-337.

Spelsberg, T., Goldberger, A., Horton, M., and Hora, J. (1987). Nuclear acceptor sites for sex steroid hormone receptors in chromatin. *J. Steroid Biochem.*, **35** : 383-390.

Suarez, A., Cologer-Clifford, A., and Simon, N. Sexual differentiation of an estrogen-sensitive regulatory system for aggression. *Eastern Psychological Association*, Boston, 1992.

Svare, B., Davis, P., and Gandelman, R. (1974). Fighting behavior in female mice following chronic androgen treatment. *Physiol. Behav.*, **12** : 399-403.

vom Saal, F. and Bronson, F. (1980). Sexual characteristics of adult female mice are correlated with their blood testosterone levels during prenatal development. *Science*, **208** : 597-599.

Weichman, B. and Notides, A. (1980). Estrogen receptor activation and the dissociation kinetics of estradiol, estriol, and estrone. *Endocrinology*, **106** : 434-439.

Weichman, B. and Notides, A. (1977). Estradiol-binding kinetics of the activated and nonactivated estrogen receptor. *J. Biol. Chem.*, **252** : 8856-8862.

Yamamoto, K. (1985). Steroid receptor regulated transcription of specificgenes and gene networks. *Ann. Rev. Genet.*, **19** : 209-252.

Young, W., Goy, R., and Phoenix, C. (1964). Hormones and sexual behavior. *Science*, **143** : 212-218.

Zoppi, S., Marcelli, M., Desylpere, J.-P., Griffin, J., Wilson, J., and McPhaul, M. (1992). Amino acid substitutions in the DNA-binding domain of the human androgen receptor are a frequent cause of receptor-binding positive androgen resistance. *Mol. Endocrinol.*, **6** : 409-415.

# Sexually Dimorphic Hypothalamic Cell Groups and a Related Pathway that are Essential for Masculine Copulatory Behavior

P. YAHR

*Department of Psychobiology, University of California, Irvine, CA, 92717 USA*

## Sexually dimorphic cell groups in the medial preoptic area

For researchers interested in the neural control of male sexual behavior, few observations have generated more excitement than the discovery that the anatomy of the medial preoptic area (MPOA) is different in males than in females. The existence of sexually dimorphic cell groups (Allen et al.,1989; Bleier et al., 1982; Commins and Yahr, 1984a; Gorski et al., 1978; Hines et al., 1985; LeVay, 1991; Swaab and Fliers, 1985; Tobet et al., 1986; Viglietti-Panzica et al., 1986), synaptic contacts (Raisman and Field, 1971, 1973), dendritic arbors (Ayoub et al., 1983; Greenough et al., 1977) and other phenotypes (De Vries et al., 1984) in an area known to be essential for the display of male sexual behavior (Sachs and Meisel, 1988) raised the hope that we might soon be able to recognize the cells that control male behavior, to determine their projections and to specify the intracellular changes that occur in response to testosterone (T).

Some of these dimorphisms have proven useful for studying hormonal effects on brain development and/or for studying neural plasticity in adulthood. It is only recently, though, that any have been directly implicated in the control of masculine behaviors. Balthazart and Surlemont (1990) have shown that the sexually dimorphic, medial preoptic nucleus in quail, designated POM, is the part of the MPOA on which T acts to stimulate copulation. They have also shown that POM is essential for T induction of this behavior. Similarly, my group has shown that two cell groups in the sexually dimorphic area (SDA) of the gerbil MPOA are essential for male sex behavior. In this chapter, I describe the gerbil SDA and summarize our data on its behavioral effects. I also review data indicating that the SDA influences sexual behavior via a projection to the retrorubral field (RRF), the site of the A8 dopaminergic cell bodies in the midbrain tegmentum (Paxinos and Watson, 1986). Finally, I discuss possible homologies between the cell groups of the SDA and cell groups in the MPOA of other species.

*M. Haug et al. (eds.), The Development of Sex Differences and Similarities in Behavior, 409–419.*
© 1993 *Kluwer Academic Publishers.*

# The cell groups of the gerbil SDA

The gerbil SDA is a set of cell groups in the caudal MPOA. Its two largest components are the medial SDA (mSDA) and the lateral SDA (lSDA). In coronal sections, the mSDA appears oblong, with its long axis oriented dorsoventrally (Figure 1). It is located just lateral to the periventricular nucleus. The lSD

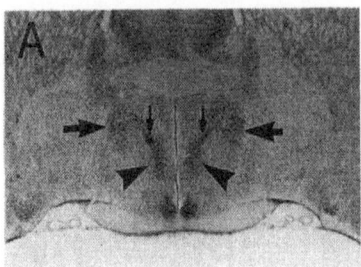 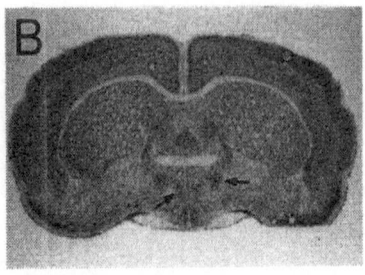

**Figure 1** A : Photomicrograph of a 60-um, thionin-stained coronal sectionthrough the SDA of a male gerbil. The arrowheads point to the lateral edges of the mSDA. The larger arrows point to the lateral edges of the lSDA. The smaller arrows point to the dorsal edges of the SDApc. B : Protein synthesis autoradiogram of a coronal section through the SDA of a male gerbil. Prepared by C. Ulibarri using procedures described in Kennedy, Suda, Smith, Miyaoka, Ito and Sokoloff (1981). Left and right arrows point to the lateral edges of the mSDA and lSDA, respectively.

appears ovoid, with its apex pointing ventrally, and is situated dorsolateral to the mSDA, near the anterior commissure. The mSDA and lSDA are connected by a bridge of cells that appears to be an extension of the lSDA rostrally and of the mSDA caudally. The mSDA, lSDA and bridge stand out clearly in males, giving the male SDA a hooked or C shape. This is true whether the SDA is visualized by Nissl staining (Figure 1A; Commins and Yahr, 1984a), acetylcholinesterase histochemistry (Commins and Yahr, 1984b) or protein synthesis autoradiography (Figure 1B; Ulibarri and Yahr, unpublished). In females, the mSDA, lSDA and bridge are less distinctive. In addition, much of the area lateral to the mSDA, i. e., the area that would be below the bridge or under the hook of the male SDA, appears to be part of the SDA in females. Inclusion of this area gives the female SDA a wing shape.

Embedded in the caudodorsal part of the male mSDA is a small, dense cell group designated the SDA pars compacta (SDApc). The SDApc is prominent bilaterally in nearly all males (Figure 1A). In contrast, we only occcasionally see the SDApc in adult females, even when they are given T (Commins and Yahr, 1984a, b; Ulibarri and Yahr, 1988).

Cells throughout the SDA accumulate T and/or its metabolites (Commins and Yahr, 1985). The adult SDA and SDApc also respond to T morphologically and histochemically (Commins and Yahr, 1984a,b; Crenshaw et al., 1992; Yahr and Stephens, 1987). The SDApc responds to T developmentally as well (Ulibarri and Yahr, 1988; Yahr, 1988).

# The SDA and male sexual behavior

Both the mSDA and lSDA are necessary for sexual behavior in male gerbils. Destroying either cell group bilaterally (Figure 2), by infusing the neurotoxin N-methyl-d,l-aspartic acid (NMA; Hastings et al., 1985), virtually eliminates

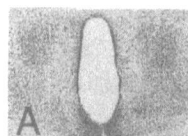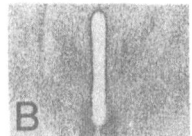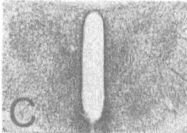

**Figure 2** : Photomicrographs of 60-um, thionin-stained sections through the gerbil SDA. Left : Cell-body lesions of the mSDA. Center : Cell-body lesions of the lSDA. Right : The SDA of a male gerbil given vehicle infusions in the SDA.

copulatory behavior in sexually experienced males (Yahr and Gregory, unpublished). Within two weeks after infusion of NMA, all males with lesions of the mSDA had stopped mounting even though they were exposed to a dose of T (5-mm Silastic capsules implanted subcutaneously) that fully maintains mating in castrated males (Yahr et al., 1979). In contrast, males infused with the phosphate-buffer vehicle continued to copulate to ejaculation. The effects of lSDA lesions were nearly as severe. Seven of eight males with these lesions stopped mounting by two weeks after lesion surgery. These data are summarized in Figure 3A.

While cell-body lesions in the mSDA or lSDA eliminate mating in T-treated males, lesions of nearby cell groups do not. As a follow-up to the study just described, we studied sex behavior in four groups of sexually experienced males. One group received bilateral infusions of NMA in either the mSDA or lSDA as before, although the dose was reduced 17 % to improve localization. Two other groups received the same infusions in the dorsal MPOA, just above the mSDA, or in the ventral MPOA, ventrolateral to the mSDA. Males in the fourth group received vehicle infusions at these dorsal or ventral sites. Again, all males were given T. As shown in Figure 3B, mSDA and lSDA lesions impaired sex behavior. Only three of nine males with these lesions mounted receptive females 2-3 weeks after surgery, and only one ejaculated. In contrast, 12 of 15 males with lesions outside the SDA copulated to ejaculation during the same period. Thus the mSDA and lSDA appear to be the most important cell groups in the caudal MPOA for the control of sex behavior. Loss of cell bodies in these areas can account for the deficits in male sexual behavior that occur after larger radiofrequency lesions of the MPOA (Yahr et al., 1985). This is the first time that specific cell groups in the mammalian brain have been causally linked to the display of male sexual behavior.

In contrast to the mSDA and lSDA, the SDApc does not appear to play a role in male sexual behavior. Some of the males that copulated to ejaculation after receiving dorsal MPOA lesions had no detectable SDApc at histology.

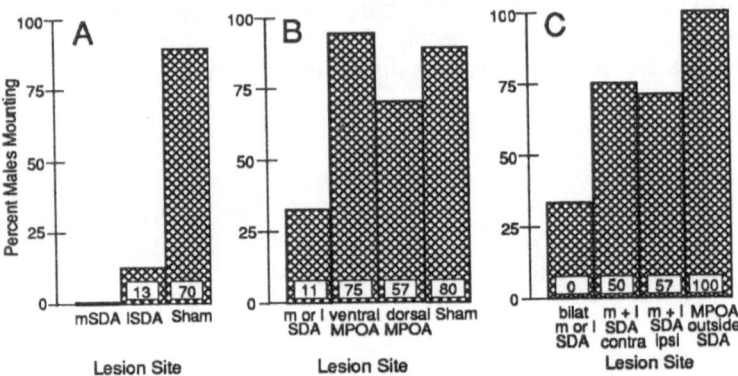

**Figure 3** : The effects of cell-body lesions of the SDA on the copulatory behavior of sexually experienced male gerbils given exogenous T. Data shown are for 2-3 weeks after surgery. The number at the base of each bar indicates the percentage of males copulating to ejaculation. A : The effects of bilateral mSDA or lSDA lesions. B : The effects of bilateral lesions in the mSDA or lSDA versus other parts of the caudal MPOA. See text for details. C : The effects of unilateral lesions of the mSDA combined with contralateral (m + lSDA contra) or ipsilateral (m + lSDA ipsi) lesions of the lSDA as compared to the effects of bilateral lesions of the mSDA or lSDA and to the effects of lesions that missed the SDA on at least one side of the brain (MPOA outside SDA).

Conversely, the SDApc was intact bilaterally in most males with lSDA lesions, but these males stopped copulating. Thus, the SDApc is neither necessary nor sufficient for the display of male sexual behavior.

# Efferents of the SDA

Having demonstrated a link between the SDA and male sexual behavior, we turned our attention to identifying neural pathways that mediate these effects. We traced the neural outputs of the SDA by injecting Phaseolus vulgaris leucoagglutinin (PHA-L) into either the mSDA or lSDA and immunocytochemically identifying the areas of the brain that contained labeled fibers (Finn et al., unpublished). Over 75 areas, from the septum to the medulla, contained labeled fibers with terminal boutons. When these terminal fields were injected with the retrograde tracers FluoroGold or rhodamine-labeled beads, as was done in over half of the cases, labeled cell bodies were consistently found in the SDA. SDA cells were not labeled, though, when retrograde tracers were applied to sites that had not been labeled during anterograde tracing or that had contained only unbranched, continuing fibers.

Both anterograde and retrograde tracing showed that the projections of the mSDA and lSDA are similar, though they often differ in size. Projections from the mSDA predominate in the forebrain, particularly in the medial hypothalamus. Projections of the lSDA predominate in the mid- and hindbrain, particularly in their lateral parts.

Many areas identified as targets of SDA efferents are also sources of SDA afferents (De Vries et al., 1988). In some cases, though, the projections appear to be unidirectional. The RRF, for example, receives a substantial projection from the SDA, particularly the ISDA, but it does not reciprocate.

# SDA-midbrain pathway essential for male sexual behavior

We began our search for pathways pertinent to male sex behavior in the midbrain tegmentum. More specifically, we were interested in the pathway from the SDA to the RRF because the RRF lies within the general area of the midbrain that had been implicated in the control of sexual behavior in male rats (Bracket and Edwards, 1984; Brackett et al., 1986) and because it was one of the few targets of SDA efferents that was not also a source of SDA afferents.

The strategy we use to identify SDA-related pathways that influence sex behavior is to lesion pathways of interest bilaterally but asymmetrically (Brackett and Edwards, 1984). The SDA is lesioned on one side of the brain and the source of SDA afferents and/or target of SDA efferents is lesioned on the other. Controls include males that are given sham operations and/or males given both lesions on the same side of the brain. Additional controls usually emerge at histology. These consist of males in which the SDA lesion, the second lesion or both destroyed less than half of their intended target(s) or missed them entirely.

In our initial study (Finn and Yahr, unpublished), sexually experienced, gonadally intact males were assigned to five groups. Four received unilateral radiofrequency lesions directed at the left or right ISDA. Two of the four also received unilateral lesions directed at the RRF contralateral or ipsilateral to the SDA lesion. The other two received lesions directed at the ventrolateral midbrain central gray (CGvl) because some of the fibers that reach the RRF from the SDA traverse it to terminate in the CGvl. The fifth group consisted of sham-operated controls. As discussed above, a sixth group of control-lesioned males was formed after histology. The data are summarized in Figure 4A. The males in which the ISDA and RRF were lesioned contralaterally showed lower levels of copulatory behavior than any of the other groups. This suggested that the SDA projection terminating in the RRF was an important one.

To pursue this lead, we reexamined the role of the SDA-RRF pathway using asymmetric cell-body lesions in T-treated males. Sexually experienced male gerbils implanted s.c. with 5-mm capsules of T were assigned to three groups. Two received unilateral infusions of NMA aimed at the mSDA and ISDA. In these males, NMA infusions were also aimed at the contra- or ipsilateral RRF. The third group received vehicle infusions at both the hypothalamic and midbrain sites. The results of this study are summarized in Figure 4B. Males in which SDA and RRF cells were lesioned contralaterally displayed almost no sexual behavior. Males with ipsilateral lesions in the same sites copulated normally, as did males in which one or both lesions missed their targets. These data verify that the projection from the SDA to the RRF is essential for male sexual behavior.

414

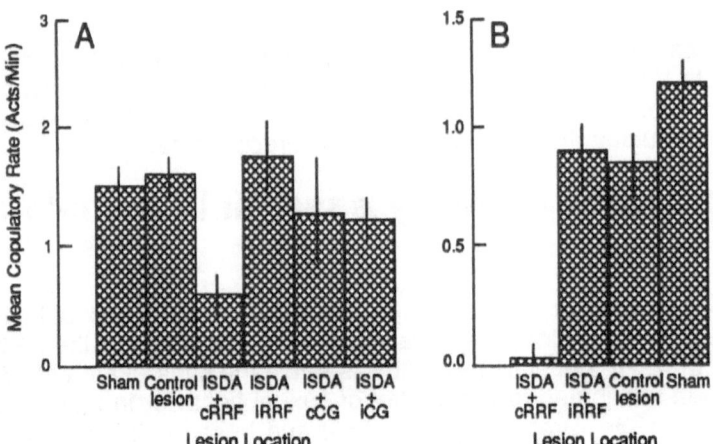

**Figure 4** Copulatory rates of sexually experienced male gerbils given lesions of the SDA and/or midbrain tegmentum. Copulatory rate indicates the total number of copulatory acts, i.e., mounts, intromissions and/or ejaculation, that the male displayed per min that he was with the female, through one ejaculation. Vertical lines denote standard errors. A : Effects of unilateral, radiofrequency lesions of the ISDA combined with contralateral (c) or ipsilateral (i) lesions of the RRF or CGvl. The control lesion group consisted of males in which the SDA lesion, the midbrain lesion, or both damaged less than 50% of their intended target(s) or missed them entirely. For males in the sham group, the electrode was lowered into the brain but no current was passed. B : Effects of unilateral, cell-body lesions of the SDA combined with contralateral or ipsilateral lesions of the RRF. The conditions for the control lesion group are the same as in A. Males in the sham group received infusions of the NMA vehicle.

# The mSDA and ISDA influence sex behavior independently

We also used the asymmetric lesion technique to determine that the mSDA and ISDA influence male sex behavior independently, not via a common pathway. Since the mSDA projects to the ISDA and vice versa (De Vries et al., 1988; Finn et al., unpublished), we had initially suspected that they influenced sexual behavior via a single pathway. However, since both project to many sites, we had to consider the alternative as well. To our surprise, the effects of the lesions favored the hypothesis that the two cell groups affect sex behavior independently (Figure 3C). Males in which the mSDA and ISDA were lesioned unilaterally and contralaterally showed as much sex behavior as males in which the two lesions were done ipsilaterally and as males with control lesions in the MPOA (Yahr and Gregory, unpublished). As before, bilateral lesions of either the mSDA or ISDA virtually eliminated copulatory behavior. Thus, despite their proximity and reciprocal connections, the mSDA and ISDA do not regulate sex behavior via their connections with each other.

## Homologous cell groups in other species

The clarity with which hypothalamic cell groups stand out in gerbils has no doubt aided our attempts to study the functions of the SDA. However, similar structure-function relationships will presumably be observed in other species when homologous cell groups are studied.

Cell groups that are likely to be homologous to the mSDA are the caudomedial POM in quail (Viglietti-Panzica et al., 1986) and a part of the medial preoptic nucleus (MPN), namely the medial MPN (MPNm), in rats (Simerly et al., 1984). The caudomedial POM, the MPNm and the mSDA are all located in the same part of the MPOA. In the case of the MPNm, data on connectivity also suggest homology to the mSDA (De Vries et al., 1988; Finn et al., unpublished; Simerly and Swanson, 1986, 1988), but data are not available on function. While the caudal MPOA is essential for the display of sexual behavior in male rats, as suggested by the effects of both electrolytic and cell-body lesions (Sachs and Meisel, 1988), no one has compared the effects of MPNm lesions with the effects of lesions elsewhere in the caudal MPOA. Recently, though, Baum and Everitt (1992) have shown that MPNm cells contain more c-fos, the product of one of the immediate early genes, after copulation than before. In the case of the quail POM, data on connectivity are not available, but functional analyses suggest homology to the mSDA. Electrolytic lesions that damage 10-50% of POM severely impair mating in sexually experienced male quail given exogenous T (Balthazart and Surlemont, 1990). Whether the quail POM also contains a cell group that is homologous to the lSDA is not clear.

Cell groups potentially homologous to the lSDA are the magnocellular MPN in hamsters (Powers et al., 1987) and the posterodorsal preoptic nucleus in rats (Simerly et al., 1984). All three are found laterally, and at least somewhat dorsally, in the caudal or midstrocaudal MPOA. Cells of the gerbil lSDA also appear large, like those of the magnocellular MPN in hamsters. Like the lSDA, the magnocellular MPN may be necessary for male sex behavior. It coincides with the part of the MPOA that was consistently damaged in male hamsters that stopped copulating after MPOA lesions (Powers et al., 1987). The posterodorsal preoptic nucleus has not been studied in regard to sex behavior, but like the MPNm, it contains more c-fos after copulation than before (Baum and Everitt, 1992).

A cell group that is probably homologous to the SDApc is the central MPN (MPNc) in rats (Simerly et al., 1984). Like the SDApc, the MPNc does not appear to be necessary for the display of masculine sexual behavior by males. The MPNc has not been specifically manipulated in studies of sexual behavior, yet since it is small and largely overlaps the sexually dimorphic nucleus (SDN) of the rat MPOA (Bloch and Gorski, 1988), it is almost certainly destroyed by lesions that destroy the SDN. Such lesions do decrease mounting behavior in female rats given T (Turkenberg et al., 1988). However, they do not disrupt sex behavior in sexually experienced male rats (Arendash and Gorski, 1983) and produce only transient deficits in naive males (De Jonge et al., 1989). Thus neither the SDN nor the MPNc can play an important role in this behavior.

Since it has been suggested that the SDN may be homologous to the third interstitial nucleus of the anterior hypothalamus (INAH-3) in humans (Allen et al., 1989; Le Vay, 1991), a cell group that is dimorphic not only in regard to sex but also in regard to sexual orientation, INAH-3 may be a homologue of the SDApc as well. Unfortunately, homology to the SDApc and/or SDN/MPNc offers little insight into the possible functions of INAH-3 at this time. While it has been claimed that the SDN regulates prolactin and gonadotropin secretion, based on the effects of lesions (Preslock and McCann, 1987), others claim (Bloch and Gorski, 1988) that the lesions produced in that study were medial to the SDN. Moreover, sexual differentiation of gonadotropin secretion can be dissociated from sexual differentiation of the rat SDN (Gorski et al., 1978) and the gerbil SDApc (Ulibarri and Yahr, 1988).

It has also been suggested (Hennessey et al., 1986) that the SDN might mediate the inhibitory effects of the MPOA on feminine sexual behavior (Powers and Valenstein, 1972). However, the MPOA lesions that facilitated lordosis in males given ovarian steroids (Hennessey et al., 1986) were much larger than the SDN/MPNc. Indeed, they appeared to include most or all of the MPNm, part of the lateral MPN (MPNl; Simerly et al., 1984) and other parts of the MPOA. This study did include males with smaller lesions that were less effective at facilitating lordosis, but the variations in effectiveness of these smaller lesions across subjects was not analyzed with respect to the damage to the SDN. The possible role of the SDApc in the inhibition of feminine sexual behavior in male gerbils has not been explored.

As noted above, neither the SDApc nor the SDN/MPNc appears to be involved in the control of masculine sexual behavior in males since lesions of these cell groups do not modify this behavior in sexually experienced males (Arendash and Gorski, 1983; Yahr and Gregory, unpublished). Based on these observations, one would predict that INAH-3 is not necessary for sexual behavior in men, whether they chose men or women as their partners.

# References

Allen, M. S., Hines, M., Shryne, J. E. and Gorski, R. A. (1989). Two sexually dimorphic cell groups in the human brain. *J. Neurosci.*, **9** : 497-506.

Arendash, G. W. and Gorski, R. A. (1983). Effects of discrete lesions of the sexually dimorphic nucleus of the preoptic area or other medial preoptic regions on the sexual behavior of male rats. *Brain Res. Bull.*, **10** : 147-154.

Ayoub, D. M., Greenough, W. T. and Juraska, J. M. (1983). Sex differences in dendritic structure in the preoptic area of the juvenile macaque monkey brain. *Science*, **219** : 197-198.

Balthazart, J. and Surlemont, C. (1990). Copulatory behavior is controlled by the sexually dimorphic nucleus of the quail POA. *Brain Res.*, **25** : 7-14.

Baum, M. J. and Everitt, B. J. (1992). Increased expression of c-fos in the medial preoptic area after mating in male rats : role of afferent inputs from the medial amygdala and midbrain central tegmental field. *Neurosci.*, **50** : 627-646.

Bleier, R., Byne, W. and Siggelkow, I. (1982). Cytoarchitectonic sexual dimorphisms of the medial preoptic and anterior hypothalamic areas in guinea pig, rat, hamster, and mouse. *J. Comp. Neurol.*, **212** : 118-130.

Bloch, G. J. and Gorski, R. A. (1988). Cytoarchitectonic analysis of the SDN-POA of the intact and gonadectomized rat. *J. Comp. Neurol.*, **275** : 604-612.

Brackett, N. L. and Edwards, D. A. (1984). Medial preoptic connections with the midbrain tegmentum are essential for male sexual behavior. *Physiol. Behav.*, **32** : 79-84.

Brackett, N. L., Luvone, P. M. and Edwards, D. A. (1986). Midbrain lesions, dopamine and male sexual behavior. Behav. *Brain Res.*, **20** : 231-240.

Commins, D. and Yahr, P. (1984a). Adult testosterone levels influence the morphology of a sexually dimorphic area in the Mongolian gerbil brain. *J. Comp. Neurol.*, **224** : 132-140.

Commins, D. and Yahr, P. (1984b). Acetylcholinesterase activity in the sexually dimorphic area of the gerbil brain : sex differences and influences of adult gonadal steroids. *J. Comp. Neurol.*, **224** : 123-131.

Commins, D. and Yahr, P. (1985). Autoradiographic localization of estrogen and androgen receptors in the sexually dimorphic area and other brain regions of the gerbil brain. *J. Comp. Neurol.*, **231** : 473-489.

Crenshaw, B. J., De Vries, G. J. and Yahr, P. (1992). AVP innervation of sexually dimorphic structures of the gerbil forebrain under various hormonal conditions. *J. Comp. Neurol.*, **322** : 589-598.

De Jonge, F. H., Louwerse, A. L., Ooms, M. P., Evers, P., Endert, E. and van de Poll, N. E. (1989). Lesions of the SDN-POA inhibit sexual behavior of male Wistar rats. *Brain Res. Bull.*, **23** : 483-492.

De Vries, G. J., De Bruin, J. P. C., Uylings, H. B. M. and Corner, M. A. (1984). *Sex Differences in the Brain, Progress in Brain Research, Vol. 61*, Elsevier, Amsterdam, New York and Oxford.

De Vries, G. J., Gonzales, C. L. and Yahr, P. (1988). Afferent connections of the sexually dimorphic area of the hypothalamus of male and female gerbils. *J. Comp. Neurol.*, **271** : 91-105.

Gorski, R. A., Gordon, J. E., Shryne, J. E. and Southam, A. M. (1978). Evidence for a morphological sex difference within the medial preoptic area of the rat brain. *Brain Res.*, **148** : 333-346.

Greenough, W. T., Carter, C. S., Steerman, C. and DeVoogd, T. J. (1977). Sex differences in dendritic patterns in hamster preoptic area. *Brain Res.*, **308** : 172-176.

Hastings, M. H., Winn, P. and Dunnett, S. B. (1985). Neurotoxic amino acid lesions of the lateral hypothalamus : a parametric comparison of the effects of ibotenate, N-methyl-d,l-asparate and quisqualate in the rat. *Brain Res.*, **360** : 248-256.

Hennessey, A. C., Wallen, K. and Edwards, D. A. (1986). Preoptic lesions increase the display of lordosis by male rats. *Brain Res.*, **370** : 21-28.

Hines, M., Davis, F. C., Coquelin, A., Goy, R. W. and Gorski, R. A. (1985). Sexually dimorphic regions in the medial preoptic area and the bed nucleus of the stria terminalis of the guinea pig brain : a description and an investigation of their relationship to gonadal steroids in adulthood. *J. Neurosci.*, **5** : 40-47.

Kennedy, C., Suda, S., Smith, C. B., Miyaoka, M., Ito, M. and Sokoloff, L. (1981). Changes in protein synthesis underlying functional plasticity in immature monkey visual system. *Proc. Natl. Acad. Sci.*, **78** : 3950-3953.

LeVay, S. (1991). A difference in hypothalamic structure between heterosexual and homosexual men. *Science*, **253** : 1034-1037.

Paxinos, G. and Watson, C. (1986). *The Rat Brain in Stereotaxic Coordinates.* Academic Press, New York.

Powers, J. B., Newman, S. W. and Bergondy, M. L. (1987). MPOA and BNST lesions in male Syrian hamsters : differential effects on copulatory and chemo-investigatory behaviors. Behav. *Brain Res.*, **23** : 181-195.

Powers, J. B. and Valenstein, E. S. (1972). Sexual receptivity : facilitation by medial preoptic lesions in rats. *Science*, **175** : 1003-1005.

Preslock, J. P. and McCann, S. M. (1987). Lesions of the sexually dimorphic nucleus of the preoptic area : effects upon LH, FSH and prolactin in rats. *Brain Res. Bull.*, **18** : 127-134.

Raisman, G. and Field, P. M. (1971). Sexual dimorphism in the preoptic area of the rat. *Science*, **173** : 731-733,

Raisman, G. and Field, P. M. (1973). Sexual dimorphism in the neuropil of the preoptic area of the rat and its dependence on neonatal androgen. *Brain Res.*, **54** : 1-29.

Sachs, B. D. and Meisel, R. L. (1988). The physiology of male sexual behavior. In : Knobil, E. and Neill, J. (Eds.), *The Physiology of Reproduction*, Raven Press, New York, pp. 1393-1485.

Simerly, R. B. and Swanson, L. W. (1986). The organization of neural inputs to the medial preoptic nucleus of the rat. *J. Comp. Neurol.*, **246** : 312-342.

Simerly, R. B. and Swanson, L. W. (1988). Projections of the medial preoptic nucleus : a Phaseolus vulgaris leucoagglutinin anterograde tract-tracing study in the rat. *J. Comp. Neurol.*, **270** : 209-242.

Simerly, R. B., Swanson, L. W. and Gorski, R. A. (1984). Demonstration of a sexual dimorphism in the distribution of serotonin-immunoreactive fibers in the medial preoptic nucleus of the rat. *J. Comp. Neurol.*, **225** : 151-166.

Swaab, D. F. and Fliers, E. (1985). A sexually dimorphic nucleus in the human brain. *Science*, **228** : 1112-1115.

Tobet, S. A., Zahniser, D. J. and Baum, M. J. (1986). Sexual dimorphism in the preoptic/anterior hypothalamic area of ferrets : effects of adult exposure to sex steroids. *Brain Res.*, **364** : 249-257.

Turkenburg, J. L., Swaab, D. F., Endert, E., Louwerse, A. L. and van de Poll, N. E. (1988). Effects of lesions of the sexually dimorphic nucleus on sexual behavior of testosterone-treated female Wistar rats. *Brain Res. Bull.*, **21** : 215-224.

Ulibarri, C. and Yahr, P. (1988). Role of neonatal androgens in sexual differentiation of brain structure, scent marking, and gonadotropin secretion in gerbils. *Behav. Neur. Biol.*, **49** : 27-44

Vigletti-Panzica, C., Panzica, G. C., Fiori, M. G., Calcagni, M., Anselmetti, G. C. and Balthazart, J. (1986). A sexually dimorphic nucleus in the quail preoptic area. *Neurosci. Lett.*, **64** : 129-134.

Yahr, P. (1988). Pars compacta of the sexually dimorphic area of the gerbil hypothalamus : postnatal ages at which development responds to testosterone. *Behav. Neur. Biol.*, **49** : 118-124.

Yahr, P., Commins, D., Jackson, J. C. and Newman, A. (1982). Independent control of sexual scent marking behaviors of male gerbils by cells in or near the medial preoptic area. *Horm. Behav.*, **16** : 304-322.

Yahr, P., Newman, A. and Stephens, D. R. (1979). Sexual behavior and scent marking in male gerbils : comparison of changes after castration and testosterone replacement. *Horm. Behav.*, **13** : 175-184.

Yahr, P. and Stephens, D. R. (1987). Hormonal control of sexual and scent marking behaviors of male gerbils in relation to the sexually dimorphic area of the hypothalamus. *Horm. Behav.*, **21** : 331-346

# Sex Differences in Human Social Behavior: Meta-Analytic Studies of Social Psychological Research

A. H. EAGLY

*Department of Psychological Sciences, Purdue University, West Lafayette, Indiana 47907-1364 USA*

The extent to which women and men differ in their characteristics and behavior is a controversial issue among psychologists and other social scientists. Debates about human sex differences and similarities often have strong political overtones because the conclusions that scientists draw from research findings can have implications for the treatment of women and men in society. Despite the obvious difficulties of addressing a scientific topic that is politicized and therefore especially vulnerable to ideological influences, a very substantial research literature that allows comparisons between men's and women's social behavior has been amassed, primarily from research by social psychologists. For a subgroup of these psychologists who are committed to using empirical research to test theories of gender and sex differences, summarizing and interpreting these investigations has become an important activity. This chapter reports these psychologists' efforts to integrate and understand studies that have compared the social behavior of women and men.

## Psychologists' typical methods of studying sex differences

The methods used to study female and male behavior must be taken into account to appropriately interpret the findings that psychologists have produced. Especially important is the experimental tradition in psychology, which allows comparisons of women's and men's behavior under the assumption that all contemporaneous factors other than sex are equivalent. Investigators attempt to hold other factors constant in order to interpret an observed behavioral difference as a sex difference and not as a difference caused by some extraneous variable that happens to be correlated with sex. As part of this strategy of holding other factors constant, investigators expose female and male subjects to equivalent stimuli. For example, in an aggression

421

*M. Haug et al. (eds.), The Development of Sex Differences and Similarities in Behavior, 421–436.*
© 1993 *Kluwer Academic Publishers.*

experiment, female and male subjects are exposed to the same eliciting stimuli. Comparisons between women and men are also usually controlled for differences in demographic characteristics such as age and social class. Moreover, experimental data are usually collected in laboratory or field settings that are relatively free of the role obligations of daily life that are associated with employment and family. Research subjects thus are observed, not in their homes or workplaces, but in a psychological laboratory or field setting that has been standardized in such a way that all subjects are exposed to the identical or near-identical stimulus situation.

Given this research strategy, psychologists sometimes make claims that may appear to violate common sense, for example, psychologists have maintained that there is no clear evidence that females are more nurturant than males (Maccoby and Jacklin, 1974). The observation underlying this claim is that female and male research subjects, when faced with the identical nurturance-eliciting stimuli, behaved very similarly. Yet the conclusion drawn about nurturance pertains not merely to the behavior that was observed in nurturance-eliciting experimental situations, but at least implicitly to people's general or underlying tendency to be nurturant. In contrast to this conclusion, observations of people in natural settings would quickly reveal that women provide more nurturance than men in family and occupational roles. Psychologists who conclude that women and men are really the same in terms of an underlying tendency to be nurturant can ascribe this real-life behavioral difference, not to a psychological sex difference, but to the assignment to women of caretaker roles that require nurturant behavior. Moreover, such reasoning implies that if men were assigned these roles, they would behave in an equally nurturant manner. Thus, psychologists' traditional emphasis on behavior in standardized experimental situations serves their goal of drawing conclusions, not merely about behavior in these specific situations, but about the more general tendencies or dispositions that cause behavior.

Psychologists also carry out a great deal of more naturalistic research that is not in this experimental tradition. Such studies most often ask participants to report on aspects of their daily lives, for example, on their friendships, their actual and potential love relationships, their marriages, and their experiences in employment. In addition, psychologists sometimes observe and record overt behaviors in natural settings where people interact in the context of their ordinary social roles. Moreover, research findings can consist of aggregate social statistics, for example, on crime, drug abuse, and mental illness. When the behaviors and reports of women and men are compared in these more naturalistic research traditions, much ambiguity surrounds the interpretation of the resulting findings. For example, sex differences in the characteristics that women and men report they prefer in mates (e.g., Feingold, 1992) or in the frequency of mental illness (e.g., Nolen-Hoeksema, 1987) might be explained by theories emphasizing biological factors, childhood socialization, employment roles, family roles, gender roles, or combinations of these factors. Psychologists have a special interest in partitioning those causes that are intrinsically sex-related in the sense that they follow from biology or early experience from those that are more arbitrarily correlated with sex because of a particular set of social arrangements. It is precisely because this task is so difficult that psychologists traditionally emphasized sex comparisons produced in experimental research in which they could observe behavior not directly under the control of occupation, family, and most of the obligations of daily life.

# Psychologists' methods of integrating research

How do psychologists draw conclusions from the research that has compared women and men? There is first of all the issue of how investigators decide whether male and female responses actually differ, regardless of what interpretation can be given to any difference that might be established. In an individual study, an investigator of course invokes a statistical analysis to determine if the difference between the women and men is unlikely to be due to chance variation and can therefore be considered statistically significant. However, general conclusions about sex differences and similarities typically depend, not on a single study, but on an evaluation of a relatively large number of empirical studies, each of which has invoked a statistical analysis. Therefore, the findings of individual studies have to be aggregated and integrated in some fashion, before a general conclusion can be drawn.

## Meta-analysis and the aggregation of sex comparisons

Traditionally this process of aggregating and integrating research findings was accomplished by recognized experts who announced conclusions based on their perception of the main trends in the findings. However, during the past fifteen years, a methodological revolution has occurred in the integration of research: psychologists have applied new methods to evaluating many questions, including the question of whether women and men differ. These methods are the quantitative techniques of research integration that are known as *meta-analysis* (Cooper, 1989; Hedges and Olkin, 1985; Rosenthal, 1991).

Meta-analysis provides explicit and statistically justified methods of drawing conclusions from empirical studies examining whether there is a sex difference in a particular class of behaviors. As a first step, the magnitude of the difference is assessed for each study in terms of its *effect size* or *d*, which expresses the finding in standard deviation units. For sex-difference findings, *d* is defined as the difference between the means of the male and female groups divided by the within-group standard deviation. (Alternatively, the magnitude of a finding can be described by the correlation between sex, a dichotomous variable, and the dependent variable of interest.).

To draw conclusions, reviewers then perform statistical analyses on the effect sizes that represent the findings of the individual studies. To answer the question of whether there is an overall difference between female and male behavior, reviewers compare the mean of the effect sizes with the no-difference baseline of 0.00. If this mean is significantly different from 0.00, the null hypothesis that there is no sex difference can be rejected, on the basis of the entire set of studies taken into account by the reviewer.

It might seem doubtful that it is necessary to invoke such a sophisticated technique as meta-analysis to answer the simple-seeming question of whether a sex difference exists at all in a set of studies. These methods would be superfluous if, for example, studies produced non-overlapping distributions of female and male responses. It is almost never the case, however, that sex differences are so large in psychological data, or, for that matter, in physical data. Even height, a physical characteristic with a large sex difference that is readily "visible to the naked eye," produces partially overlapping distributions of women and men. Yet sex differences in psychological data almost always are considerably smaller in magnitude than this height sex difference in part because psychological characteristics are assessed by methods that are less direct and less reliable than those that can be used to assess physical differences. Under these circumstances, many sex-difference findings may fail to reach statistical significance in individual studies, given that investigators' sample sizes are often not very large. Nonetheless, the sex difference may be quite reliable when a research literature is evaluated as a whole by meta-analytic techniques.

Meta-analytic reviews of research have thus become routine in efforts to address the basic question of whether women and men differ psychologically and behaviorally. This popularity reflects in part a growing general preference among psychologists for a method of integrating research that is more systematic that the informal or *narrative* methods that were previously used and that were not based on any clear rules for drawing conclusions. Yet meta-analysis is particularly valuable for comparing the sexes in part because the extremely large numbers of studies that are often available for integration make narrative reviewing especially difficult and unreliable. Moreover, because of the potential for statistical conclusion-drawing to restrain reviewers' own biases and preferences at least to some extent, it is especially helpful method to invoke in politically sensitive research areas.

## Earlier narrative integrations of sex comparisons: the no-difference consensus

These meta-analytic efforts to integrate sex-difference research should be viewed in the context of prior efforts to perform this same task without the benefit of quantification. Particularly influential among psychologists was Maccoby and Jacklin's (1974) narrative review of the empirical evidence concerning sex differences in many of the traditional areas of psychological research. These authors' quite skeptical conclusions about the existence of human sex differences should themselves be viewed in the context the easy acceptance of sex differences by earlier generations of psychologists on the basis of extremely flawed and unscientific evidence (see Rosenberg, 1982; Shields, 1975). Furthermore, even Maccoby and Jacklin's limited acknowledgements of sex differences were questioned by subsequent reviewers in the 1970s (e.g., Frodi et al., 1977). The conclusions of the 1970s reviews were widely generalized by textbook authors and other psychologists to suggest that there is little scientific evidence for sex differences in any human social behavior except for aggression. Even though Maccoby and Jacklin actually reserved judgment about whether women and men differ in several classes of social behavior, the general conclusion accepted by many in the scientific community was that sex differences are few in experimental studies in which women and men are observed under identical conditions.

## Meta-analyses that challenged the no-difference consensus

This verdict was premature, in part because Maccoby and Jacklin (1974) had concentrated on studies of children and made use of only a proportion of the available research on adults. Moreover, just as these 1970s verdicts were meeting widespread acceptance, the initial applications of meta-analytic techniques raised serious questions about the view that sex differences are few and far between in the experimental research literatures that are relevant to understanding social behavior. Aggregated meta-analytically, research findings suggested that the sexes differed after all when the criterion was whether the mean of the effect sizes calculated for individual studies differed from 0.00. For example, Hall (1978) showed that the ability to decode nonverbal cues, a capacity that no doubt facilitates social sensitivity, is superior in women compared with men. Cooper (1979) meta-analyzed the same sample of conformity studies examined by Maccoby and Jacklin and found, contrary to their conclusion, a tendency for women to conform more than men in one type of experimental setting--namely, group-pressure conformity paradigms. Confirming Cooper's conclusions, Eagly and Carli (1981) found that women, compared with men, agreed more with other people in a larger sample of conformity and persuasion studies, although evidence for this sex difference was strongest in group-pressure conformity studies. This conformity sex difference has been given differing interpretations: women's greater conformity may reflect their efforts to support others and maintain group harmony, whereas men's greater nonconformity may provide a means for them to attract attention to themselves and consequently exert leadership (see also Eagly et al., 1981).

Meta-analyses of other large research literatures in experimental social psychology followed in rapid succession and established that male and female social behavior differs in a number of respects. Gradually it became apparent that these observed differences are not particularly surprising, but conform to people's general ideas about how the sexes differ, in other words, the findings are gender stereotypic. Specifically, research on nonverbal behaviors was examined meta-analytically, primarily by Hall and her colleagues (e.g., Hall, 1984; Hall and Halberstadt, 1986; Stier and Hall, 1984). These reviews established, for example, that women are better nonverbal encoders as well as better decoders, that is, better than men at both sending and receiving messages nonverbally. In social situations, women smile and laugh more than men, use their faces and bodies more expressively, show more involvement with others' behavior, touch other people more, and approach them more closely. Women also report greater empathy for others' emotional experiences, although empathy sex differences are less clear with indicators tapping physiology or nonverbal reactions (Eisenberg and Lennon, 1983). In general, these sex differences appear consistent with the widespread belief that women are more socially skilled, emotionally sensitive, and expressive than men, as well as more concerned with personal relationships.

Meta-analyses examining whether the sexes behave differently in experiments on task-oriented groups also found several relatively consistent effects (see Wood and Rhodes, 1992). In verbal behavior in group discussions, women act friendlier than men and agree more with other group members (Anderson and Blanchard, 1982; Carli, 1982). In contrast, men, more than women, contribute behaviors that are strictly oriented to accomplishing the task that the group was assigned (Anderson and Blanchard, 1982; Carli, 1982; Lockheed, 1985). In addition, all-female groups perform better than all-male groups, compared with the baselines provided by their performance as individuals, when group tasks require complex social interaction, presumably because women's superior repertoire of positive interpersonal behavior facilitates performance in this situation (Wood, 1987). In groups that are initially leaderless, men are more likely than women to emerge as leaders, whereas women are slightly more likely to emerge as social facilitators (Eagly and Karau, 1989). When allocating rewards, men take more for themselves than women do and are somewhat more likely to allocate via an equity rule (Carli, 1982). These several findings on sex differences in group behavior are generally consistent with the commonly-held belief that women are more concerned than men about the social aspects of interaction and others' feelings, whereas men are more focused than women on task completion and other relatively tangible group outcomes.

Other quantitative reviews have investigated sex differences in prosocial and antisocial behavior elicited in experimental studies conducted in laboratory and field experiments. Men are somewhat more helpful than women in the kinds of short-term interactions with strangers that have been widely studied by social psychologists and labeled *helping behavior* (Eagly and Crowley, 1986). The stereotypic quality of this finding can be appreciated once it is recognized that helping behavior, as construed in this particular research tradition, encompasses primarily nonroutine acts of rescuing others from danger and everyday polite behaviors (e.g., opening a door for someone, picking up something he or she has dropped). These forms of helping might be labeled heroic and chivalrous. Female-stereotypic forms of helping, namely, acts of caring for others and tending to their needs, primarily in close or long-term relationships, were not examined in such studies. Men also act more aggressively than women in experimental settings, and this sex difference is larger for aggression that produces physical harm or pain than for aggression that produces psychological or social harm (Eagly and Steffen, 1986).

In a meta-analysis examining leadership style, Eagly and Johnson (1990) were able to examine both laboratory experimental studies of college students and organizational studies of managers. In laboratory studies, comparisons between the sexes suggested gender-stereotypic sex differences, with women's leadership style being more interpersonally oriented, less task-oriented, and more democratic than men's. In contrast, in organizational studies of women and men who occupied the same managerial role, only the tendency for women to be more democratic (and less autocratic) than men was maintained.

Outside of the tradition of experimental social psychology, quantitative reviewers have integrated comparisons between the sexes in other research areas that provide insights about social behavior. For example, Feingold (1991, 1992) examined mate selection preferences reported in questionnaire studies as well as revealed by advertisements in personals columns. This review established that women placed more emphasis on potential mates' socioeconomic status, ambitiousness, character, and intelligence, whereas men placed more emphasis on physical attractiveness. Also, quantitative reviewers have shown that women report higher levels of life satisfaction and happiness than men do (Wood et al., 1989), yet exhibit higher levels of many mental illnesses, especially depression (Nolen-Hoeksema, 1987).

In contrast to these numerous quantitative reviews, other domains of social behavior in natural settings have been surveyed in the 1980s and early 1990s using traditional, narrative methods. In these more informal reviews as well, claims that women and men differ abound, for example, in the nature of their friendship and close relationships (e.g., Hendrick, 1988), their tendencies to give and receive social support (e.g., Vaux, 1985), and their modes of coping with stress (e.g., Gove and Colten, 1991). Finally, other discoveries of sex differences based on more qualitative research also attracted attention, in particular, Gilligan's (1982) work on moral reasoning and several authors' analyses of managerial style (e.g., Loden, 1985; Helgesen, 1990; Rosener, 1990).

# Reactions to meta-analytic generalizations that the sexes differ

Very quickly after the publication of the first wave of these meta-analytic studies, some psychologists raised questions about the validity of the new generalizations. Conclusions that human social behavior is gender-stereotypic of course violated the skeptical conclusions about sex differences that had been recently incorporated into psychology textbooks largely on the basis of Maccoby and Jacklin's (1974) narrative reviews. Moreover, the new reviews contradicted the appealing view that sex differences exist only in the minds of perceivers, the view that they are "mere stereotypes." The idea that stereotypes are necessarily inaccurate, reflected in Allport's (1954, p. 187) definition as a stereotype as "an exaggerated belief associated with a category," enjoyed widespread acceptance among social scientists. Research comparing the sexes had seemed to provide an excellent opportunity to show that people believe in group differences in the absence of real differences.

Doubting that the generalizations arising from meta-analytic scholarship could be valid, critics raised a number of issues. For example, one potential source of invalidity is a publication bias in favor of significant findings, which could have excluded null findings from scientific journals. Yet publication bias is probably a less serious problem for research on sex differences than on most other topics because comparisons between women and men are very frequently peripheral to the main hypotheses of studies of social behavior; therefore, their direction and significance have little to do with the publishability of studies (Eagly, 1987; Hall, 1984). More plausible is the idea that biases in the findings available to reviewers derive mainly from investigators' own values and attitudes and could encourage or discourage the inclusion of sex comparisons in research reports.

Another potential validity problem is that meta-analysts might ignore study quality, thereby mixing together many poor studies with better studies to produce distorted generalizations (e.g., Basow, 1986). Yet meta-analysts generally do take study quality into account. Studies that are uninterpretable are excluded at the outset, and reviewers typically code the remaining studies on numerous quality-relevant features. These features are then related to the effect sizes to determine whether the difference between the sexes is affected by each component of study quality. Moreover, in meta-analytic calculations, studies are very often weighted according to one important aspect of their quality, the reliability of their findings (see Hedges and Olkin, 1985).

A different issue is whether meta-analyses have established that differences between the sexes are in fact extremely small (e.g., Deaux, 1984; Doyle, 1985). Although this magnitude issue needs careful evaluation in every quantitative review, it is important to realize that sex-difference findings are *not* particularly small compared with other research findings in psychology (see Eagly, 1987, pp. 116-118). If sex-difference findings are dismissed as trivially small, the great majority of the other findings described in social and personality psychology textbooks must be dismissed as trivial also.

Although these and other questions have been raised about meta-analytic findings, generalizations based on quantitative aggregations of studies have distinct advantages over findings of single studies (see Eagly, 1986, 1987). There is of course no such thing as a perfect empirical study: studies suffer from various imperfections and necessarily have the limitation of being based only on a particular sample of subjects, settings, and occasions. Yet the biases present in individual studies would often tend to cancel one another when findings are aggregated, with the result that the aggregated finding would have more satisfactory validity. Moreover, conclusions based on aggregated findings are more generalizable because they arise from a considerably broader range of persons, settings, and occasions than do single studies.

Finally, some psychologists regard the new wave of sex-difference research unfavorably, not because its validity might be flawed, but because they fear that discoveries of sex differences will have negative implications for women (see

Baumeister, 1988) or that such findings implicate biology and thus imply that biology is destiny. Such writers manifest the tendency that Hare-Mustin and Marecek (1988) termed *beta bias*, a preference for ignoring or minimizing differences. Yet the argument that reports of sex differences cause women to be viewed as inferior to men rests on the simplistic argument that masculine qualities are more favorably evaluated than feminine ones, a proposition that research on gender stereotypes has shown is false (see Eagly and Mladinic, 1989; Eagly et al., 1991). Moreover, the idea that sex differences necessarily implicate biology is also false because theories that emphasize environmental factors provide powerful alternatives to biological theories. More scientifically responsible than *beta bias* (or its opposite, *alpha bias*, a preference for exaggerating differences) is an attitude of openness to empirical findings. Scientists should allow empirical research to shape their views about the presence or absence of sex differences and the magnitude and implications of such differences (see Eagly, 1990).

# Testing theories of sex differences in human social behavior

There was something of a hiatus in the development of theories about sex differences during the period when psychologists doubted the existence of these phenomena. Now, based on the meta-analytic scholarship of the past fifteen years as well as on other evidence, the sometimes powerful effects of gender on human behavior once more have captured psychologists' attention. There is again something to explain. Psychologists have amassed evidence that the sexes differ in many aspects of their behavior, even in experimental research settings that elicit behavior in such a way that it is not directly under control of family or occupational roles. Given this state of scientific knowledge, the relatively simple question of *whether* sex differences exist has thus evolved into the more theoretically interesting question of *why* these differences occur. Theories of psychological sex differences range from those that emphasize biological factors or childhood experience to those that place a much stronger emphasis on environmental factors that impact on adults.

If psychologists confine themselves merely to explaining the overall pattern of sex differences in psychological research, it is difficult to provide rigorous tests of theories. Indeed, in the hands of dedicated theorists, the sex differences noted in earlier in this chapter can no doubt be explained from the perspective of several different theories. Therefore, to provide more challenging tests of theories of sex differences, they are increasingly expected to explain, not just overall sex differences in classes of behaviors, but the patterning of these differences across studies (and therefore across social settings). It is thus important to understand that for any class of behaviors such as aggression, some studies produce large differences, most produce smaller differences, and a few may yield reversals of the overall direction. To be a serious competitor in contemporary discourse on psychological sex differences, theories must produce hypotheses, not merely about the overall direction of differences, but about their variation across the studies in a research literature.

Examining inconsistencies in sex-difference findings is a central feature of many of the meta-analyses that have been noted in this chapter. Reviewers invoke meta-analytic tests of homogeneity to assess whether a set of studies, judged by their effect sizes, can be considered to have consistent outcomes, that is, outcomes sampled from a common population. If the hypothesis of homogeneity is rejected, the reviewer has the task of explaining why different studies produced different findings. As a first step, the reviewer examines the relations between characteristics of the studies and studies' findings. These relations are often relevant to testing theories of sex differences.

## Social role theory of sex differences

There are several strong candidates for accounting for sex differences in social behavior: the sociobiological perspective that features principles of human evolution and the biology of reproduction (e.g., Buss, 1987), the "separate cultures" idea that people learn rules for social interaction from experience in largely sex-segregated peer groups in childhood (e.g., Maccoby, 1990; Maltz and Borker, 1982), and status theories that emphasize the higher status that follows from being male rather than female in society (e.g., Ridgeway and Diekema, 1992). Although a general review of such theories is beyond the scope of this paper, one theory will be noted in some detail, in order to illustrate the steps that psychologists now take to test their theories in the context of the large existing research literatures that provide theory-relevant findings.

Eagly (1987) proposed that sex differences could be accounted for in terms of gender roles, defined as those shared expectations about appropriate conduct that apply to individuals solely on the basis of their socially identified sex. Research on gender stereotypes has consistently documented the existence of different expectations for men's and women's attributes and social behavior (e.g., Broverman et al., 1972; Deaux and Lewis, 1983; Williams and Best, 1982). Factor analytic studies of gender stereotypes (e.g., Broverman et al., 1972; Eagly and Steffen, 1984) have shown that the content of most of these expectations that are relevant to social behavior can be summarized in a very general way in terms of differences on two dimensions, the communal and the agentic (Bakan, 1966). Women are expected to possess high levels of communal attributes, including being friendly, unselfish, concerned with others, and emotionally expressive. Men are expected to possess high levels of agentic qualities, including being independent, masterful, assertive, and instrumentally competent.

These gender-role expectations are assumed to arise from the distribution of women and men into different specific social roles, especially family and occupational roles. Women and men are believed to possess attributes suited for the roles that they typically occupy (Eagly, 1987; Eagly and Steffen, 1984; Williams and Best, 1982; Yount, 1986). Particularly important is the assignment of childrearing and other domestic work primarily to women and the tendency for women and men to carry out different types of paid employment in a largely sex-segregated economy. The distinctive communal content of the female gender role is assumed to derive from the domestic role and from occupational roles filled disproportionately by women (e.g., secretary, teacher, nurse). Likewise, the distinctive agentic concept of the male gender role is assumed to derive from men's typical roles in the society and economy.

Role theory assumes that sex differences in social behavior are in part caused by the tendency of people to behave consistently with their gender roles. It also acknowledges that an individual's personal history of enacting social roles is an indirect cause of sex differences because these experiences help define the person's repertoire of skills and attitudes. Sex-differentiated prior experiences cause men and women to have somewhat different skills and attitudes, which then cause them to behave differently. This role-theory account of the causes of sex differences in summarized in Figure 1.

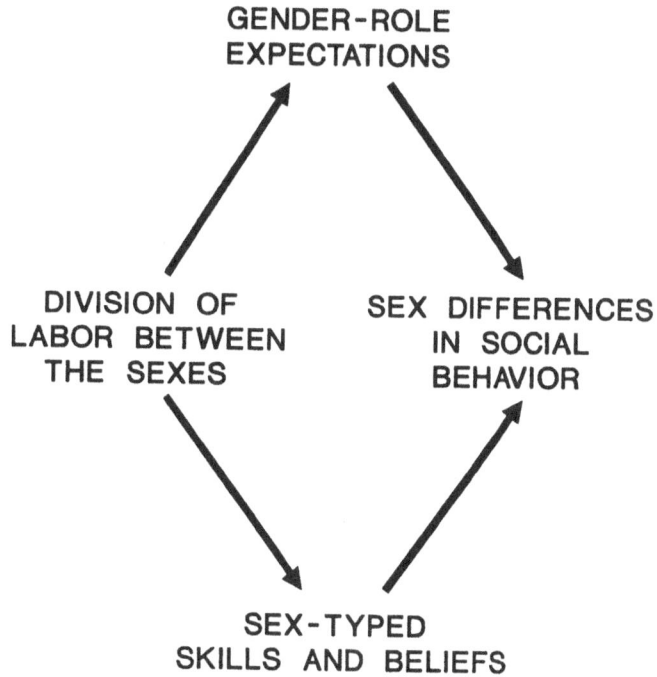

**Figure 1** Social role theory of sex differences in social behavior.

## Social role theory and the prediction of inconsistencies in sex differences

It is noteworthy that so many of the overall sex differences established in meta-analyses are consistent with the role theoretic perspective. The normative expectations that women should be communal and men agentic are almost uniformly consistent with the findings reported in this paper's brief survey of quantitative reviews of sex differences--the meta-analyses of conformity, nonverbal behavior, group interaction and performance, leadership, helping, and aggression. However, because many of these differences are no doubt compatible with other theoretical perspectives as well, the ability of the theory to explain inconsistencies across studies provides a more rigorous test of its adequacy than its ability to explain the overall direction of the difference in various behaviors. To account for these inconsistencies, the theory should suggest *moderator variables*, that is, social settings and subject groups for which the sex difference is attenuated and other settings and groups for which the difference is accentuated.

Illustrative of this moderator-variable approach is social role theory's hypothesis that variability in sex differences can derive from situational differences in the salience of gender-role expectations. For example, the presence of an audience is likely to enhance sex differences because other people are ordinarily perceived as supporting social norms. Furthermore, as Deaux and Major (1987) have also maintained, an audience may increase the salience of people's self-assessment of their own behavior in terms of normative standards. A second potential moderator arises in role theory's emphasis on sex-differentiated skills and abilities. Variability in sex-difference outcomes may derive from the extent to which performance of the specific behavior examined in a study requires communal qualities and the extent to which it requires agentic qualities: highly communal actions should draw disproportionately on skills and interests of women and consequently accentuate sex differences in the female direction. For the same reasons, highly agentic activities are likely to accentuate sex differences in the male direction.

Meta-analyses that have employed this moderator-variable approach have garnered considerable support for these (and other) social role predictions. For example, in research on helping behavior, an audience of by-standers was present in many studies (particularly in the field experiments) but absent in many others; this variation in studies' methods provided an excellent opportunity for testing the proposition that sex differences are larger in the presence of an audience. Eagly and Crowley (1986) anticipated that the general tendency for men to be more helpful to strangers would, like other sex differences derived from normative expectations, be enhanced by an audience. Indeed, audience presence was associated with stronger sex differences.

The extent to which the relevant behavior represents agentic or communal concerns also accounted for variability in sex differences in helping studies (Eagly and Crowley, 1986). For example, greater helping by men than women was accentuated when helping required an assertive intervention (e.g., bystander intervening in an emergency situation) rather than a more acquiescent response (e.g., a monetary contribution in response to a request for a charity donation). The agentic or communal nature of the task assigned to the group also proved important in explaining sex differences in group performance (Wood, 1987). In this meta-analysis the tasks assigned to groups were categorized as requiring relatively complex interpersonal activity versus predominantly task-oriented activity. As noted in the summary of sex-difference research, all-female groups performed especially well, in comparison with their performance as individuals, at tasks that required complex social interaction. In addition, all-male groups showed a nonsignificant tendency to perform well, again in comparison to individual performance, at tasks requiring high levels of task-oriented activity. Finally, Eagly and Karau (1989) found that the tendency for men to emerge as group leaders weakened with tasks that required complex social interaction or that researchers had identified as in some sense feminine. These findings thus illustrate the ability of social role theory to produce detailed predictions about the conditions under which women and men differ in their social behavior.

# Conclusion

During the past fifteen years, meta-analytic reviews of the findings of research comparing the social behavior of the sexes in experimental settings have challenged the prior consensus that women and men behave equivalently (or nearly so) in these settings and that the sexes are therefore equivalent in the tendencies that underlie social behavior. Instead, an overall pattern of stereotypic sex differences has been identified, and the magnitude of these differences appears to be typical of other research findings in psychology. Because of this new knowledge, the 1990s should witness a flourishing of psychological theories of gender and sex differences. To be convincing, such theories will have to do more than explain the overall pattern of human sex differences. Theories will be confirmed or disconfirmed based on their ability to account for the patterning of sex-differentiated behavior across social settings. Moreover, theories of sex differences must take into account both the experimental research literatures of social psychology and the rapidly growing nonexperimental research literatures that reveal the gendered aspects of behaviors in everyday life.

# References

Allport, G. W. (1954). *The Nature of Prejudice*, Addison-Wesley, Reading, MA.

Anderson, L. R. and Blanchard, P. N. (1982). Sex differences in task and social-emotional behavior. *Basic Appl. Soc. Psychol.*, **3** : 109-139.

Bakan, D. (1966). *The Duality of Human Existence: An essay on Psychology and Religion*, Rand McNally, Chicago.

Basow, S. A. (1986). *Gender Stereotypes: Traditions and Alternatives* (2nd ed.), Brooks/Cole, Monterey, CA.

Baumeister, R. F. (1988). Should we stop studying sex differences altogether? *Amer. Psychol.*, **42** : 756-757.

Broverman, I. K., Vogel, S. R., Broverman, D. M., Clarkson, F. E. and Rosenkrantz, P. S. (1972). Sex-role stereotypes: a current appraisal. *J. Soc. Issues*, **28** : 59-78.

Buss, D. M. (1987). Sex differences in human mate selection criteria: an evolutionary perspective. In : Crawford, C., Smith, M. and Krebs, D. (Eds.), *Sociobiology and Psychology: Ideas, Issues and Applications*, Erlbaum, Hillsdale, NJ, pp. 335-351.

Carli, L. L. (1982). *Are women more social and men more task-oriented? A meta-analytic review of sex differences in group interaction, reward allocation, coalition formation, and cooperation in the Prisoner's Dilemma game*, Unpublished manuscript, University of Massachusetts, Amherst.

Cooper, H. M. (1979). Statistically combining independent studies: a meta-analysis of sex differences in conformity research. *J. Personal. Soc. Psychol.*, **37** : 131-146.

Cooper, H. M. (1989). *Integrating Research: A Guide for Literature Reviews* (2nd ed.), Sage, Newbury Park, CA.

Deaux, K. (1984). From individual differences to social categories: analysis of a decade's research on gender. *Amer. Psychol.*, **39** : 105-116.

Deaux, K. and Lewis, L. L. (1983). Components of gender stereotypes. *Psychol. Doc.*, **13** : 2583.

Deaux, K. and Major, B. (1987). Putting gender into context: an interactive model of gender-related behavior. *Psychol. Rev.*, **94** : 369-389.

Doyle, J. A. (1985). *Sex and Gender: The Human Experience*, Brown, Dubuque, IA.

Eagly, A. H. (1986). Some meta-analytic approaches to examining the validity of gender-difference research. In : Hyde, J. and Linn, M. C. (Eds.), *The Psychology of Gender: Advances Through Meta-Analysis*, Johns Hopkins University Press, Baltimore, pp. 159-177.

Eagly, A. H. (1987). *Sex Differences in Social Behavior: A Social-Role Interpretation*, Erlbaum, Hillsdale, NJ.

Eagly, A. H. (1990). On the advantages of reporting sex comparisons. *Amer. Psychol.*, **45** : 560-562.

Eagly, A. H. and Carli, L. L. (1981). Sex of researchers and sex-typed communications as determinants of sex differences in influenceability: a meta-analysis of social influence studies. *Psychol. Bull.*, **90** : 1-20.

Eagly, A. H. and Crowley, M. (1986). Gender and helping behavior: a meta-analytic review of the social psychological literature. *Psychol. Bull.*, **100** : 283-308.

Eagly, A. H. and Johnson, B. T. (1990). Gender and leadership style: a meta-analysis. *Psychol. Bull.*, **108** : 233-256.

Eagly, A. H. and Karau, S. J. (1991). Gender and the emergence of leaders: a meta-analysis. *Psychol. Bull.*, **60** : 685-710.

Eagly, A. H. and Mladinic, A. (1989). Gender stereotypes and attitudes toward women and men. *Pers. Soc. Psychol. Bull.*, **15** : 532-558.

Eagly, A. H., Mladinic, A. and Otto, S. (1992). Are women evaluated more favorably than men? *Psychol. Women Quart.*, **15** : 203-216.

Eagly, A. H. and Steffen, V. J. (1984). Gender stereotypes stem from the distribution of women and men into social roles. *J. Personal. Soc. Psychol.*, **46** : 735-754.

Eagly, A. H. and Steffen, V. J. (1986). Gender and aggressive behavior: a meta-analytic review of the social psychological literature. *Psychol. Bull.*, **100** : 309-330.

Eagly, A. H. and Wood, W. (1991). Explaining sex differences in social behavior: a meta-analytic perspective. *Pers. Soc. Psychol. Bull.*, **17** : 306-315.

Eagly, A. H., Wood, W. and Fishbaugh, L. (1981). Sex differences in conformity: surveillance by the group as a determinant of male nonconformity. *J. Personal. Soc. Psychol.*, **40** : 384-394.

Eisenberg, N. and Lennon, R. (1983). Sex differences in empathy and related capacities. *Psychol. Bull.*, **94** : 100-131.

Feingold, A. (1991). Sex differences in the effects of similarity and physical attractiveness on opposite-sex attraction. *Basic Appl. Soc. Psychol.*, **12** : 357-367.

Feingold, A. (1992). Gender differences in mate selection preferences: a test of the parental investment model. *Psychol. Bull.*, **112** : 125-139.

Frodi, A., Macaulay, J. and Thome, P. R. (1977). Are women always less aggressive than men? A review of the experimental literature. *Psychol. Bull.*, **84** : 634-660.

Gilligan, C. (1982). *In a Different Voice: Psychological Theory and Women's Development*, Harvard University Press, Cambridge, MA.

Gove, S. and Colton, M. E. (1991). Gender, stress, and distress. In : Eckenrode, J. (Ed.), *The Social Context of Coping,* Plenum, New York, pp. 139-163.

Hall, J. A. (1978). Gender effects in decoding nonverbal cues. *Psychol. Bull.*, **85** : 845-875.

Hall, J. A. (1984). *Nonverbal Sex Differences: Communication Accuracy and Expressive Style*, Johns Hopkins University Press, Baltimore, MD.

Hall, J. A. and Halberstadt, A. G. (1986). Smiling and gazing. In : Hyde, J. S. and Linn, M. C. (Eds.), *The Psychology of Gender: Advances Through Meta-Analysis*, Johns Hopkins University Press, Baltimore, MD, pp. 136-158.

Hare-Mustin, R. T. and Marecek, J. (1988). The meaning of difference: gender theory, postmodernism, and psychology. *Amer. Psychol.*, **43** : 455-464.

Hedges, L. V., and Olkin, I. (1985). *Statistical Methods for Meta-Analysis*, Academic Press, San Diego, CA.

Helgesen, S. (1990). *The Female Advantage: Women's Ways of Leadership*, Doubleday/Currency, New York.

Hendrick, C. (1988). Roles and gender in relationships. In : Duck, S. W. (Ed.), *Handbook of Personal Relationships*, Wiley, Chichester, UK, pp. 429-448.

Lockheed, M. E. (1985). Sex and social influence: a meta-analysis guided by theory. In : Berger, J. and Zelditch, M. Jr. (Eds.), *Status, Rewards, and Influence: How Expectancies Organize Behavior*, Jossey-Bass, San Francisco, pp. 406-429.

Loden, M. (1985). *Feminine Leadership or How to Succeed in Business without Being One of the Boys,* Times Books, New York.

Maccoby, E. E. (1990). Gender and relationships: a developmental account. *Amer. Psychol.*, **45** : 513-520.

Maccoby, E. E. and Jacklin, C. N. (1974). *The Psychology of Sex Differences*, Stanford University Press, Stanford, CA.

Maltz, D. N. and Borker, R. A. (1982). A cultural approach to male-female miscommunication. In : Gumperz, J. J. (Ed.), *Language and Social Identity*, Cambridge University Press, New York, pp. 196-266.

Nolen-Hoeksema, S. (1987). Sex differences in unipolar depression: evidence and theory. *Psychol. Bull.*, **101** : 259-282.

Ridgeway, C. L. and Diekema, D. (1992). Are gender differences status differences? In : Ridgeway, C. L. (Ed.), *Gender, Interaction, and Inequality*, Springer-Verlag, New York, pp. 157-180.

Rosenberg, R. (1982). *Beyond Separate Spheres: Intellectual Roots of Modern Feminism*, Yale University Press, New Haven, CT.

Rosener, J. B. (1990). Ways women lead. *Harvard Bus. Rev.*, **68** : 119-125.

Rosenthal, R. (1984). *Meta-Analytic Procedures for Social Research*, Sage, Beverly Hills, CA.

Shields, S. (1975). Functionalism, darwinism, and the study of women. *Amer. Psychol.*, **30** : 739-754.

Stier, D. S. and Hall, J. A. (1984). Gender differences in touch: an empirical and theoretical review. *J. Personal. Soc. Psychol.*, **47** : 440-459.

Vaux, A. (1985). Variations in social support associated with gender, ethnicity, and age. *J. Soc. Issues*, **41** : 89-110.

Williams, J. E. and Best, D. L. (1982). *Measuring Sex Stereotypes: A Thirty-Nation Study*, Sage, Beverly Hills, CA.

Wood, W. (1987). Meta-analytic review of sex differences in group performance. *Psychol. Bull.*, **102** : 53-71.

Wood, W. and Rhodes, N. (1992). Sex differences in interaction in task groups. In : Ridgeway, C. L. (Eds.), *Gender, Interaction, and Inequality*, Springer-Verlag, New York, pp. 97-121.

Wood, W., Rhodes, N. and Whelan, M. (1989). Sex differences in positive well-being: a consideration of emotional style and marital status. *Psychol. Bull.*, **106** : 249-264.

Yount, K. (1986). A theory of productive activity: the relationships among self-concept, gender, sex-role stereotypes, and work-emergent traits. *Psychol. Women Quart.*, **10** : 63-88.

## Notes

Much of the research by Eagly and collaborators reported in this chapter was supported by grants from the National Science Foundations Grants (most recently BNS-8807495). The chapter was written while the author was a Visiting Professor at the University of Tübingen supported by a grant from the Deutsche Forschungsgemeinschaft.

# The Psychobiology of Sexual Orientation

## B. A. GLADUE

*Department of Psychology, Laboratory of Psychoendocrinology, North Dakota State University, Fargo, ND 58105 USA*

From a sexological point of view regarding creation, in the beginning there was sex, and then sometime afterwards there was sexual orientation. While no one disputes that sex is a biological manifestation, the origins of sexual orientation, whether it is homosexual or heterosexual continue to be debated with some enthusiasm. Whether something so significant in the life of a human, the sex of sexual partner, is truly a matter of free will or choice is questionable. The current debate regarding explanations for differences in sexual orientation is marked by often rancorous disagreements about the extent, if any, of biological factors. In both popular media and in scholarly journals, the issue is pondered: "Is homosexuality (as well as lesbianism) to be understood by natural science, or is diversity in sexual orientation based solely upon social and cultural opportunities, circumstances, and/or outright individual choice?

This "nature" vs "nurture" argument has been raised on a wide range of issues associated with sex differences and similarities as well as within- sex differences in behavior for over a hundred years, and although most parties realize it is a foolish simplistic dichotomy, positions are staked out nonetheless, and the "biological" vs "socio-cultural" camps continue their assaults. The argument is silly, of course, because ALL behavior of a living things has a biological basis. Beginning with genetics, through to embryology, anatomy, physiology and neuroscience, the "explanation" for any behavior, even one as seemingly complex as sexual partner preference, must have biological factors in its development and display. The real questions facing students of sexual orientation are HOW, WHEN, and WHAT kinds of influences do biological processes play in the manifestation of a behavior not too long ago characterized as a "deviant choice"? And despite assertions that the evidence isn't very clear or compelling (in the beginning of our understanding a process, is the situation ever so obvious and clear?) contemporary researchers in human psychobiology of sexuality has moved from "is it biological?" kinds of questions to explorations into specifics: "what particular biological interactions are involved, in what systems, and when". This paper will review some of the latest findings regarding biological influences in the development of sexual orientation.

*M. Haug et al. (eds.), The Development of Sex Differences and Similarities in Behavior, 437–455.*

# Genetic evidence

Since a noticeable diversity in human sexual expression and orientation has existed for some time, it is surprising that only a handful of relevant behavioral genetics studies have been conducted, most only during the past two decades. The earliest study (Kallman, 1952) sparked interest by its report of a 100% concordance rate for homosexuality among monozygotic (MZ) twin brothers compared to a 15 % concordance rate for dizygotic (DZ) twin males. In addition to methodological problems with that study and with genetics studies of sexual orientation in general, (for review, see Pillard et al., 1981) others failed to find such a high rate of concordance, often reporting *discordance* of sexual orientation among twin pairs (Zuger, 1976; Friedman et al., 1976; McConaghy and Blaszczynski, 1980) as well as striking concordances in MZ twins (Eckert et al., 1986). Interest in exploring possible heritable components in sexual orientation continued with the work of Pillard and colleagues, culminating in several reports showing a strong familial connection to male homosexuality (Pillard et al., 1982; Pillard and Weinrich, 1986). Additional evidence from other groups (Blanchard and Sheridan, 1992; Buhrich et al., 1991) supports the notion for an inherited influence upon the development of homosexuality in men.

The most compelling genetic study to date comes from Bailey and Pillard (1991). In this study of 161 homosexual men (115 proband twins and 46 probands with adoptive brothers; probands had a total of 174 relatives of interest), a series of heritability estimates employing genetic mathematical modelling approaches found statistically significant higher concordance for MZ twins than DZ twins. Concordance rates for MZ twins were 52 % (29/56 twin pairs), 22 % (12/54) for DZ twins, and only 11 % (6/57) for the adoptive brothers. Further, estimated heritability of sexual orientation ranged from 0.31 to 0.74 (that is, 31 to 74 % of the phenotypic variance associated with homosexuality can be accounted for genetically: for a detailed description of models and assumptions employed, see Bailey and Pillard, 1991). The authors note that in these models, all of the heritability estimates were statistically significant, but that the impact of shared environmental differences was not statistically significant (accounting for only 0 to 23 % of phenotypic variance).

Another approach to exploring genetic components of sexual orientation is to compare the incidence of homosexuality and heterosexuality in brothers of homosexual men (and sisters of lesbian women). Several studies have found that siblings of homosexual men (non-twin brothers) are more likely to be themselves homosexual than when compared to comparison groups of heterosexual men (Pillard and Weinrich, 1986; Bailey et al., 1981). And from a related demographic perspective, Blanchard and Sheridan (1992) found that the sibling sex ratio for homosexual men was significantly greater than that of heterosexual men and women. This is an interesting, if unexpected, replication of work done by Kallman (1952) and Lang (1960) since one psychodynamic argument often used to "explain" homosexuality is that men reared with a lot of sisters are apt to acquire "feminine characteristics" including sexual interest in men. Given that this and other large-scale demographic studies (Slater, 1962;

Hare and Moran, 1979) show that homosexual men are more likely to have an excess of brothers than sisters, and be born earlier in the series, the "social feminization" argument seems especially thin.

Taken as a whole, these findings are not likely to be the last word in genetic or demographic studies (nor should they be). Refinements in experimental methodology paired with behavioral genetic modelling will no doubt yield more and more compelling evidence for familial and heritable aspects of homosexuality in men. While there is no evidence for a "gene" coding for homosexuality, Bailey and Pillard (1991) present several important points. First, they note that their data and model assume that major genes for homosexuality are unlikely, but that a multifactorial threshold model is worth considering. Assuming that homosexuality is influenced by constitutional factors, then heritable variations in brain development may account for the diversity in sexual orientation. Or, variations in physical appearance of the offspring may lead to differential parental treatment with a similar outcome. In either case, in this model, genetics may not absolutely predetermine one's sexual orientation, but influence biological processes which then interact with other biological and non-biological (social, cultural, environmental) aspects of the individual's life to establish a sexual orientation. Nonetheless, the current evidence from recent genetic studies shows that there is reason to believe in a heritable component of something as fundamental as sexual partner preference.

While evidence for a genetic influence upon psychosexual development seems, at the very least, likely, the question still remains regarding how such heritable factors manifest themselves in the developing human. As Bailey and Pillard (1991) put it "what, exactly, is inherited?" That is, what might be the consequential influences of genes upon the anatomy and physiology of an organism throughout its developmental critical periods and lifespan?

Current thinking about the developmental psychobiology of sexual orientation has been influenced heavily by findings in the general area of anatomical, physiological and behavioral sex dimorphism. The exceptionally large and detailed literature on animal behavior ackowledges sex differences in brain areas and physiological systems involved in sexual behavior, differences thought to be established by key hormone interactions during critical developmental time frames. The dominant explanatory model, shaped from this work, is the Neurohormonal Theory of Sexual Differentiation. Based upon findings from decades of animal experimentation (reviewed by Goy and McEwen, 1980), this theory argues that the developing CNS is "masculinized" by exposure to androgens (and/or its metabolites estradiol and dihydrotestosterone) during critical periods of development, without which the animal's brain (and subsequent behavior) is "feminized". Since the bulk of the data in support of this notion are derived from experiments with small mammals (rats, hamsters, rhesus monkeys, and so forth), some have argued that an extension to humans is unwarranted (Gooren, 1990). However, experiments with non-human primates show that hormonal organizing influences upon behavior can be very subtle but no less lasting and meaningful, and occur without any overt effects on genitalia (Goy et al., 1988).

Several laboratories have uncovered a variety of sex differences in brain anatomy, neuroendocrinology, gonadal functioning, and behavior in humans as well as in animals. And while some of these findings remain slightly controversial, the overwhelming evidence supports the existence of fundamental biological sex differences. Using these sex differences as a referential framework for understanding the biology of homosexuality, has led investigators to look for corresponding within-sex differences associated with sexual orientation.

The extension of the "Neurohormonal" theory of sexual differentiation to sexual orientation has not been without controversy. In this theoretical extension, crucial sex steroids act upon the brain during prenatal and postnatal development which then behaviorally masculinizes and defeminizes the brain during sexual differentiation with ultimate influences upon one's sexual orientation. There have been many reviews of the literature on this topic (some might quibble that there are more reviews than empirical tests of the hypothesis!), all concluding, at least, that the evidence is not yet compelling enough to state that human psychosexual development is shaped in as similar and as predictable a path as found in other mammals. Nonetheless, the theory is useful, in that it offers a starting point to compare in homosexual and heterosexual men the neuroendocrine, neuroanatomical, and neuropsychological processes for which clear sex differences have been demonstrated. In this regard, we may find clues as to how "genetics" may impact the developing person.

# Hormonal evidence

Much has been said and written about the influence of gonadal hormones upon sexual orientation. In simple terms, the argument has been made, and subsequently dispatched, that "male hormone" levels would be lower in homosexual men compared to heterosexual men, presumably because homosexual men had "female-like" (i.e., low) circulating T levels. Aside from the silliness of hormonal nomenclature in what constitutes a "male" or "female" hormone (for an excellent discussion of this topic, see Whalen, 1984), the idea that levels of T are a marker for homosexuality or heterosexuality has been generally discarded. Peripheral levels of sex steroids in a given person, or group of persons is unrelated to their sexual orientation. In 25 out of 31 studies comparing circulating testosterone levels in homosexual and heterosexual adult men, no convincing (i.e., statistically significant) differences were found. In 3 studies, homosexual men had lesser testosterone (T) levels, in 3 other studies homosexual men had greater T levels than heterosexual men (for extensive review listing, see Gladue, 1988, 1990; Gooren, 1988; Gooren et al., 1990). Given that circulating T levels vary considerably among men, and reflect current historical conditions of a given male (diet, exercise, health status, drug usage, etc.) there is no logical reason to expect a difference in T level merely on the basis of sexual orientation.

While it is extremely unlikely that adult sex hormone levels have any relationship to adult sexual partner preference, there is some argument that perinatal hormone levels have an organizing effect upon the developing nervous system, with the result that the nervous system may have later behavioral predispositions (reviewed in Gladue, 1990). Described earlier, this Neurohormonal Theory of Sexual Differentiation assumes that key endocrine interactions with brain tissue during formative critical periods of development "organize" brain tissue and subsequent behavior toward particular directions, patterns, and developmental pathways. Much of our understanding about sexual differentiation and sex-dimorphic behavior is influenced and driven by this theory. And, for the most part, it has held up well over the years, particularly with regard to non-human animal models, and to some degree, with data collected in humans (see Reinisch et al., 1991 for an excellent and thorough review of this complex literature).

Where the main contention occurs is the application of this theory, or variations of this theory, toward sexual orientation. Gooren (1988) has argued that the evidence for a neuroendocrine predisposition toward homosexuality is unsubstantiated by the data. Dörner and co-workers (1987 have taken quite an opposite position. And Gladue (1988, 1990) notes that evidence exists to at least consider the general hypothesis empirically testable. All groups cite studies from their laboratory to support their positions, and, the issue remains unresolved. The main disagreement centers around what, if any, connection can be made between the development and functioning of the hypothalamic-pituitary-gonadal axis in men who vary according to sexual orientation. Let us briefly consider the evidence.

In 1975, Dörner and colleagues reported that a single intravenous injection of estrogen can elevate the circulating level of luteinizing hormone (LH) above initial values in homosexual but not heterosexual men.

Those authors concluded that a positive-feedback response to estrogen shown by those homosexual men reflected a predominately "female-differentiated" brain, and this neuroendocrine response pattern reflected a neural and endocrine "predisposition" toward female-like behavior, specifically an erotic attraction toward men. At the time, the finding was remarkable, and the consequential reasoning by this group that homosexual men had a "female" hypothalamus seemed overly simplistic and an excessive interpretation of the data, especially given methodological problems with the study. Despite the criticisms and skepticism, however, it was nearly a decade before another laboratory attempted an experimental re-evaluation of Dörner's extraordinary findings (Gladue et al., 1984). In that study, Gladue et al. (1984) found that lifelong homosexual men had a neuroendocrine (in this case, LH) response to estrogen intermediate to that of heterosexual men and heterosexual women. In addition to replicating Dörner's basic finding, these authors obtained data suggesting that the pituitary response to estrogen might be mediated by some gonadal process, since testosterone responses to the estrogen challenge were also different in homosexual and heterosexual men. The authors concluded that the data while not direct evidence for an atypical neuroendocrine development in homosexual men, were also not inconsistent with such a hypothesis. In any event, the "LH response to estrogen" feedback pattern was touted by some as a biological marker for homosexuality, by others as at least an indicator for a biological basis for homosexuality. A number of studies from other laboratories soon followed.

The first attempt to replicate Gladue et al. (1984) study, was by Gooren (1986). With a larger sample of heterosexual and homosexual subjects of both sexes, Gooren found no significant sexual orientation difference in LH responsiveness to estrogen. Further, Gooren has since argued that the wide range of variation in the response pattern is more likely due to testicular steroidogenesis differences among groups of men, and that sexual orientation *per se*, is irrelevant (Gooren, 1988). Gooren further suggests that various factors (viral testicular infections, drugs, alcohol, body weight, and age) can alter the funtioning of the hypothalamic-pituitary-gonadal axis in men, especially in response to estrogen treatment (Gooren, 1988).

Later studies on the "neuroendocrine response pattern" in homosexual and heterosexual men have yielded mixed results. A smaller study by Gladue (1990) found a "positive LH response to estrogen" in currently exclusively homosexual men reporting prior bisexual fantasy and activity, and no such response pattern in a smaller group of currently exclusively heterosexual men reporting prior bisexual fantasy. Another group (Hendricks et al., 1989) attempted to expand upon the Gladue et al. (1984) and Gooren (1986) protocols by administering a range of estrogen doses to homosexual and heterosexual men. However, so few homosexual men were tested at any dose (ns varied from 3 to 5 subjects per group) that insufficient power was available for a meaningful test of the hypothesis.

While the evidence for a "neuroendocrine predisposition to homosexuality" is not as clear as deemed by Dörner and colleagues (1987), the situation is also not as unsubstantiated as argued by Gooren. To date, only a few carefully designed and executed neuroendocrine response pattern studies have been published, and the results are mixed. What is interesting about these studies is that they explore, in the adults, endocrine processes associated with brain regions thought to have been differentially affected during development. Perhaps the data from neuroendocrine studies can be better appreciated and evaluated in the context of studies on neuroanatomical differentiation of those brain regions likely responsible for neuroendocrine functioning. It is the connection between neuroanatomy and sexual differentiation/orientation that we now consider.

# Neuroanatomical evidence

Ever since sex differences in physiology and behavior were connected to influences of gonadal hormones on brain tissue (see Goy and McEwen, 1980 for review), the search was on for neuroanatomical sex differences that might be involved in the mediation of such behavioral differences. The earliest discoveries were at the ultrastructural level using animal models [size of neuronal nuclei (Pfaff, 1966), synaptic patterns in hypothalamus (Raisman and Field, 1971), and dendritic branching patterns (Greenough et al., 1977), and regions of the preoptic area (POA) of the hypothalamus (Gorski et al., 1978)]. Inevitably, the search began for such structural differences in human brains.

Early investigations in sex dimorphic human neuroanatomy focused on sex-related variations in brain weight (Wada et al., 1975; Peters, 1991 and Hofman and Swaab, 1991 for reviews). Other groups studied fiber tracts connecting the two cerebral hemispheres. Sex differences in areas of the corpus callosum were found (de LaCoste-Utamsing and Holloway, 1982), although there is a continuing argument about the reliability and significance of these differences (Kertesz et al., 1987; Weis et al., 1989; Clarke et al., 1989) or whether such differences in callosal structure are meaningfully related to sex differences in behavior (McGlone, 1980; Witelson, 1989; Byne et al., 1988; for review, see Hofman and Swaab, 1991).

Deeper within the human brain, sex differences have been reported for the anterior commissure (AC), a fiber tract connecting temporal lobes from each brain hemisphere. The AC has been shown to be, on average, 12 % larger in females than in males (Allen and Gorski, 1991), even though the males' brains were larger. In that same study, the authors report that the massa intermedia (MI), a structure crossing the third ventricle that connects the left and right thalami was present in more women than men. And in those persons having a MI, the structure was, on average, 53 % larger in women than in men (Allen and Gorski, 1991). One suspects that such significant differences are functionally consequential, and the authors note that such anatomical sex differences in structures connecting the two hemispheres may underlie sex differences in cognition and cerebral lateralization.

Still deeper within the brain, several laboratories have demonstrated sex differences in structures of the nervous system thought to be involved with reproduction. Swaab and Fliers (1985) described a sexually dimorphic nucleus of the preoptic area of the human brain, in which the volume of this cell group was 2.5 fold larger in men than in women, with 2.2 fold as many cells in men than in women. Shortly thereafter, Allen et al. (1989) identified sexually dimorphic cell groups within the same region (POA). One of these cell groups, which they describe as the Interstitial Nuclei of the Anterior Hypothalamus, Number 3 (INAH-3), was 2.8 fold larger in male brains than in the female brain, independent of age. Since the studied brain region influences gonadotropin secretion, maternal behavior, and sexual behavior in many mammalian species, the authors suggested that functional sex differences of the hypothalamus may be related to sex differences in neural structure. Elsewhere in the brain, a sex difference has been reported for the bed nucleus of the stria terminalis (Allen and Gorski, 1990), in which the nucleus in men is 2.5 fold larger than in women. In animals, the bed nucleus is involved in such sexually dimorphic activities as aggression, sexual behavior and neuroendocrine functioning, with an implication that a comparable relationship between structure and function exists in humans.

Taken as a group, these findings of sex differences in hypothalamic tissues are nothing short of remarkable. Only a decade ago, the idea that men and women had anatomically different brains seemed not only politically inappropriate, but preposperous, bordering on some kind of "new phrenology". And while there seems to be minor disagreement among laboratories about the exact geographic boundaries of these sexually dimorphic regions (especially the

SDN-POA), the replicated findings of such hypothalamic and extra-hypothalamic sex differences in humans set the stage for the next step: a search for within sex differences in brain areas associated with differences in sexual orientation.

The first group to compare the sexually dimorphic nucleus of the POA (SDN-POA) in heterosexual and homosexual men found no difference (Swaab and Hofman, 1990). In a study comparing homosexual men who died of AIDS (n = 10), heterosexual men who died of AIDS (n = 4) and heterosexual men dead from other causes (n = 18), the SDN-POA was similar in nucleus volume and total cell number. However, in that same study, there was a substantially larger (1.7 x volume, 2.1 x cell number) suprachiasmatic nucleus (SCN) in homosexual men compared to the other two groups. The SCN is associated with controlling and generating coordinated hormonal, physiological and behavioral rhythms. Although the SCN was not reported to be a sexually dimorphic structure (i.e., no difference in volume or cell size between men and women), previous research had shown that the SCN has a different "shape" in men and women. Swaab et al. (1985) and Hofman et al. (1988) described the SCN in women as having an elongated shape, while in men it appeared more spherical. In their report of a larger SCN in homosexual men, Swaab and Hofman (1990) also noted that the rostrocaudal axis of the SCN was longer in homosexual men than in heterosexual men, while no differences were found in maximal cross-sectional area of the nucleus. The authors conclude that "homosexuals have a more elongated SCN than heterosexuals" (Swaab and Hofman, 1990), a shape very similar to that which they previously reported for women. Thus, while Swaab and Hofman (1990) argue that the SDN-POA data do not support the hypothesis that homosexual men have a "female hypothalamus", the same cannot be said for the SCN.

Shortly thereafter, LeVay (1991) replicated the earlier finding by Allen et al. (1989) of a sex difference in the INAH-3: heterosexual men had a substantially larger INAH-3 than did heterosexual women, about twice the size. The more interesting and novel finding by LeVay was that the INAH-3 in heterosexual men was also significantly larger by the same magnitude compared to the size of that region in homosexual men. Thus, LeVay (1991) concluded that "INAH-3 is dimorphic not with sex but with sexual orientation, at least in men" (p. 1035). The issue of whether such sex dimorphisms in neuroanatamy are a cause or a consequence of behavior has been raised by some observers. For the most part, it seems more likely that the INAH-3 is formed early in life and has later influences upon sexual behavior, rather than the reverse, a point stressed by LeVay (1991, p. 1036).

Finally, Allen and Gorski (1992) have reported that the anterior commissure of homosexual men was 18 % larger than in heterosexual women and 34 % larger than that of heterosexual men. They suggest that this notable anatomical difference might underlie differences in cognitive functioning and brain lateralization differences reported among men differing in sexual orientation (see below for a discussion of those neuropsychological studies). In any case, this series of remarkable advances and observations in human neuroanatomy add weight to the biological bases for sexual behavior differences in general, and sexual orientation in particular. At the very least, these findings should prompt further inquiries by other laboratories. And, if replicated, these data will sharpen our focus on how sexual differentiation operates, and what impacts these biological processes have on such complex behavioral patterns as sexual partner preference.

# Neuropsychological evidence

In addition to possible neuroanatomical and neuroendocrine differences between men and women, many researchers report significant sex differences in certain cognitive skills, primarily in the dimension of spatial abilities (for review, see Halpern, 1986). The origins for sex differences in spatial ability are hotly debated. One position holds that cognitive differences between men and women are a consequence of different experiences and expectations produced by socialization (Signorella and Jamison, 1986). An alternative position argues that biological factors (i.e., differential development of relevant neural and information processing pathways) may be the critical determinants for sex differences in cognition (Kimura and Harshman, 1984; also, see McCormick and Witelson, 1991). Of course, similar psychosocial and biological arguments have been raised to account for differences in psychosexual development (sexual orientation). And within the past decade, a flurry of studies from various research groups have yielded evidence that, within sex, there are differences in spatial ability associated with differences in sexual orientation.

One of the earliest reports, by Wilmott and Brierley (1984) found that scores obtained by homosexual men on the Wechsler Adult Intelligence Scale (WAIS) performance IQ measure (reflecting, in part, spatial ability) were lower than those of heterosexual men but comparable to those of heterosexual women. Later, Sanders and Ross-Field (1986) noted that homosexual men underperformed heterosexual men on two measures of spatial ability, a water level horizontality task, and the Vincent Mechanical Diagrams Test.[1]

Subsequently, our laboratory found that homosexual men underperformed heterosexual men on a critical measure of spatial ability, the Mental Rotations Task (MRT), and on a Water Level Task, a measure of horizontality (Gladue, et al., 1990). In addition, homosexual women also underperformed heterosexual women on the Water Level Task. Like Sanders and Ross-Field, we found that homosexual men were comparable to heterosexual women on these measures.

This basic finding has since been explored by two other groups. Using the same protocol as Gladue et al. (1990), Tkachuk and Zucker (1991) found mean MRT scores of heterosexual men to be significantly higher than that of homosexual men. And McCormick and Witelson (1991), using a slightly different set of tests (the Spatial Relations subtest of the Primary Mental Abilities battery, and the Spatial Relations subtest of the Differential Aptitude Test Battery), found that homosexual men underperformed relative to heterosexual men, but were still scoring at higher levels than heterosexual women. These authors also noted that, in their studies on handedness, the prevalence of non-consistent righthandedness (non-CRH) among homosexual men (48 % non-CRH) was greater than that found in the general population (35 % non-CRH) (McCormick and Witelson, 1990, 1991). Taken as a whole, these spatial ability and handedness data, suggest possible neurobiological and neuropsychological factors related to the development of sexual orientation in men.

# Other types of evidence

Aside from the neuroanatomical, neurohormonal, and neuropsychological elements associated with the psychobiology of sexual orientation, there are other, often complimentary, lines of research that contribute to our understanding of the determinants of sexual orientation. Some of these findings are supplemental to those described above; in other cases, the data often appear to contradict prevailing hypotheses of the origin of sexual orientation.

## Congenital adrenal hyperplasia (CAH) studies

CAH is an inherited, recessive disorder of adrenal steroid formation in which girls are prenatally exposed to virilizing sex hormones. Affected girls are born with partial or fully masculinized genitalia, which can be normalized with surgical intervention. And postnatal hormonal replacement therapy counters the main effects of excessive androgen production. Several studies have shown that such girls, prenatally exposed to masculinizing hormones, have higher rates of homosexuality/bisexuality (Money et al., 1984), as well as childhood toy preferences and play behavior similar to that of boys (Berenbaum and Hines, 1992). In addition, such CAH girls have "male-like" spatial abilities as very young children (Berenbaum, unpublished observation) and as adolescents (Resnick et al., 1986). Curiously, Money and Lewis (1982) presented findings that among CAH men, the incidence of homosexuality was less than that of the general population, suggesting that the development of heterosexuality might itself require androgen in men.

## Maternal stress

Animal studies have shown that maternal stress can result in altered fetal hormone and enzyme activity, causing a temporary deficit in fetal androgen production. The behavioral consequence of this in animals has been demasculinized and feminized behavior in the affected offspring (Ward, 1984). Applying this principle to humans, Dörner et al. (1980) proposed that mothers of homosexual men would have been under greater stress during pregnancy than mothers of heterosexual men. Two groups have reported evidence in support of such a notion (Dörner et al., 1983; Ellis et al., 1988), while other groups have argued against the hypothesis (Schmidt and Clement, 1990; Bailey et al., 1991). However, Bailey and colleagues (1991) did note that, like Ellis et al. (1988), some stress-relevant (stress-prone?) features of the mothers pregnancy were associated with reports of childhood effeminacy in those sons. A combination of methodological problems, statistical analyses and interpretations of data overhang all of these studies, and any clear conclusion is not possible at this time.

## Prenatal hormone manipulation of "at-risk" pregnancies

One of the ways in which prenatal hormonal influences upon sexual behavior development has been studied is to consider the behavior of offspring born to mothers who were treated with various drugs during pregnancy. Most of these "at-risk" pregnancies were therapeutically assisted with synthetic progestins (either androgen- or progesterone-based), synthetic estrogens, such as diethylstilbestrol (DES), or a combination of estrogens and progestins. As reviewed by Reinisch et al., (1991), the data suggest masculinizing influences of androgen-based synthetic progestins and DES, whereas progesterone-based molecules appear to have had feminizing or demasculinizing influences upon behavior. The authors reviewed 19 studies, of which 5 specifically addressed sexual orientation in some way. Of these, one study reported a higher incidence of homosexual fantasy and behavior in women prenatally exposed to DES (Ehrhardt et al., 1985), a molecule that has been shown in animal models to behaviorally masculinize/defeminize.

# A comment on biological theories of sexual orientation

Over the past several decades, discussions about the origins of diversity in sexual orientation often degenerated into a fruitless debate about the absolute mode of causation being either "nature" or "nurture". Yet even scholars typically associated with a strong "socio-cultural" leaning regarding human behavioral diversity agreed that heredity and endocrinology must play crucial roles (Mead, 1961; for an excellent overview of this debate as it occured mid-century, see Diamond, 1965). Most observers now argue for, at least in principle, a multifactorial scheme toward understanding human psychosexual development, a so-called "biopsychosocial" approach. Incorporating genetic, endocrine, and neural developmental factors along with life-span social-learning components of behavioral development would appear to have "something for everyone". But even within this scheme, there is substantial and rancorous debate about the framework of action for biological factors. Simply stated, how do we make sense of the biological data regarding sexual orientation?

What we are faced with is an array of impressive data regarding the psychobiology of sexual orientation, but no single theoretical model that satisfactorily includes all of these data. However, we keep trying. So far, we have moved from a simplistic psychobiological view of sex and gender (where men and women represent discrete non-overlapping bundles of anatomical and behavioral characteristics), to a "continuum" model where sex and sexual orientation are cast on a bipolar male-female line. In this bipolar continuum homosexual men presumably fall somewhere between heterosexual men and women, while lesbians theoretically fall somewhere between heterosexual women and men. Influenced by the Neurohormonal Organization of Sexual Differentiation Theory, the continuum is a helpful model. Some of the neuroanatomical data seem to fit this schema: homosexual men have INAH-3 cell size and volume intermediate to that of heterosexual men and women. And while the SCN is larger in homosexual men, it has a "female- like" sex-dimorphic shape. Some of the neuroendocrine data fit here as well: an LH response pattern intermediate to that of heterosexual men and women was observed in homosexual men, although other researchers fail to find this pattern. And some of the neuropsychological data fall on this continuum: spatial abilities of homosexual men are either intermediate to that of heterosexual men and women, or are more "female-like".

But not every characteristic and trait thought to be sex-dimorphic fits neatly into this model. For example, the model may be appropriate for male homosexuals, but less so for female homosexuals. For example, according to the continuum model, lesbians would exhibit "male-like" aggressive behavior and spatial abilities, whereas gay men would be less aggressive than heterosexuals. In both cases, the evidence doesn't support such simplistic sex-reversals (Gladue et al., 1990; Gladue, 1991): in fact, lesbians appear to be more "female-like" on measures of spatial ability, and less physically aggressive than their heterosexual counterparts. As I have argued elsewhere, it may well turn out that a different set of processes is associated with the development of sexual orientation in women than in men, and that lesbian women may represent the more "female" region of such masculine-feminine continua (Gladue et al., 1990). [There is some precedence for this notion based on animal experiments, where typical "female" sexual behavior may require a small amount of endocrine-brain interaction during critical periods (Döhler, 1991) and the absence of such hormone results in a hyper-exagerrated female behavioral pattern (Clemens and Gladue, 1978; Gladue and Clemens, 1982).] In any event, for some behaviors, the Neurohormonal Organization hypothesis model may be a useful working hypothesis, but for other behaviors, substantial modifications in the model may be required.

In other cases, especially syndromes of atypical endocrine exposure such as CAH, with prenatally high levels of androgens, enough to masculinize genitalia, there are less severe behavioral consequences. Although CAH women are more likely to report homosexual and bisexual imagery and activity, and exhibit less stereotypical female behaviors and interests, they do not show the severity of response one might expect from such a major endocrine exposure during critical periods of development. Elsewhere, others have found that while prenatal exposure to DES may be capable of masculinizing erotic behavior in women (Ehrhardt et al., 1985), another study of DES women from that group shows that such treatments had no effect on masculinizing gender-role behavior of girls or women (Lish et al., 1991). Thus, we may need to re-examine the Prenatal Neurohormonal Theory of Sexual Orientation and the "sex-dimorphic continuum" with a special eye toward understanding its broad relevance and applicability to both sexes. To be sure, the number of studies exploring the psychobiology of lesbians is appallingly small. And until we expand our inquiries to explore neuroanatomical, neuroendocrine, and neuropsychological processes in homosexual women, our "continuum" is missing some key points.

We now have a set of findings from many laboratories suggesting that human sexual orientation has a genetic basis, and that certain brain areas and neuroendocrine processes known to be androgen-dependent and/or sex-dimorphic appear to differ in homosexual and heterosexual men, and that there are corresponding neuropsychological disparities as well. When we have a large enough set of studies of human sexual orientation and its relationship to a wide range of sexually dimorphic behaviors, we may be able to construct a "biosocial" model in which different events occuring at different times are "weighted" for their impact on the development of sexual orientation. Rather than a simple linear "cascade" model, in which A triggers B which triggers C, and so forth, an interactive variable weights model may better fit the data. Associated with this "weighted" model is the notion that not all men and women arrive at their sexual orientation following the same path. A continual and humbling reminder of the complexity (even enormity) of the task for a Theory of Sexual Orientation Development, is that heterosexuals, like homosexuals, vary in their psychosexual milestones of genital, neuropsychological, erotic and reproductive development. We need to consider each of the likely key biological factors and how they, in turn, influence the individuals psychosocial development.

## Metaphors and conclusion

Trying to assemble all of the data from the studies cited above, and scores of other related inquiries, into one Grand Theory of the Development of Sexual Orientation has been extremely difficult. As two long-time explorers of this discipline have noted with dry understatement, *"In contemporary sexology, little is settled regarding the determinants of gender identity, gender role, and sexual orientation"* (Zucker and Green, 1992, p.126). Others have been more circumspect, taking an excessively cautious tone. For example, Gooren et al. (1990) state a case that *"it can be concluded that at present no evidence exists for a relationship between a hormonally regulated sexual differentiation of the human CNS and the development of sexual orientation or gender identity"* (p. 190), and later, *"In light of all the evidence...it is questionable whether the concept of homosexuality as a form of pseudohermaphroditism of the brain is tenable. That certain prenatal biological factors facilitate a homosexual orientation later in life cannot yet be discounted, but irrefutable evidence is presently lacking."* (p. 191).

Both of these quotes represent an honest scholarly concern that sexual orientation, especially homosexuality in either men or women, may not be influenced by biological factors, or that, at the very least, the evidence is insubstantial. Thus, despite an accumulating body of evidence, in some cases, replicated by numerous research groups, strongly suggesting, at least in part, some combination of biological factors to be involved in the development of sexual orientation, the issue remains, for many, an "open question". Others who may be fundamentally opposed to any incorporation of modern biology into an understanding of human behavioral complexity, will not be swayed by evidence, however compelling, and will no doubt cling to their belief until, as the philosopher and historian of science Thomas Kuhn (1962) once opined, they no longer walk the earth in argumentative opposition.

## A metaphor

In some criminal jurisprudence proceedings, in which the state lays claim against an individual, a person cannot be found guilty, or a criminal action not sanctioned unless the evidence supports "proof beyond reasonable doubt".

In many ways, trying to "prove" that homosexuality, like heterosexuality, is biologically based, is like those crime dramas, where everyone, the police, the lawyers, the citizens, and of course, the reader or viewer "know" what is going on: they just have to prove it beyond a reasonable doubt in a court of law. And sometimes, even a compelling and convincing body of evidence, however it may circumstantial, may not provide such proof, if a major "contrary" piece of evidence raises a reasonable doubt. On the other hand, one could start from the position that homosexuality is a matter of "free will", "lifestyle choice", "parental identification with mother", social reinforcement, or other psychosocial explanations. In this position, there are few, if any, biological influences predisposing one toward homosexuality. In that case, employing our legal metaphor, biological evidence, especially many pieces of it from various quarters, should be the basis for "reasonable doubts" about non-biological theories of psychosexual development. Hence, we end up with an intellectual stalemate, where everyone waits for more evidence, before subscribing to a working hypothesis or theory.

For a different approach to this metaphor, consider civil jurisprudence proceedings, such as may be brought by one citizen against another, where the burden of proof is less stringent. In these cases, one need only bring a "preponderance of evidence" to support a claim. In those cases, competing arguments are presented with evidence in support of each, and the argument with the most weight (and believability) prevails (usually). Typically, this is the case for most scientific debate: the weight of evidence in support of competing arguments shapes how we approach an understanding and interpretation of a phenomenon. Using this approach, one can only conclude that, while imperfect, and while still in search of a perfect set of data that will yield uncontestable findings, the evidence to date grows in support of the notion that the development of sexual orientation, both heterosexuality and homosexuality, is early and critically based upon a myriad of biological factors. What remains is to search for a better understanding "beyond a reasonable doubt". After that, we can get on with the task of understanding more of the complexity of human behavioral and sexual interactions.

# References

Allen, L. S., Hines, M., Shryne, J. and Gorski, R. A. (1989). Two sexually dimorphic cell groups in the human brain. *J. Neurosci.*, **9** : 497-506.

Allen, L. S. and Gorski, R. A. (1990). A sex difference in the bed nucleus of the stria terminalis of the human brain. *J. Comp. Neurol.*, **302** : 697-706.

Bailey, J. M. and Pillard, R. C. (1991). A genetic study of male sexual orientation. *Arch. Gen. Psychiatry*, **48** : 1089-1096.

Bailey, J. M., Willerman, L. and Parks, C. (1991). A test of the maternal stress theory of human male homosexuality. *Arch. Sex. Behav.*, **20** : 277-293.

Berenbaum, S. and Hines, M. (1992). Early androgens are related to childhood sex-typed toy preferences. *Psychol. Sci.*, **3** : 203-206.

Blanchard, R. and Sheridan, P. M. (1992). Sibling size, sibling sex ratio, birth order, and parental age in homosexual and nonhomosexual gender dysphorics. *J. Nerv. Ment. Dis.*, **180** : 40-47.

Buhrich, N., Bailey, J. M. and Martin, N. G. (1991). Sexual orientation, sexual identity, and sex-dimorphic behaviors in male twins. *Behav. Genet.*, **21** : 75-96.

Byne, W., Bleier, R. and Houston, L. (1988). Variations in human corpus callosum do not predict gender: a study using magnetic resonance imagery. *Behav. Neurosci.*, **102** : 222-227

Clarke, S., Kraftsik, R. Van der Loos, H. and Innocenti, G. (1989). Forms and measures of the adult and developing corpus callosum: is there sexual dimorphism? *J. Comp. Neurol.*, **280** : 213-230.

Clemens, L. G. and Gladue, B. A. (1978). Feminine sexual behavior in rats enhanced by prenatal inhibition of androgen aromatization. *Horm. Behav.*, **11** : 190-201.

Diamond, M. (1965). A critical evaluation of the ontogeny of human sexual behavior. *Quarterly Rev. Biol.*, **40** : 147-175.

Döhler, K. D. (1991). The pre-and postnatal influence of hormones and neurotransmitters on sexual differentiation of the mammalian hypothalamus. *Int. Rev. Cytology*, **131** : 1-57.

Dörner, G., Docke, F., Götz, F., Rohde, W., Stahl, F. and Tonjes, R. (1987). Sexual differentiation of gonadotrophin secretion, sexual orientation and gender role behavior. *J. Steroid Biochem.*, **27** : 1081-1087.

Dörner, G., Geier, T., Ahrens, L., Krell, L., Munx, G., Sieler, H., Kittner, E. and Muller, H. (1980). Prenatal stress as possible aetiogenic factor of homosexuality in human males. *Endokrinologie*, **75** : 365-368.

Dörner, G., Schenk, B., Schmiedel, B. and Ahrens, L. (1983). Stressful events in prenatal life of bi- and homosexual men. *Exptl. Clin. Endocr.*, **81** : 83-87.

Eckert, E. D., Bouchard, T. J., Bohlen, J. and Heston, L. L. (1986). Homosexuality in monozygotic twins reared apart. *Brit. J. Psychiatry*, **148** : 421-425.

Ehrhardt, A. A., Meyer-Bahlburg, H. F. L., Rosen, L. R., Feldman, J. F., Veridiano, Z. P., Zimmerman, I. and McEwen, B. S. (1985). Sexual orientation after prenatal exposure to exogenous estrogen. *Arch. Sex. Behav.*, **14** : 57-77.

Ellis, L., Ames, M. A., Peckham, W. and Burke, D. (1988). Sexual orientation of human offspring may be altered by severe maternal stress during pregnancy. *J. Sex Res.*, **25** : 152-157.

Friedman, R. C., Wollensen, F. and Tendler, R. (1976). Psychological development and blood levels of sex steroids in male identical twins of divergent sexual orientation. *J. Nerv. Ment. Dis.*, **163** : 282-288.

Gladue, B. A. (1988). Hormones in relationship to homosexual/bisexual/heterosexual gender orientation. In : Sitsen, J. M. A. (Ed.), *Handbook of Sexology, Vol. 6, The Pharmacology and Endocrinology of Sexual Function*, Elsevier, Amsterdam, pp. 388-409.

Gladue, B. A. (1990). Hormones and neuroendocrine factors in atypical human sexual behavior. In : Feierman, J. R. (Ed.), *Pedophilia: Biosocial Dimensions*, Springer-Verlag, New York, pp. 278-298.

Gladue, B. A. (1991). Aggressive behavioral characteristics, hormones, and sexual orientation in men and women. *Aggr. Behav.*, **17** : 313-326.

Gladue, B. A. and Clemens, L. G. (1982). Development of feminine sexual behavior in the rat: androgenic and temporal influences. *Physiol. Behav.*, **29** : 263-267.

Gladue, B. A., Beatty, W. W., Larson, J. and Staton, R. D. (1990).Sexual orientation and spatial ability in men and women. *Psychobiol.*, **18** : 101-108.

Gladue, B. A., Green, R. and Hellman, R. E. (1984). Neuroendocrine response to estrogen and sexual orientation. *Science*, **225** : 1496-1499.

Gooren, L. G. (1986). The neuroendocrine response of luteinizing hormone to estrogen administration in heterosexual, homosexual and transsexual subjects. *J. Clin. Endocrinol. Metab.*, **63** : 583-588.

Gooren, L. G. (1988). An appraisal of endocrine theories of homosexuality and gender dysphoria. In : Sitsen, J. M. A. (Ed.), *Handbook of Sexology, Vol. 6. The Pharmacology and Endocrinology of Sexual Function*, Elsevier, Amsterdam, pp. 410-424.

Gooren, L. G., Fliers, E. and Courtney, K. (1990). Biological determinants of sexual orientation. *Ann. Rev. Sex Res.*, **1** : 175-196.

Gorski, R. A., Gordon, J. H., Shryne, J. E. and Southam, A. M. (1978). Evidence for a morphological sex difference within the medial preoptic area of the rat brain. *Brain Res.*, **148** : 333-346.

Goy, R. W. and McEwen, B. S. (1980). *Sexual Differentiation of the Brain.*, Basic Books, New York.

Goy, R. W., Bercovitch, F. B. and McBrair, M. C. (1988). Behavioral masculinization is independent of genital masculinization in prenatally androgenized female rhesus macaques. *Horm. Behav.*, **22** : 552-571.

Greenough, W. T., Carter, C. S., Steerman, C. and DeVoogd, T. J. (1977). Sex differences in dendritic branching patterns in hamster preoptic area. *Brain Res.*, **126** : 63-72.

Halpern, D. F. (1986). *Sex Differences in Cognitive Ability*, Erlbaum, Hillsdale, NJ.

Hare, E. H. and Moran, P. A. (1979). Parental age and birth order in homosexual patients: a replication of Slater's study. *Brit. J. Psychiatry*, **134** : 178-182.

Hendricks, S. E., Graber, B. and Rodriguez-Sierra, J. F. (1989). Neuroendocrine responses to exogenous estrogen: no differences between heterosexual and homosexual men. *Psychoneuroendocrinology*, **14** : 177-185.

Hofman, M. A., Fliers, E., Goudsmit, E. and Swaab, D. F. (1988). Morphometric analysis of the suprachiasmatic and paraventricular nuclei in the human brain. *J. Anat.*, **160** : 127-143.

Hofman, M. A. and Swaab, D. F. (1991). Sexual dimorphism of the human brain: myth and reality. *Exp. Clin. Endocrinol.*, **98** : 161-170.

Kallman, F. J. (1952). Twin and sibship study of overt male homosexuality. *Amer. J. Human Genet.*, **4** : 136-146.

Kertesz. A., Polk, M., Howell, J. and Black, S. (1987). Cerebral dominance, sex and callosal size in MRI. *Neurology*, **37** : 1385-1388.

Kimura, D. and Harshman, R. A. (1984). Sex differences in brain organization for verbal and non-verbal functions. In : DeVries, G. J., DeBruin, J. P. C., Uylings, H. B. M. and Corner, M. A. (Eds.), *Sex Differences in the Brain Progress in Brain Research, Vol. 61,* Elsevier, Amsterdam, pp. 423-441.

Kuhn, T. (1962). *The Structure of Scientific Revolutions,* University of Chicago Press, Chicago.

Lacoste-Utamsing, C. and Holloway, R. (1982). Sexual dimorphism in the human corpus callosum. *Science,* **216** : 1431-1432.

Lang, T. (1960). Die homosexualitat als genetisches problem. *Acta Genet. Med. Gemellol.,* **9** : 370-381.

LeVay, S. (1991). A difference in hypothalamic structure between heterosexual and homosexual men. *Science,* **253** : 1034-1037.

Lish, J. D., Ehrhardt, A. A., Meyer-Bahlburg, H. F. L., Rosen, L. R., Gruen, R. S., and Veridiano, N. P. (1991). Gender-related behavior development in females exposed to diethylstilbestrol (DES) in utero: an attempted replication. *J. Amer. Acad. Child Adol. Psychiat.,* **30** : 29-37.

McConaghy, N. and Blaszczynski, A. (1980). A pair of monozygotic twins discordant for homosexuality: sex-dimorphic behavior and penile volume responses. *Arch. Sex. Behav.,* **9** : 123-131.

McCormick, C. M. amd Witelson, S. F. (1991). A cognitive profile of homosexual men compared to heterosexual men and women. *Psychoneuroendocrinology,* **16** : 459-473.

McCormick, C. M. and Witelson, S. F. (1990). Sexual orientation and functional hemispheric asymmetry. *Neuroendocr. Lett.,* **12** : 300.

McGlone, J. (1980). Sex differences in human brain asymmetry: a critical survey. *Brain Behav. Sci.,* **3** : 215-263.

Mead, M. (1961). Cultural determinants of sexual behavior. In :Young, W. C. (Ed., *Sex and Internal Secretions, 3rd Ed.,* Williams and Wilkins, Baltimore, MD.

Money, J. and Lewis, V. (1982). Homosexual/heterosexual status in boys at puberty: idiopathic adolescent gynecomastia and congenital virilizing adrenocorticism compared. *Psychoneuroendocrinology,* **7** : 339-347.

Money, J., Schwartz, M. and Lewis, V. G. (1984). Adult erotosexual status and fetal hormonal masculinization and demasculinization 46, XX congenital virilizing adrenal hyperplasia and 46 XY androgen-insensitivity syndrome compared. *Psychoneuroendocrinology,* **9** : 405-414.

Peters, M. (1991). Sex differences in human brain size and the general meaning of differences in brain size. *Can. J. Psychol.,* **45** : 507-522.

Pfaff, D. W. (1966). Morphological changes in the brains of adult male rats after neonatal castration. *J. Endocrinol.*, **36** : 415-416.

Pillard, R. C., Poumadere, J. and Carretta, M. (1982). A family study of sexual orientation. *Arch. Sex. Behav.*, **11** : 511-520.

Pillard, R. C., Poumadere, J. and Carretta, M. (1981). Is homosexuality familial? A review, some data, and a suggestion. *Arch. Sex. Behav.*, **10** : 465-475.

Pillard, R. C. and Weinrich, J. D. (1986). Evidence of familial nature of male homosexuality. *Arch. Gen. Psychiat.*, **43** : 808-812.

Raisman, G. and Field, P. M. (1971). Sexual dimorphism in the preoptic area of the rat. *Science*, **173** : 731-733.

Reinisch, J. M., Ziemba-Davis, M. and Sanders, S. A. (1991). Hormonal contributions to sexually dimorphic behavioral development in humans. *Psychoneuroendocrinology*, **16** : 213-278.

Resnick, S. M., Brenebaum, S. A., Gottesman, I. I. and Bouchard, T. J. (1986). Early hormonal influences on cognitive functioning in congenital adrenal hyperplasia. *Develop. Psychol.*, **22** : 191-198.

Sanders, G. and Ross-Field, L. (1986). Sexual orientation and visuospatial ability. *Brain and Cognition*, **5** : 280-290.

Schmidt, G. and Clement, U. (1990). Does peace prevent homosexuality? *Arch. Sex. Behav.*, **19** : 183-187.

Signorella, M. L. and Jamison, W. (1986). Masculinity, femininity, androgyny, and cognitive performance : a meta-analysis. *Psychol. Bull.*, **100** : 207-228.

Slater, E. (1962). Birth order and maternal age of homosexuals. *Lancet*, **1** : 69-71.

Swaab, D. F. and Fliers, E. (1985). A sexually dimorphic nucleus in the human brain. *Science*, **228** : 1112-1115.

Swaab, D. F. , Fliers, E. and Partiman, T. S. (1985). The suprachiasmatic nucleus of the human brain in relation to sex, age, and senile dementia. *Brain Res.*, **342** : 37-44.

Swaab, D. F. and Hofman, M. A. (1990). An enlarged suprachiasmatic nucleus in homosexual men. *Brain Res.*, **537** : 141-148.

Tkachuk, J. and Zucker, K. J. (1991). *The Relation Among Sexual Orientation, Spatial Ability, Handedness, and Recalled Childhood Gender Identity in Women and Men*. Paper presented at the meeting of the International Academy of Sex Research, Barrie, Ontario.

Wada, J. A., Clarke, R. and Hamm, A. (1975). Cerebral hemispheric asymmetry in humans. *Arch. Neurol.*, **32** : 239-246.

Ward, I. L. (1984). The prenatal stress syndrome: current status. *Psychoneuroendocrinology*, **9** : 3-11.

Weis, S., Weber, G., Wenger, E. and Kimbacher, M. (1988). The human corpus callosum and the controversy about a sexual dimorphism. *Psychobiol.*, **16** : 411 - 415.

Whalen, R. E. 1984. Multiple actions of steroids and their antagonists. *Arch. Sex. Behav.*, **13** : 497-502.

Wilmott, M. and Brierley, R. (1984). Cognitive characteristics and homosexuality. *Arch. Sex. Behav.*, **13** : 311-319.

Witelson, S. F. (1989). Hand and sex differences in the isthmus and genu of the human corpus callosum. *Brain*, **112** : 799-835.

Zucker, K. J. and Green, R. (1992). Psychosexual disorders in children and adolescents. *J. Child Psychol. Psychiat.*, **33** : 107-151.

Zuger, B. (1976). Monozygotic twins discordant for homosexuality: report of a pair and significance of the phenomenon. *Comprehensive Psychiatry*, **17** : 661-669.

# Alternative Conceptions of Sex (and Sex Differences)

R.H.  UNGER

*Department of Psychology, Montclair State College, Russ Hall, Upper Montclair, N.J. 07043, USA*

## Sexual dimorphism : the biological critique

The apparently simple word "sex" is used to refer to our reproductive category, physiological properties, both reproductive and nonreproductive behaviors, and, in human beings, our sense of who we are. Recently, feminist scholars have introduced the term "gender" to refer to the social aspects of relationships between the sexes. Terminological distinctions have not, unfortunately, eliminated conceptual confusion in this area (Unger and Crawford, In press). A core problem is the tendency to view various aspects of sex (and even gender) in terms of simple dichotomies. Nevertheless, exceptions can be found for even our most fundamental biological distinctions. Because sex is usually viewed from the perspective of mammalian physiology, the characteristics of the egg producer - female - and the sperm producer - male - are often thought of as fixed and universal.  However, a number of fish species change sex (Diamond, this volume).

Not all vertebrates have two sexes. Recently, researchers have begun to examine the reproductive physiology and behavior of an all-female species of whiptail lizards (Crews, 1987b). In this species, there are no males and the females reproduce by means of parthenogenesis. Offspring derive from unfertilized eggs which contain the same genes as their single parent. Although male individuals and their sperm have been lost, reproductive behaviors characteristic of both sexes such as mounting, copulation, attractivity, and receptivity have been retained. Furthermore, ovarian hormones influence the extent to which both male-like and female-like behaviors will be exhibited. The pseudo-male behaviors facilitate reproduction much as male courtship behavior does in species with two sexes.

The biological categories of male and female are not as exclusive as we may have thought. As noted above, females in at least one all-female species show the complete range of behaviors associated with males in related species.  In another species, the spotted hyena, females exhibit the sexual anatomy and behavioral aggressiveness usually associated with males (Frank et al., 1991). In still a third species, the bighorn sheep, the sexes do not appear to differ in either form or behavior (Hubbard, 1990).

*M. Haug et al. (eds.), The Development of Sex Differences and Similarities in Behavior, 457–476.*
© 1993 *Kluwer Academic Publishers.*

These so-called oddities demonstrate the extent of the variability between species in terms of sex differences in both anatomy and reproductive behavior. I chose these extreme examples in order to demonstrate that one can find examples of almost any kind of pattern one is looking for by picking the appropriate animal. We lack, however, a theoretical framework for choosing which animal model is the most appropriate one for comparisons with human beings.

# Limits on the relationship between physiology and behavior

Generalizations about sexual dimorphism may lead us to believe that the mechanisms that connect sexual anatomy, physiology, and behavior are more invariant than has been found to be the case. For example, gamete production, sex hormone secretion, and mating behavior are correlated in many vertebrates, but not all. As Crews (1987a) has pointed out, species that exhibit a disassociated reproductive tactic - a time interval between gametogenesis and mating - call into question the universality of a functional association between hormonal production and mating behavior. This relationship is further challenged by species such as cats and some primates for whom sexual experience may be a more potent contributor to sexual activity following castration than is hormonal status (Michael et al., 1973 ; Rosenblatt and Aronson, 1958).

Preconceived beliefs about sexual dimorphisms may cause us to emphasize stability and consistency and to ignore the role of other factors in the expression of supposedly sexually differentiated behaviors. In many species, the capacity for both male and female behaviors is retained in both sexes. Hormones only alter their threshold of activation. Whether and how much these behaviors will be expressed depends upon a number of other factors. It is the existence of these variables which challenge our notions about simple male-female dichotomies.

Questions about the extent and kind of behavioral differences between males and females are controversial ones. There is little doubt that exposure to perinatal androgens alters the behaviors of animals of either sex in many species. However, many feminist critics would argue whether we should term such changes as "male-like" or "masculinizing" rather than by some more neutral term (Longino, 1990; Spanier, 1991). Other critical questions include: does the masculinizing effect of androgens extend to behaviors that are not directly associated with reproduction? And, to what extent are such effects, if they exist, irreversible? Can they be changed through the experience and environment to which the organism is exposed? In other words, to what degree are sex-related differences in behavior biologically determined? Surprisingly, this is not as easy a question to answer as one might believe.

Behavioral dimorphism is an even more controversial distinction than is anatomical or biochemical dimorphism. Use of a term meaning "two bodied" masks the fact that behavioral dimorphisms are, at best, relative rather than absolute.

*"Few behavioral responses are dimorphic in an absolute sense. In many cases, both sexes display a given behavior pattern. It is the relative difference in frequency, intensity, or context associated with the display of a particular behavior pattern that is termed a sex difference. A behavioral dimorphism is therefore a relational construct, an expression of statistical comparison, and not a directly observable phenomenon "(Goldfoot and Neff, 1987, pp. 179 - 180).*

Thus, although any animal may display the behavior of the other sex, it is much more likely that it will display behaviors characteristic of its own sex. These behavioral effects are not limited to those directly associated with reproduction such as mounting in males and sexual receptivity in females. Recent evidence suggests, however, that sex-related behaviors are relatively easily modified.

# Environmental modification of sex-related behaviors

The most interesting studies are on primates because they are genetically most similar to ourselves. Researchers interested in nonreproductive dimorphisms in primates have concentrated upon three major categories of behavior. These behaviors are: aggression and rough-and-tumble play (more characteristic of males than females) and nurturance (grooming and care-giving, more characteristic of females than males).

There is clear evidence from experimental studies of primates that rough-and-tumble play, at least, may be influenced by the level of androgens circulating in the fetal bloodstream. For example, researchers have injected pregnant rhesus monkeys with testosterone and observed its effect upon their offspring. They found that the female offspring showed levels of play intermediate between that of normal males and normal females (Goy, 1970). These females also engaged in more chasing and threatening behavior than normal females did. Other studies have also shown that prenatal exposure to androgens appears to induce higher levels of physical activity in both primate and human females (Ehrhardt and Meyer-Bahlburg, 1981).

Recent studies indicate that the environment is also important in influencing the level of these activities in both sexes. For example, Goldfoot and Neff (1987) investigated the level of rough-and-tumble play exhibited by juvenile female rhesus monkeys living in five-member groups. Females living in all-female groups display a very low frequency of this form of play. However, it is considerably higher in females in one-male, four-female groups and lower again in females living in two-male, three female groups. The researchers suggest that males initiate the activity and select male partners for it. When no male partner is available, they engage a female in rough-and-tumble play and she reciprocates.

Isosexual rearing also influenced the extent to which male and female rhesus monkeys engage in mounting and presenting behaviors (Goldfoot et al., 1984). The effect of rearing was greater for heterotypical than homotypical behaviors.

In other words, for males, presenting was more affected; whereas for females mounting was more affected by single-sex rearing. Behaviors related to reproduction were more influenced than rough and tumble play. These studies support two major points. First, even in animals, social manipulations modify some behaviors known to be influenced by perinatal hormones. Second, different behaviors (even in the same species) vary in terms of how responsive they are to social modification. Another study (Gibber, 1981) looked at sex differences in the parenting of rhesus monkeys. She found that both males and females looked at, approached, and picked up stranded newborn monkeys in an adjacent cage with an attached passageway to an equal extent. However, when both a male and a female were in the testing cage, females displayed virtually all the parenting behavior observed. Many of the males who had showed nurturant responses when alone appeared to be inhibited by the presence of an adult female. If the researcher had tested these animals only in mixed sex pairs, she might have concluded a much greater sex difference in the tendency to take care of infants.

Some sex-related differences may originate from factors correlated with, but not dependent on genetic sex. One such confounding factor in primate groups is dominance. For example, males mount much more frequently than females do (98% versus 25% of each sex), but males are usually more dominant in groups. High dominant males mount more than low dominant males and most of the females who do mount are high ranking. In groups with no males, a statistically higher percentage of females mount than in mixed-sex groups (Goldfoot and Neff, 1987). These observations support the idea that some social factor related to dominance rank affects mounting in both sexes.

It is not clear what factors underlie dominance in primates. Among baboons, for example, the highest ranking males do not have the highest level of testosterone in their bloodstreams. Their testosterone levels are, however, more resistant to being lowered by stress than those of less dominant males (Sapolsky, 1987). An important question is which comes first. Is their high social position determined by their unique physiological status? Or, does their high rank confer physiological protections not available to lower status males?

A few studies suggest that testosterone levels are affected by peer interactions as well as the other way around. For example, Rose et al., (1972) found that testosterone levels rose in male monkeys when they were exposed to receptive females who gave them sexual access. When the same monkeys were exposed to a set of males who did not allow them to establish dominance, their testosterone levels fell below pre-test levels and rose again when they were returned to the presence of the receptive females.

In a field study where a coalition of younger males displaced the dominant male, Sapolsky (1987) found that during the succeeding three month period of social instability, the six equally dominant males showed more testosterone suppression from stress than usually found among high ranking baboons. He also observed a correlation not found during any other season. High ranking males were the most aggressive, started the most fights, and had the highest levels of testosterone in their bloodstream. This finding suggests that the endocrine aspects of dominance may be as sensitive to the behavioral features as much as the other way around.

# The relationship between hormones and behavior in humans

## Some caveats

Since it is unethical to inject people with hormones to see what effect it has on their sexual differentiation, clinical cases in which the various components of sex are discordant is one way to explore the nature of the relationships between the biological and psychological aspects of sex in human beings. However, the use of clinical case material carries with it additional problems and generalizations between anomalous and normal development may be as perilous as generalizations between animals and humans.

For example, people for whom the multiple determinants of sex do not coincide may be more sexually flexible or plastic than other people (Diamond, 1965). It may be easier for them to shift their sexual identities than it is for people whose sex is consistent. Also, individuals who come for clinical treatment may not be a representative sample of people with the same anomalies. People who seek or are sent for clinical treatment are often more adversely affected than others with the same organic characteristics. We cannot know how many people in the nonclinical population also possess their biological properties.

Explanation of causality in individuals with anomalous sexual development is also made more difficult because of the important role that culture and learning play in our behavior. Humans display a level of self consciousness and awareness that is not important when considering animal behavior. It is possible, therefore, to explore variables such as physical appearance and body image which are largely irrelevant in animal studies.

We can also expect from studies of animals that biological and environmental variables may affect different kinds of sex-related behaviors in different ways. Baker (1980) has made a distinction between gender-role behavior (traits such as aggression or nurturance), gender identity (whether the person perceives himself or herself to be male or female), and sexual orientation. Each of these categories may present a different pattern of sexual discordance. They may be influenced by a different mix of biological and social variables.

## The adrenogenital syndrome

Females with the adrenogenital syndrome (the endogenous form is also known congenital adrenal hyperplasia or CAH) have been found to identify firmly as girls and women. However, researchers have found differences between this group and control girls who had not been exposed to excessive androgens before birth (either matched normal females, unaffected siblings, or clinical controls). Girls with the syndrome are reported to show more intense active outdoor play, increased association with male peers, and long-term identification as a tomboy by both themselves and others. All of these behavioral differences are considered to be related to their high level of energy expenditure (Erhardt and Meyer-Bahlburg, 1981).

They also differed from control girls by displaying a lower level of parenting concerns. They engaged in less doll play and baby care and showed less interest in rehearsing the roles of wife and mother versus having a career. However, none of their behaviors would be considered abnormal for a female in our culture. They were not any more aggressive than girls from the control populations nor did they show a "male-like" cognitive profile ; i.e., a consistent advantage in spatial-perceptual over verbal abilities (Ehrhardt and Meyer-Bahlburg, 1981).

Despite their childhood depiction as tomboys and their avid interest in high school sports, none of these young women pursued sports as a career or even as a major pastime (Money and Mathews, 1982). As these young women reach adulthood, researchers appear to disagree about their feminine identification and heterosexual orientation. In one follow-up study of young women who had been studied during adolescence, Money and Mathews (1982) reported that none of these women had a history of difficulty in establishing friendships or dating relationships with men. Four of their subjects had married. In contrast, Hurtig and Rosenthal (1987) reported a consistent pattern of delay in dating and sexual relationships as well as signficant changes in gender identity as measured by the greater tendency of CAH girls to draw male figures first and differentiate them more.

It is difficult to draw conclusions about the causal relationship between prenatal hormones and sex-related behaviors from these data. For example, persistent relationships between physical activity levels in childhood and adolescent behaviors have been reported. Moreover, studies of adolescent boys and girls prenatally exposed to high levels of progestens - which were expected to have a demasculinizing effect - report only chance differences from comparisons groups (Ehrhardt et al., 1984; Kester, 1984). And, although those young women who were exposed to DES had a significantly higher level of homosexuality or bisexuality than untreated controls, 75% of them were exclusively or nearly exclusively heterosexual (Ehrhardt et al., 1985).

In sum, the connection between physiological events and behavior in these individuals does not appear to be particularly strong. Their sexual identity and orientation appear, in general, to follow the sex of rearing. All of these adolescents have been reported to score within one standard deviation of the norms for individuals in their age group. Some sex-related behaviors, such as those associated with a high degree of energy expenditure, may show parallels with animal studies, but even these effects do not appear to persist until adulthood. These studies rule out any rigidly deterministic effect of prenatal hormones on sex-related behaviors.

## The testicular feminization syndrome

The testicular feminization syndrome would appear to be a parallel hormonal disorder to the adrenogenital syndrome since individuals with this anomaly are genetic males who are partially or completely insensitive to testosterone. Since this is a rare disorder, there have been relatively few studies of their behavior. Money and Ehrhardt (1972) surveyed the clinical data on ten such individuals and reported that they show a high preference for traditionally feminine roles. Eighty percent preferred the role of homemaker over an outside job; 100 percent reported having dreams and fantasies of raising a family; 80 percent reported playing primarily with dolls and other girls' toys. They rated themselves as high in affectionateness and as fully content with the female role.

Since these individuals are exposed to no more estrogen than normal females, it is difficult to hypothesize hormonal causality for their high level of traits associated with feminine stereotypes. Their characteristics are, however, consistent with an interpretation based on the mediation of gender by physical appearance which will be discussed more fully below. For example, adults with this syndrome tend to be found in occupations that put a high premium on an attractive female appearance such as modeling, acting, and prostitution. They are said to present an unusually attractive appearance.

## Five alpha-reductase deficiency

The newest syndrome in which theories about social/biological effects may be examined is five alpha-reductase deficiency. Like testicular feminization, it is an inherited condition (due to a recessive rather than a sex-linked gene). Affected individuals lack an enzyme which aids in the conversion of testosterone to dihydrotestosterone. Dihydrotestosterone is the androgen that induces fusion of the scrotum and the growth of the penis. Thus, these individuals are born with normal testes and male internal structures combined with a clitoris-like penis and an incomplete or absent scrotum which may resemble the labia of females. Their external genitalia are quite similar to the ambiguous structures of females who have been exposed to prenatal androgens (Rubin et al., 1981). When modern scientific methods for determining sex are unavailable, they may be identified and raised as girls.

Males with five alpha-reductase deficiency are, however, masculinized at puberty when their normal testes pour large amounts of testosterone into their systems. This testosterone produces deepening of the voice, enlargement of the penis and testicles, erections, and ejaculation from a urethral orifice at the base of the penis (Imperato-McGinley and Peterson, 1976; Peterson et al., 1977). Such individuals would appear to provide a perfect test case for examining the effect of socialization versus biological factors in sexual identity since they are biological males who have been raised as females throughout childhood. The interesting question is : what happens to their sexual identity when their sex of rearing and their physical properties become discordant at this relatively late point in their lives? How reversible is sexual identity?

These questions are not as easy to answer as they might appear. For example, Imperato-McGinley and her colleagues (Imperato-McGinley et al., 1979) studied a group of 38 related individuals with the disorder in a rural region of the Dominican Republic. In this inbred group, five alpha-reductase deficiency is so common that it has a name *guevedoce* or "penis at twelve." The researchers claimed that the first nineteen cases of this disorder were reared unambiguously as girls. More recent cases have been recognized early and treated as special.

What is surprising about these studies is reports of the striking ease with which such individuals shifted from female to male at puberty. The researchers stated that seventeen individuals successfully changed to a male identity and fifteen married. These findings suggest a much later capacity for sex identity reversal than studies on other sexual anomalies would indicate is possible. The researchers believe that affected individuals were able to make the shift because their brains had been masculinized before birth. They argue that so-called male brains were able to overcome easily many years of female socialization.

The biologically determinist conclusions of these researchers have, however, been challenged. Researchers who conducted an intensive analysis of Imperato-McGinley's own data suggested that the shift from female to male identity was not as simple as it first appeared. They noted, for example, that she described these individuals as realizing that they were different from other girls sometime between the ages of seven and twelve (Rubin et al.,1981). This realization took place shortly after the age at which children in their culture are encouraged to segregate by sex for play and domestic tasks. They shifted to a masculine gender identity over several years and began sexual intercourse with females at the same age as those affected males who had been raised as boys.

It is not clear, moreover, whether these children were indeed raised unambiguously as females. Their genitalia, while not male, were certainly not normally female. Photographs of the external genitalia of three of the prepubescent subjects revealed marked labioscrotal fusion in two cases, absent labia minora in all three cases, and phalluses ranging from an enlarged abnormal clitoris to a small incomplete penis. *"Even cursory inspection of the genitalia should have revealed the abnormal configuration of these organs to any observer, especially to the mother"*. (Rubin et al., 1981, p. 1322). No one, however, asked the mothers whether they had noticed anything or what others thought the genital anomalies meant. There is little individual privacy in this society and any physical abnormality would be likely to be noticed by many people in such a relatively small, isolated group.

This case illustrates how one cannot ignore the role of culture in the differentiation of sexual identity even in situations where development differs drastically from the norm. A recent study of another isolated population - in New Guinea - with five alpha-reductase deficiency (Herdt and Davidson, 1988) illustrates how cultural categories may influence sexual identification. Like the group in the Dominican Republic, the genetic abnormality is common enough to have received a colloquial name. In fact, this society actually has three linguistic terms for sex : male, female, and an ambiguous compound word which the researchers translated as "male-like thing/adult person, masculine." The latter term emphasizes the transformational quality of change. This belief in the modifiability of sex is also indicated by the pidgeon word used to describe hermaphroditic individuals "Turnim-man."

Herdt and Davidson argue that male pseudohermaphrodites represent a third sex in their society. They are usually recognized at birth because of anomalies in their genitals. Their data on 14 individuals with the disorder indicate that nine were reared ambiguously as males and five as females. Those raised as females changed to a male role at adulthood, but under circumstances of social trauma. For example, two such individuals were rejected after marriage by their husband when he discovered they had small penises. None of them were initiated into the men's cults. They switched roles to "pass" as males under a great deal of external public pressure because there was no place to hide or to be female. The shift was facilitated by the availability of a third sexual category.

The researchers ask: "How do we interpret this scandal-induced halting outcome twenty years after birth?" It is hard to see strong support for the suggestion that either male hormones or a brain masculinized *in utero* led to the change in sexual identity. These individuals opted out of a confining village situation if possible because there was no place for exposed unmarried female-like individuals. It is understandable that they would switch to the male role to adapt better to a male-dominated society once their defects were known. Such considerations may have also played a role in the identity switch within a sex-traditional rural Dominican society.

In contrast, eight such individuals in the United States who were raised as females and who experienced testosterone-induced activation at puberty prior to medical intervention, apparently maintained female gender-identity despite disfiguring pubertal virilization (Rubin et al., 1981). Researchers have reported similar results for females with adrenogenital syndrome who were misassigned as males at birth (Money and Ehrhardt, 1972). Psychosexual identity appears to be formed in the early years of childhood. It depends typically on the sex of rearing even when this is in contrast to some of the biological factors of sex. Once formed, it cannot be easily reversed despite ugly virilization in a "girl" at puberty or breast development and erectile inadequacy in a "boy." Individuals in our culture who develop doubts about their sexual identity typically take years to change sex and go through a gradual readjustment to their changing body image and societal reactions to it (Ehrhardt and Meyer-Bahlburg, 1981).

# The relationship between hormones and behavior in normal humans

The evidence for a relationship between hormones and behaviors in biologically normal individuals is also ambiguous. For example, researchers have failed to find any connection between maternal stress during pregnancy and either gender nonconformity in childhood or adult homosexuality (Bailey et al., 1991). Maternal stress has been hypothesized to delay the surge of testosterone necessary for sexual differentiation of the brain. These results are consistent with findings indicating that prenatal progesterone had no effect on males' gender identity, rough and tumble play, interest in sports, or visual spatial skills (Kester, 1984).

A simple hormonal explanation for hypothetical sex-related differences in mathematics performance is also unlikely. Some researchers (Benbow and Benbow, 1984; Benbow, this volume) have found a link between left-handedness, nearsightedness, and allergies in a population of mathematically talented youth which they believe to be due to testosterone suppression of the growth of the left hemisphere during fetal life. However, these connections may not generalize beyond this highly unusual population. For example, a recent meta-analysis which examined 100 studies of mathematical performance representing the testing of nearly four million students, found sex-related differences favored females in samples of the general population and grew larger, favoring males, only in selected samples of precocious individuals (Hyde et al., 1990). Other recent studies have found no difference in the absolute levels of mathematical performance as a function of either sex or handedness among eighth graders and no relationship between spatial abilities and mathematical performance in standard dominant girls (Casey et al., 1992).

As will be discussed later in this paper, theories about biological determinism must take into account the sociocultural environment as it is mediated by parents and peers. For example, cross-cultural studies in Taiwan, Japan, and the United States have found that, as early as the first grade, children and their mothers believed that boys were better in math (Lummis and Stevenson, 1990). The world of computers is stereotypically male (Unger and Crawford, 1992). It is also largely solitary (Braun et al., 1986). It is possible to conjecture that precocious children are socialized toward mathematical achievement because of the way their external characteristics influence their interactions with parents and peers. It is not necessary to conjecture biological causality.

# Beyond nature and nurture: The role of appearance

To resolve the controversy over whether the sex of rearing is of paramount importance in psychosexual identification, one may look at intensive case studies of sexually anomalous individuals. But, such cases also do not resolve any traditional "nature-nurture" conflict. Close examination of these cases reveals the impossibility of separating the biological characteristics of humans from the social consequences of these characteristics. One of the more obvious, but frequently ignored, truisms in the study of the biological bases of behavior is that one cannot remove organisms from their environment. We often ignore the fact, however, that the organism's body structure (and in the case of humans, social reactions to that structure) forms part of their environment.

## Case studies from the literature on sexual anomalies

There is considerable data in the research literature to suggest that physical appearance and body image may mediate gender identity and sex-related behaviors. One well-known case is that of the twin whose penis was destroyed and who was raised as a female (Money and Ehrhardt, 1972). Data on behavior during childhood suggested that stereotypically masculine and feminine characteristics were more under the control of socially mediated factors than biological ones (Money and Ehrhardt, 1972). This case and two other cases of sex reassignment reported by Money (1974) appeared to provide strong evidence that most traditional gender differences are socially learned.

However, when the twin was seen at age thirteen by a new set of psychiatrists, they reported her to be beset by problems (Diamond, 1982). These reports emphasized problems with peers due to her lack of feminine appearance and her aspirations for a masculine occupation. She has since reverted to a male role (Diamond, this volume) and no longer supports the thesis that sexual identity is primarily dependent on social learning during a critical period of early childhood.

Stoller (1985) has also provided details about a case that may illuminate some of the issues involved in the controversy about sexual identity and gender in individuals with hormonal anomalies (in this case, five alpha reductase deficiency). Stoller regards the case as evidence for the biological determination of sexual identity because the individual identified as a male despite a female upbringing. He also notes, however, that Mary was a first child born to a feminine mother who found the child *"too active, too forceful, and too ungraceful"* (p. 66).

Appearance at adolescence seems to have been particularly important for this individual too. Stoller states that on meeting her at age fourteen, *"I found 'her' grotesque as a girl: though 'her' mother had attempted to have 'her' dress properly for the doctor, it was a bad masquerade...it was clear that this child was living an impossible existence as a girl"* (p. 67). Mary who became Jack described her adolescence as *"the ugly duckling days...being ridiculed because I was different. That was the hardest part, the worst part"* (p. 71) He/she notes that before puberty as a model tomboy, *"I had a lot of playmates and not particularly bad memories. I still wore pants and cowboy boots and played army and did all the things I wanted to"* (p.72). These individuals had difficulty maintaining a gender identity that conflicted with bodily norms that are considered desirable for a member of their sex in our society. It is significant that girls with CAH who were virilized showed higher masculinity scores than their nonvirilized counterparts (Hurtig and Rosenthal, 1987). It should not be surprising that relatively unattractive individuals might reject a female role.

## Physical appearance and gender norms

In recent years, behavioral scientists have conducted hundreds of studies verifying that physical appearance variables are reliably perceived and systematically affect social attitudes, attributions, and actions (Cash, 1990). Recent meta-analyses confirm that a "beauty is good" stereotype exists for individuals of both sexes (Eagly et al., 1991). This stereotype is sometimes stronger than stereotypes based on gender and appears to be present within the first ten milliseconds that a person is perceived (Locher et al., In press).

Beauty is not only seen as good, but also provides information about socially appropriate gender-typing as well as other forms of behavioral and social deviance (Unger et al., 1982). A number of studies have shown, for example, that attractive women are seen as more feminine and attractive men are seen as more masculine than their less attractive counterparts (Gillen, 1981; Major and Deaux, 1981; Unger, 1985). Attractiveness norms are more rigidly applied to females than to males in our society (Cash, 1990). Thus, lack of attractiveness can be a major stigma for females.

## Physical attractiveness and puberty

The effects of physical appearance appear to become more salient during adolescence. Puberty is the period in which differences in self esteem between girls and boys emerge. Dissatisfaction with how one looks begins during puberty and is linked to rapid and normal weight gain that is part of growing up (Attie and Brooks-Gunn, 1989). Boys perceive their bodies significantly more positively than girls in terms of overall body image (Tobin-Richards et al., 1983). Pubertal girls, as compared to boys, were less proud of their bodies, felt more poorly developed in terms of adult body structure, and wished they were thinner. Perceptions about weight produced the largest differences between males and females of any measure and were more salient for girls than for boys.

Since there is a great deal of individual variation in the timing of the events of puberty it is possible to use such individual differences to examine the impact of social beliefs on psychological functioning. For example, the "long lithe look" is more attainable by girls who enter puberty later than the average age. Early maturing girls, on the other hand, weigh more and are slightly shorter than their late maturing peers even when pubertal growth is complete (Brooks-Gunn, 1987). Early maturers have poorer body images related to weight and are more concerned about dieting than late maturers (Attie and Brooks-Gunn, 1989). In contrast, boys who mature early tend to perceive themselves more positively than boys who are either on-time or late (Tobin-Richards et al., 1983).

These within- and between-sex interactions are probably due to societal stereotypes linking attractiveness and gender. Adult masculinity has unambiguous positive connotations whereas adult femininity carries with it a double bind (Unger and Crawford, 1992). Early maturity in girls appears to offer advantages in terms of popularity with the opposite sex. But, it is also predictive of lower levels of academic achievement. These girls may not yet be ready emotionally for heterosexual behavior and may have difficulty coping with sexual demands from older and/or more experienced partners.

## Physical appearance, gender identity, and the goodness-of-fit model

There is considerable evidence to suggest that stereotypes that "what is beautiful is good" are more detrimental to homely persons than they are beneficial to attractive individuals (Hatfield and Sprecher, 1986). Individuals who cannot conform to our society's demands for feminine attractiveness would, therefore, be at particular risk during adolescence when these standards become salient. Data from the case studies discussed earlier fit this pattern.

Several researchers interested in human development have recently proposed a goodness-of-fit model to account for this kind of reciprocal interaction between biological and contextual factors. They suggest that just as people bring their unique characteristics to a particular setting, there are specific demands that are placed on them by significant persons in their social setting. If their attributes are incongruent with social demands, a negative adjustment may result. This model would help to explain sex-related differences in psychological adjustment associated with individual differences in the rate of maturation.

Lerner and Jovanovic (1990) have used this model to explain why physically unattractive early adolescents of both sexes had fewer positive peer relationships and scored lower on standardized adjustment tests. Such effects would, of course, be magnified for individuals whose physical deviations make it even more difficult for them to be socially accepted.

## Changing identity: transsexuals and gender-benders

Another way to examine the effect of body image on sexual identity is to look at a group of people who firmly believe that they were born with the bodies of the wrong sex. This phenomenon is known as transsexualism or gender dysphoria. To all appearances, the transsexual has acquired the wrong sexual identity and once acquired, this identity appears to be unchangeable. Many transsexuals maintain that they have been discontented with their identity from earliest childhood. No form of psychological therapy has been easily able to influence their belief.

Grimm (1987) estimates that there are 30,000 transsexuals worldwide, 10,000 of whom live in the United States. Male-to-female transsexuals outnumber female-to-male transsexuals by at least four to one, perhaps by as much as eight to one. Many researchers believe that the reason for this disparity is because primarily androcentric cultures are less accepting of variant male role behaviors. Thus, men who deviate in some ways may come to feel that they are not men at all. For example, it is perfectly acceptable for women to wear pants, carry briefcases, and enjoy sports. However, a man who likes dresses, would prefer to carry a purse, and enjoys needlepoint would have a great deal more difficulty even in today's society.

Transsexuals do not transcend traditional male-female dichotomies. Male-to-female transsexuals, in particular, often adopt an exaggerated stereotypical version of feminine dress and behavior. They wear more elaborate clothing and make-up than most women. The medical establishment appears to encourage such stereotyping since the more feminine the appearance and behavior of the applicant, the more likely his request for surgery will be granted (Raymond, 1979).

Surgical treatment of transsexuals actually confirms traditional social constructions of maleness and femaleness. It opts for massive, permanent changes in the body rather than acceptance of the idea that roles and bodies may be independent. It ignores the possibility that the connection between biology and behavior is imposed by the cultural standards for each sex.

The outcome of such surgery is currently a matter of controversy. Some studies of postoperative transsexuals have found high levels of satisfaction with the surgery and the new life (Blanchard et al., 1985). However, not all studies report such positive outcomes. Post-surgical appearance appears to be the most important predictor of psychological adjustment. Physical factors that make is difficult for them to "pass" as members of their adopted sex or which continue to remind them of their reassigned status are associated with continued psychological difficulties (Ross and Need, 1989).

An interesting study of women who are sometimes mistaken as men (Devor, 1987) also illustrates how appearance may alter gender identity. These women do not pass as men in a consistent or purposeful fashion. They have clear female identities, but because of their tallness, body build, and nonverbal behaviors are often mistaken for men or boys during brief encounters of an impersonal and public nature.

Although these women are not transsexuals, they may tell us something about the social pressures that produce gender dysphoria in our society. All of them reported as girls that they enjoyed physical activity and that they were tomboys throughout their early years. The majority played mostly with boys or were loners. About half came from homes where their fathers acted as though they would have preferred them to be sons. Many of these women were tall...only one was smaller than the average North American woman. This combination of behavioral preferences and physical characteristics appears to have led them to become "gender benders."

Body image may play a greater role in the development of gender identity than we had previously believed. For example, Green and his associates (Green et al., 1982) found virtually no differences in familial characteristics between 50 traditional and 49 nontraditional girls ages 4 to 12. The mothers of nontraditional girls, however, reported more than the other mothers that adults comment that their daughters would make handsome boys. Green (1974) has previously reported that physical attractiveness in childhood is sometimes associated with the development of a feminine gender identity in boys.

## Cultural constructions of gender

There is no clear evidence of a biological basis for cross-sex identity (Bolin, 1987; Diamond, this volume). Recently, feminist scholars have begun to look at transsexualism in terms of violation of the rules by which sex and gender are constructed in our society. Transsexualism tests the extent to which a culture takes definitions of sex and gender for granted.

Kessler and McKenna (1978), for example, argue that gender is constructed and maintained by social interactions. Some aspects of gender identity may be learned rather easily. In fact, transsexuals do not undergo surgical manipulations to change their sex until they have satisfied their physicians that they have successfully passed as a member of the other sex for a long time. In most encounters, others accept the sex by which one presents oneself. Since the so-called natural connection between sex and gender is rarely questioned, people assume that the signals associated with gender in our society (such as clothing, hairstyle, and nonverbal behaviors) also define biological sex. The presence or absence of sex-appropriate genitalia is assumed.

These studies suggest that gender (in terms of body identity and self-awareness) can produce sex (conceptualized as differentiated behavior) just as easily as the other way around. Surgical treatment of transsexualism, in fact, treats bodies as more modifiable than behavior. Examination of how well one's body fits into sex-related social categories allows us to transcend traditional biological/environmental dichotomies. In this kind of model, individual characteristics produced by biological constraints are acted on by developmental and social factors. Socially consistent variables (such as the connection between attractiveness and attributions about gender) can be disting.

Typically the gender socialization of children takes a number of years (Unger and Crawford, 1992). Recent studies have indicated a major impact of the peer environment during childhood (Maccoby, 1988; Thorne and Luria, 1986). We can apply a goodness-of-fit model to parental and peer responses to children's gender-inappropriate behaviors as well as to appearance. For example, Lewis (1987) has shown that children's gender-inappropriate toy play at age two was predictive of socially problematic behaviors at age six only if their earlier play did not fit their mothers' gender schema. Such a model would help explain why only some individuals question their gender.

We must also recognize that attributions involving sex and gender are also culturally specific. People in this society do not question that sex is a dichotomy. However, not all cultures agree with Western society's notion that all people are either men or women. Earlier in this paper I discussed some alternative sexual categories such as "turnim-man" associated with biological anomalies. However, the idea that various societies can and do construct alternative genders, independent of a person's physical body, is difficult for members of our culture to conceive. One such category used by some northwestern American Indian societies is the Berdache. A similar category known as the Xanith exists in some traditional Arab societies (Wikan, 1977). These individuals are biological males who adopted the clothes and some of the roles of the other sex and who had sexual relations with other men. They may, however, revert to the male role without sanction, or switch back and forth between roles.

Attempts to classify such individuals as hermaphrodites, homosexuals, transvestites, or transsexuals fail because their behavior fits none of these ethnocentric norms (Williams, 1987). Difficulties arise because scholars cannot agree whether sexual preference, dress, gender role, or even identity are core characteristics. For example, the Berdache do not appear to question their biological maleness and they do not always cross dress. Homosexuality in their society is not always associated with being a member of this social category. These individuals differ from gay men in our own society because sex between two berdaches is not socially sanctioned.

Williams (1986) has recently published a book based on an extensive participant-observer study of the Berdache. He concludes that American Indians

472

are not biologically reductionist nor bipolar in their gender system. He sees the Berdache as a third, alternative gender.

This kind of analysis attempts to deconstruct our conception of sex and gender. It provides an alternative to assumptions about a stable core to which one simply adds deviations to broaden the picture. Instead, it argues that the margin is itself culturally specific. Other societies validate the gender variance that our society denigrates as deviance (Brod, 1987).

It is clear that there are a great many sources of variability associated with the apparently simple word "sex". As noted at the beginning of this paper, however, sex is used to refer to our reproductive category, physiological properties, reproductive and nonreproductive behaviors, and, in human beings, our sense of who we are, physically and psychologically. It also refers to a system of categories that differ from one culture to another. We will probably never be able to determine one single variable that causes a person to be male or female. The language of dimorphism leads us into searching for causal dichotomies. How would our analyses be affected if we used the concept of "many sexes" rather than just two?

# References

Attie, I. and Brooks-Gunn, J. (1989). The development of eating problems in adolescent girls: A longitudinal study. *Develop. Psychol.*, **25**, 70-79.

Bailey, J. M., Willerman, L., and Parks, C. (1991). A test of the maternal stress theory of human male homosexuality. *Arch. Sex. Behav.*, **20**, 277-293.

Baker, S. W. (1980). Biological influences on human sex and gender. *Signs*, **6**, 80-96.

Benbow, C. and Benbow, R. (1984). Biological correlates of high mathematical reasoning ability. In : DeVries, G.J., De Bruin, J.P.C., Uylings, H.B.M. and Corner, M.A. (Eds.), Progress in Brain Research, vol. 61, *Sex Differences in the Brain*, Amsterdam: Elsevier Press, pp.

Blanchard, R., Steiner, B. W. and Clemmensen, L. H. (1985). Gender dysphoria, gender reorientation, and the management of transsexualism. *J.Coun. Clin. Psychol.*, **53**, 295-304.

Bolin, A. (1987). Transsexualism and the limits of traditional analysis. *Amer. Behav. Sci.*, **31**, 41-65.

Braun, C. M., Goupil, G., Giroux, J. and Chagnon, Y. (1986). Adolescents and microcomputers : sex differences, proxemics, task and stimulus variables. *J. Psychol.*, **120**, 529-542.

Brod, H. (1987). Cross-culture, cross-gender: Cultural marginality and gender transcendence. *Amer. Behav. Sci.*, **31**, 5-11.

Brooks-Gunn, J. (1987). The impact of puberty and sexual activity upon the health and education of adolescent girls and boys. *Peabody J. Educ.*, **64**, 88-112.

Casey, M. B., Pezaris, E. and Nuttall, R. L. (1992). Spatial ability as a predictor of math achievement : the importance of sex and handedness patterns. *Neuropsychologia*, **30**, 35-45.

Cash, T. F. (1990). The psychology of physical appearance. In: Cash, T.E. and Pruzinsky, T. (Eds.), *Body images: Development, Deviance, and Change,* New York, Guilford, pp. 51-79.

Crews, D. (1987a). Diversity and evolution of behavioral controlling mechanisms. In : Crews, D. (Ed.), *Psychobiology of Reproductive Behavior : an Evolutionary Perspective,* Englewood Cliffs, N. J.: Prentice-Hall, pp.

Crews, D. (1987b). Functional associations in behavioral endocrinology. In : Reinisch, J.M., Rosenblum L.A. and Sanders, S.A. (Eds.), *Masculinity/Femininity: Basic Perspectives,* New York: Oxford University Press, pp. 83-106.

Devor, H. (1987). Gender blending females: women and sometimes men. *Amer. Behav. Sci.,* **31,** 12-40.

Diamond, M. A. (1965). A critical evaluation of the ontogeny of human sexual behavior. *Quart. Rev. Biol.,* **40,** 147-175.

Diamond, M. A. (1982). Sexual identity, monozygotic twins reared in discordant sex roles and a BBC follow-up. *Arch. Sex. Behav.,* **11,** 181-186.

Eagly, A. H., Ashmore, R. D., Makhijani, M. G. and Kennedy, L. C. (1991). What is beautiful is good, but... : a meta-analytic review of research on the physical attractiveness stereotype. *Psychol. Bull.,* **110,** 109-128.

Ehrhardt, A. A. and Meyer-Bahlburg, H. F. L. (1981). Effects of prenatal sex hormones on gender-related behavior. *Science,* **211,** 1312-1318.

Ehrhardt, A. A., Meyer-Bahlburg, H. F. L., Feldman, J. F. and Ince, S. E. (1984). Sex-dimorphic behavior in childhood subsequent to prenatal exposure to exogenous progestagens and estrogens. *Arch. Sex. Behav.,* **13,** 457-477.

Ehrhardt, A. A., Meyer-Bahlburg, H. F. L., Rosen, L. R., Feldman, J. F., Veridiano, N. P., Zimmerman, I. and McEwen, B. S. (1985). Sexual orientation after prenatal exposure to exogenous estrogen. *Arch. Sex. Behav.,* **14,** 57-75.

Frank, L. G., Glickman, S. E. and Licht, P. (1991). Fatal sibling aggression, precocial development, and androgens in neonatal spotted hyenas.*Science,* **252,** 702-704.

Gibber, J. R. (1981). *Infant-directed behaviors in male and female rhesus monkeys.* Unpublished doctoral dissertation. Department of Psychology, University fo Wisconsin-Madison.

Gillen, B. (1981). Physical attractiveness: A determinant of two types of goodness. *Person. Soc. Psychol. Bull.,* **7,** 277-281.

Goldfoot, D. A. and Neff, D. A. (1987). Assessment of behavioral sex differences in social contexts: perspectives from primatology. In: Reinisch, J. M., Rosenblum, L. A. and Sanders S. A. (Eds.), *Masculinity/Femininity : Basic Perspectives,* New York, Oxford University Press.

Goldfoot, D. A., Wallen, K., Neff, D. A., McBrain, M. C. and Goy, R. W. (1984). Social influences on the display of sexually dimorphic behavior in rhesus monkeys : isosexual rearing. *Arch. Sex. Behav.,* **13,** 395-412.

Goy, R. W. (1970). Early hormonal influences on the development of sexual and sex-related behavior. In: Schmitt, F. O. (Ed.),*The Neurosciences: Second Study Program,* New York, Rockefeller University Press, pp. 199-207.

Green, R. (1974).*Sexual Identity Conflict in Children and Adults,* New York: Basic Books.

474

Green, R., Williams, K. and Goodman, M. (1982). Ninety-nine "tomboys" and "non-tomboys": behavioral contrasts and demographic similarities. *Arch. Sex. Behav.,* **11**, 247-266.

Grimm, D. E. (1987). Toward a theory of gender : transsexualism, gender, sexuality, and relationships. *Amer. Behav. Sci.,* **31**, 66-85.

Hatfield, E. and Sprecher, S. (1986). *Mirror, Mirror...the Importance of Looks in Everyday Life,* Albany, New York : Suny Press.

Herdt, G. H. and Davidson, J. (1988). The Sambra "Turnim-man": sociocultural and clinical aspects of gender formation in male pseudohermaphrodites with 5α-reductase deficiency in Papua New Guinea. *Arch. Sex. Behav.,* **17**, 33-56.

Hubbard, R. (1990). *The Politics of Women's Biology,* New Brunswick: Rutgers University Press.

Hurtig, A. L. and Rosenthal, I. M. (1987). Psychological findings in early treated cases of female pseudohermaphroditism caused by virilizing congenital adrenal hyperplasia. *Archiv. Sex. Behav.,* **16**, 209-223.

Hyde, J. S., Fennema, E. and Lamon, S. J. (1990). Gender differences in mathematical performance: a meta-analysis. *Psychol. Bull.,* **107**, 139-155.

Imperato-McGinley, J. and Peterson, R. E. (1976). Male pseudohermaphrodism : the complexities of male phenotypic development. *Amer. J. Med.,* **61**, 251 - 272.

Imperato-McGinley, J., Peterson, R. E., Gautier, T. and Sturla, E. (1979). Androgens and the evolution of male-gender identity among male pseudohermaphrodites with 5 alpha-reductase deficiency. *New Engl. J. Med.,* **300**, 1233-1237.

Kessler, S. J. and McKenna, W. (1978). *Gender: An Ethno-Methodological Approach,* New York: Wiley.

Kester, P. A. (1984). Effects of prenatally administered 17-alpha-hydroxyprogesterone caproate on adolescent males. *Archiv. Sex. Behav.,* **13**, 441-455.

Lerner, R. M. and Jovanovic, J. (1990). The role of body image in psychosocial development across the lifespan : a developmental contextual perspective. In : Cash, T.F. and Pruzinsky, T. (Eds.), *Body Images: Development, Deviance, and Change,* New York: Guilford.

Lewis, M. (1987). Early sex role behavior and school age adjustment. In : Reinisch, J.M., Rosenblum, L.A. and Sanders, S.A. (Eds.), *Masculinity/Femininity: Basic Perspectives,* New York: Oxford University Press, pp. 202-226.

Locher, P., Unger, R. K., Sociedad, P. and Wahl, J. (In press). At first glance: accessibility of the physical attractiveness stereotype. *Sex Roles.*

Longino, H. E. (1990). *Science as Social Knowledge: Values and Objectivity in Scientific Inquiry,* Princeton: Princeton University Press.

Lummis, M. and Stevenson, H. W. (1990). Gender differences in beliefs and achievement: a cross-cultural study. *Develop. Psychol.,* **26**, 254-263.

Maccoby, E. E. (1988). Gender as a social category. *Develop. Psychol.,* **24**, 755-765.

Major, B. and Deaux, K. (1981). Physical attractiveness and masculinity and femininity. *Pers. Soc. Psychol. Bull.,* **7**, 24-28.

Michael, R. P., Wilson, M. I. and Plant, T. M. (1973). Sexual behavior of male primates and the role of testosterone. In : Michael, R.P. and Crook, J. H. (Eds.), *Comparative Ecology and Behavior of Primates,* New York: Academic Press, pp. 235-313.

Money, J. (1974). Prenatal hormones and postnatal socialization in gender identity differentiation. In : Cole, J.K. and Dienstbier, R. (Eds.), *Nebraska Symposium on Motivation 1973,* Lincoln: University of Nebraska Press, pp.

Money, J. (1987). Propaedeutics of diecious G-I/R: Theoretical foundations for understanding dimorphic gender-identity/role. In: Reinisch, J.M., Rosenblum, L.A. and Sanders, S.A. (Eds.), *Masculinity/Femininity : Basic Perspectives,* New York : Oxford University Press, pp. 13-28.

Money, J. and Ehrhardt, A. (1972). *Man and Woman, Boy and Girl,* Baltimore: Johns Hopkins University Press.

Money, J. and Mathews, D. (1982). Prenatal exposure to virilizing progestins: an adult follow-up study on 12 young women. *Arch. Sex. Behav.,* **11**, 73-83.

Peterson, R. E., Imperato-McGinley, J., Gautier, T. and Sturla, E. (1977). Male pseudohermaphrodism due to steroid 5 alpha-reductase deficiency. *Amer. J. Med.,* 62, 170-191.

Raymond, J. (1979). *The Transsexual Empire: The Making of the She-Male,* Boston: Beacon Press.

Rose, R., Gordon, T. and Bernstein, I. (1972). Plasma testosterone levels in the male rhesus: influences of sexual and social stimuli. *Science,* **178**, 643- 645.

Rosenblatt, J. S. and Aronson, L. R. (1958). The decline of sexual behavior in male cats after castration with specific reference to the role of prior sexual experience. *Behavior,* **12**, 285-338.

Ross, M. W. and Need, J. A. (1989). Effects of adequacy of gender reassignment surgery on psychological adjustment: A follow-up of 14 male-to-female patients. *Arch. Sex. Behav.,* **18**, 145-153.

Rubin, R. T., Reinisch, J. M. and Haskett, R. F. (1981). Postnatal gonadal steroid effects on human behavior. *Science,* **211**, 1318-1324.

Sapolsky, R. M. (1987). Stress, social status, and reproductive physiology in free-living baboons. In: Crews, D. (Ed.), *Psychobiology of Reproductive Behavior: An Evolutionary Perspective,* Englewood Cliffs, N. J.: Prentice-Hall, pp. 291-322.

Spanier, B. B. (1991). Lessons from "Nature": Gender ideology and sexual ambiguity in biology. In: Epstein, J. and Straub, K. (Eds.), *Body Guards,* New York: Routledge, pp. 329-350.

Stoller, R. J. (1985). *Presentations of Gender,* New Haven: Yale University Press.

Thorne, B. and Luria, Z. (1986). Sexuality and gender in children's daily worlds. *Soc. Prob.,* **33**, 176-190.

Tobin-Richards, M. H., Boxer, A. M. and Petersen, A. C. (1983). The psychological significance of pubertal change: sex differences in perceptions of self during early adolescence. In: Brooks-Gunn, J. and Petersen, A.C. (Eds.), *Girls at Puberty,* N. Y.: Plenum, pp. 127-154.

Unger, R. K. (1985). Personal appearance and social control. In: Safir, M., Mednick, M. T., Izraeli, D. and Bernard, J. (Eds.), *Women's Worlds: From the New Scholarship,* New York: Praeger, pp. 142-151.

Unger, R. K. and Crawford, M. (1992).*Women and Gender: A Feminist Psychology,* New York: McGraw Hill.

Unger, R. K. and Crawford, M. (In press). Sex and gender: the troubled relationship between terms and concepts. *Psychol. Sci.*

Unger, R. K., Hilderbrand, M., and Madar, T. (1982). Physical attractiveness and assumptions about social deviance: Some sex by sex comparisons. *Pers. Soc. Psychol. Bull.,* **8**, 293-301.

Wikan, U. (1977). Man becomes woman: transsexualism in Oman as a key to gender roles. *Man,* **12**, 304-319.

Williams, W. L. (1986). *The Spirit and the Flesh: Sexual Diversity in American Indian Culture,* Boston: Beacon Press.

Williams, W. L. (1987). Women, men, and others: beyond ethnocentrism in gender theory. *Amer. Behav. Sci.,* **31**, 135-141.

# Dimensions of Human Sexual Identity : Transsexuals, Homosexuals, Fetishists, Cross-Gendered Children and Animal Models

## R. GREEN

*Department of Psychiatry and Biobehavioral Sciences, UCLA School of Medicine, 760 Westwood Plaza, Los Angeles, California 90024-1759 USA*

Unpacking complex sexual behavior into its components permits examination and manipulation that may reveal origins, activators, and mechanisms. With animal sexual behavior, Beach (1979) advocated this strategy, an approach that has been richly rewarded.

In 1974 in *Sexual Identity Conflict in Children and Adults,* I defined human sexual identity as embracing three elements. They were 1. core morphological or anatomic identity - the individual's self-concept as male or female, 2. gender role behavior - behaviors more commonly expressed by males or females - (culturally defined masculinity and femininity), and 3. sexual orientation - erotic interest in same-sexed, other-sexed, or both-sexed persons. As described next, this three-part concept discriminates three patterns of atypical sexual identity - transsexualism, transvestism, and homosexuality.

The "uncomplicated" transsexual male, discontent being male from childhood's earliest years, show extensive cross-gender behavior from those years and later is erotically interested in males. The converse is true for the female transsexual. Thus, transsexuals are atypical on components 1, 2, and 3 of sexual identity.

By contrast, "pure" transvestites are always anatomically male. They are content being male but periodically cross-gender dress with accompanying genital arousal. Their sexual orientation is directed toward females. Thus, transvestites are atypical on component 2 only.

By contrast, "pure" homosexuals, male or female, are content in the anatomic sex in which they were born, are usually within conventional limits of masculinity and femininity, but are sexually drawn to persons of their own sex. Thus, they are atypical on component 3 only.

These three elements of sexual identity implicate perplexing aspects of human psychosexual differentiation. Consider, first, transsexuals. As if the "conventional" transsexual were not enough of a conundrum (using Jan, nee

*M. Haug et al. (eds.), The Development of Sex Differences and Similarities in Behavior, 477–486.*
© 1993 *Kluwer Academic Publishers.*

James Morris' autobiography title), not all transsexuals with an anatomic self-concept of th eother sex, and manifesting the gender role of the other sex, are erotically attracted to persons of their own anatomic sex. In other words, not all males who want to become women are attracted to males, and not all females who demand to become men are attracted to females. Many males, after becoming women, live as lesbians. Some females, after becoming men, live as gay men. Why ?

A psychodynamic interpretation for men becoming lesbians is grounded in the classic Freudian theory of castration anxiety and the feared female *"vagina dentata"*. Before penectomy, the male was erotically drawn to females but was fearful of castration as the consequence of penile-vaginal intercourse. The transsexual male masters this anxiety by taking control of the castration process.

Having overcome this source of fear, the postoperative transsexual is able to participate sexually with a female. A behaviorist view of the phenomenon sees learned anxiety from sexual encounters with a female in the preoperative state causing impotence. When the postoperative transsexual need no longer fear impotence after penectomy, sexual involvement with females can proceed.

I have evaluated several post-surgical male transsexuals who were sexually active with females, some having been active with women before surgery (and thus fulfilling neither psychological formulation), and some who became sexually interested in women only after sex reassignment.

Fewer examples of females becoming homosexual men are reported and no developmental theory has been advanced to explain its occurrence. Nine female transsexuals were recently described from the Netherlands who were sexually interested in males after being reassigned as male. For most, their discontent being female preceded their sexual attraction toward men (Coleman et al., 1992). Other reports have emanated from England (Clare and Tully, 1989). Twenty years ago, I evaluated a female who was married to a man but whose identity was as a "gay man" (unpublished).

Transvestites are another puzzle for understanding male-female differentiation. When the definition of transvestism includes erotic arousal to cross-dressing, it is nearly exclusively a behavior of males. Why ? One theory, an anatomic one, suggests that the association of cross-dressing by the heterosexual male (often beginning in adolescence), with a fantasy of the self as female, produces an erection. This penile arousal provides immediate pleasurable feedback. The immediacy of sexual pleasure in the male promotes a conditioned response to cross-dressing. Another theory, a sociological one, sees the more forbidden nature of male cross-dressing as the source of erotic arousal.

Another unsettling issue with transvestism is that it may evolve into transsexualism. Over the course of years some transvestites experience a change from intermittent fetishistic cross-dressing and living as otherwise conventional heterosexual men to frequent or regular cross-dressing, without penile arousal, and with the desire to become women. Some also report erotic interest in men.

479

The typically atypical person, the male homosexual (human sexuality's "standard deviation"), is also problematic, theoretically. He has a male identity and masculine behavior, but a female erotic pattern. Why did one element of the system cross-over from male to female ? And, sometimes, two elements cross over. Some male homosexuals are behaviorally feminine and some female homosexuals are behaviorally masculine.

My 15 year study with cross-gendered behaving boys highlights these asymmetries in sexual identity differentiation. It also poses issues for animal research.

We studied 66 boys who, when first evaluated at ages 4-12, preferred to be girls, and behaved like girls. From their second and third year these boys showed a preferential interest in dressing in girls or women's clothes. When genuine items were unavailable, they improvised feminine attire : bath towels became skirts, father's t-shirts became dresses. When their mothers were asked about the frequency of their son's cross-dressing, the typical response was, "As often as you let him". Their favorite or frequently played with toy was a female-type dress-up doll, such as Barbie. Their preferred playmates were girls. When assuming roles in "house" games or imitating characters from media, they were women or girls. Most of these boys had verbalized their wish to be girls. These cross-gendered boys and their parents were demographically matched with conventionally gender-behaving boys and their parents.

Both groups were periodically reevaluated. The sexual identity of two-thirds of the two groups was determined about 15 years later. In adolescence or young adulthood, with one exception (from the cross-gendered group), the boys were content being male. With two exceptions (again, from the cross-gendered group), the boys were essentially masculine. However, three-fourths of the previously cross-gendered boys were homosexual or bisexual. Only one in the contrast group was bisexual. He was the monozygotic previously masculine twin of a previously cross-gendered boy who was now also bisexual (but more homosexual than the previously masculine twin).

Thus, with regard to the components of sexual identity, although it is difficult to determine whether core identity in one group shifted from female (or was always male), gender role behavior did change (feminine to masculine), and for 3/4, sexual orientation was discrepant from components 1 and 2 (Green, 1974, 1987).

Can we explore non-human behaviors to understand these boys ? Homosexual behavior among male primates may be more prevalant within groups of "peripheralized males". These males are characteristic of free-living troops of Rhesus monkeys and baboons. It has been suggested that my cross-gendered boys are "peripheralized males" (Goy and Goldfoot, 1875). If so, what innate and experiential factors influence their peripheralization ? Elsewhere (Green, 1987), I have discussed at length the influences on atypical sexual identity development in boys. Here I will summarize.

Evidence is good that prenatal androgen levels influence behaviors characterized as rough-and-tumble play, toy preference, and sex of preferred playmates. Evidence is good that interest in newborns, or a surrogate activity, doll play, is affected by prenatal androgen. Data from young female monkeys hormonally manipulated by androgen injections to the pregnant mother (tomboy monkeys) and the human experiment of nature, congenital adrenal hyperplasia (tomboy girls) support this conclusion (Young et al., 1964; Ehrhardt and Baker, 1974 ; Berenbaum and Hines, 1992).

Perhaps cross-gendered boys had lower than typical prenatal androgen levels. Their interest in rough-and-tumble play is low, their interest in doll play is high, and their preferred peer group is female.

Perhaps this posited endocrine difference also organizes hypothalamic or other brain nuclei to influence erotic attraction. Could it affect the size of the human INAH-3 nucleus which appears to be sex-dimorphic and may be related to sexual orientation (Levay, 1991)? Are tomboy monkeys not only behaviorally masculinized, but hypothalamicaly masculinized as well ? Is their INAH-3 (or a comparable area modified ? If prenatal androgen affects the organization of INAH-3, then both early life cross- gender behaviors and later life erotic ones may be age-appropriate expressions of this influence. Peer group interaction is critical for the development of primate sexual behavior. Depriving young Rhesus monkeys of both peer play experience and maternal comfort disrupts sexual behavioral development, whereas providing peer interaction only permits its expression (Harlow, 1965). Peer group gender composition distinguishes pre-homosexual boys from pre-heterosexual boys in our 15 year prospective study. By retrospective report it may also distinguish pre-heterosexual and pre-homosexual girls.

Whereas most children by 4-5 years congregate in same-sex groups, the pre-homosexual child's peer group is heterosocial. With cross-gendered boys, their disinterest in rough-and-tumble play, coupled with their interest in doll play, affects their early peer group composition. It promotes a heterosocial experience. This integration into a heterosocial group could affect later erotic interests. Boys in a female peer group could affect later erotic interests. Boys in a female peer group could be adopting the socio-sexual norms of that group culture. Thus, boys would model those who will primarily be interested in males. The converse could operate with females.

These observations and speculations promote questions for animal researchers. Are there young non-human primates that spontaneously congregate in opposite-sex peer groups ? If so, what else distinguishes them behaviorally and/or endocrinologically ? Are they cross-sex identified on component 1 of sexual identity ? Are there indicators of component 1 in non-human primates that could be quantified and compared ?

Peer group composition in non-humans could be amenable to experimental manipulation. Is there an influence on sexual behavior when a young primate is, by design, the only one of its sex in a group of young animals ?

Consider, too, primate juvenile rehearsal at sex play. If the "odd" male or female socialized in an opposite-sex peer group witnesses opposite-sex peers interacting in sexual rehearsals with animals of the "odd" animal's own sex, will this influence that "odd" animal to adopt the pattern of his peers ? (In other words, will the male with a female peer group shown a sex interest in males ?).

Yet another powerful psychosexual influence on humans is the early father-son experience. In our 15 year study of cross-gendered and masculine boys, significant differences emerged in shared father-son time during the first five years. Beginning in the second year, feminine boys as a group reportedly shared less time with their fathers. Furthermore, looking only at the feminine boys, there was an inverse relation between the extent of early father-son time and later homosexual orientation. Less father-son time was associated with more homosexual ratings on the Kinsey scale of sexual orientation.

Father-son data were sliced an additional time. In each instance where the feminine boy had a brother, he was masculine. When the extent of father-feminine son time was compared with time shared by the father with the masculine brother, fathers and cross-gendered brothers shared less.

But determining cause and effect in the early father-son experience is problematic. Some fathers lost interest in interacting with their sons because the boy's interests were not in tune with his, but resonated from earliest years with those of mother (perhaps a reflection of low prenatal androgenization). Other fathers, by contrast, were rarely available for their sons before, and as, cross-gender behavior emerged.

Why should early father-son experience be correlated with later sexual orientation ? A deficiency in father-son shared time is seen as promoting early cross-gender behavior and later same-sex romantic interests from both learning theory and psychodynamic perspectives. Father (or other adult male) unavailability is seen as depriving the male child of a model for identification with, and learning of, male-type behaviors. Father-absent boys tend to score in a more feminine direction on psychological tests of masculinity and femininity (Hetherington, 1966). A psychodynamic speculation whereby cross-gendered boys mature into homosexual men is that they are starved for affection from males. Not only was their relationship with their father remote, but they were also rejected by other boys.

Can this variable be studied with the non-human primate ? Early primate parent interaction with children is usually mother-infant. But, if male and female monkeys were raised by fathers only (with technological help for feeding), would their behaviors be affected ? How will fathers compare to mothers and terry cloth surrogates on influencing social and sexual development ? Will both male and female children be more masculine ?

The variable of father-son contact or experience is difficult to evaluate in the non-human. It is not only time shared that is important to humans, it is the symbolic nature of the relationship as well. Further, when young Rhesus monkeys are allowed peer and mother contact only, they develop heterosexual behaviors. And, they develop nearly normally with peer play only (Harlow, 1965). So, where is the influence of poppa primate ?

Some other research questions whose answers could inform about sexual identity :

Could a mother monkey be tricked into believing that her male newborn is female? Could genital-modifying surgery change her interactions with the infant so as to affect the child's later behavior? How would peers interact with this female-appearing male? Would the postnatally castrated and penectomized male interact socially more as a male or as a female ? Would he be a "sissy"?

Can gender-atypical juvenile play in the primate be promoted by hormonal manipulation other than with prenatal testosterone given to the female (the "tomboy" model) ? Will anti-androgen given prenatally to the male change sex-dimorphic juvenile behaviors ? Will stress during pregnancy to the monkey's mother change her hormone levels or the behavior of offspring ? Work with rodents has generated a "prenatal stress" theory of homosexual orientation in human males. Stressing pregnant rats promotes more female-type behavior in male offspring, presumably through interference with prenatal androgen production and/or metabolism, perhaps in its time of peak activity, perhaps via the interference of adrenal stress hormones. Studies with humans have been inconsistent. Some find that the mothers of male homosexuals recall more severe stress during pregnancy than the mothers of male heterosexuals (Dörner, 1976), others find no difference (Bailey, 1991). Can the pregnancy stress experiments of mice and (some) men be adapted to the primate?

Another perplexing aspect of human psychosexual development is fetishistic behavior in males. Fetishism is genital arousal to inanimate objects. Fetishes run the gamut. More common varieties include high-heeled shoes and underwear, more uncommon ones include safety pins, or the handle bars of 10-speed English racing bicycles. Fetishes are believed by behavior therapists to be a conditioned or learned association between the object and pleasurable penile arousal.

So, some thoughts about fetishism in animals. Can non-humans develop fetishes ? Penile erections and thrustings are present in Rhesus monkeys and chimpanzees from infancy. They occur in a variety of situations in which the general level of excitement is high. If a monkey had a spinally implanted electrode that induced erection, and stimulation of the electrode accompanied atypical visual stimuli, could atypical arousal patterns be conditioned ? One atypical stimulus that is not a fetish could be a con-specific same-sex animal. Would stimulation of female sexual areas produce a fetish in the non-human female ? Would it help if the electrodes were implanted within the brain in areas that elicit genital arousal in the manner of Maclean's work two decades ago with the squirrel monkey (Maclean, 1973) ?

Another endocrine research thought. In the human male, there is a surge in testosterone between 3 weeks and 3 months. What does it do ? If the early postnatal testosterone surge in the non-human primate is blocked, what is the effect on sexual behavior ? On hypothalamic nuclei ?

Mature sexual behavior patterns in higher mammals are most difficult to manipulate experimentally. Erwin and Maple (1976) described bisexual behavior in two male Rhesus monkeys. They had been reared in cages with social access only to their mothers for the first 8 months. Shortly after weaning, they were paired with each other, and allowed exclusive and continuous social contact until 27 months. From 30 to 33 months, they had exclusive social access to 1 year old males. A 37 months, the males were paired with females, with which they remained for 6 months. After separation from the females, they were housed alone until 54 months. Then they were reunited for 30 minutes and paired with an unfamiliar male for 30 minutes. At 66 months each male was reunited with the female, and was paired with an unfamiliar female. Two months later, the males were simultaneously introduced into a test cage which contained an unfamiliar receptive adult female.

What happened sexually after this dizzying social calendar?

At their reunion at 27 months, the males mounted each other, in turn, possibly with anal intromission. There was considerable pelvic thrusting. Both males mounted the male 1 year olds and thrust against them, without penetration. Simultaneous masturbation between the older pairs was observed. When paired with females, both males copulated normally.

At their reunion after two years of separation, they immediately mounted each other. Mounts were long. The males achieved anal intromission. Both males, while mounted, exhibited behavior typical of females when they are mounted - reaching back, supporting the male, and facing him with lipsmacking. No ejaculation occurred. There were no aggressive or threatening gestures. When reunited later at 63 months, again there was anal intromission and thrusting.

Both males also exhibited a high rate of sexual behavior with both familiar and unfamiliar females. The sexual *preference* of these males was determined by releasing them into a cage with an unfamiliar, sexually receptive female. The two males immediately made contact *with each other*, rather than with the female. When the female approached the males who were embracing each other, she was slapped and bitten.

Another manipulation of early peer group experience with Stumptail monkeys did not change sexual preference, although social preference may have been modified. Three feral-born males were obtained at about 3 years. They were then housed together for 9 years. During tests preceding those for sexual behavior, the males more often approached and spent time in proximity to a female than to a familiar male. In sexual tests, all three males ejaculated with female partners. One ejaculated, without intromission, with male partners. The same male did not achieve intromission with females. The second time that the males were tested with females, they approached and mounted them more than male partners. However, males groomed male partners longer (Slob and Schenck, 1986). It would be of interest to repeat this study with laboratory bred monkeys that did not have three years of natural juvenile sexual play.

Also in Archives, we published an account by Chevalier-Skolnikoff (1974) of the sexual behaviors of Stumptail monkeys demonstrating the capacity for same-sex activity by both males and females. In captivity, 23 female-female interactions were observed out of 143 sexual interactions. Females mounted females higher up on the back than is characteristic of the typical male mount. They thrust the same number of times as males. In three sessions the female mounter displayed the behavioral features of orgasm displayed by males. Male-male pairings were also recorded. Their variety of sexual positioning is of interest to students of human sexuality. It included a male mounting a male from the rear and taking the mountee's penis into his mouth, a male mounting the male with the mountee manually stimulating the mounter's penis, two males, while placed buttocks to buttocks, each manipulating the penis of the other, and two males mutually mounting with mutual oral-genital stimulation.

The pigmy chimpanzee, Bonobo, could be another useful primate model. Male-male oral-genital sex, and mutual same-sex masturbation are readily observed in captivity. Can these homoerotic behaviors be experimentally increased or reduced ?

Interpreting these same-sex sexual-appearing behaviors is problematic, however. The debate is long-running on distinguishing "sexual" behaviors in primates from social hierarchial ones. Nevertheless, one feature observed by investigators regarding same-sex primate contact is that "homosexual" interactions most commonly involve two animals with a long history of previous association. Another is the absence of threats or other agonistic antecedents to these events (Beach, 1979).

The work of Slob and co-workers on sexual preference in rodents is of major interest in that it is the rare example of endocrine manipulation associated with a change in sexual preference. Female Wistar rats treated neonatally with testosterone (T) but not with dihydrotestosterone (DHT), and later with T, show a preference for estrous females over males. Males castrated neonatally and given testosterone propionate, dihydrotestosterone propionate, or oil, on days 0-10 postnatally and then given DHT, DHT plus estrogen, or T in adulthood are also sexually modified. When given the choice between an estrous female versus a non-estrous female, and an estrous female versus a male, they did *not* show a sexual partner preference. However, after sexual contact with an estrous female, they preferred her over a non-estrous female. Removal of the hormone implant, followed by T administration, resulted in males preferring estrous females, but neonatally DHT- or oil-treated males had a lower preference for females than TP-treated or control males.

Males were also treated perinatally to prevent aromatization of testosterone to estradiol by ATD (1, 4, 6-androstatriene -3, 17-dione). Neonatally ATD-treated males showed less preference for an estrous female than controls or prenatally treated ATD males. Thus, neonatal availability of estrogen (from T) may help organize the male's preference for an estrous female (Brand and Slob, this Volume).

In closing, let me sound a political note. I direct your attention to the broader significance of this work.

Research on sexual identity, especially sexual orientation, is controversial. The impact of the research is in the eyes of the beholder.

Some of us concerned with legal protection of persons with an atypical sexual identity whose behaviors are not injurious to others see innate contributors to these behaviors as positive. Currently 44 American states permit civil discrimination on the basis of sexual orientation and 23 criminalize homosexual conduct (Green, 1992). In American constitutional law, disadvantaged minority groups may receive special legal protection if their prejudiced behavior is "immutable". As a legal term of art, "immutable" means that the behavior is inborn or otherwise essentially unchangeable. Reduced to a simple analogy, if homosexual orientation is the sexual equivalent of left-handedness, homosexuality could be protected legally. Left-handed persons cannot be discriminated against in employment or housing. They do not go to jail for masturbating with the wrong hand.

On the other side of this political debate are those who see demonstrations of biological origins of sexual identity as a blueprint fo prevention - genocide against homosexuals.

More optimistic souls, of whom I am one, see reforms evolving socially and legally with the increasing acceptance of the concept of sexual privacy. This change should obviate any later medical interest in extinguishing a pattern of benign sexuality, even if the technology were to evolve.

We are not building the atomic bomb. But, we must remain sensitive to the political and social ramifications of our work.

# References

Bailey, J., Willerman, L. and Parks, C. (1991). A test of the maternal stress theory of human male homosexuality. *Arch. Sex. Behav.,* **20** : 277-293.

Beach, F. (1979). Animal models for human sexuality. In : Sachar, E. (Ed.), *Sex, Hormones and Behaviours,* Elsevier, Amsterdam, pp. 113-132.

Berenbaum, S. and Hines, M. (1992). (See paper this conference by Hines for up-to-date citations).

Brand, T. and Slob, A. (1991). (See paper this conference by Slob for up-to-date citations).

Chevalier-Skolnikoff, S. (1974). Male-female, female-female, and male-male sexual behavior in the Stumptail monkey, with special attention to the female orgasm. *Arch. Sex. Behav.,* **3** : 95-116.

Clare, D. and Tully, B. (1989). Transhomosexuality or the dissociation of sexual orientation and sex objects choice. *Arch. Sex. Behav.,* **18** : 531-536.

Coleman, E., Bockting, W. and Gooren, L. (1992). Homosexual and bisexual identity in sex-reassigned female-to-male transsexuals. *Arch. Sex. Behav.,* **22** : 35-48.

Dörner, G. (1976). *Hormones and Brain Differentiation,* Elsevier, Amsterdam.

Ehrhardt, A. and Baker, S. (1974). Fetal androgens, human central nervous system differentiation, and behavior sex differences. In : Friedman, R., Richart, R. and Van de Wiele, R. (Eds.), *Sex Differences in Behavior,* Wiley, New York, pp. 33-51.

Erwin, J. and Maple, T. (1976). Ambisexual behavior with male-male anal penetration in male Rhesus monkeys. *Arch. Sex. Behav.,* **5** : 9-14.

Goy, R. and Goldfoot, D. (1975). Neuroendocrinology : animal models and problems of human sexuality. *Arch. Sex. Behav.,* **4** : 405-420.

Green, R. (1987). *The "Sissy Boy Syndrome" and the Development of Homosexuality,* Yale University Press, New Haven.

Green, R. (1974). *Sexual Identity Conflict in Children and Adults,* Basic Books, New York, Gerald Duckworth, London.

Green, R. (1992). *Sexual Science and the Law,* Harvard University Press, Cambridge, MA.

Harlow, H. (1965). Sexual behavior in the rhesus monkey. In : Beach, F. (Ed.), *Sex and Behavior,* Wiley, New York, pp. 234-265.

Hetherington, E. (1966). Effects of paternal absence on sex-typed behavior in negro and white preadolescent males. *J. Person. Soc. Psychol.,* **4** : 87-91.

LeVay, S. (1991). A difference in hypothalamic structure between heterosexual and homosexual men. *Science,* **253** : 1034-1037.

Maclean, P. (1973). New findings on brain function and sociosexual behavior. In : Zubin, J. and Money, J. (Eds.), *Contemporary Sexual Behavior,* The Johns Hopkins University Press, Baltimore, pp. 53-71.

Slob, A. and Schenck, P. (1986). Heterosexual experience and isosexual behavior in laboratory-housed male stumped-tailed macaques. *Arch. Sex. Behav.,* **15** : 261-268.

Young, W., Goy, R. and Phoenix, C. (1964). Hormones and sexual behavior. *Science,* **143** : 212-218.

# Index

# List of participants

**G. M. Alexander** Department of Psychiatry and Biobehavioral Sciences, UCLA School of Medicine, 760 Westwood Plaza, Los Angeles, CA 90024-1759, USA

**Y. Arai** Department of Anatomy, Juntendo University School of Medicine, Hongo, Tokyo 113, JAPAN

**C. Aron** Institut d'Histologie, 4, rue Kirschleger, 67085 Strasbourg, FRANCE

**J. Balthazart** Université de Liège, Laboratoire de Biochimie Générale et Comparée, 17, Place Delcour (bât. L1), B-4020 Liège, BELGIQUE

**M. J. Baum** Department of Biology, Boston University, 2, Cummington Street, Boston, MA 02215, USA

**C. P. Benbow** Department of Psychology, Iowa State University, Ames, IA 50011-3180, USA

**P. F. Brain** School of Biological Sciences, University College of Swansea, Swansea, SA2 8PP, Wales, UK

**C. Brinton** Department of Anatomy, University of Hawaii, School of Medicine, 1960 East-West Road, Honolulu, HI 96822, USA

**L. G. Clemens** Department of Zoology, Michigan State University, Natural Science Building, East Lansing, MI 48824, USA

**J. F. Debold** Department of Psychology, Tufts University, Medford, MA 02155, USA

**M. Diamond** Department of Anatomy, University of Hawaii, School of Medicine, 1960 East-West Road, Honolulu, HI 96822, USA

**K. D. Döhler** Pharma Bissendorf Peptide GmbH, Karl-Wiechert Allee 3, 3000 Hannover 61, GERMANY

**A. H. Eagly** Department of Psychological Sciences, Purdue University, West Lafayette, IN 47907, USA

**B. Fadem** UMD New Jersey, Medical Science Building, Rm. E-561, 185 South Orange Avenue, University Heights, Newark, NJ 07103-2714, USA

**S. J. C. Gaulin** Department of Anthropology, University of Pittsburgh, Pittsburgh, PA 15260, USA

**B. A. Gladue** Department of Psychology, North Dakota State University, Fargo, ND 58105, USA

**R. Green** Department of Psychiatry and Biobehavioral Sciences, UCLA School of Medicine, 760 Westwood Plaza, Los Angeles, CA 90024-1759, USA

**A. Guillamon** Universidad Nacional de Education a Distancia, Departamento de Psicobiologia, P.O. Box, Apartado n° 50.487, Madrid, SPAIN

**M. Haug** Université Louis Pasteur, Laboratoire de Psychophysiologie, URA 1295, 7, rue de l'Université, 67000 Strasbourg, FRANCE

**M. Hines** Department of Psychiatry and Biobehavioral Sciences, UCLA School of Medicine, 760 Westwood Plaza, Los Angeles, CA 90024-1759, USA

**F. J. Johnson** Department of Biological Sciences, University of Southern California, HEDCO Neurosciences Building 115, Los Angeles, CA 90089-2520, USA

**J. Juraska** Department of Psychology, University of Illinois, 603 E. Daniel Street, Champaign, IL 61820, USA

**M. Kail** Université René Descartes (Paris V), Laboratoire de Psychologie Expérimentale, URA 316, 23, rue Serpente, 75OO6 Paris, FRANCE

**E. B. Keverne** University of Cambridge, Sub-Department of Animal Behaviour, Madingley, Cambridge CB3 8AA, UK

**J. Lapolice** Université du Québec à Trois Rivières, Laboratoire de Neuropsychologie, C.P. 500, Trois-Rivières, Québec G9A 5H7, CANADA

**G. Laviola** Fisiopatologia O.S., Istituto Superiore di Sanita, Viale Regina Elena 299, OO161 Roma, ITALY

**W. H. Meck** Department of Psychology, Columbia University, New York, NY 10027, USA

**J. Mos** Duphar B.V., Department of Pharmacology, P.O. Box 900, 1380 DA Weesp, THE NETHERLANDS

**K. L. Olsen** Neuroendocrinology Program, National Science Foundation, Rm 321, 1800 G. Street, Washington, DC 20550, USA

**P. Palanza** Università Degli Studi di Parma, Dipartimento di Biologia e Fisiologia Generali, Sezione Zoologia, Viale delle Scienze, 43100 Parma, ITALY

**L. F. Petrinovich** Department of Psychology, University of California, Riverside, CA 92521, USA

**R. Poole** Science Magazine, 4909 North 17th Street, Arlington, VA 22207, USA

**M. P. Safir** Department of Psychology, University of Haïfa, Haïfa 31905, ISRAEL

**S. Segovia** Universidad Nacional de Education a Distancia, Departamento de Psicobiologia, P.O. Box, Apartado n° 50.487, Madrid, SPAIN

**J. P. Signoret** INRA, Station de Physiologie de la Reproduction, URA 1291, Centre de Recherches de Tours, 37380 Nouzilly, FRANCE

**N. G. Simon** Center for Molecular Bioscience and Biotechnology, Mountaintop Campus 111, Lehigh University, Bethlehem, PA 18015, USA

**A. K. Slob** Department of Endocrinology and Reproduction, Faculty of Medicine and health Sciences, Erasmus University, P.O. Box 1738, 3000 DR Rotterdam, THE NETHERLANDS

**R. Unger** Department of Psychology, Montclair State University, 124 Russ Hall, Upper Montclair, NJ 07043, USA

**C. Wagner** Institute of Animal Behavior, Rutgers University, 101 Warren Street, Newark, NJ 07102, USA

**R. E. Whalen** Department of Psychology, University of California, Riverside, CA 92521, USA

**C. L. Williams** Department of Psychology, Barnard College of Columbia University, 3009 Broadway, New York, NY 10027, USA

**M. L. Xavier** Instituto de Anatomia do Pr. J. A. Pires de Lima, Faculdade de Medicina, Alameda Pr. Hernâni Monteiro, Porto 4200, PORTUGAL

**P. Yahr** Department of Psychobiology, University of California, Irvine, CA 92717, USA